Ambulatory
Geriatric
Care

Ambulatory Geriatric Care

Thomas T. Yoshikawa, M.D.

Assistant Chief Medical Director
Office of Geriatrics and Extended Care
U.S. Department of Veterans Affairs
Adjunct Professor of Health Care Sciences
The George Washington University School of Medicine and Health Sciences
Washington, D.C.

Elizabeth Lipton Cobbs, M.D.

Assistant Professor of Medicine and Health Care Sciences
Director, Division of Aging Studies and Services
The George Washington University School of Medicine and Health Sciences
Washington, D.C.

Kenneth Brummel-Smith, M.D.

Director, Geriatric Clinics
Portland Veterans Affairs Medical Center
Associate Professor
Department of Medicine and Family Medicine
Oregon Health Sciences University
Portland, Oregon

With 29 illustrations

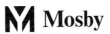 Mosby

St. Louis Baltimore Boston Chicago London Philadelphia Sydney Toronto

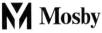
Dedicated to Publishing Excellence

Editor: Stephanie Manning
Assistant Editor: Laura DeYoung
Project Supervisor: Barbara Merritt
Designer: David Zielinski
Editing and Production: Monotype Composition Company, Inc.

Copyright © 1993 by Mosby–Year Book, Inc.

Printed in the United States of America

Mosby–Year Book, Inc.
11830 Westline Industrial Drive
St. Louis, Missouri 63146

Library of Congress Cataloging-in-Publication Data

Ambulatory geriatric care / [edited by] Thomas T. Yoshikawa, Elizabeth
 Lipton Cobbs, Kenneth Brummel-Smith.
    p. cm.
  Includes bibliographical references and index.
  ISBN 0-8016-6543-4
  1. Geriatrics. 2. Ambulatory medical care. 3. Health promotion.
I. Yoshikawa, Thomas T. II. Cobbs, Elizabeth Lipton. III. Brummel-
Smith, Kenneth.
  [DNLM: 1. Ambulatory Care—in old age. 2. Geriatric Assessment.
3. Geriatrics. 9303]
RC952.A78 1993
618.97—dc20
DNLM/DLC   92-48425
for Library of Congress   CIP

93 94 95 96 97 GW/MY 9 8 7 6 5 4 3 2 1

CONTRIBUTORS

Zail S. Berry, M.D., M.P.H.
Department of Health Care Sciences
Division for Aging Studies and Services
George Washington University
Washington, D.C.

Patricia Lanoie Blanchette, M.D., M.P.H.
Associate Professor of Medicine and
  Public Health
Director, Geriatric Medicine Program
John A. Burns School of Medicine
University of Hawaii
Honolulu, Hawaii

Peter A. Boling, M.D.
Associate Professor of Internal Medicine
Director, Home Care Program
Medical College of Virginia
Richmond, Virginia

Kathy S. Brenneman, M.D.
Director, Geriatric Medicine
Washington Hospital Center
Washington, D.C.

Kenneth Brummel-Smith, M.D.
Acting Chief, Division of Geriatrics
Portland VA Medical Center
Portland, Oregon

Amanda Clark
Department of OB/GYN, Urogynecology
  Section
Oregon Health Sciences University
Portland, Oregon

Elizabeth L. Cobbs, M.D.
Director, Division for Aging Studies and
  Services
Department of Health Care Sciences
George Washington University Medical
  Center
Washington, D.C.

Jeffrey L. Cummings, M.D.
Neurobehavior Unit
VA Medical Center West Los Angeles
Los Angeles, California

John J. Danner, M.S.W.
Director, Independent Living Services
Clinical Gerontology Service
Rancho Los Amigos Medical Center
Downey, California

Carole E. Deitrich, R.N.C., M.S., G.N.P.
Associate Clinical Professor
School of Nursing
University of California, San Francisco
San Francisco, California

Rebecca Elon, M.D., M.P.H.
Assistant Professor
Johns Hopkins University School of
  Medicine
Johns Hopkins Geriatric Center
Francis Scott Key Medical Center
Baltimore, Maryland

Helene Emsellem, M.D.
Department of Neurology
George Washington University Medical
  Center
Washington, D.C.

Bruce Ferrell, M.D.
Assistant Professor of Medicine and
  Geriatrics
UCLA School of Medicine
Associate Director for Clinical Programs
GRECC VA Medical Center
Sepulveda, California

Mary Elina Ferris, M.D., M.S. Ed.
Associate Professor of Family Medicine
Loma Linda University School of
  Medicine
Clinical Associate Professor of Family
  Medicine
University of Southern California School
  of Medicine
Director, Family Practice Residency
Glendale Adventist Medical Center
Glendale, California

Mary Kane Goldstein, M.D.
Director of Graduate Medical Education
GRECC VA Medical Center
Palo Alto, California

Keith Gross, M.D.
Clinical Instructor in Medicine
  (Dermatology)
UCLA School of Medicine
Los Angeles, California
Division of Dermatology
Harbor-UCLA Medical Center
Torrance, California

Arnold Gurevitch, M.D.
Professor of Clinical Medicine
  (Dermatology)
UCLA School of Medicine
Los Angeles, California
Chief, Division of Dermatology
Harbor-UCLA Medical Center
Torrance, California

Jeffrey E. Halter, M.D.
Division of Geriatric Medicine
University of Michigan
Ann Arbor, Michigan

Arthur E. Helfand, D.P.M.
Professor and Chairman
Pennsylvania College of Podiatric
  Medicine
Adjunct Professor, Podiatric Medicine
Jefferson Medical College
Thomas Jefferson University
Philadelphia, Pennsylvania

Kenneth W. Hepburn, Ph.D.
Geriatrics Section
Department of Family Practice and
  Community Health
University of Minnesota
Minneapolis, Minnesota

**Helen Higby, R.N.C., M.S.,
G.N.P.**
School of Nursing
University of California, San Francisco
San Francisco, California

Gordon A. Ireland, Pharm. D.
VA Medical Center
Jefferson Barracks Division
St. Louis, Missouri

Dennis Jahnigen, M.D.
Section of Geriatrics
Department of Internal Medicine
Cleveland Clinic Foundation
Cleveland, Ohio

Joseph Keenan, M.D.
University of Minnesota Medical Center
Minneapolis, Minnesota

David Law, M.D.
Professor of Medicine
George Washington University
Deputy ADCMD for Hospital Based
  Services
Department of Veterans Affairs
Washington, D.C.

Barry Lebowitz, M.D.
Chief, Mental Disorders of the Aging
  Research Branch
National Institute of Mental Health
Rockville, Maryland

Susan M. Lillie, O.T.R.
Coordinator, Adaptive Driving
Evaluation Program
Santa Clara Valley Medical Center
San Jose, California

Enid Light, Ph.D.
Mental Disorders of the Aging Research
  Branch
National Institute of Mental Health
Rockville, Maryland

David Lipshitz, M.D., Ph.D.
GRECC VA Medical Center
Little Rock, Arkansas

Patrick M. Lloyd, D.D.S., M.S.
Associate Professor, Department of
  Prosthodontics
Director of Geriatrics
Marquette University School of Dentistry
Milwaukee, Wisconsin

Robert Luchi, M.D.
VA Medical Center
Houston, Texas

Kenneth W. Lyles, M.D.
Clinical Director, GRECC
Durham VA Medical Center
Associate Professor of Medicine
Duke University Medical Center
Durham, North Carolina

Joanne Lynn, M.D.
Center for the Evaluative Clinical
  Sciences
Dartmouth Medical School
Hanover, New Hampshire

Scott L. Mader
Assistant Professor of Medicine
Case Western Reserve University
ASOC/Geriatrics and Extended Care
Cleveland VA Medical Center
University Hospitals of Cleveland
Cleveland, Ohio

Michael E. Mahler, M.D.
Neurobehavior Unit
VA Medical Center West Los Angeles
Los Angeles, California

James W. Mold, M.D.
Director, Geriatrics Division
Department of Family and Community
  Medicine
Associate Professor
University of Louisville Medical School
Louisville, Kentucky

Edward Mongan, M.D.
Chief of Medicine
Rancho Los Amigos Medical Center
Downey, California

John E. Morley, M.D.
Dammert Professor of Gerontology
Division of Geriatric Medicine
St. Louis University School of Medicine
Director, GRECC VA Medical Center
St. Louis, Missouri

Linda A. Morrow, M.D.
GRECC VA Medical Center
West Roxbury, Massachusetts

Laura Mosqueda, M.D.
Geriatric Health, Education and Research
  Center
Rancho Los Amigos Medical Center
Downey, California

Thomas Mulligan, M.D.
Associate Professor, Internal Medicine
Medical College of Virginia
Associate Chief of Staff for Geriatrics and
  Extended Care
Division of Geriatric Medicine
Hunter Holmes McGuire VA Medical
  Center
Richmond, Virginia

Pamela Nagami, M.D.
Department of Internal Medicine
Southern California Permanente Medical
  Group
Kaiser Medical Center
Woodland Hills, California

Joseph Oliveira, M.S.
Research Assistant
Stanford University, Palo Alto California
GRECC VA MC, Palo Alto, California

Robert Palmer, M.D., M.P.H.
University Hospitals of Cleveland
Cleveland, Ohio

Hiep Pham, M.D.
Division of Geriatrics
University of South Florida Medical
  School
Tampa, Florida

Michael Plopper, M.D.
Clinical Director, Senior Programs
Mesa Vista Hospital
Sharp Cabrillo Hospital
San Diego, California

Richard Reed, M.D., M.P.H.
Department of Family Practice and
  Community Health
University of Minnesota
Minneapolis, Minnesota

David B. Reuben, M.D.
Multicampus Division of Geriatric
  Medicine and Gerontology
UCLA School of Medicine
Los Angeles, California

Bruce E. Robinson, M.D.
Division of Geriatrics
University of South Florida Medical
  School
Tampa, Florida

**Laurence Z. Rubenstein, M.D.,
M.P.H.**
Director, GRECC Sepulveda VA Medical
  Center
Associate Professor of Medicine
UCLA School of Medicine
Los Angeles, California

Douglas W. Scharre, M.D.
Neurobehavior Unit
VA Medical Center West Los Angeles
Los Angles, California

**Robert M. Schmidt, M.D.,
M.P.H., Ph.D., F.A.C.P.**
Director, Health Watch Program,
  California Pacific Medical Center
Professor, Center for Preventive
  Medicine and Health Research
San Francisco State University
San Francisco, California

Herbert C. Sier, M.D.
Division of Geriatric Medicine
Lutheran General Hospital
Park Ridge, Illinois
Clinical Assistant Professor of Medicine
University of Chicago
Chicago, Illinois

Eila C. Skinner, M.D.
Department of Urology
University of Southern California School
  of Medicine
Los Angeles, California

Barbara A. Soniat, M.S.W., Ph.D.
Assistant Professor
Director, Geriatric Assessment and Case
  Management Program
Division of Aging Studies and Services
George Washington University
Washington, D.C.

**Leah Ellenhorn Stromberg,
M.S.W., L.C.S.W.**
Clinical Social Work Supervisor
Rancho Los Amigos Medical Center
Downey, California

George E. Toffet, M.D.
VA Medical Center
Houston, Texas

Joan Teno, M.D., M.S.
Center for the Evaluative Clinical
  Services
Dartmouth Medical School
Hanover, New Hampshire

John Walsh, M.D.
Section of Gerontology
VA Medical Center
Portland, Oregon

Angela Walther, M.D.
Office of Geriatric Medicine
University of Cincinnati College of
  Medicine
Cincinnati, Ohio

Richard E. Waltman, M.D.
Allenmore Medical Center
Tacoma, Washington

Gregg Warshaw, M.D.
Department of Family Medicine
University of Cincinnati College of
  Medicine
Cincinnati, Ohio

Adrian J. Williams, M.D.
Pulmonary Division
VA Medical Center West Los Angeles
Los Angeles, California

Thomas T. Yoshikawa, M.D.
Office of Geriatrics and Extended Care
Department of Veterans Affairs
Washington, D.C.

To our spouses, Catherine Yoshikawa,
Philip Green, and Karen Brummel-Smith,
whose love and support made this book possible.

FOREWORD ─────────────────

This volume on ambulatory care for elderly persons fills a major need. Most textbooks of geriatric medicine, while typically providing guidance for understanding and treating the major diseases faced by older persons, rarely addresses the much more common aspects of care as seen when the older person comes to her or his doctor's office or a clinic with everyday questions and problems.

This book takes up these everyday issues in careful, easily understood detail— from preventive, screening, and health maintenance measures to careful multifaceted evaluation, to management of the wide range of conditions that may occur. It also provides important perspectives on such topics as rehabilitation, the roles of nurses, social workers, and managing legal, ethical, and financial issues.

The editors have assembled a group of authors who are well-informed and experienced professionals, qualified to give up-to-date advice. In my judgment, the contents of this book are sound and should provide very practical, readily accessible guidance to almost any physician or other health professional involved in ambulatory care of older persons.

T. Franklin Williams, M.D.
Professor of Medicine Emeritus, University of Rochester
Attending Physician, Monroe Community Hospital

PREFACE

The field of Geriatrics has grown rapidly during the past 10 years. In recognition of this, special board examinations are now offered in Geriatric Medicine and Geropsychiatry. In concert with this accelerated maturation of the field of Aging there has been a major shift in the approach to the care of patients. Health care of elderly patients has evolved with an increasing emphasis on maintaining and restoring patient function, through a network of interdisciplinary practitioners. An increased focus on outcomes and individual patient preferences of goals of care guides clinical decision-making. In addition, clinical care is now practiced predominately in an ambulatory setting rather than in the traditional acute hospital environment.

Unfortunately, much of the training of physicians still occurs solely in inpatient medical centers. Thus, it is not surprising that the majority of the currently available textbooks of Geriatrics (or Geriatric Medicine) focus on the care of elderly patients primarily from an inpatient perspective. Recently, several quality textbooks have been written on care of geriatric patients in nursing homes. But, there is a pressing need for a reference source on the care of older adults in an outpatient setting. *Ambulatory Geriatric Care* is written to meet the needs of clinicians who care for elderly patients in an ambulatory or office setting.

Ambulatory Geriatric Care is organized into four main sections. The first section focuses on principles of geriatric care in an ambulatory setting. Important topics such as establishing appropriate goals of care, managing caregiver stress, accessing community resources, utilizing advance directives of care, treating the dying patient, and prescribing drugs appropriately receive special attention. How the physician can set up an office with attention to the special needs of older patients, and the interdisciplinary roles of nurses and social workers in this setting are also discussed.

The second section provides an in-depth review of the important aspects of assessment within a variety of clinical and social circumstances. Practical and useful assessment tools for clinical evaluation and management are discussed, as well as evaluating patients for surgery, driving, and nursing home placement. A chapter on the assessment of safety issues in the home is also included in this section.

The third section emphasizes successful aging through health maintenance and preventive measures. The chapters address such subjects as nutritional recommendations, exercise, and preventive interventions. An important but often neglected subject of social and spiritual contributors to successful aging is also included.

The final and largest section of *Ambulatory Geriatric Care* is devoted to the management of common clinical problems of elderly patients that are typically encountered in the office setting. These chapters encompass medical conditions pertaining to specific systems, including the genitourinary, neuropsychiatric, musculoskeletal, endocrinological, cardiovascular, gastrointestinal, and pulmonary systems, as well as specific problems of weight loss and obesity, vision, sleep, oral health, sexual dysfunction, anemia, pain, gynecological disorders, and the skin. Each chapter is organized in a similar format, i.e., clinical relevance, clinical manifestations, diagnostic approach, and intervention to facilitate easy and quick accessibility to key information.

Each chapter begins with a section on "Key Points" which allows the clinician to quickly summarize/review the essential information written in the chapter. In addition to references a suggested reading list is provided. The text is written to provide maximum information that is clinically useful in the fewest words possible.

The authors of *Ambulatory Geriatric Care* include both clinicians who practice geriatric medicine in the outpatient setting and nationally recognized experts in the field of Aging. The editors of *Ambulatory Geriatric Care* are geriatricians with backgrounds in clinical practice, research, training and education, policy development, and administration. By distilling the knowledge and experience of these contributors and editors in the collaborative tradition of geriatric medicine, we hope to provide office-based practitioners the most current, accurate and useful information on providing health care to older adults. Our ultimate goal is to improve the health and quality of life of our most cherished population—the elderly person.

Thomas T. Yoshikawa, M.D.
Elizabeth L. Cobbs, M.D.
Kenneth Brummel-Smith, M.D.

ACKNOWLEDGMENT _____

We would like to express our appreciation to Joan Bennett, John Michiuk, and Dr. Elizabeth Cobbs' colleagues at the Division for Aging Studies and Services at George Washington University Medical Center.

We extend our gratitude to the staff at the Geriatric Health, Education and Research Center at Rancho Los Amigos Medical Center, its Director, Bryan Kemp, Ph.D., and the patients they serve for their support.

We wish to thank the Department of Veterans Affairs for their long and continued support for programs in geriatrics and long-term care.

CONTENTS _____

PRINCIPLES OF AMBULATORY GERIATRIC CARE

CHAPTER 1

Goals of care

JOANNE LYNN

KEY POINTS
- Health care is optimal when it yields the best possible outcomes for the patient.
- The usual "fix-it" model is inadequate for geriatric medicine.
- The best possible outcome for an elderly patient must be defined by the patient's preferences and values. Most treatments are only partially effective and carry both burdens and benefits, and reasonable persons differ in evaluating these.
- Good decision making requires that the possible futures of the patient be characterized to the extent possible and understood by the decision makers.

CONVENTIONAL FIX-IT MODEL

When a patient comes to a physician with one or more health problems, the physician usually seeks to make a diagnosis that labels the etiology and physiology underlying the complaints. Treatment is determined by the diagnosis because it is linked to a professional judgment of how to address the medical abnormality. Success is judged by whether treatment restores a target abnormality toward normal (e.g., shrinking a tumor, returning a high serum sodium toward normal, or eliminating a pathological bacterium from the bloodstream). This might be called the "fix-it" model of health care decision making.

The patient's role is quite limited in this scheme, as illustrated by the usual case presentation at a medical conference: The patient's unique situation is encapsulated by presenting age, sex, and, sometimes, occupation and marital status. The body of the case is the physiology, usually presented as the results of examinations and tests. The goal of the presentation is to determine the etiology of abnormal symptoms and signs, explain abnormal physiological findings, and allow these facts to determine an optimal plan of treatment. The composite likely outcome of treatment and its likely impact on how the patient will live are scarcely mentioned. The role of the patient is quite narrow; generally, the patient assents to the prescribed treatments. The patient is allowed to refuse a treatment, but such a course is seen as aberrant, unwise, and not entirely understandable.

Death is the most extreme physiological abnormality, and some providers assume that delaying death is always a good outcome in health care decision making. The patient who refuses life-sustaining treatment thus is sure to be troubling to the provider because the patient is declining the accepted goals of health care.

The fix-it model is often adequate in acute, single-etiology disease. The child who falls from an apple tree and breaks an arm has a single dysfunction that merits a straightforward, highly beneficial treatment and leads to a complete recovery of normal health and function.

This is not the usual case, however, in the ambulatory practice of geriatric medicine. Indeed, the ordinary elderly patient who comes to the physician's office is coping with multiple chronic diseases and partially effective treatments, all of which have profound and lasting effects upon the patient's life. The fix-it model becomes woefully inadequate as a framework for health care decision making with medical conditions of the elderly person which tend to be chronic and never completely fixable. A model that focuses instead on seeking the best *outcome* for each patient requires the physician to assume a creative and personal role in constructing the array of treatment options available for that patient. The physician and patient (or surrogate) then collaborate to choose the best available plan of care according to that patient's individual values and preferences.

IMPROVED OUTCOME AS THE GOAL OF CARE[2]

In the usual case of geriatric ambulatory care, health care providers must consider that the patient's life is profoundly shaped by the illness and its treatment over an extended period of time. Various possible treatment plans can affect the patient's life differently, and it is common that patients differ in how they evaluate the effects of each plan of care.

The patient who is terrified of pain might refuse a plan of care that a more stoic individual would prize. The patient who is concerned with physical self-image might be devastated by a mutilating surgery that another person would largely ignore. Such differences are widespread and have led to the establishment of a more comprehensive model of good decision making. This model requires, first and foremost, that the patient's current situation be well understood. Then, the physician must predict the likely outcomes without specific treatment, be creative in imagining the possible alternative treatment strategies, and predict the likely outcomes with each major treatment strategy.

With this information, the choice, with rare exception, should be the one that reflects the patient's values and preferences. The best possible outcomes are not defined as such by the medical professions, or even by the society at large, but by the patient. Given the chance, people do evidence substantial differences. Some patients with prostatic hypertrophy will choose surgery and others watchful waiting, depending upon personal priorities in restoring function and personal assessments of the impact of various side effects.[1] The woman with breast cancer will choose a more radical surgery if long-term risks are important and disfigurement is of little concern. Another woman with the same disease but different values for long-term risks and self-image might choose the most limited surgical procedure available. Some people with long-term serious illnesses welcome the opportunity to die; others want to fight longer.

Therefore, the first obligation of the physician is to *gather enough information* to forecast likely outcomes. The second obligation is to *project all possible plans of care* that might improve those outcomes. Third, the physician must *forecast the likely outcomes* with each major alternative plan of care. The physician must then *collaborate with the patient* (or an appropriate proxy, if the patient cannot) to choose the plan of care that offers the best outcomes. The requirement for a patient's input about the decision arises not because of informed consent law, but because the definition of "best possible outcomes" is subjective, varying widely among people. *Since the patient's evaluation of likely outcomes is of overriding importance, the patient's involvement is essential in order to determine what will count as the best possible outcomes.*

Health care practice often falls short in the early phases of this process because careful thought is not given to the range of possible plans of care and likely outcomes. Treatments are introduced, then are assumed to be rather routinely indicated, and, thereafter, the possibilities of abstaining from their use or trying something different are not considered. Many physicians assume that a dying patient who is not eating must be given artificial hydration and nutrition, that a set of gangrenous toes is an obvious indication for amputation, or that an obstructed biliary tree mandates placement of a drainage stent. The outcomes of foregoing these treatments are scarcely considered. Yet, in some cases like these, the course offered without treatment is actually more desirable to some patients than the course with treatment. Some patients live a long time with gangrene of one or two toes, which causes no discernable distress. Dying without correcting abnormal nutrition and hydration may well be more comfortable for a patient than any available treatment.

Plans of care often need to be constructed creatively to be maximally helpful to older patients. If a patient greatly fears hospitalization, perhaps the chemotherapy can be given as an outpatient procedure. If the patient abhors the notion of long-term artificial nutrition, perhaps a trial of treatment would be more acceptable. Inability to follow a plan of care is not to be treated as aberrant noncompliance but as an essential element for health care providers to consider in forecasting the future and deciding to pursue a plan of care.

Health care providers have misconceptions about additional constraints on the decision-making process. They may fear that involving the patient and trying to make the care plan fit the patient's preferences is difficult and may frighten or otherwise harm the patient. However, patients commonly welcome the chance to be involved in their care plans and rarely are inappropriately distraught in dealing with the situation. Obviously, good counseling skills and sensitivity are always helpful in negotiating these emotionally weighty issues.

PLANS OF CARE THAT CANNOT BE OFFERED

There are very few conceivable plans of care that cannot be offered. Physicians cannot provide a plan of care that offers illegal killing such as homicide or assisted suicide. They cannot offer to violate laws intended to protect the public health. They cannot provide treatment that is not available to a patient because of funding and other policy constraints in the health care system.

This list of plans of care that cannot be offered is very short. The first, illegal killing, does not often arise as a pressing issue, despite current public interest. Few people who are offered adequate symptom relief are interested, and, because such action is illegal, its implementation is barred.

The second, the protection of the public health, is more commonly an issue. Some cases are firmly decided by governing law, for example, the requirement for treatment of a contagious disease. However, in the care of elderly patients, some cases are quite troubling to health care providers. Is it, for example, reasonable to sedate or restrain some nursing home residents because their loud crying or invading the privacy of other residents is terribly disruptive to others' well-being? At some point, the outrageous behavior of one person should be coercively controlled for the well-being of all, but the threshold for that determination can be very difficult to establish.

Finally, care plans that are extremely expensive are commonly encountered in the care of chronically ill and elderly persons. Everything from false teeth to nursing home beds is in short supply and cannot readily be obtained for a patient who has scant personal resources. The patient might be well served by having the services of a home health aide for 2 hours a day. If that benefit is not available through a public program and the patient cannot pay, the services should not ordinarily be suggested.

Potential outcomes must be described within these constraints. The physicians's goal is to characterize all of the major plans of care that *could* be implemented, envision their outcomes, and collaborate with the patient in choosing the most desirable course of action.

STARTING AND STOPPING TREATMENTS

Providers sometimes think that they cannot stop a treatment once it has been started; this is a serious error.[3,5] The likely outcomes are known with greater precision after, rather than before, a trial of therapy. Sometimes, a trial of treatment is required before the patient's future can be estimated. Some patients who undergo a trial of treatment derive unexpected benefits when the treatment turns out to be unusually effective. Without such a trial, they would have lost the chance for benefit. The case for stopping treatment will usually be clearer than the case for not starting treatment. If one cannot stop an overwhelmingly burdensome treatment, there will be an unfortunate barrier to initiating that treatment.

For many clinicians, stopping a treatment is more troubling than failing to start because it requires clinicians to be explicit about considerations that are morally and emotionally difficult and usually left unsaid. Stopping a treatment also requires documentation that usually can be avoided if the treatment is not initiated. Morally and legally, however, it is just as serious to avoid implementing a treatment that would have been the patient's best option as it is to avoid stopping a treatment that no longer serves the patient well. As a practical matter, potentially harmful treatments should be initiated as time-limited trials of treatment, with planned times for reevaluation and a commitment to stop if burdens accrue and benefits do not.

Some clinicians feel that certain treatments, such as basic nursing care or intravenous hydration, must always be used. Yet some patients would not be well served by the most benign interventions. A patient near death with severe multiple myeloma may have so many fractures that changing the sheets is too painful to be justified. A patient who fights the restraints needed to keep a feeding tube in place and whose dementia is severe might be best served by spoon feeding, even if it is predicted to be nutritionally inadequate. There is no mode of treatment that can be said to be required in every case.

It cannot always be an appropriate goal to prolong life. Virtually all people believe that some outcomes would be worse than death. The conditions that are held to be worse than death ordinarily include some combination of physical pain, separation from loved ones, cognitive disability, short prognosis, and family burden. However, reasonable persons differ substantially in their opinions about which outcomes are so undesirable that they would prefer death. Some, for example, would accept even quite severe pain, while others would find death a welcome relief from pain.

Many older persons would rather not undergo a troubling course of care that has many risks, unpleasant side effects, and the certain outcome of spousal impoverishment. Health care decision making must allow the patient to choose a shorter length of life and hope for a better outcome in terms of function, symptoms, or some other attribute.

COUNSELING PATIENTS ABOUT OUTCOMES AND THE FUTURE

With improved understanding of the efficacy of many treatments, the clinician often has information available to predict the outcomes of disease and the benefits and risks of various treatments. Decisions such as the choice to treat systolic hypertension in elderly persons may be made with consideration of fairly precise estimates of the potential benefits and adverse reactions.[4]

Clinicians need to explain these risks in a manner that elderly patients and their families can understand. Patients who have intolerable side effects from antihypertensive medications, or who choose to live with the risk of adverse sequelae from hypertension, may reasonably forgo specific medical treatment. Ongoing commitment by the physician to locate the best available data, in the literature and medical community, is essential in order to provide the most accurate portrayal of potential treatments and outcomes.

Despite their importance, probabilities for outcomes may be a difficult concept for patients to understand. The 1 patient out of 100 who suffers an adverse event may be comforted little by knowing that this was a rare event. Despite this tension of applying the aggregate information to the individual patient, information about probabilities allows patients and providers to put risk and adverse consequences in the proper perspective. Patients often assume that intermediate probabilities for serious adverse consequences are certain to happen (if the patients are relatively fatalistic) or *not* to happen (if the patients are optimistic). Sometimes biases can be overcome by counseling methods that relate these risks to ordinary examples such as the chances of having a winning baseball team or having a new marriage end in divorce. The clinician might correlate the patients' risks to the probability of their being struck by lightning. Another useful counseling technique for clinicians considering prevention strategies is to tell the patient how many patients would have to be treated to prevent one adverse event. Sometimes telling patients detailed stories about what has happened to other patients makes the issues easier to understand than if they were expressed only in statistical form.

Patients and family often can establish their own framing of the best and worst outcomes. Questions like "What is the best that you think is likely to happen, without it coming as a surprise?" or "What is the worst outcome that you think might happen to you, without it coming as a surprise?" serve to establish a range of likely outcomes that are within the patient's realm of reality. Likewise, patients and families can relate stories gathered from waiting room conversations, popular literature, and family experiences. These stores are helpful for discussion, including the degree to which they are typical.

CONCLUSION

Medical textbooks usually focus upon diagnosis and treatment, with treatment following the diagnosis, in the fix-it model of decision making. Descriptive research is often insufficient to characterize the outcomes of elderly persons with diseases and conditions that have varied possible courses of care. Despite the relatively high incidence of amputation, for example, there are no descriptions in the medical literature of the course of elderly persons who do not have amputation. The clinical course of demented patients who do not have feeding tubes, in comparison with the course of those who have artificial feeding, has never been described.

Of overriding importance to patients are the outcomes of their health care decisions. Each physician must expand the framework for decision making when working with elderly patients, discarding the simplistic fix-it model that disregards patients' circumstances and preferences and developing the ability to formulate health care options creatively. Skill in the process of collaboratively choosing treatment options with patients and surrogates would enable physicians to secure preferred outcomes for their elderly patients.

REFERENCES

1. Barry MJ et al: Watchful waiting vs immediate transurethral resection for symptomatic prostatism: the importance of patients' preferences, *JAMA* 259:3010, 1988.
2. Lynn J, DeGrazia D: An outcome model of medical decision making, *Theoretical Med* 12:325, 1991.
3. President's Commission for the Study of Ethical Problems in Medicine and Biomedical and Behavioral Research: *Deciding to forego life-sustaining treatment*, Washington, DC, 1983, US Government Printing Office.
4. (SHEP) Cooperative Research Group: Prevention of stroke by antihypertensive drug treatment in older persons with isolated systolic hypertension: final results of the systolic hypertension in elderly program (SHEP), *JAMA* 265:3255, 1991.
5. The Hastings Center: *Guidelines on the termination of treatment and the care of the dying*, Bloomington, 1987, Indiana University Press.

SUGGESTED READINGS

Laupacis A, Sackett DL, Roberts RS: An assessment of clinically useful measures of the consequences of treatment, *N Engl J Med* 318:1728, 1988.
Sox HC Jr et al: *Medical decision making*, Boston 1988, Butterworths.
The Coordinating Council on Life-Sustaining Medical Treatment Decision Making by the Courts: *Guidelines for state court decision making in authorizing or withholding life-sustaining medical treatment*, Williamsburg, Va, 1991, The National Center for State Courts.

CHAPTER 2

The office visit

KATHY S. BRENNEMAN

KEY POINTS
- Adaptation of the traditional office visit improves the ability of the physician to serve the health care needs of frail elderly patients.
- The office environment should be suitable for functionally impaired elderly persons.
- Trained office staff contribute significantly to the success in meeting the special needs of elderly patients.
- Preappointment data collection may save time for the physician but cannot replace the interview process.
- Special data organization, including a prioritized problem list, is helpful in caring for complex problems of elderly patients.
- Establishing individual patient preferences, goals of care, and advance directives with patients and surrogates are important components of outpatient care for elderly patients.

The initial office visit of an elderly patient with complex problems can be an overwhelming experience for both the primary care physician and the patient. The busy practitioner may feel frustrated by the older patient who, because of impaired mobility, arrives late for the appointment and then presents a constellation of symptoms and concerns, regimen of multiple medications, and lengthy past medical history.

Traditional medical education has led physicians to evaluate patients by identifying a chief complaint, followed by a history of the present illness, review of past medical and surgical events, social and family history, review of systems, and physical examination. An initial office visit of approximately 45 to 60 minutes is typically allotted. Using this format to evaluate a 90-year-old patient with weakness, hearing loss, and dysmobility, in addition to multiple past medical problems, results in an unsatisfactory formulation of the patient's problems and frustration for the patient and physician

9

alike. Thoughtful restructuring of the office environment and visit can lead to adaptations that accommodate the needs of the elderly patient who is coping with multiple problems that are acute, chronic, and affect overall health and function.

OFFICE ENVIRONMENT

Access to the office may be the first barrier that older people face when they visit their physicians. An office setting that features wide or automatic doors, wheelchair ramps, well-lit entryways, and parking that allows easy access to the building is ideal.

Office design can have an important impact on the ease with which efficient care can be provided for the elderly person. The office suite should provide adequate space for wheelchairs, walkers, and canes. The floor should be free of throw rugs, cords, and other obstacles. Solid colors and vertical lines hinder the depth perception of older people and should not be used in stairs or hallways. A bright horizontal stripe on steps or a horizontal contrast in a patterned carpet can help reduce the risk of falls. Chairs should be selected that provide sufficient support for patients to arise from the chairs without assistance. Firm high seats and arm rests are desirable features. A handicapped bathroom is highly desirable, featuring enough space for a wheelchair, an elevated toilet seat, strategically placed grab bars, and a wheelchair-accessible sink. While these features may not always be immediately available, it is important for physicians to consider these and other features of accessibility when they change office spaces or remodel existing facilities.

Older persons with impaired mobility from arthritis or other causes may have difficulty climbing onto a traditional examination table. Examination tables historically have been built to enhance the physicians' comfort at the expense of the patients'. An electrically operated table can be easily lowered and raised, benefiting both patients and physicians. A table that adjusts the position of patients greatly aids physicians in obtaining proper positioning of their patients for physical examinations.

The quality of communication between physicians and patients is enhanced by office environments that permit optimal auditory and visual function and allow elderly persons to be comfortable. Many elderly people cope with chronic hearing deficits. Background music decreases the ability of hearing-impaired persons to understand spoken words. Patients who have difficulty processing information may have difficulty maintaining concentration during an interview if there is excessive office noise or music. Effective communication is facilitated by keeping background noise to a minimum, ensuring that patients are using their usual assistive hearing devices, and by having interviewers face the patients.

Older patients face a plethora of aging-related changes and diseases that can affect vision. (See Chapter 55, Eye Disorders.) Therefore, it is important that the office suites, hallways, and bathrooms be well lit. Patients should be encouraged to wear their glasses when visual acuity is tested or a cognitive screening test is performed.

Physicians should avoid sitting directly in front of glass where glare may interfere with patients' ability to see.

Since the care of frail elderly patients frequently involves multiple caregivers, the ideal office suite includes a small conference room that accommodates a physician, patient in a wheelchair, and two or three others. The ability to simultaneously interview several individuals involved in a patient's care can substantially expedite history taking. Additionally, relatives who do not actually participate in the patient's personal care may wish to be included in discussions and decisions affecting the patient's care. When the physician reviews the findings and diagnoses of a patient, the ability to gather all concerned individuals together is necessary to efficient practice and eliminates additional phone calls to other family members and repeated explanations of the patient's condition. Family meetings to discuss decision making and advance directives are frequently necessary. Conference rooms also can function as a resource center and small library and can be used for displaying community information, pamphlets, and other educational materials.

ROLE OF THE RECEPTIONIST

The receptionist is likely to be the patient's initial contact with the physician's practice, and, for this reason, the receptionist should have a clear understanding of the office procedure best suited for the elderly patient. Successful communication should be established from the outset. The receptionist should convey information regarding what can be expected during the initial evaluation, the patient's or surrogate's responsibilities, and the financial structuring of the practice.

With training and experience, the receptionist may elicit the concerns that precipitated the patient's visit. This information establishes the priorities of the first visit and ensures that the most important issues are addressed. For an elderly person with many complex medical problems, the receptionist may need to explain that more than one visit could be required to complete the initial assessment. The patient and family should know that substantial time may be devoted to exchanging and gathering information during the initial visit. A complete history and examination may require more than one visit. A comprehensive functional assessment may be accomplished only over time through a series of visits. Reassurance that all problems will be addressed in time is helpful to patients and families.

The receptionist should instruct the patient or surrogate to bring past medical information to the first visit. Medical records from hospitals or other physicians should be requested in advance. The patient or family should be encouraged to bring all medications, including eye drops and over-the-counter remedies such as laxatives.

A cognitively impaired elderly person should always be accompanied by a caregiver, preferably an individual who is familiar with the issues relevant to the patient's health and functional capacity. A primary surrogate or contact person should be identified for a patient who has substantial cognitive impairments. The primary contact person should be identified by the receptionist when the first appointment is made.

In an effort to minimize forgotten visits, the receptionist may devise a system to call the patient or contact person and confirm appointments shortly before the scheduled date. Additionally, office personnel should assist with transportation arrangements if the patient is unable to make arrangements.

PREAPPOINTMENT DATA COLLECTION

Data collection before the patient's initial office visit is frequently used to gather insurance information, emergency contacts, telephone numbers, and addresses. Some practitioners expand this effort and request the patient or caregiver to provide written information about medical and surgical history, medications, family history, activities of daily living, social history, and review of systems. This allows the patient or caregiver to reflect on the history, symptoms, and concerns, in detail, before the visit. Collection of data before an office visit permits the patient to obtain addresses and telephone numbers of other physicians and gather correct information regarding dates of those visits, increasing the likelihood that the clinician receives appropriate, detailed, and accurate past medical information.

However, preappointment data collection does not eliminate the need for face-to-face history taking with the patient. The data sheets should be reviewed in person with the patient or caregiver so that information can be explored and clarified. The preappointment data forms permit a quick survey of the information and early prioritization of the patient's problems. Having the broad spectrum of information available at the beginning of the office visit may help eliminate a patients's end-of-appointment disclosure of information that would mandate immediate attention.

Some clinicians find that the sheets for preappointment data collection are overly structured and prefer to gather information in person from the patients or surrogates. Allowing patients to tell their stories provides insight into the patients' values, mental status, family interaction, and general function. A patient who is unable to give an adequate history and maintain concentration, or who looks to relatives for answers or denies all problems, creates an overall impression for the physician that directs the subsequent portion of the evaluation. In addition, the interview process itself is therapeutic for many patients. The physician should avoid the temptation to shuffle papers or talk to the families instead of the patients. Elderly patients appreciate physicians who listen to them.

THE FIRST VISIT

For many frail older patients, it is not possible to accomplish comprehensive evaluation in one office visit. The traditional model of a *complete* history and physical examination carried out in one episode often must be discarded in favor of an initial visit that is flexible and designed to serve the diverse needs of the individual patient.

As Sir William Osler said, "Listen to the patient, he'll give you the diagnosis." The first visit, therefore, should be a time for beginning a relationship with the patient and initiating data collection. The elderly patient may have an extensive medical history and multiple current health concerns. A comprehensive evaluation and correlation of symptoms and signs is likely to take time.

Efficient time management is an ongoing priority in any physician's practice. Most clinicians find ways to use their skills of observation throughout their contact with the patient during the visit. For example, after giving the patient directions to the examination room, the physician may observe the patient's ability to stand with or without assistance. Noting the characteristics of the patient's gait and mobility begins the neurological examination.

Using the information from the form for preappointment data collection or from the initial portion of the interview, the physician decides the priorities of the visit. For example, the evaluation of a patient with memory loss requires a detailed mental status examination that uses cognitive and affective assessment tools. A discussion of assessment tools commonly used in the evaluation of elderly patients is found in Chapter 13.

Data organization in the medical record

Regardless of the methods for data collection, a system for organizing the data is necessary. If a form for preappointment data collection is used, this information must be reviewed. Each clinician develops a system for managing information that allows meaningful organization and speedy retrieval of key elements of data. The accompanying box illustrates the content and format of such a system that allows organization of information that is especially relevant in the initial evaluation of an elderly patient.

INITIAL EVALUATION OF GERIATRIC PATIENT

Primary reason for visit
Current medical problems
Past medical history
Past surgical history
Current medications
Medication allergies
Vaccine status
• Influenza
• Pneumococcus
• Tetanus

Social issues
• Living status (apartment, married, etc.)
• Driving
• Smoking
• Drinking alcohol

Moreover, the practitioner may listen attentively and still record data under various categories as the patient talks. This method permits patients to tell diffuse stories in their own words, while the physician records information in a meaningfully organized fashion.

An additional tool that saves time during follow-up visits or unscheduled visits and calls is an information sheet listing the patient's name and telephone number, surrogate and telephone number, pharmacy number, and associated providers such as visiting nurses or case managers. A current record of health problems and medications should be recorded and updated at regular intervals (Figure 2-1) so that the physician can tell, at a glance, what services the patient is receiving.

Review of systems

The traditional review of systems can be modified to incorporate some of the common syndromes and problems that older patients exhibit. This information may be included in the preappointment data but should be carefully reviewed with the patient. The patient's responses are enhanced by careful selection of terms and modification of questions to fit that patient's background and level of understanding.

Revising the review of systems to include the common syndromes affecting older patients enables the physician to discover many underreported conditions. Important, potentially remediable areas of concern that physicians and patients often ignore include sensory changes, falls, sexual function, incontinence, driving safety, and memory loss. Evidence of sensory changes should be sought routinely since vision, hearing, taste, and smell frequently diminish with age, causing substantial impact on the function and well-being of an older person. Loss of vision is associated with an increase in falls, while decreased taste and smell can contribute to weight loss. Falls are underreported by older persons and can lead to significant injuries. Sexual function often is not discussed in the physician's office but may have great impact on the quality of an older person's life. Incontinence also deserves an evaluation for treatable causes. (See chapters that also discuss each of the above topics.)

Problem list

A prioritized list of problems should be established at the time of the initial visit. Prioritization is best accomplished in partnership with the patient or surrogate to seek consensus on the goals of care and determine which problems warrant additional evaluation. (See Chapter 1.) This technique highlights elements of the patient's overall condition and function that can be improved or, at least, stabilized. Outcomes of improved function or comfort may be more important than laboratory parameters reflecting disease activity. When cure is impossible, priorities of care may focus on preventing further disability from the disease. For example, a diagnosis of multi-infarct dementia precludes hope for repair of preexisting brain damage; however,

PATIENT INFORMATION SHEET

Date _____

Name _____   Phone _____

Surrogate _____   Phone _____

Advance directives _____

_____

Allergies _____

Pharmacy number _____

Other providers _____

Problem list

1. _____   6. _____

2. _____   7. _____

3. _____   8. _____

4. _____   9. _____

5. _____   10. _____

Medications	Dose/Frequency	Date prescribed

Figure 2-1 Example of information sheet for elderly patients. These data are useful as quick references for follow-up visits, unscheduled visits, or calls by patients and families.

adequate blood pressure control, avoidance of centrally acting antihypertensive medications, and daily doses of aspirin may prevent further infarcts and additional morbidity.

Formulating a list of problems for an elderly patient with functional impairments requires the physician to extend the focus of the health assessment outside the medical realm into psychological and social aspects of the patient's life. Solutions to deficits in one aspect of function may require considerations in other domains. For example, an older person with hemiparesis and poststroke depression may require psychotherapy and antidepressant medication (psychological realm), as well as transportation to and from church (social realm) to achieve maximum functional recovery.

After completing the problem list, physicians and patients, or their surrogates, collaborate regarding plans of care that are most likely to have significant positive impact on the patients' status. The importance of cooperative mutual decision making is emphasized. The patients and their families are more likely to comply with evaluation and treatment plans if they concur with the formulation of the problem. Disagreement between physicians and patients or families about the significance of the patients' signs and symptoms is likely to result in failed trials of treatment.

An attempt to evaluate and address too many of a patient's problems at once may be overwhelming for the patient, family, and physician. Patients who have not received medical attention for a prolonged period (as is sometimes the case with previously vigorous older persons who proudly avoided doctors) may resist making and keeping subsequent appointments. The complexities and priorities of each older patient must be weighed by the clinician. Unless a particular condition is life threatening, it may be more effective for a clinician to evaluate and treat such a patient slowly and comprehensively. Like patients from any other age group, elderly persons must perceive that there is a problem before they will be motivated toward change. Compliance with the physician's recommendations is more likely to occur if the patient or surrogate fully understands the issues and agrees with the approach to care. A partnership for health care necessitates concordance between physician and patient.

Advance directives and surrogate decision makers

In addition to a prioritized list of problems, a special section in the medical record should document discussion of advance directives and reflect designated surrogate decision makers. (See Chapter 9.) Copies of legal documents certifying guardians, forms for durable power of attorney, and other important documents should be kept together in a readily accessible area of the chart. Progress notes reflecting discussions with patients or surrogates about the goals of care and the patients' preferences for limitations on care may be kept in this section. These notes should be dated, and the names and roles of those participating in the discussion should be recorded. Periodic update and verification is advisable.

FOLLOW-UP VISITS

Continuity is a particularly important element of an effective care plan since many elderly persons are coping with chronic diseases and disabilities. While discreet problems such as infections and injuries may arise and subsequently resolve, many problems will endure, to some degree, throughout the relationship of the patient and physician. Attending to prevention, minimizing the impact of disabilities, and promoting function are often recurrent themes of subsequent office visits.

When addressing recurrent problems, the physician and patient should plan the agenda for the next encounter at the termination of the office visit. This information should be recorded in the progress notes and reviewed by the physician and the patient at the beginning of the next visit. The timing of visits is an important consideration when physicians manage chronic health difficulties. For example, an older patient with severe anxiety about various health issues may benefit from brief weekly visits until the crisis is resolved and the anxiety is reduced to a tolerable level. An overabundance of phone calls between visits may signal the need for an increase in the frequency of office visits for a time.

Efficiency is a high priority for most practitioners, and it is aided by prospectively establishing time allotments for visits. Informing patients about these allotments may help the physician set limits for difficult and complex patients. Usually, this helps the office run smoothly.

REFERRALS

Patients and families appreciate information on community resources and services pertaining to older persons. Visiting nurses, home health aides, social workers, and lawyers who specialize in issues affecting elderly persons are frequently requested. Lawyers should be familiar with estate planning for cognitively impaired patients, advance directives, and issues of surrogacy. Many communities offer resource consultants who specialize in various issues concerning older adults.

Patients and families often ask for information regarding adult day care programs, community agencies that help Alzheimer's patients and families, rehabilitation facilities, assisted living residences, and nursing homes. Many programs and facilities publish brochures or newsletters that can be displayed and made available in the physician's office. An informed receptionist or nurse can assist patients and families with this information.

SUGGESTED READINGS

Branch L., Nemeth K: When elders fail to visit physicians, *Med Care* 23:11, 1985.

Fahs M et al: Primary medical care for elderly patients Part II: results of a survey of office-based clinicians, *J of Comm Health* 14:2, 1989.

Malone M, Allison J: How *not* to practice geriatrics, *Geriatr* 45:12, 1990.

CHAPTER 3

Principles of prescribing medications

GORDON A. IRELAND

KEY POINTS
- Consideration of nonpharmaceutical management should always precede medication selection.
- The choice of medication therapy should be based on the patient's expected quality of life.
- Physiological changes of aging necessitate adjustments of medication dose and/or dosage.
- Patient and/or family education regarding disease and therapy is of utmost importance.
- Regular monitoring should be conducted for evidence of therapeutic benefit and adverse reactions with regard to the patient's quality of life.

Prescribing medications to geriatric patients should occur only after a thorough consideration of all possible nonpharmacological therapies—only then should medications be used. For example, the management of anxiety and/or depression may be accomplished by changing the patient's environment or living conditions or correcting the underlying cause. Insomnia may be managed by changing the patient's daily sleep pattern. The patient in a long-term care facility who cannot sleep at 9 PM may not need a sedative but may be managed by rooming with another patient who also likes to stay up later.

When prescribing medications for the elderly patient, a physician should consider three general factors: the therapeutic goal, potential adverse effects, and patient's quality of life.[1] The therapeutic goal should be one that is realistically achievable. The goal may not be to cure, as in a young patient, but to control the disease and maximize the patient's quality of life. In fact, for the geriatric patient, quality of life may be the most important issue. The therapy should produce the best quality of life possible. This may be achieved by the physician's analysis of the therapeutic benefits along with possible adverse reactions. The clinical feature of adverse effects in geriatric patients may be different in severity and presentation from those seen in younger patients and, therefore, may go unrecognized as an adverse effect and be treated by additional medications.[6] Any change in clinical status of a patient that is associated chronologically with a medication change, even a small change such as the time of day the dose was administered, should be viewed as an adverse effect until proved otherwise. The interplay of therapeutic goal and adverse effects often has a narrow margin for older patients.

PHARMACOLOGY

Definition

Pharmacology is the study of the preparation, characteristics, effects, and uses of drugs. *Pharmacokinetics* refers to properties of a drug that determine or affect the absorption, distribution, and clearance (metabolism and excretion) of that drug. *Pharmacodynamics* is the study of factors or properties (frequently host factors) that determine or affect the action of a drug.

Physiological changes of aging

The aging process produces many physiological changes that affect the activity of medications.[3] The pharmacokinetic parameters affected by the physiological changes of aging are listed in the box on p. 20.

Absorption. The effects on absorption may be separated into two general categories: the extent of absorption and the rate of absorption. Research data suggest that the extent of absorption does not change significantly with aging.[7] It appears that an older patient absorbs the same amount of medication from an oral dose as a younger patient. However, the rate of absorption for most medications decreases with aging. This decrease in rate may produce a slower onset of action and a lower peak effect. Older patients being treated for an acute problem that needs rapid action should be allowed approximately twice the time to reach the desired effect as in younger patients. For example, in patients treated for insomnia, drowsiness occurs in 15 to 30 minutes in a young patient following an adequate dose of a sedative, whereas in an elderly patient it may take 45 to 60 minutes. It is important to allow adequate time for the desired effect before giving the elderly patient a second dose. If the second dose is given too rapidly, the patient may experience toxicity when both doses eventually exhibit their full activity. Orders for prn medications should be written to alert the user or administrator of this effect. Poor nutrition may also contribute to decreased rate of absorption. (See Nutritional Status for further discussion of this topic.)[3]

Distribution. During the aging process, the distribution of body content may change. The percentage by weight that is made up of fat may increase and total body water may decrease.[3] These two factors may differ from patient to patient because of many factors, including basic nutrition and hydration. The *volume of distribution* (Vd)

PHARMACOKINETIC PARAMETERS AND THE
PHYSIOLOGICAL CHANGES OF AGING

Absorption
- Increased gastric pH
- Decreased gastrointestinal blood flow
- Gastrointestinal mucosal changes
- Delayed gastric emptying time
- Decreased gastrointestinal motility

Distribution
- Decreased lean body mass
- Increased percentage body fat
- Decreased total body water
- Decreased cardiac output★

Metabolism
- Decreased cardiac output★
- Decreased viable liver cells
- Decreased function of the oxidation pathway
- Decreased amounts of liver metabolic enzymes

Excretion
- Decreased cardiac output★
- Decreased number of functioning nephrons
- Decreased glomerular filtration rate

★Some data indicate cardiac output is unchanged with age in healthy older adults.

of a medication is determined by the relationship between the amount of body fat, body water, and the solubility of the medication in each compartment. For example, the effect of lipid-soluble drugs (e.g., benzodiazepines) may be longer in duration for for individuals with higher body fat content. Because of interpatient variability in body fat and water, it is difficult to predict the Vd of a drug with accuracy in individual geriatric patients. Since the dose of a medication needed to produce a plasma concentration is directly proportional to the size of the Vd, it is, therefore, difficult to predict an accurate dose. Starting with a low dose and increasing the dose, as clinical and adverse effects allow, is the safest and most effective way to prescribe medications in elderly patients.[2]

Clearance. Clearance is the elimination of the medication from the body by metabolism (primarily liver), excretion (primarily kidney), or a combination of both.[7] Clearance by liver metabolism may be decreased or remain unchanged with aging, depending on the specific pathway through which the chemical is metabolized. Research indicates that medications metabolized by the oxidation pathway may have age-related decreased rates of clearance, even though all commonly used liver function tests are normal.[3] Such medications should be administered less frequently, or another medication should be chosen that has the same therapeutic effect but uses a different metabolic pathway. Dalmane (flurazepam), for example, a sedative commonly pre-scribed in hospitals, is metabolized by the oxidation pathway and has been shown to have a half-life as long as 2 weeks in the geriatric patient. Its use has been associated with morning falls in elderly patients who may remain lethargic into the afternoon after a dose of Dalmane the previous evening. The other metabolic pathways have not been shown to be significantly affected by the aging process.[3] Malnutrition and hypothyroidism, problems common to the geriatric population, may cause a decrease in rate of metabolism by all pathways, even though liver function studies may prove normal.

Clearance by renal excretion is decreased in essentially all patients age 65 years and older.[7] Although the decrement in clearance varies from patient to patient in the same age group, the decrease in the excretion rate worsens as age increases. Creatinine clearance values are good estimates of glomerular filtration and when studied over a large population, a linear relationship exists between the creatinine clearance and the medication elimination rate constant; but for each creatinine clearance determined, the medication excretion rate may vary widely from poor to good clearance. The ability of the kidneys to clear a medication may be estimated by calculating the creatinine clearance. This measurement, though only an estimate of glomerular fil-tration rate, is better than any readily available measurement for the determination of liver medication clearance. The dosing interval will often be greater than that used in younger patients when treating an older patient with a medication primarily cleared through the kidneys.

Since the absorption, distribution, and clearance of medications administered to elderly patients are not easily or accurately determined, the practitioner is urged to obtain blood concentrations of medications for which therapeutic parameters have been established.[7] For chronically administered oral medications, the most repro-ducible blood level occurs immediately before a dose after steady state has been achieved (i.e., after five half-lives of a continuous dose). For parenteral or short-term oral medications, blood levels may be drawn at various times depending on the medication and the type of pharmacokinetic information desired. However, it is essential to know the amount of the dose, the time the dose was given, and the time the blood level was drawn before a meaningful interpretation of the level may be made.

Pharmacodynamics. The physiological changes of aging not only affect pharma-cokinetic parameters but also pharmacodynamic factors.[3] Changes in pharmacody-namics are possibly produced by variable receptor sensitivity, changes in numbers of receptors, or a combination of the two. These changes may be the reason why two patients with the same pharmacokinetic parameters react with different intensities to the same medication or why geriatric patients experience different, or more severe, adverse effects than younger patients (e.g., the mental confusion associated with histamine-2 antagonists). The pharmacodynamic changes may also explain why older patients may experience paradoxical reactions to certain medications (e.g., excitation rather than sedation when given phenobarbital or diphenhydramine).

With all these potential variables in pharmacokinetics and pharmacodynamics affecting medication therapy in geriatric patients, it is important to heed the adage "start low and go slow."[7] The incidences of toxicities and side effects are less frequent and less severe when the initial doses are as low as possible, and changes are made in small increments and patients closely monitored.

FACTORS TO CONSIDER IN PRESCRIBING DRUGS

Multiple medications

Polypharmacy or *polymedicating* is common in the geriatric population.[3] Multiple studies have shown that persons 65 and older take an average of five to seven medications daily. While some patients may need five or six medications to control their diseases and improve their quality of life, the majority do not. Evidence suggests that incidences of falls and other adverse effects increase significantly when elderly patients take more than four medications. Compliance also becomes more difficult as the number and dose of medications increase. The indications for continuing each medication should be evaluated on a periodic basis (e.g., every 6 to 12 months). Since the average older person has multiple chronic diseases (see the box below)[5], multiple medications seem like a rational mode of therapy. This rationale fades as quality of life becomes more important than curing all of the patient's diseases. In fact, some therapeutic modalities for the younger patient may not be effective in the geriatric patient because of the physiological changes of aging that have occurred in the diseased organ. For example, the therapeutic effect of digoxin in the treatment of congestive heart failure is of questionable benefit since the inotropic mechanism seems to have little positive effect on the aging cardiac muscle.

Patients with multiple diseases may be seen by several medical specialists. Specialists may contribute to polypharmacy since these clinicians have specialty medications with which they are familiar, and they may feel uncomfortable commenting on another specialist's therapy. A primary care physician should coordinate the care

---

DISEASES COMMON TO THE GERIATRIC POPULATION*

Arthritis (55%)
Cardiac disease (50%)
Hypertension (43%)
Vascular disease (40%)
Chronic pain (30%)
Pulmonary disease (25%)
Peptic ulcer disease (25%)
Cancer (25%)

---

*Age 65 years and older.

plan for the patient after considering the advice of all specialists by maintaining detailed and frequent communication with the specialists and the patient to prevent polypharmacy.

Nutritional status

Medications may be affected by the nutritional status of the patient.[3] Although there currently is a minimum amount of supporting data, poor nutrition may decrease the rates of gastrointestinal absorption, transfer across tissue membranes, and cellular enzymatic reactions. These changes may decrease absorption, distribution, and clearance and, ultimately, the effectiveness of medication therapy.

Hydration also is an important factor in medication effectiveness. An adequate amount of water in the gastrointestinal tract is necessary for a medication's dissolution and absorption and the prevention of medication-induced constipation; a normal blood volume is essential for optimal distribution and the prevention of medication-induced orthostatic hypotension; interstitial fluid is necessary for good intercellular transport of medications; and good blood flow is necessary for optimal liver metabolism and renal excretion of medications. Patients should be continuously reminded of the importance of good nutrition and hydration.

Cognitive impairment

Although cognitive impairment may be associated with age-related disorders and specific diseases, it also is a common result of an adverse effect from medications.[3] The impairment may not be easily recognizable but may be noticeable to the patient as a slowness in mental recall. A mental status evaluation at baseline should be administered (e.g., Folstein Mini Mental State Test) and repeated if a medication-induced change is suspected. It is important to always consider medications as the cause of a change in an elderly patient's mental status.

Economic status and generic brands

Economic constraints should be considered in all therapeutic regimens. Generic medications may decrease the cost to the patient. A number of potential problems regarding generic medications need to be addressed. First, not all generic brands have the same bioavailability under all administering circumstances. Switching from one generic to another generic may cause the patient to experience swings in therapeutic control or encounter varying amounts of adverse effects. It is important to stay with one generic brand that is acceptable to both patient and practitioner. The patient should ask to have a prescription filled with the same generic brand, once a suitable generic medication has been identified. Practitioners also may write a "no substitution" prescription for a specific generic brand. Second, compliance may become a problem if the patient is not adequately educated about the differences in shape and color among generic preparations. Many elderly patients remember to take their medications by color (e.g., the blue pill three times a day; the pink pill two times a day; the white pill once a day). If the next refill of the blue pill is white, the white pill is pink, and the pink pill is green, it is understandable how therapeutic regimens could be disrupted with potentially serious results.

Support systems

Many support systems are available to help elderly patients manage their medications successfully. Neighbors and families may be educated in observation techniques and medication administration. Visiting nurses or other agencies may be employed. Medication dispensing boxes that are filled on a weekly basis may be used to aid in the patient's compliance. It is important to maintain a list of available services in the patient's geographical area and advise the patient about the availability and usefulness of those services.

PRINCIPLES FOR PRESCRIBING DRUGS

The choice of medication should be made after the potential end point of therapy and desired quality of life are determined. The choice should not be made solely on the basis of the disease state to be treated, but also should include such factors as the route of administration, pharmacokinetics and pharmacodynamics of the medication, potential patient compliance, and economics of therapy. The goals in drug selection are to achieve maximum therapeutic benefit with the least adverse effects, the best compliance, and the least economic impact on the patient.

In addition to the common routes of drug administration (i.e., oral tablet, capsule, or liquid and intravenous, intramuscular, or subcutaneous injection), other routes should be considered such as transdermal patch, rectal suppository, or inhalant, depending on availability, clinical circumstances, effectiveness, patient tolerance, functional capacity, and expense.

The dose and dosage should be chosen on the basis of the pharmacokinetics of the medication. Practitioners should remember that the rate of absorption decreases and the half-life increases for most medications excreted by the kidneys or by the oxidation pathway in the liver. In the treatment of chronic diseases, medications administered once or twice a day will aid in the patient's compliance with therapy. For example, when second-generation oral hypoglycemic agents are used, the longer half-life of glyburide gives it a potential advantage over glipizide. Glyburide may be dosed one time a day, whereas glipizide usually needs to be dosed two times a day.

Education of the patient and caregiver is immensely important for successful achievement of a desired outcome from a drug prescription. Compliance in all patient populations depends on well-educated patients, whether living at home, in hospital, or in a long term-care facility. Education should involve all aspects of therapy, including nonpharmaceutical modalities. The goal of each medication used should be stated along with the approximate time frame in which these goals may be realized. Pertinent potential adverse effects must be addressed, including information about what the patient should do if adverse effects occur. The education process should be repeated at every visit by all the patient's health care practitioners. All instructions for correct administration of the medications, and any other important information, should be in written form for the patient to review as necessary.

The patient's and caregiver's understanding of educational information should be evaluated, and, if their understanding is inadequate, other means of insuring compliance must be instituted. A visiting nurse, pharmacist, or neighbor might fill dispensing trays and monitor the compliance of the patient. Patients should be instructed to bring all of their medications with them for each visit with their physicians so that a thorough therapeutic, adverse effect, and compliance evaluation may be made. Timely monitoring of patient therapy is essential for geriatric patient care.

REFERENCES

1. Bulpit CJ, Fletcher AE: Drug treatment and quality of life in the elderly, *Clin Geriatr Med* 6(2):309, 1990.
2. Cooper JM: Reviewing geriatric concerns with commonly used drugs, *Geriatrics* 44(12):79, 1989.
3. Diggory P et al: Medicine in the elderly, *Postgrad Med J* 67:423, 1991.
4. Hussar DA: Drug interactions in the older patient, *Geriatrics* 43(Sup):20, 1988.
5. Jinks MJ, Raschko RR: A profile of alcohol and prescription abuse in a high-risk community-based elderly population, *DICP Ann Pcol* 24:971, 1990.
6. Lamy PP: Adverse drug effects, *Clin Geriatr Med* 6(2):293, 1990.
7. Reidenberg MM: Drug therapy in the elderly: the problem from the point of view of a clinical pharmacologist, *Clin Pharmacol Ther* 42(6):677, 1987.

SUGGESTED READINGS

Bulpit CJ, Fletcher AE: Drug treatment and quality of life in the elderly, *Clin Geriatr Med* 6(2):309, 1990.
Lamy PP: Adverse drug effects, *Clin Geriatr Med* 6(2):293, 1990.

CHAPTER 4

Rehabilitation

KENNETH BRUMMEL-SMITH

KEY POINTS

- Primary physicians have a crucial role in rehabilitation of the older patient.
- Consider a rehabilitation intervention for any patient with a history of recent loss of function.
- The principles of rehabilitation include stabilization of the primary disorder, prevention of secondary disabilities, treatment of functional defects, and promotion of adaptation.
- Refer those patients with ambulation and transfer problems to a physical therapist for evaluation.
- Refer patients with self-care deficits and instrumental activities of daily living (IADL) deficits to an occupational therapist.
- Referrals to allied health therapists should include the patient's diagnosis, medical restrictions, if any, and the instructions "Please evaluate and treat."
- A wide assortment of assistive devices is available for those in need; however, proper evaluation of a patient's needs and training the patient to use the device will ensure compliance.
- Prevention of secondary disabilities continues for the person's lifetime.

Rehabilitation is a process whereby persons with disabilities are assisted in recovering lost or diminished functional abilities. In many ways, geriatrics and rehabilitation are intimately related. When caring for geriatric patients, even in the office setting, the physician is frequently confronted by an array of medical conditions, most of which have no cure. Under these circumstances, there should be a shift in the focus of care from eradicating illness to optimizing function. Rehabilitation interventions provide the mechanism for physicians to optimize a patient's functional abilities.

The primary care physician plays a crucial role in rehabilitation, regardless of the setting of care. In office settings, many rehabilitation interventions may be initiated by the primary physician. Physicians are often called upon to approve or prescribe assistive devices. The physician also must be aware of the risks of rehabilitation interventions and ameliorate them. Other important activities include consultations with allied health care providers such as social workers, physical and occupational therapists, or home health care providers. This relationship is usually a multidisciplinary one, and communications are achieved by phone calls and written reports. Unfortunately, the luxury of a regular interdisciplinary team meeting is not available to most office-based physicians.

Rehabilitation is also closely tied to comprehensive assessment. (See Chapter 12.) Assessment provides the clinical information on which decisions can be made regarding care. Despite many medical and social interventions, direct functional interventions are most often associated with rehabilitation. Retraining in activities of daily living (ADL) and instrumental activities of daily living (IADL), providing assistive devices for use in the home, or enhancing strength and endurance of the patient are all the purview of rehabilitation.

When physicians manage patients who require rehabilitation, it is important for them to become familiar with some definitions. The World Health Organization has proposed the use of the terms impairment, disability, and handicap for discussing these issues. An *impairment* refers to a disorder that is experienced at the organ system level. The usual state of aging is associated with many impairments such as arthritis and decreases in renal function or muscle strength. If the impairment is severe enough to decrease the person's ability to function, that is called a *disability*. Rehabilitation is primarily oriented toward disabled persons and helps them eradicate, reduce, or adapt to their disabling conditions. When people are prevented from expressing their full potential as independently functioning individuals, they have been *handicapped*; hence, there are no handicapped people, only handicapping societies. Terms such as *crippled, wheelchair bound,* or *invalid* should be avoided because they are disrespectful and demeaning.

PRINCIPLES OF REHABILITATION

While the basic principles of rehabilitation are the same, regardless of a patient's age, the application of those principles is modified when physicians care for an older person. (See box on p. 28.)

Stabilization of the primary disorder is often difficult and elusive in geriatrics. The best approach uses functional interventions simultaneously with attempts at medical stabilization.

Preventing secondary complications or disabilities (see box p. 28) is also different for older persons. Such problems develop more often, more rapidly, and are more

---

PRINCIPLES OF REHABILITATION

Stabilize the primary disorder
Prevent secondary disabilities
Treat functional deficits
Promote adaptation
• Person to disability
• Environment to person
• Family to person

SECONDARY DISABILITIES SEEN IN REHABILITATION

Anorexia	Incontinence
Confusion	Pneumonia
Contractures	Pressure sores
Deconditioning	Shoulder problems
Dependency	Venous thrombosis
Depression	

---

difficult to treat than in younger persons.[4] The occurrence of one of these disabilities can lead to a significant setback in the rehabilitation process.

Treatment of functional deficits is the foundation of rehabilitation. Therapy often includes muscle reeducation, strengthening, and endurance training, as well as learning novel ways to carry out well-established activities. There is little evidence that the recovery of lost functional abilities is inherently different in older persons. However, the treatment of such persons may differ. Older persons may learn at a slower pace, require more repetitions to learn new physical activities, and require a longer time to build strength.[1]

The development of multiple areas of adaptation is also a key goal in rehabilitation. The person must adapt to a new disability. For some older persons, adapting to disabilities is especially difficult. The environment also must be adapted to the person. Older houses, for example, may be more difficult to adapt because doorways often need to be widened. Two-story houses are common in gentrified neighborhoods. Access to the second floor can be difficult for the elderly person. Finally, the family must adapt to the disabled person. An overly supportive family may promote dependency by helping the disabled person too much. Conversely, the demands on the family, many of whom are elderly themselves, may lead to neglect or even abuse of the disabled person.

OUTPATIENT REHABILITATION FOR COMMON GERIATRIC PROBLEMS

Stroke

Stroke is the most common condition for which geriatric patients receive rehabilitation. While most rehabilitation interventions occur in the acute facility or skilled nursing home, primary physicians see many patients in the office where questions are raised about continued or new rehabilitation interventions. The physician also is often involved in home rehabilitation efforts after a patient is discharged from a health care facility.

Although most gains from rehabilitation come during the first 6 months after the stroke, there is often a role for rehabilitation long after this time period. For instance, the person may not have received any intensive rehabilitation and may still need a significant amount of training. A person may never have learned about certain assistive devices or self-care skills. There also may have been spontaneous improvements that were not initially recognized such as clearing of an impaired sensorium. Finally, there may have been a recent diminution of self-care skills because of intercurrent illnesses. Any new development that indicates a recent decline in the patient's functioning or reason to expect further improvement with rehabilitation should be seen as an opportunity for reevaluation.

Monitoring patients for secondary disabilities should continue for the rest of their lives. (See the box on p. 28.) The most important secondary disabilities in outpatient stroke patients are pressure sores, contractures, subluxation of the shoulders (sometimes with associated hand-shoulder syndrome), and deconditioning. Pressure sores are seen primarily in immobilized patients, but it is important to be aware that leg braces sometimes cause pressure areas. Contractures are often seen in the wrists, hip adductors and flexors, knees, and ankles. Periodic range of motion examinations are needed to identify patients who have contractures. Patients with contractures should be referred to a therapist for stretching exercises and serial casting if the limitation of range is interfering with function. Subluxation of the shoulder is frequently overlooked in primary care.[6] The superior margin of the humerus can be palpated as an indentation approximately 1 to 2 cm below the acromioclavicular joint. The morbidity of this complication is the development of moderate to severe pain, or worse, the hand-shoulder syndrome (reflex sympathetic dystrophy). This syndrome is characterized by edema, erythema, and slight temperature increase in the involved upper extremity. The main therapeutic approach is physical therapy. While standard analgesics and nonsteroidal antiinflammatory drugs (NSAIDs) are appropriate, other interventions such as corticosteroids, or sympathetic nerve blocks, may be required.[9] Deconditioning should be suspected in any patient who has had a prolonged period of bed rest. The patient usually exhibits an exaggerated blood pressure and heart rate in response to exercise (with no other associated problems such as congestive heart failure). Endurance is also severely limited. Physical therapists can be very helpful in designing an exercise program, but the duration of recovery for the patient will probably be twice that of the time spent at bed rest.[10]

Perhaps one of the most important complications the primary physician can diagnose is depression. For most older people, their primary physicians function as their psychiatrists. Emotional conditions influence outcomes as much as physical deficits such as weakness or sensory loss.[7] Unfortunately, patients' emotional conditions are often overlooked in clinical practice. In addition, patients with left hemisphere strokes seem particularly prone to depression.[2]

Ensuring that patients have necessary equipment and assistive devices is often the responsibility of the primary physician. If the patient has never had a home assessment, then either the physician or a health care professional from a visiting nurses' association can perform this vital service. The array of equipment that is available is discussed below.

Hip fracture

With the advent of diagnosis related groups (DRGs), patients with hip fractures are leaving the hospital sooner and are less ambulatory. If they go to a nursing home, they also are liable to stay there for a prolonged period of time.[3] Both of these adverse effects are probably due to rehabilitation that is provided less intensively. Whether rehabilitation occurs in patients' homes or at outpatient clinics, patients regain their function as well as if they had received untested rehabilitation.

Patients who have had a compression screw or hip prosthesis inserted can begin ambulation training in the first week after the surgery. Pain management is crucial to allow for full exercise tolerance. This is important to prevent deconditioning and thrombosis complications. Physical therapy can be very helpful in gait training.[5] A cane is helpful to "unweight" the affected side. It should be cut to length so that when the arm hangs at the side, the crook of the cane comes to the wrist. An intact rubber tip is needed. The patient should use the cane in the hand opposite the hip fracture. Patients with poor balance probably will need a walker. Many communities have exercise groups for older persons in senior centers or YMCAs.

Complications may occur during the ambulatory care period; the major ones are infections and loosening of the prosthesis. Infection of a prosthesis should be suspected in any patient with unexplained fever, pain, or decreases in prior levels of functioning. Diagnosis of prosthetic septic arthritis is made by aspirating the joint for a culture. Loosening is usually attended by pain felt immediately when standing up but then diminishing once standing for a short period of time. On radiographs, areas of radiolucency can be seen around the hardware. Some patients may need replacement, although many benefit from a nonsurgical approach by using pain medications, walking devices, and bed exercises.

Arthritis

The cornerstone of arthritis management is pain management. An in-depth discussion of these conditions is found in Chapter 40. Intraarticular injections of corticosteroids and anesthetics can be very helpful and enable the patient to exercise and maintain mobility.

The primary roles of rehabilitation are strengthening of the muscles, maintaining range of motion, and training in joint protection techniques. Patients should be assessed by physical and occupational therapists. A daily home exercise program should be established, including "ranging," lying prone for 10 to 15 minutes to prevent hip and knee flexion deformities, and strengthening exercises. Patients must distinguish between too much stress on the joints and not enough exercise. Occupational therapists can prescribe a variety of adaptive equipment such as can openers, dressing sticks, button hooks, and reachers.

Movement disorders

Parkinson's disease is one of the most common neurological conditions seen in aging patients. While inpatient rehabilitation efforts have not proved beneficial to this disorder, outpatient treatment may be more effective. Group treatment programs seem to be the most effective. Balance and gait training should be taught. Dancing seems to help some people more than standard training programs. Physicians can remind patients of the "mantra": Consciously use the head-up-shoulders-back posture to counteract the body position in Parkinson's disease.

THE USE OF ASSISTIVE DEVICES

Physicians should be familiar with common assistive devices used in rehabilitation. Devices can be used to assist with ADL (see box on p. 32) or IADL and to modify the patient's environment. Therapists can be very helpful in deciding which devices are most appropriate for a particular patient and in training patients about the use of such devices. There are excellent catalogs that demonstrate these devices.[8]

Devices for IADL

Especially for women, their ability to return to cooking is seen as a major step in rehabilitation. Even if it is only preparation of light meals, independent cooking also can reduce the cost of care significantly. A wide variety of can and bottle openers is available for those with limited hand strength. Special grips exist as aids for pouring from milk cartons or opening boxes. Cutting boards are available that permit single-handed cutting. A stool with casters enables those who have limited endurance to rest while they cook.

```
┌────────────────── AIDS FOR ACTIVITIES OF DAILY LIVING (ADL) ──────────────┐
│                                                                            │
│   **Feeding**                          **Bathing**                         │
│   Rocker knives                        Tub bench                           │
│   Cutting boards                       Shower hose                         │
│   Plate retainers                      Grab bars                           │
│                                        Long-handled brush                  │
│   **Dressing**                                                             │
│                                        **Grooming**                        │
│   Button hooks                         Tilt mirror                         │
│   Velcro closures                      Built-up handles                    │
│   Tilt mirrors                                                             │
│   Reachers                             **Safety**                          │
│                                                                            │
│   **Toileting**                        *Lifeline* service                  │
│                                        Remote control lights               │
│   Grab bars                            Telephone dialers                   │
│   Arm frames                           Stair rails                         │
│   Raised seats                         Removal of throw rugs               │
│                                                                            │
└────────────────────────────────────────────────────────────────────────────┘
```

Communication is also important for older patients' independence. Simple devices such as pen holders, large-dial telephones, and magnifying lenses can be very useful. Although computers are primarily used by younger disabled persons at this time, the future holds even greater promise for computer-assisted communication, shopping, and environmental control for the elderly persons.

The important role of recreation in older people's lives must not be forgotten. From simple items such as large-print cards, card holders, and automatic shufflers, to games with large pieces, knitting machines, and interesting tools such as bowling ball ramps and pool cue holders, the patients' desires and interests should be the only limiting factors.

Mobility aids

Many types of assistive devices are available to promote mobility. (See the box on p. 33) Canes are the simplest devices but should be used only by patients with relatively good coordination and balance. A four-pronged (quad) cane adds stability and is useful for patients who have had a stroke. Patients with arthritis of the wrist have difficulty in using standard canes or walkers, and the addition of forearm troughs aid in their use. There are special walkers that can be used to go up stairs and hemiwalkers that are used mainly by stroke survivors. Because walkers require the use of both hands, an attached bag is useful to carry objects. Most older patients do best with a front-wheeled walker because it is easy to propel and stable if patients lean on it. Pickup walkers (i.e., those without wheels) should not be used by patients with Parkinson's because these walkers may promote backward falls.

MOBILITY AIDS

Canes

Standard
Quad
Hemi

Walkers

Pickup
Front-wheeled
Four-wheeled
Stair-climbing

Wheelchairs

Many types and sizes
Adapted door handles
Key holders

Wheelchairs are frequently used by older persons, even when they can ambulate. This is especially true when they wish to go long distances such as at shopping malls. The types of wheelchairs available are almost infinite. All patients who are prescribed a wheelchair should be evaluated by a physical therapist. The correct height and width must be determined. The patients should be assessed to determine whether leg rests, seat cushions, brake lock extensions, or arm troughs will be required.

HOME MODIFICATIONS

While modifications to the home can make the difference between independence and dependency, tact must be used when suggestions are made to older people about changing their "castles." It is also wise to make only a few suggestions at one time and depend on the continuing relationship to allow for later changes. Most of the changes that are beneficial occur in bathrooms, kitchens, and entryways. One of the most important, and most difficult changes, is to widen doorways to allow access with a walker or wheelchair. This is especially true for persons living in mobile homes. Walkers are about 24 inches wide, though some are narrower. Wheelchairs are 24 to 30 inches wide. Most doorways are 27 to 30 inches wide. If the tolerance is close, some width can be gained by removing the door or installing a special hinge that allows the door to swing out and lay flat against the wall.

General accessibility can be gained by replacing doorknobs with handles, removing throw rugs, and providing good lighting. If a ramp is necessary, there must be 12 inches of run for every 1 inch of rise. Rails should be placed on all stairs, preferably on both sides. Some people prefer to remove sliding doors to make closets more accessible.

REFERRALS TO CONSULTANTS

The primary physician often consults with other specialists when confronted with rehabilitation issues. The physiatrist (a specialist in physical medicine and rehabilitation) is particularly helpful in determining whether the patient could benefit from a brace or prosthesis, analyzing abnormal gait or movement patterns, or designing specialized rehabilitation programs. A physiatry consultation is also useful when physicians manage patients with spasticity problems and perform electromyographic examinations.

Physical and occupational therapy consultations are frequently used in rehabilitation. Physical therapists are primarily involved with the patient's mobility, endurance, strength, and flexibility. Occupational therapists attend to the patient's coordination, self-care, and home and community skills. Leisure activities are also addressed. Physical and occupational therapists can be of benefit to the patient whose safety is of concern.

Other specialists may be needed during the course of rehabilitation. A social worker may be required for a number of reasons. Speech and language pathologists can develop communication programs, teach the patient how to use alternative communication techniques, and evaluate and treat swallowing disorders. Home rehabilitation nurses provide in-depth family training and assessment.

REFERENCES

1. Brummel-Smith K: Rehabilitation. In Cassell CK, Reisenberg DE, Sorensen LB, Walsh JR, eds, *Geriatric medicine*, New York, 1990, Springer-Verlag.
2. Clothier J, Grotta J: Recognition and management of poststroke depression in the elderly, *Clin Geriat Med* 7:493, 1991.
3. Fitzgerald JF, Moore PS, Dittus RS: The care of elderly patients with hip fracture: changes since implementation of the prospective payment system, *N Eng J Med* 319:1392, 1988.
4. Gillick MR, Serrell NA, Gillick LS: Adverse consequences of hospitalization in the elderly, *Soc Sci Med* 16:1033, 1982.
5. Goldstein TS: *Geriatric Orthopedics: rehabilitative management of common problems*, Gaithersburg, Md, 1991, Aspen.
6. Kelly JF: Stroke rehabilitation for elderly patients. In Kemp B, Brummel-Smith K, Ramsdell JW, eds, *Geriatric rehabilitation*, Boston, 1990, College-Hill Press.
7. Kotila M et al: The profile of recovery from stroke and factors influencing outcome, *Stroke* 15:1039, 1984.
8. Sammons catalog 1991: your complete source of rehabilitation and ADL products, Brookfield, Ill, 1991, Fred Sammons Inc.
9. Schwartzman RJ, McLellan TL: Reflex sympathetic dystrophy: a review, *Arch Neurol* 44:55, 1987.
10. Siebens H: Deconditioning. In Kemp B, Brummel-Smith K, Ramsdell JW, eds, *Geriatric rehabilitation*, Boston, 1990, College-Hill Press.

SUGGESTED READINGS

Brummel-Smith K: Rehabilitation. In Cassell CK, Reisenberg DE, Sorensen LB, Walsh JR, eds, *Geriatric medicine*, New York, 1990, Springer-Verlag.

Kemp B, Brummel-Smith K, Ramsdell JW: *Geriatric rehabilitation*, Boston, 1990, College-Hill Press.

CHAPTER 5 _____

Home care

KENNETH W. HEPBURN
JOSEPH M. KEENAN

KEY POINTS

- Home care has become the foundation of this country's community-based long-term care system.
- The physician, as a member of the home care team, provides continuity of patient care and medical consultation and supervision.
- The physician serves as the most important link between the patient and the home care system and, therefore, must be knowledgeable about the available services.
- Home care incorporates the patient's and family's preferences, psychosocial supports of family and friends, and familiar environment of the home.
- The physician's home visit is a powerful affirmation of the patient-doctor relationship and is greatly appreciated by patient and family.
- The main tools of the home visit are the "black bag," good office systems and support, and the physician's art and ingenuity.
- Physicians should charge for management services related to home care.

It is appropriate that a textbook about ambulatory geriatrics should include a chapter on home care, even though many home care patients do not fit the usual description of the ambulatory patient. Home care has traditionally been an important part of ambulatory care. In recent decades, however, physicians have decreased their involvement in home care, shifting their provision of medical services almost exclusively to the office and institutional settings. Home care is still primarily managed as part of physicians' office practices, and, more than 90% of physician-delivered services in the home are for older persons.

MODERN HOME CARE

What distinguishes modern home care is the development of a cadre of professionals, primarily in nursing but also in social work and the therapy disciplines (occupational, physical, respiratory, and speech therapies), who are skilled in the assessment and management of complex illness in the home setting. Modern home care includes the traditional chronic care nursing services, as well as personal care provided by aides and other attendants (the majority of home care remains low-tech chronic care and personal services). Many home care nurse clinicians have come from the hospitals' intensive care or nurse supervisor ranks, some with training in specialty areas of care such as infectious diseases, oncology, or cardiology. The pressures of diagnosis related groups (DRGs) for earlier hospital discharges have created increased demand for all of the therapy disciplines in the home setting. Physical and occupational therapies are especially appropriate in the home because of the obvious advantage of targeting treatment to the patient's actual living environment.

Modern home care tends to be more of a team effort than traditional home care. Home care professionals all work with the medical supervision of a physician, but they do function with relatively greater autonomy than their hospital-based counterparts. Because of the greater array of services and complexity of care available in the home, a new professional function has evolved—the case manager. (See Chapter 8.) Any member of the home care team may function as the case manager, but it is typically appropriate for the nurse or social worker to provide that service. The physician's medical supervision and continuity of care and case management are discussed below.

Modern home care can be characterized further by safe, easy-to-use, technological innovations that extend the range of what is medically feasible in the home. Perhaps most notable has been the development of reliable, portable infusion systems. All types of infusions given to a medically stable patient can be administered in the home, usually with a 50% or greater cost savings than in the hospital setting. Included in an ever-growing list of successful home infusions are blood products and other biologicals, hydration fluids and parenteral nutrition, chemotherapy, antibiotics, narcotics, heparin, terbutaline, and even dobutamine for severe heart failure. Epidural morphine infusion for long-term pain management can be provided with a totally implanted pump and infusion system. Medication refill and flow rate programing are done transdermally at the bedside. Other complex therapies adapted for the patient's home include dialysis and ventilator-dependent patient care. For the heavy-care patient, a special bed (Independent Care Unit[3]) has been designed that has a flotation mattress to prevent skin breakdown and incorporates a shower, whirlpool, and toilet to facilitate total care (Fig. 5-1).

Innovations in diagnostic equipment and sophisticated monitoring systems have improved the safety and quality of care for frail homebound patients. In most larger urban areas, plain x-ray and ultrasonography services are available. Even more widely available are the usual diagnostics of the ambulatory setting such as routine cultures

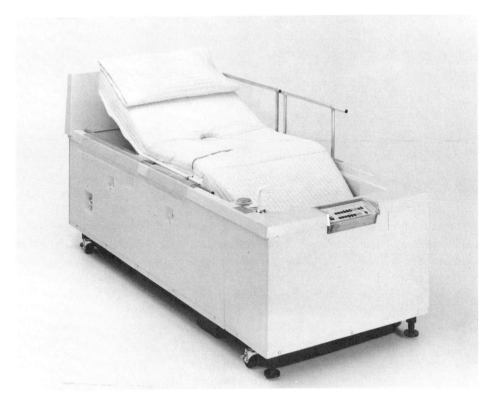

Figure 5-1 The Independent Care Unit is solid-state, electronically controlled, and has a combination flotation bed (pressure controlled mattress), whirlpool (foot end), shower (plastic panels go up on sides), and toilet. Center section can be retracted to expose a waste unit that has warm-water bidet cleansing and warm-air drying features.

and blood and urine testing. Electrocardiograms, glucometry, and oximetry are available at bedside, and vital signs and cardiac rhythms can be monitored by telemetry. Medication reminders help forgetful patients with pill schedules. Motion detectors with infrared beams and trouble-alert systems summon help in the event of more serious problems. Although there may be an appropriate limit to the use of technology for monitoring older persons at home, these devices provide the safety needed to complement the efforts of a part-time caregiver, thereby fostering independence of the elderly persons and delaying or perhaps even preventing their nursing home admission.

PHYSICIAN'S ROLE IN HOME CARE

Home care is clearly indicated as the treatment of choice for a growing number of illnesses ranging from the chronic care of disabled, frail, elderly persons, to post-hospital rehabilitation and the complex care of persons with acquired immunodeficiency syndrome (AIDS). If the patient is medically stable and has adequate, family, caregiver support, many acute diseases, especially those requiring infusion therapy, can be successfully—and economically—managed at home with less risk of nosocomial problems. Although home care can save costs of third-party payors, it often entails greater costs for the families and patients. Some services reimbursed in the hospital may not be covered at home. When care is provided at home, the costs to caregivers, in time and lost employment opportunities, can be considerable.

As modern home care gains stature as the standard of care for more illnesses and is no longer seen merely as an acceptable alternative to hospitalization physicians will be obliged to increase their involvement. In the team approach to modern home care, the physician plays a critical role. Medicare legally requires a physician to participate in the planning and supervision of home care. Active medical direction and supervision should enhance home care provided by professionals other than physicians. Another team member may function as case manager, but the physician, who has a primary relationship with the patient and family, provides continuity of care. The physician often can best validate the plan of care, even though others provide it.

Physician's home visits

Physician's home visits will be an important and necessary part of care, especially with the projected increases in home management of frail elderly persons and home treatment of acute illnesses. Home visits allow the physician to assess significant changes in condition, make major changes in the care plan, or judge the effectiveness or appropriateness of employing a complex in-home intervention (e.g., infusion therapy). Home visits can play a key role in supporting a patient's or family's belief in the efficacy of a home-based approach to care.

Assessment. As a member of the modern home care team, the physician will be expected to provide in-home assessment and personal supervision of home care patients with complex medical problems. The physician's diagnostic acumen and practice of the art of medicine—the gracious and respectful meeting of the patient and family in their milieu—are still the most important aspects of a home visit. Better diagnostic and therapeutic options available in the home have improved the quality of home assessment and made transport of a home care patient to the office or emergency room unnecessary and possibly inappropriate.

In-home assessment of elderly patients gives a more accurate picture of their health problems and needs. A study using blind comparison of home assessment versus office assessment for the same group of geriatric patients provided evidence of the efficacy of home assessments.[1] The authors found that home assessments uncovered an average of two additional significant medical problems, resulting in five additional orders to the care plan. Further, scores on cognitive function assessment in the home were significantly better than in the office, and the medication list compiled in the home identified an average of four more drugs than those obtained in the office.[1,3]

Assessments in the home go beyond scrutinizing the medical problems of the patient. They include evaluation of psychosocial supports, caregiver competence and motivation, and adequacy of the home environment, as well as patient function within that environment. Other members of the home care team can be helpful in conducting these assessments. If complex or intensive care plans are anticipated, it is advisable to teach these routines in the home setting so that all of the potential barriers to successful care, including caregiver well-being and performance, can be directly assessed. Similarly, only direct assessment—observing the patient and caregiver functioning in the actual home setting—permits a full appreciation of the environmental variables and allows reasonable adjustment of environmental barriers in the care plan.

Examination in the home can be challenging. Most bedrooms have poor lighting, and it can be awkward to examine a patient in a low, wide bed. An excellent solution to the poor lighting problem, especially for performing procedures or vaginal speculum examinations, is an adjustable focus headlamp. Such a lamp not only provides lighting comparable to the office treatment room, but it also allows the examiner's hands to remain free while redirecting the light. A home care strategy that experienced physicians report is to pad and use the kitchen table as an examination table. The kitchen is often the room in the house with the best lighting and usually has running water nearby. The height of the kitchen table approximates that of an office examination table, and it provides good access to the patient for procedures or examinations. Privacy is also an issue in some homes and may require that family members leave the examining area for a period of time.

The accompanying box lists some of the items that most physicians include in their house call bags. It is easy to see, even from this incomplete list, why some physicians who frequently visit homes have begun to stock vans almost like mobile offices. The instruments and therapeutics obviously vary with the physicians' anticipated needs of the home visits. Physicians who make regular home visits can use office staff to prepare the specific diagnostic or treatment setups for the home visits that are planned for that day. Office staff can also restock disposable items in the house call bag, on a regular basis, just as they do for office examination rooms.

House call bag. The house call bag can be the traditional black leather, rigid, multicompartment bag or case; size depends on number of compartments and capacity desired. Less expensive but adequate alternatives include a briefcase, plastic toolbox, photographic equipment bag, fishing tackle box, sports bag, or, for the bicyclist doctor, a backpack. Physicians may want to use a relatively compact, lightweight bag for their usual house call equipment needs and a second, larger, soft-sided, duffel bag for bulkier dressing materials and procedure setups. Any contaminated materials or specimens should be carried in a bag that can be easily washed and disinfected.

———— WHAT TO INCLUDE IN THE HOUSE CALL BAG ————

Examination instruments and materials

Standard
- Stethoscope
- Sphygmomanometer
- Percussion hammer
- Tuning fork
- Ophthalmoscope or otoscope with disposable specula
- Nasal speculum
- Cerumen loop
- Tongue blades and Q-tips
- #15 blade and scalpel (disposable) for paring corns and calluses
- Nonsterile examining gloves
- Examining lubricant
- Sterile examining gloves

Optional
- Vaginal speculum with ring forceps, single-toothed tenaculum, and disposable endometrial biopsy kit
- Pelvic examination skis—two 4 ft long, 1 in × 5 in oak boards with heel holes cut in the ends to be positioned under the mattress, extending out from bedside to facilitate pelvic examination
- Anoscope or sigmoidoscope—suction and irrigatiton may be improvised with a basin, 50 ml syringe with tapered adapter, and 2 ft of ⅜ in flexible polyvinylchloride (PVC) tubing
- Minor biopsy or laceration repair setup
  Kelly clamp, mosquito clamp
  Small pickup with teeth
  Pickup without teeth
  Small needle holder
  #15 blade and scalpel
  Iris scissors
  Sterile aperture drape (disposable)
  Medicine cup and cotton balls
  Suture materials and other instruments
- Sterile urinary catheterization setup with appropriate catheter

Dressing materials

Standard
- Suture scissors, pickups, Kelly clamp
- Cotton balls
- 1 in and 2 in adhesive tape
- 2 in × 2 in and 4 in × 4 in gauze pads
- Alcohol and povidone swabs
- Soiled dressing bag (plastic Ziplock)
- Contaminated sharps container
- Tincture of benzoin, 2 oz

Optional
- Elastic bandages, 2 in, 3 in, and 4 in
- Stockingette and plaster bandage material to fashion splints
- Gelcast (Unna boot) material
- Sterile (0.9 normal) saline, 500 ml for irrigation or intravenous (IV) use

Medications

Standard
- Lidocaine 1%, 50 ml
- Epinephrine 1 ml vials, 1:1000 for subcutaneous or intramuscular injection
- Atropine 0.4 mg (1 ml ampule)
- Prochlorperazine 2 ml (5 mg/ml) in disposable syringe
- Diazcpam 2 ml (5 mg/ml) in disposable syringe
- Terbutaline 2 ml (1 mg/ml) for subcutaneous injection
- 50% glucose solution
- Glucagon 1 unit (1 mg)
- Trinitroglycerin tablets (0.4 mg), 1 bottle
- Disposable syringes (2½ ml and tuberculin) and 27-gauge, 25-gauge, and 22-gauge needles

Optional
- All other drugs and preparations as anticipated
- Intravenous infusion supplies—peripheral venous access catheters or needles, IV tubing, 500 ml (plastic bottle) 5% dextrose in water with 0.25 normal saline

---

WHAT TO INCLUDE IN THE HOUSE CALL BAG—cont'd

Diagnostic equipment
- Sterile specimen container (urine, sputum)
- Phlebotomy supplies—vacuum tubes, tourniquet, sterile needles, and vacuum tube holder
- Transport culture tube
- Stool occult blood cards
- Urine diagnostic dipsticks (blood, glucose, ketones, protein, pH)

Optional
- Glucometer and supplies
- Portable electrocardiogram machine
- Ear oximetry unit
- Tonometer and anesthetic eye drops

Physicians who perform tests, procedures, or dressing changes that involve contamination of instruments with body fluids or disposable supplies must handle and dispose of these materials as they would in the hospital or office. Families also should be taught appropriate handling of contaminated materials and to arrange for proper disposal, especially of "sharps," through a home care agency or physician's office.

Physicians who carry injectable medications in their house call bag must protect them from exposure to extreme temperatures if a bag is left for extended periods in the physician's car. It is helpful if office staff routinely check for and replace outdated vials. If a multidose vial of medication requires refrigeration, a single dose can be drawn just before the planned home visit. Narcotics and controlled drugs require special care and should be taken out of the call bag and placed in a locked area between home visits. Physicians should maintain a log of any narcotics administered from their personal call bag stocks. Some physicians prefer, for their own personal safety, to make it widely known that they carry no drugs with any illicit or street value. Patients that require significant narcotics for ongoing pain management are best supplied through pharmacy prescriptions.

Scheduling visits and responding to calls. Physician's offices have developed efficient systems of patient management that can be beneficially applied to a home care practice. Most home care patients are medically stable, and home visits can be scheduled electively. The office receptionist should learn the physician's preference for scheduling of most routine visits. Physicians with large home care practices may even benefit from geographic clustering of visits. The receptionist should make a reminder call on the day of the home visit and, if necessary, confirm the time and availability of the family caregiver. Chronic home care patients should receive routine notices from the office practice for periodic screening and health maintenance.

Effective and timely communication with patients, caregivers, and other members of the home care team is critical for a successful home care practice. Calls from caregivers or home care professionals should be screened for urgency by the office triage nurse. The office receptionist or triage nurse should schedule a time with the caller for the physician to call back. Scheduling calls promotes timely care management and prevents "telephone tag." Physicians should make every effort to take calls immediately, if a home care team member calls from the home of a patient about a problem. The opportunity for additional physician-directed assessment or immediate change in care plan will be missed if the return call is delayed. Guidelines for the specific circumstances that warrant an immediate call-back response depend, in part, on the rapport that the physician has with home care team members. These circumstances may change as the physician and other team members develop experience and confidence in each other's patient assessment and management styles.

Medical records. Medical record maintenance and documentation of home care is essential and, as in other areas of health care, comprises an important part of communication. Home visits, family visits, family and team conferences, and significant telephone consultations all warrant a chart entry. In particular, the chart should reflect discussions with patients and caregivers about the risks or benefits associated with home care, and that the caregivers have been instructed in—and were willing and able to carry out—their roles. Advance directives should be solicited and documented.

FUNDING SOURCES FOR HOME CARE

Home care, more than any other area of health care, has a complex and confusing system of payment for services. Like long-term care, many services are not covered by insurance or public funding and the family or patient pays for those services. Physicians need to learn the general guidelines for Medicare and Medicaid home care eligibility, as well as some of the services that are available through other funding sources. However, these guidelines have changed frequently in the past and are likely to continue changing. Thus, physicians may rely on other members of the home care team who are informed about current changes and can advise patients on available resources and funding options.

The accompanying box lists the Medicare guidelines for home care eligibility. Medicare coverage for home care has been limited primarily to the convalescent and postacute care needs of patients and does not cover chronic maintenance or personal care, unless there is an ongoing need for intermittent skilled care of a homebound patient. Health maintenance organizations that provide a Medicare option for managed care are required to offer comparable coverage of services. Medicare allows expanded home hospice benefits for terminally ill patients, persons diagnosed by a physician as having less than 6 months' life expectancy. These patients and their caregivers are eligible for additional in-home services, including respite care and coverage of medications needed for comfort.

Medicaid coverage for home care varies considerably since benefits are determined by each state. Most states also have received a 2176 Waiver from the federal government, allowing them greater range and flexibility of benefits. States can provide

_____ HOME CARE MEDICARE GUIDELINES _____

All of these conditions must be met for home care services to be covered by Medicare.

Medicare Part A

1. Patient must be under the care of a physician and the plan of treatment must be established and supervised by the physician.
2. Patient must be homebound.
   - Needs assistance to leave home
   - Requires considerable and taxing effort to leave home
   - Medical condition may contraindicate leaving home
   - Most occasions of leaving home would be brief and usually for health reasons
3. A skilled service is required on a part-time or intermittent basis.
   - Inherent complexity of services or condition of patient requires professionally trained person such as a nurse, or physical, speech, or occupational therapist
   - The services are defined as noncustodial or nonmaintenance; thus, a patient's services are covered only if they are demonstrated to facilitate progress to a higher level of functioning

   - *Intermittent* has been redefined by the Medicare Catastrophic Coverage Act of 1988 to mean those services that are required less than 7 days a week; however, up to 38 consecutive days of needed services may be covered (effective January 1, 1990)
   - Nonskilled personal care services may be covered if they are part of a care plan that involves skilled intermittent care
4. Provider must be a participating Medicare-certified home care agency.

Medicare Part B

   Durable medical supplies may be covered if the devices allow an impaired individual to remain comfortably at home.
   - Must be prescribed by physician
   - Physician must state the specific diagnosis necessitating the device, prognosis, and projected use of the device
   - Medicare covers 80% of the cost to purchase or rent the devices (whichever is cheaper), after the Part B deductible has been met

Modified from Health Insurance for the Aged Act, Public Law 89-97, Section 101-102, 79 Stat. 286, 290-91 (1985, codified as amended at 42 USC Section 1395-1395xx (1982); and Medicare Catastrophic Coverage Act of 1988, Public Law 100-36. U.S. Congress.

significant home care support for individuals who are poor and assessed as sufficiently frail and likely to need nursing home admission in the near future. Up to 75% of the expected cost of nursing home care may be used for care and services that allow patients to remain in the community.

Other services may be available from a variety of sources to supplement the home care medical plan. Support for home care services is offered to veterans through the Department of Veterans Affairs' hospital-based home care program. Some states have used Social Services Block Grant (Title XX) funding to provide community-based services for older persons. Area Agencies on Aging provide important services for frail elderly persons in the community such as Meals-on-Wheels, transportation, and even home repair and improvement services in some areas. Churches, service organizations, and other voluntary groups often provide important support and social services for the frail elderly and their caregivers. Since these services vary greatly by locality and change frequently, it may be best to consult a hospital discharge planner or a home care team social worker to provide current advice or availability.

PHYSICIAN'S REIMBURSEMENT

Surveys of physicians for their attitudes about home care have revealed widespread dissatisfaction with reimbursement as one of the major barriers to greater involvement in home care. Approximately one half of the family physicians and internists responding to the 1990 AMA national survey indicated that they would do more home visiting if reimbursement was better.[2] As of January 1992, the Health Care Financing Administration has opted to increase the relative value units associated with physicians' home visits. (See the box on p. 45 for home visits' Current Procedural Terminology (CPT) codes.) As a result, Medicare reimbursement for a home visit will be two to three times more than the average amount covered for that service in 1991. The full fee increase will be phased in over a four-year period (1992 to 1996). This fee structure is still less than most physicians consider adequate for the time spent on a home visit, but it is clearly a step in the right direction.

A more important reimbursement issue for most physicians is the lack of compensation for their supervisory and case management roles for home care provided by others. The 1990 AMA survey found that physicians spend, on average, 3 to 4 hours per week performing telephone calls and paperwork associated with home care referrals.[2] With the rapidly growing population of frail elderly persons who live in the community, the time physicians spend supervising home care will surely increase.

Currently, supervising and case management are not compensated at all. Current procedural terminology (CPT) codes have been developed for these services (see the box on p. 46); but, to date, Medicare has refused to recognize these codes as reimbursable services. Physicians are encouraged to use these codes to establish a profile of charges for case management and conferencing services. Private insurers have recognized the benefit of these services and some have begun reimbursing for charges submitted under these codes.

The improved reimbursement for a physician's home visit is a positive step, but it appears that a greater amount of the physician's time for modern home care will be spent supervising the home care team. The issue of adequacy of reimbursement is worsening and could pose a serious barrier to the appropriate future development of, and access to, home care. Without adequate compensation, physicians will be forced to limit their involvement in home care. Since Medicare law requires the physician's supervision of all home care, lack of the physician's involvement could seriously jeopardize availability of these important services for the frail elderly in the community.

CURRENT PROCEDURAL TERMINOLOGY
(CPT) CODES FOR HOME SERVICES

The following codes are used to report evaluation and management services provided in a private residence. Typical times have not yet been established for this category of services.

New patient

99341—Home visit for the evaluation and management of a new patient, which requires three key components
- A problem-focused history
- A problem-focused examination
- Medical decision making that is straightforward or of low complexity

Counseling and coordination of care with other providers or agencies are provided consistent with the nature of the problems and the patient's and family's needs. Usually, the problems are of low severity.

99342—Home visit for the evaluation and management of a new patient, which requires three key components
- An expanded problem-focused history
- An expanded problem-focused examination
- Medical decision making of moderate complexity

Counseling and coordination of care with other providers or agencies are provided consistent with the nature of the problems and the patient's and family's needs. Usually, the problems are of moderate severity.

99343—Home visit for the evaluation and management of a new patient, which requires three key components
- A detailed history
- A detailed examination
- Medical decision making of high complexity

Counseling and coordination of care with other providers or agencies are provided consistent with the nature of the problems and the patient's and family's needs. Usually, the problems are of high severity.

Established patient

99351—Home visit for the evaluation and management of an established patient, which requires at least two of three key components
- A problem-focused interval history
- A problem-focused examination
- Medical decision making that is straightforward or of low complexity

Counseling and coordination of care with other providers or agencies are provided consistent with the nature of the problems and the patient's and family's needs. Usually, the patient is stable, recovering, or improving.

99352—Home visit for the evaluation and management of an established patient, which requires at least two of three key components
- An expanded problem-focused interval history
- An expanded problem-focused examination
- Medical decision making of moderate complexity

Counseling and coordination of care with other providers or agencies are provided consistent with the nature of the problems and the patient's and family's needs. Usually, the patient is responding inadequately to therapy or has developed a minor complication.

99353—Home visit for the evaluation and management of an established patient, which requires at least two of three key components
- A detailed interval history
- A detailed examination
- Medical decision making of high complexity

Counseling and coordination of care with other providers or agencies are provided consistent with the nature of the problems and the patient's and family's needs. Usually, the patient is unstable or has developed a significant complication or a significant new problem.

CURRENT PROCEDURAL TERMINOLOGY (CPT) CODES
FOR PHYSICIANS' CASE MANAGEMENT SERVICES

Physicians' case management is the responsibility of physicians for directing care of a patient and coordinating and controlling access to, or initiating and supervising, other health care services needed by the patient.

Team conference

99361—Medical conference by a physician with interdisciplinary team of health professionals or representatives of community agencies to coordinate activities of patient care (patient not present); approximately 30 minutes.
99362—Same as 99361 except requiring approximately 60 minutes.

Telephone calls

99371—Telephone call by a physician to patient for consultation or medical management or for coordinating medical management with other health care professionals (e.g., nurses, therapists, social workers, nutritionists, physicians, pharmacists); simple or brief (e.g., to report on tests or laboratory results, clarify or alter previous instructions, integrate new information from other health professionals into the medical treatment plan, or adjust therapy).
99372—Intermediate telephone call (e.g., to provide advice to an established patient on a new problem, initiate therapy that can be handled by telephone, discuss test results in detail, coordinate medical management of a new problem for an established patient, discuss and evaluate new information and details, or initiate new plan of care).
99373—Complex or lengthy telephone call (e.g., counseling session with anxious or distraught patient, detailed or prolonged discussion with family members regarding seriously ill patient, communication necessary to coordinate complex services of several different health professionals working on different aspects of the total patient care plan).

REFERENCES

1. Altkorn DL et al: Recommendation for a change in living situation resulting from an outpatient geriatric assessment: type, frequency and risk factors, *J Am Geriatr Soc* 39:508, 1991.
2. Keenan JM et al: A national survey of the home visiting practice and attitudes of family physicians and internists, Unpublished data.
3. Ward WH et al: Cognitive function testing in comprehensive geriatric assessment: comparison of cognitive test performance in residential and clinic settings, *J Am Geriatr Soc* 38:1088, 1990.

SUGGESTED READINGS

Steel K: Home care for the elderly: a new institution, *Arch Intern Med* 151:439, 1991.
Keenan JM, Fanale JE: Home care: past and present, problems and potential, *J Am Geriatr Soc* 37:1076, 1989.
Council on Scientific Affairs: Home care: the 1990s, *JAMA* 263:1241, 1990.

CHAPTER 6

Caregiver stress

BARRY LEBOWITZ
ENID LIGHT

KEY POINTS

- Most older persons are supported by a system of family and informal caregiving.
- This caregiving is provided willingly and is the source of great personal and emotional reward.
- At the same time, caregiving represents a significant risk factor to the health and well-being of the principal caregiver, usually a spouse or an adult daughter.
- Caregiving provides a model of chronic stress in which a broad range of physical, emotional, and behavioral sequelae have been traced.
- Clinicians need to be aware of the potential for caregiver stress and develop approaches to treatment that will address the need of both patient and caregiver.
- Interventions include educating and counseling caregivers, encouraging use of support groups and community services, providing respite services, and managing the health-related consequences of caregiver stress.

BACKGROUND

Two myths regarding the social and the family environment of older persons have been widely held. The first myth portrays older people as living in abandonment and social isolation. The second myth purports widespread violence, neglect, and abuse directed toward the older person by family members. Two decades of empirical research have consistently shown that family and social support is widespread, available, positive, and, in fact, normative in our society.[3]

The family is the major resource for older persons in need of ongoing care and support. The number of people involved in a regular caregiving relationship with older persons in the United States has been estimated to be from 2.2 to 3 million people. Within ethnic and minority communities in the United States, research has

47

shown that family support and caregiving are even more deeply established than in the majority of white communities, and that use of formal support services is seen as a last resort where family and friends are unavailable or inaccessible.[11]

The regular assistance provided to an older person ranges from household tasks such as cooking, cleaning, shopping, and bill paying, to personal care in the activities of daily living such as bathing, dressing, and toileting. Typically, long-term care plans for community-dwelling older persons include community-based services that provide meals, assisted living, recreation, respite and adult day care. Aggressive outreach, comprehensive assessment, and vigorous case management may all be important to maintaining the older person in the community, but at the core of the long-term care plan for the elderly person is the family.

THE CAREGIVER'S ROLE

Research and clinical experience have revealed that the sharing of caregiving responsibilities among members of the family is neither efficacious nor desirable. Ideally, a single individual assumes the chief caregiving responsibility for a dependent older adult. This individual is most typically a spouse, or if no spouse is available, then an adult child. Although men and women assume these caregiving responsibilities, it is usually the wife or the adult daughter who assumes the role and responsibility of caregiving.[4]

Older wives who are caring for their disabled husbands frequently report feeling overwhelmed by the volume and range of responsibilities they face. There is too much to do and not enough time to do it all. The need for respite care (i.e., temporary relief to the family caregiver through in-home care during the day or overnight care by a surrogate caregiver) is consistently and repeatedly expressed by these women. However, when respite care services are made available, few who are eligible actually take advantage of them. Clinicians should encourage caregivers to accept respite services.

Older husbands who are caring for their disabled wives, a smaller yet significant group, report the need for knowledge and training about various household and personal care tasks. The current cohort of older men traditionally has taken responsibility for few household chores such as cooking, cleaning, and laundry. While these husbands are willing to take on various caregiving responsibilities, they simply do not have the expertise necessary to accomplish them. Educational materials such as books, videotapes, and classes may be helpful. Caregiver support groups allow these caregivers to learn from the experiences of others.

It is not unusual to find many older female caregivers who have long histories of caregiving responsibilities, some stretching 30 years or longer. Many women have cared for their children, older mothers, middle-aged husbands who have had heart attacks or strokes, and older husbands who have had various late-onset diseases. In particular, the mothers of mentally ill or mentally retarded children who have grown old must cope with ongoing needs for substantial care and parental involvement.

In ethnic and minority communities there is a well-established pattern of involvement of the grandparent generation in child care and other aspects of family maintenance and support. Careers of caregiving for this cohort of older women often run parallel to careers in the paid work force.

Women and men bearing principal caregiving responsibilities for one or both disabled parents manage their duties differently. Sons typically arrange to purchase the care required for their parents. Adult daughters, however, are confronted with myriad conflicting and competing demands. Jobs, husbands, children, and parent caregiving all combine to produce the so-called sandwich generation of women who are caught in the middle.[4] These conflicting demands are serious and intense but typically are resolved by a reduction in job involvement. Some women actually leave the paid labor force to provide care to a disabled parent. Others remain in their paid jobs but significantly alter the terms and conditions of their employment by reducing their work hours from full- to part-time and refusing promotions or other opportunities for advancement that would have required greater commitments of their time or responsibilities to travel. A referral for counseling to address life changes caused by one's having to care for a disabled family member would be appropriate for caregivers of this type.

Regardless of the illness or disability, the caregiving experience has many universal features, as are listed in the accompanying box[2] below. Education about the nature of the patient's illness and changes that can be anticipated for the patient's caregiving needs may be extremely helpful to the caregiver. Caregivers may be reluctant to seek help. The clinician should suggest services that reduce the caregiver's burden and foster the caregiver's ability to cope successfully. Adult day care for an ambulatory patient with dementia, for example, may be an appropriate alternative to full-time care by a family member.

COMMON ELEMENTS OF THE CAREGIVER'S ROLE

Burden of increased dependency and support needs by the impaired person
Management of disruptive or emotional behaviors of the impaired person
Curtailment of social activities and free time
Loss of privacy
Disruption of regular daily schedules
Insufficient help from informal and formal sources
Disruption of family relationships and roles
Anticipatory bereavement

CONSEQUENCES TO THE CAREGIVER

While there are many difficulties and tremendous sacrifices associated with caregiving, individuals who function in a caregiving relationship with an older person may derive many rewards and benefits. In particular, the fulfillment of obligations or responsibilities, satisfaction derived from making a significant contribution to a loved one, and maintenance of a bond of affection and support often are regarded as highly positive and rewarding in a caregiving relationship.

At the same time, the stress of providing long-term care for a disabled elderly person has been well documented, which has led to concern about the potential adverse consequences for the caregiver. The caregiver of a patient with Alzheimer's disease has been called the hidden victim of the disease.[17]

Caregiving for an Alzheimer's patient requires extraordinary levels of care because of the severe emotional, behavioral, and cognitive deficits that are the hallmarks of this disease. Caregiving for an Alzheimer's patient may necessitate unremitting vigilance so that the patient does not pose a threat to self or others. In addition, caregivers face unpredictable disruptions to circadian rhythms (e.g., frequent nighttime awakenings at unpredictable hours) and regular functions (e.g., meals, exercise). Physical demands of the caregiver include providing heavy personal care to the patient (e.g., diapering, feeding, bathing). Caregivers also experience a loss of social interactions and are faced with managing the emotional and behavioral manifestations of the disease (e.g., wandering, aggression, hypersexuality, sundowning, agitation). Meanwhile, caregivers are watching a loved one, with whom they have shared their lives, deteriorate and lose their selfhood.[14] Because of the nature of Alzheimer's disease and its impact on the caregiver, studies examining the emotional states of caregivers do not necessarily reflect the consequences of caregiving for patients with other disorders. There is insufficient information to generalize from these studies to the overall impact of caregiving.

Caregivers as a group are reluctant to use formal health and social services, in general, and mental health services, in particular. When caregivers do avail themselves of these services, they do so infrequently and, typically, not until the last year of the patient's life.[8] Clinicians may play an important role by encouraging caregivers to take advantage of these services and other community resources to aid them in coping successfully with their caregiving roles.

Stress-related symptoms

Studies of caregivers have documented that caregivers, as a group, consistently report higher levels of stress than do non-caregivers.[7] At the same time, it has been noted that family caregivers, as a group, underreport symptoms of stress on global self-report instruments.[10,18] This study suggests that the number and severity of stress-related symptoms described in the literature may not actually reflect the full extent of such problems. Despite this underreporting by family caregivers, a wide range of stress-related symptoms has been reported by caregivers in general. The more common symptoms include irritability, fatigue, headaches and other somatic symptoms, high levels of anger, anxiety, hostility, guilt, hopelessness and helplessness, and feelings of loss of control or inability to cope. Clinicians should anticipate and seek these clues to caregiver stress.

Caregivers are not a homogeneous group; they are caregivers by chance. They differ in age, life experiences, genetics, social, economic, and psychological resources, environment (e.g., urban versus rural, house versus apartment), and their relationships and experiences with the recipients of care. It is not surprising that caregivers differ in the number and severity of stress-related symptoms that they report. Since it is likely that constellations of factors, rather than individual factors by themselves, are associated with promoting or reducing the effects of caregiver stress, investigators hope to discern particular patterns or profiles of caregivers who are at risk.

Depression and its symptoms

Between 30% and 50% of all caregivers will experience high levels of depressive symptomatology at some time during the course of caregiving.[5,6,13] There is evidence that there are several subsets of caregivers (e.g., those who develop anxiety disorders, clinical depression, and depressive symptoms) for whom the development of these psychiatric disorders is directly associated with the chronic stress of caregiving.

It is difficult to predict which caregivers will be the most vulnerable to psychiatric symptoms. Differences in psychiatric symptoms among caregivers based on factors such as gender, family relationships, and living arrangements have been reported. Women over 60 years of age have the highest levels of reported depression and depressive symptoms. In general, female caregivers have higher reported levels of depression and anxiety than male caregivers; spouses who are caregivers have higher levels of psychiatric morbidity than children who are caregivers; and older caregivers have higher reported levels of psychiatric morbidity than do younger caregivers.

Recognition and diagnosis of depression and its symptoms in caregivers are important because they are potentially treatable with psychological and pharmacological strategies. Family, behavioral, and cognitive therapies are among the treatments that have been adapted to the specific circumstances of depressed caregivers. Successful outcomes of these interventions for depressed caregivers have been reported in both research and clinical literature.[6,15]

Anger and abuse

Recently, caregivers have reported elevated rates of anger.[1,6] Many caregivers have expressed concern about their potential for committing violence against their impaired relatives who have Alzheimer's disease. While the number of caregivers who report having committed violence against a cognitively impaired family member is low (around 1%), close to one fifth of the caregivers are concerned about their potential for violence, which underscores the extreme stress that many caregivers feel and the profound need for interventions to alleviate stress and anger. Clinicians must be alert to the potential for abuse by caregivers and recognize signs and symptoms when they occur. Strategies to recognize and alleviate the source of caregiver stress are critically important to prevent abuse. Referrals for counseling or support groups may be the key component of a long-term plan that provides an appropriate outlet for caregiver anger.

Physical consequences of caregiving

There is a substantial body of research linking stress to physical illness. Given the chronic stressors involved in caring for an Alzheimer's patient, it is likely that caregivers may be vulnerable to the development or exacerbation of physical illnesses. Poor health of caregivers is one of the most frequently cited reasons for institutionalizing patients with Alzheimer's disease. Specific illnesses of the caregiver that have led to institutionalizing a family member are heart attacks, diabetes mellitus, strokes, peptic ulcers, fractures, and illnesses associated with exhaustion.[9,16]

There is growing evidence that stress affects the immune function in caregivers.[12] Caregivers have significantly poorer immune systems (i.e., lower percentages of total T lymphocytes and helper T lymphocytes) than matched non-caregiver controls.[12] Recently, longitudinal data demonstrated that suppressed functioning of the immune system continues over time.[13] In addition, caregivers reported more respiratory tract infections in the preceding 6 months than controls, as well as increases in the number of illness episodes, days of illness, and visits to a physician. The longitudinal data additionally suggest that although caregiving status can change and psychiatric symptoms do improve, the immune system may not completely recover. One explanation for this is that the chronic stress of caregiving may cause a loss of the immune system's plasticity in older caregivers.

Different strands of evidence suggest that the stress associated with the burden of caregiving represents a significant risk factor for the development and exacerbation of disease. The clinician should be aware of the risk for stress-related illnesses and should treat or refer caregivers when their symptoms first appear.

INTERVENTIONS

Clinicians in ambulatory care settings should recognize that patients are usually supported by a highly functional family system that is available to provide care. Caregiving can cause stress-related problems and disorders for the family caregiver. These problems can have negative consequences for the elderly patient. Many caregivers are themselves elderly, for example, spouses or 70-year-old children caring for parents who are in their 90s. Regardless of age, caregivers are vulnerable to life changes and stress-related symptoms that can compromise effective treatment and management of patient care. The primary care clinician is in a unique position to recognize these symptoms and institute early assessment and management.

Education about the nature and anticipated course of the patient's illness is an extremely effective and important intervention to prevent and minimize stress to the caregiver. Key information about the disease process allows the caregiver to focus on the patient's current needs and long-term plans for care.

Most communities offer *counseling services* for caregivers, caregiver *support groups* for a variety of medical conditions, and *services in the home* for help with the patient's personal care, housekeeping, laundry, shopping, and cooking. Caregivers may be reluctant to use these services. Many family caregivers resist accepting outside help because they feel that they should provide the necessary care themselves. *Referrals* to these services by the clinician enable reluctant caregivers to accept help, counteracting values and beliefs that families have the exclusive obligation to provide care for disabled family members. Encouraging caregivers to use community services may significantly alleviate caregivers' burdens and stress.

Respite services can provide in-home relief for the caregiver, temporary placement of the patient out of the home to free the caregiver for vacations or periods of rest, and adult day care programs. Respite programs may be provided by a family member, an institution, or the community. Regularly scheduled respites can provide long-term hope for caregivers. The clinician should be alert to the caregiver's need for a period of relief from the daily caregiving responsibilities and should make appropriate suggestions and referrals.

Clinicians sometimes encounter situations in which the patient's needs exceed the capacities of the family caregiving system. A caregiver's feelings of guilt about placing a relative in a nursing home can preclude this option, even if a nursing home is the most appropriate place for care. The clinician's endorsement of nursing home placement, when necessary for optimal care, can be important to alleviate the caregiver's sense of guilt.

THE FUTURE

Although aging-in-place is the prevailing pattern for most older persons, a significant proportion have relocated to retirement communities in the Sun Belt or elsewhere. These communities tend to be geographically distant from family. Though bonds of affection and support develop in these new communities, it is unknown how supportive these bonds can be for elderly people with chronic disabling conditions. It is conceivable that family support may not be accessible due to barriers of distance. Specialized service agencies that deal with long-distance caregiving have been established and seem to be attracting a growing clientele.

Although fears about the dissolution of the family are misplaced, the number of divorced persons, blended families, single parents, and other forms of relationships strains the prevailing norms of family-based caregiving. Based on history and current experience, it is expected that caregiving will remain a fundamental dimension of family life in the United States, though the form is likely to evolve and develop. This should be an important focus for future research on new dimensions and aspects of caregiving. Those who are involved in planning and providing clinical care for geriatric patients should be aware of the potential contribution of family caregivers, sensitive to any challenges to the health and well-being of these caregivers, and alert to the context of caregiving within our changing society.

REFERENCES

1. Anthony-Bergstone CR, Zarit SH, Gatz M: Symptoms of psychological distress among caregivers of dementia patients, *Psychol Aging* 3:245, 1988.
2. Biegel DE, Sales E, Schulz R: *Family caregiving in chronic illness*, Newbury Park, Calif, 1991, Sage.
3. Brody EM: *Women in the middle: their parent care years*, New York, 1990, Springer.
4. Brody EM: Parent care as normative family stress, *Gerontologist* 25:19, 1985.
5. Coppel DB et al: Relationships of cognitions associated coping reactions to depression in spousal caregivers of Alzheimer's disease patients, *Cognitive Ther Res* 9:253, 1985.
6. Gallagher D et al: Prevalence of depression in family caregivers, *Gerontologist* 29:449, 1989.
7. George LK, Gwyther L: Caregiver well-being: a multidimensional examination of family caregivers of demented adults, *Gerontologist* 26:3, 1986.
8. Gwyther L: Service delivery and utilization: research directions and implications. In Light E, Niederehe G, Lebowitz BD, eds: *New directions in Alzheimer's disease and family stress*, New York, Springer, (in press).
9. Haley WE et al: Psychological, social, and health consequences of caregiving for a relative with senile dementia, *J Am Geriatr Soc* 35:401, 1987.
10. Haley WE, Brown SL, Levine EG: Experimental evaluation of the effectiveness of group intervention for dementia caregivers, *Gerontologist* 27:376, 1987.
11. Harper MS, ed: *Minority aging: essential curricula content for selected health and allied health professions*, Washington, DC, 1990, US Government Printing Office.
12. Kiecolt-Glaser JK et al: Chronic stress and immunity in family caregivers of Alzheimer's disease patients, *Psychosom Med* 49:523, 1987.
13. Kiecolt-Glaser JK, Glaser R: Caregivers, mental health and immune function. In Light E, Niederehe G, Lebowitz BD, eds: *New directions in Alzheimer's disease and family stress*, New York, Springer, (in press).
14. Mace N, Rabins P: *The 36-hour day*, Baltimore, 1981, Johns Hopkins University Press.
15. Mittleman M et al: Efficacy of multicomponent individualized treatment to improve the well being of Alzheimer's caregivers. In Light E, Niederehe G, Lebowitz BD, eds: *New directions in Alzheimer's disease and family stress*, New York, Springer, (in press).
16. Snyder B, Keefe K: The unmet needs of family caregivers for frail and disabled adults, *Soc Work Health Care* 10:1, 1985.
17. Zarit SH, Orr NK, Zarit JM: *The hidden victims of Alzheimer's disease: treatment and family stress*, New York, 1985, New York University Press.
18. Zarit SH, Toseland RW: Current and future direction in family caregiving research, *Gerontologist* 29:481, 1989.

SUGGESTED READINGS

Light E, Niederehe G, Lebowitz BD, eds: *New directions in Alzheimer's disease and family stress*, New York, Springer, (in press).
Mace N, Rabins P: *The 36-hour day*, Baltimore, 1981, Johns Hopkins University Press.

CHAPTER 7

Role of nursing

HELEN HIGBY
CAROLE E. DEITRICH

KEY POINTS
- The role of the nurse in ambulatory care of the older adult is comprehensive and multifaceted, emphasizes health and maintenance of the patient's functional ability, and crosses multiple health care settings.
- Historically and philosophically, gerontological nursing has espoused the precepts of primary care of the older adult as fundamental to the specialty practice.
- Gerontological nursing is developing as a research-based practice.
- Advanced practice nurses caring for older adults in community health care settings should be reimbursed for their services.
- Advanced practice nurses caring for older adults should be able, legally, to practice within the full range of their capabilities.

Nursing aligns with other health care professionals in affirming the primary goals of ambulatory care for the older adult patient (i.e., the promotion of health, maintenance of function, prevention of disease and disability, and detection and management of illness). Achieving these goals, however, is often not as straightforward as it may appear. First, it is difficult to generalize treatment and approaches to continuing care because, as sociological studies indicate, heterogeneity increases with age and chronological and biological age are rarely matched. Second, in a typical ambulatory practice, the health care provider (HCP) must manage the extraordinarily variable health statuses of older adults, ranging from the healthy and fully functioning to the acutely ill and institutionalized. Older adults are best distinguished from each other, then, on the basis of functional abilities rather than age, diagnosis, or setting, and assessment of these abilities should be an ongoing task in ambulatory care.

In a busy office or clinical practice, the attention given to patients often focuses on the detection and treatment of disease rather than functional assessment and health maintenance activities or eduation and support of the patient and caregiver in long-term care. Interventions to promote healthy behavior, regain or maintain the ability to function, and sustain quality of life are often overlooked. To meet the challenges of health promotion and maintenance of function for elderly patients, a thorough multidisciplinary approach that considers the complex interaction of social, psychological, economic, cultural, and biomedical factors is essential. The emphasis nursing has placed, currently and historically, on health promotion, maintenance, and education complements the emphasis of medicine on diagnosis and treatment of disease. Together, nursing and medicine have provided comprehensive quality care for the older adult. The nurse, in the role of case manager, also has provided continuity of care across treatment and home settings of the older adult.

NURSES IN AMBULATORY CARE

Traditionally, nurses in an ambulatory setting such as a clinic or an office have undertaken numerous tasks, many of which had little to do with nursing but were directed toward the smooth, efficient operation of the setting. Often these "nurses" are not actually licensed personnel, but rather office-trained secretarial help or certified medical assistants who draw blood, do laboratory work, take blood pressures, assist with procedures, or help patients to dress and undress. Ambiguous labeling, confusion in responsibilities and use of professional nurses for nonprofessional tasks in an ambulatory setting result in the failure to utilize registered nurses to meet the broader goals of geriatric care.

The mandate of Healthy People 2000,[1] with its emphasis on quality of life, not simply longevity, might have been written with the professional ambulatory care nurse in mind. The focus on promoting health, preventing disease, and coping with the consequences of chronic illness characterizes the goals of nursing and suggests broader utilization of registered nurses. Additionally, the increasing cadre of master's-prepared nurses, collectively described by the term *advanced practice nurses*, offers yet another resource in this arena. Two such advanced practice nurses are the gerontological clinical nurse specialist (GCNS) who has specialized education and clinical experience in gerontology and the gerontological nurse practitioner (GNP) who is a specialist in gerontology and primary care.

The doctorally prepared nurse, specializing in gerontology, is an emerging role that offers still another resource. Besides bringing advanced clinical skills to an ambulatory practice, these nurses are skilled in theoretical and clinical research and contribute to the sciences of gerontology and nursing, as well as provide research-based clinical practice and administration. Because they analyze research critically, they also discriminate between effective new treatment modalities that should be introduced in the clinical setting and those interventions that do not yet warrant use.

The various roles among different levels of professional nurses are exemplified in the following scenario:

The patient is a 70-year-old woman with one chronic illness, osteoarthritis, who is fully ambulatory and has no specific complaints. Although she is relatively sedentary, smokes half a pack of cigarettes per day, drinks two to three alcoholic drinks per day and has a history of both osteoporosis and coronary artery disease in her first degree relatives, she is considered "essentially well." She takes aspirin for arthritic pain but no other medications. She has never had hormone replacement therapy or taken calcium supplements.

The patient's income is adequate, and she has sufficient psychosocial support, social interaction, and, overall high satisfaction with her life. Her major stressor is a spouse who is becoming frail and needs more attention at home. The patient sustains a hip fracture and needs to be hospitalized. Despite successful surgery, she experiences confusion and incontinence, and a small decubitus ulcer develops. A stay in a nursing home follows for physical therapy, rehabilitation, wound care, and incontinence assessment and management. Upon returning home, she receives office-initiated home visits that provide additional care for dressing changes and monitoring of functional capabilities, until she regains sufficient function to come to the office and resume previous activities. Meanwhile, the spouse's care has been taken over temporarily by a family member and a home health agency.

Role of the registered nurse

The health care needs of the woman in the above scenario, hereafter referred to as the index patient, are multidimensional and multilevel. The potential for the primary HCP to lose continuity and coordination of care during any one of the transitions is very high. Social stressors and potential risks for illness or disability were present before the woman's hip fracture, and the need for health and functional monitoring and assistance were necessary, even after the patient returned home. In the usual course of office visits, the registered nurse (RN) may act as first contact for this patient, performing the usual tasks, such as vital signs, but also eliciting important historical data, particularly a psychosocial and functional assessment and medication review. Questions about changes in function, physical activity, vigor, social contacts, and pleasure in usual activities must be asked specifically. Indeed, older adults are known to underreport symptoms or report only physical symptoms, believing that only symptoms interest a busy HCP. The office RN also could be involved with the index patient in a program of education about health risk factors and behavior changes to reduce those risk factors and improve well-being.

The office RN may also act as the first contact by telephone for the index patient when she returns home and regains her prior activity level. Screening the patient by telephone can help with decisions that need to be made about caregiving, rehabilitative education, or alterations in home care, with the RN serving as a conduit for information between the patient and primary HCP. All of these nursing activities should be formally documented within the ambulatory setting and should not be excluded from the patient's data base, medical records, and treatment plans.

Role of the gerontological nurse practitioner

Because the GNP performs direct patient care management and maintains a caseload of patients, the GNP may already be the index patient's primary HCP. Initially, the management of stable chronic illnesses and self-limiting acute illnesses, promotion of health, prevention of disease, and counseling and education about caregiving activities represent the spectrum of health care needs of the index patient and are within the scope of practice of the GNP. Although this patient is not sick, per se, there are many incipient threats to her function and well-being. The need for promoting the health of older adults is especially important. While people 65 years and older can expect to live longer than ever before, they cannot necessarily expect to do so actively and independently or with a high quality of life.[1] The commonly held belief that activities for promoting health and preventing disease are futile for older adults grows out of a societal myth regarding the inevitable decline of aging. (See Chapters 21 and 22.) The GNP should be the major HCP who teaches and counsels patients and family members about health and how to prevent diseases and disabilities.

Additionally, there are psychosocial issues that the GNP explores. Much of the stress of caring for a failing spouse is related to physical exhaustion, social isolation, and lack of information about what needs to be done. The time-consuming activities of anticipatory guidance and helping the index patient to prepare herself by examining her resources and coping skills is essential. It is documented in a study by the Office of Technology Assessment[2] that nurse practitioners (NP) see fewer patients than physicians because the content of the NPs interaction focuses on such matters, as described above, that require additional time and cannot be quickly resolved.

Upon the patient's admission to the hospital, the physician and nursing staff are responsible for the patient's direct management. To facilitate continuity of care, the GNP can meet and examine the patient, collaborate with the nursing staff for care planning, and be actively involved with physicians and consultants in the hospital. Some NPs seek hospital admitting privileges because of their need to maintain personal contact with their patients and provide continuity of care during the acute phase of an illness. The GNP can facilitate the transition between inpatient and outpatient settings and follow the index patient to the nursing home setting and back home. The role of the GNP could be as a liaison between the skilled nursing facility and the home health agency, while the ambulatory practice helps to interpret and coordinate medical care. The GNP within the ambulatory practice also may do home visits to assess and monitor the index patient's rehabilitation. A GNP may be employed by the skilled nursing facility or home health agency to provide primary and supervisory care for the index patient and coordinate care with the practice. This facility-based GNP would provide services according to standards of practice determined by the facility and the scope of practice of the NP.

Role of the gerontological clinical nurse specialist

A hospital that has a gerontological clinical nurse specialist (GCNS) offers an added resource for comprehensive long-term care. The GCNS, responsible for groups rather than individual patients, helps nurses with prehospitalization and posthospitalization nursing care planning. The GCNS is especially skilled in recognizing and managing the unique presentation of illnesses in older adults and the modifications necessary for their management, particularly preventing complications of hospitalization such as loss of function and excessive disability. The GCNS often functions as a specialist in both the acute care hospital and long-term care institutions, attending to specific problems such as wound care, incontinence, dementia, rehabilitation, functional assessment, and planning for necessary community resources when the patient is discharged. These skills are also invaluable to the GCNS for working with home care nurses and informal caregivers.

Role of the home health nurse

Home care is provided by skilled RNs who are competent in managing the high-tech aspects of home care such as total parenteral nutrition (TPN) and respirators, as well as the more routine care such as monitoring medications and complicated wounds. However, RNs often have no special training in geriatrics, and much assistance can be provided by the GNP who can also monitor patients at home. The GNP, through awareness of the index patient's preexisting health needs and hip fracture care, can coordinate the formal and informal support services.

Role of the doctorally prepared nurse in gerontology

Although the direct practice role of a nurse who has a doctor of philosophy (PhD) or doctor of nursing science (DNS) degree is similar to the GNP or GCNS, the additional skills and functions of the RN at this level allow clinical expertise to be directed by innovative, self-determined, research-based hypotheses for practice. The index patient may be included in a program involving innovative treatment modalities for hip fracture patients who are recuperating at home, rather than at a nursing home, or a program examining cost-effectiveness of home care versus institutional care. Although the scientist is interested in the outcome of the research, the nurse is interested in the health needs of the individual, and a course of long-term management that incorporates both aspects is planned.

Another indirect but significant contribution of doctorally prepared nurses is the education of professional nurses and other health care professionals in gerontological nursing. As in medicine, the specialties of geriatrics and gerontology are still developing, and currently there are few educators.

EDUCATION AND CERTIFICATION OF NURSES

As shown in Table 7-1, there are many different levels of nursing practice, with varying degrees of autonomy, and various types of licensure. Understandably, nurses want to be identified correctly by their credentials and practice their skills to their fullest capabilities. A brief description of the major nursing categories may clarify these levels of nursing practice. The licensed vocational nurse (LVN) or licensed practical nurse (LPN) is a licensed nurse who has graduated from a one-year program. LVNs and LPNs perform many functional tasks such as taking vital signs, preparing patients for procedures, and giving medications. Physicians may specially train such staff to do activities unique to their practice (e.g., geriatrics).

The registered nurse (RN) is a licensed professional who has completed a 2-year associate degree (AD), a 3-year diploma, or a 4-year bachelor of science in nursing (BSN) program and successfully passed state boards. Because of their more comprehensive education, nurses with BSNs may take additional responsibility for patient care, physical assessments, and decision making about psychosocial and physiological parameters. They also function more independently in telephone triage, patient education, and behavior modification programs.

Table 7-1   Nursing educational preparation and functional role

Type of nursing	Years of education	Function/role
Licensed Vocational Nurse/Licensed Practical Nurse (LVN/LPN)	1	Technical assistance
Registered Nurse (RN)		Functional assessment, history and physical examination, patient education
Associate Degree (AD)	2	
Diploma	3	
Bachelor of Science in Nursing (BSN)	4	
Master of Science in Nursing (MSN)		
Gerontological Nurse Practitioner (GNP)	RN + 2	Primary health care
Gerontological Clinical Nurse Specialist (GCNS)		Specialty care (both GNP and GCNS do assessments, teaching, counseling, clinical precepting)
Doctoral Degree		
Doctor of Philosophy (PhD) or	RN	Master's level skills, research,
Doctor of Nursing Science (DNS)	BSN	research-based practice,
	MS + 4	professional education

The advanced practice specialist in gerontological nursing has 1 to 3 years of additional education, which further distinguishes the GCNS from the GNP. While the capabilities of these specialists may be similar, there are a few important differences.

First, the GNP is a practitioner licensed as an RN, but the GNP is allowed to perform services traditionally within the scope of medicine, according to specific regulatory laws within each state. Standardization of competence is determined within many states' regulatory laws that require national and/or state certification to practice as an NP. At present, the GCNS remains a professional designation that does not require certification or regulatory legislation to practice, although many are certified in their specialty areas.

Second, the setting and focus of practice for these two types of specialists may differ. GNPs practice more frequently in ambulatory settings, and their scope of practice emphasizes primary, preventive, and long-term health care. They practice in a more independent environment and are more likely to coordinate and manage older adult patients across the spectrum of outpatient and long-term care settings. GCNSs usually work in institutional settings as employees and focus on particular conditions of patients, such as acute confused mental states, wound care, and functional assessments, as well as discharge planning. The autonomy of the individual practitioner depends on the particular role or job description; however, the education and training of these two advanced practice specialists may vary considerably. The knowledge and skills of a given clinician depend on the master's program, its emphasis, type and length of clinical experience, and, especially, the nurse's individual initiative and interest.

Doctorally prepared nurses have the clinical expertise of the master's level RN and receive 4 years or more of additional education and skills in formulating and implementing research in gerontological nursing. The capabilities and contributions to practice, beyond the skills of the advanced practice nurse that are outlined above, have already been discussed.

MAXIMIZING NURSING'S CONTRIBUTIONS TO GERIATRIC CARE

Although significant growth and progress is occurring for nurses in gerontological care, there are still issues that must be addressed and negotiated to enable nurses to reach their fullest potential as primary HCPs. A primary issue is reimbursement for services rendered, a necessity for all HCPs who work in ambulatory settings, especially during fiscally constrained times. Currently, nurse practitioners can be reimbursed for services in nursing homes, and certain categories of nurse practitioners are eligible for Medicaid reimbursement in ambulatory settings. But there should be universal reimbursement for the services of the advanced practice nurse, as is for other licensed health professionals.

The need for a team approach in geriatric care cannot be overstated; however, among the team members there are overlapping skills and functions. It is important to define responsibilities and the decision-making process to prevent redundancy of efforts. True collaboration is reciprocal and dynamic, changing as the needs of the patient and the situation change. Such fluidity is difficult to achieve in a hierarchial system, and such an arrangement is best avoided. Also to be avoided is the parallel practice, where the physician and nurse practitioner maintain separate caseloads with minimal collaboration. Teams are formed by professionals with complementary skills, and the most beneficial outcome for the older adult results from teamwork.

In addition, the advanced practice nurse legally should be able to perform functions traditionally handled by other health professionals, specifically physicians and pharmacists. Many states allow some form of prescriptive privileges for NPs so that they may provide the most cost-effective treatment for their patients without labor-intensive and expensive redundancy in care. However, these privileges are often limited or nonexistent in some states, preventing the NPs from practicing the full scope of their capabilities. Also, many states, or regions within states, exclude outpatient-based advanced practice nurses from hospital privileges. This restricts the NP from providing continuity of care during the patient's transition from community to acute hospital and back to the community. Advanced practice nurses perform indispensable, though still untapped, roles in the care and management of older adults. There is a need to expand their roles in the ambulatory setting.

REFERENCES

1. US Department of Health & Human Services, Public Health Service: Healthy people 2000: national health promotion and disease prevention objectives, DHHS Pub No PHS 91-50212, Washington, DC, 1990, US Government Printing Office.
2. US Congress, Office of Technology Assessment: Nurse practitioners, physician assistants, and certified nurse midwives: a policy analysis, Health Technology Case Study 37, OTA-HCS-37, Washington, DC, 1986, US Government Printing Office.

SUGGESTED READINGS

Phillips LRF: The elderly, the nurse, and the challenge. In Corr DM, Corr CA, eds: *Nursing care in an aging society*, New York, 1990, Spring.
Stone JT, Chenitz WC: An overview of gerontological nursing. In Chenitz EC, Stone JT, Salisbury SA, eds: *Clinical gerontological nursing*, Philadelphia, 1991, W.B. Saunders.

CHAPTER 8

Social work, case management, and community support

BARBARA A. SONIAT

KEY POINTS
- Comprehensive assessments in the ambulatory practice of geriatric medicine often derive substantial benefit from a social worker's assessment of psychological, social, cultural, and financial factors.
- Social workers are well prepared to assess the strengths and weaknesses of the caregiving system and contribute to the formulation of an effective treatment plan for the frail elderly patient.
- Social worker interventions such as individual, family, and group therapy, may enhance the success of the medical treatment plan for elderly patients.
- Social workers are especially knowledgeable about community resources that can help elderly patients cope successfully with functional impairments.
- Frail or functionally impaired elderly persons living in the community may benefit from case management services provided or arranged by the social worker.
- Clinicians should seek ways to incorporate the services of a social worker into the practice of ambulatory geriatric medicine, either by direct affiliation or referral.

In the ambulatory practice of geriatric medicine, clinicians often care for patients with a broad range of functional impairments resulting from their acute and chronic illnesses. Optimal health care of the functionally impaired geriatric patient requires an interdisciplinary perspective that uses a biopsychosocial model to approach diagnosis and treatment. Clinical social workers make important contributions to the comprehensive assessment and management of the elderly patient, either as a member of an interdisciplinary geriatric team or as a consultant. The contributions of social workers to the ambulatory care of geriatric patients include skills in psychosocial and family assessments; psychosocial treatment planning; therapeutic interventions with individuals, families, and groups; case management; and accessing community services for geriatric patients and their families.

ASSESSMENT

Frail elderly patients present to their health care providers myriad issues ranging from complaints about specific somatic symptoms to broad concerns about declining functional capacities. Comprehensive geriatric assessments seek to integrate the multiple interrelated spheres that impact the function and well-being of the older adult. In addition to biomedical data, information is collected about the patient's psychological function, network of social support, and economic resources to achieve a comprehensive understanding of factors affecting the patient's functional capacity. Social workers are well equipped to contribute to the assessment of elderly patients by collecting and interpreting data related to the patient's emotional and psychological health, values, family and caregiver dynamics, and sociocultural and economic circumstances.

Psychological assessment

Social workers are skilled at interviewing patients and formulating a psychological data base. A psychological assessment provides information about the individual's personality and cognitive abilities, history of stress-related events, and past coping styles. In particular, the patient's history of coping with illness and disability may provide important insight about how the patient will manage current and future medical problems.

A patient's emotional response to a medical illness can promote or hinder the ability to cope successfully. Social workers are skilled at identifying communication deficits and in recognizing the meaning that a specific diagnosis or disability may have for an individual.

Values assessment

The social worker's relationship with the patient can provide opportunities to focus assessment interviews on the patient's values and beliefs. The values domain of the biopsychosocial assessment reflects the patient's fundamental spiritual convictions. Knowledge of the patient's motivations, fears, religious tenets, and beliefs about death aids the formulation of appropriately individualized medical treatment plans. Individual preferences and expectations for functional capacity and health care interventions also provide a foundation for developing, in advance, directives for future health care decisions.

Family and caregiver issues

Research evidence consistently indicates that families provide most of the care for chronically ill persons.[5] Studies also show that caregiving can result in tremendous burden and stress for the caregivers.[1] (See Chapter 6.) Attention to the needs of caregivers can have a major impact on the durability of a caregiving system and consequently for patient outcome. It has been shown that caregiving factors are better predictors of the need for institutional placement of elderly patients than are the patients' health and disability factors.[3] Thus, the social worker's role in assessing the involvement and capacity of the informal support network is a critical component of the overall patient assessment. Assessment of the emotional and practical impact of patients' functional disabilities on their families and informal support systems is necessary to determine if additional resources are needed.

Cultural issues

The social worker's contribution to comprehensive assessment also can provide significant insight about cultural and social class issues that may impact treatment. Educated in cultural and family theory, social workers can help to dispel erroneous assumptions about appropriate roles for family members and concerned others in an individual patient's care, as these issues may be at least partially defined by culture. The formulation of acceptable care plans often depends on creating roles that are culturally acceptable to patients and families. Social workers are knowledgeable about such sociocultural factors and can contribute to formulation of successful care plans by sharing this knowledge with clinicians and interdisciplinary health care teams.

Economic issues

The crisis of medical illness in an elderly person may bring to light other factors that affect functioning and the quality of life such as inadequate housing, transportation, poverty, and poor social supports. The social worker is well equipped to assess these areas and help patients and families to devise economically feasible strategies for coping.

Evaluation of insurance and financial resources can have important implications for treatment options. Information about what the patient can afford is essential to formulating potential treatment plans. Patients and families become frustrated when they cannot afford the treatments and care alternatives that are recommended. Many care options for chronic illnesses are not covered by health insurance plans. The social worker helps formulate feasible treatment options by establishing the patient's eligibility for free or low-cost care options that may be available through public or private agencies such as subsidies for housing, additional help in the home, or partial care outside the home (e.g., adult day care).

DIRECT SOCIAL WORK INTERVENTIONS

Once a comprehensive assessment of the elderly patient with complex health problems is complete, attention turns to issues of management and treatment. As mentioned above, social workers frequently make important contributions in formulating treatment plans that are acceptable to patients and families and within the realm of economic feasibility. In addition, social workers provide a variety of interventions such as individual and group counseling, case management, and access to appropriate services from community resources, which improves the outcomes of care for elderly patients with complex health problems.

Counseling

Therapeutic and supportive counseling by a clinical geriatric social worker is frequently beneficial to patients and families. Common issues for elderly persons and families include coping with loss, increased dependency, changes in family functioning, caregiver stress, and decisions about long-term care needs. If appropriate, a plan for individual counseling by the clinic's social worker or through referral to an outside social work practitioner should be included in the patient's care plan.

Group counseling can be a powerful mechanism to help patients cope with common problems and is a cost-effective approach to provide therapeutic and supportive counseling for patients suffering from a variety of emotional and mental health problems.[2] In addition to therapeutic groups, support and self-help groups are effective in addressing many problems encountered in geriatric clinic populations.[4]

Geriatric patients are often referred and accompanied to clinic visits by their family members. Underlying family dynamics may confuse and complicate assessment, care planning, and treatment of the patient. Families may bring unresolved issues and conflicts that have to be understood and addressed to effectively treat the patients. Families are sometimes required to assume new roles and make decisions in areas that are unfamiliar to them. These situations can create intense anxiety, stress, uncertainty, and conflict.

The social worker recognizes the impact of the patients' problems on the family system and recommends resources for help such as therapeutic and supportive counseling, information, and referrals, or educational interventions to help family members understand and manage their relatives' problems effectively. Family support and self-help groups have been incorporated into the programs of many geriatric clinics and can be a cost-effective way to provide information, education, and support for family caregivers. Should nursing home placement become necessary, the social worker possesses both the practical information and the clinical skills to help patients and families work through the crisis of institutionalization.

Case management

Case management refers to the comprehensive coordination of care that is particularly useful for community-dwelling, functionally impaired persons at high risk for further functional decline. A case manager assumes responsibility for coordinating and monitoring the implementation of the care plan. Social workers often provide or arrange case management services for elderly patients who are unable, either temporarily or continually, to independently coordinate the multiple aspects of their health care needs. High-risk patients who benefit from case management include those who have multiple medical problems, inadequate family or other informal social support, limited economic resources, and impairments of cognition or mobility that interfere with their ability to function independently.

Case management services are particularly important for patients who need support to comply with their medical recommendations. Complying with medical recommendations can be difficult for patients who do not have adequate informal supports. Case managers may serve as the link between the clinician's office and the patient's home environment. By providing the clinician with information about the patient's home situation and informal support network, the case manager aids in formulating a treatment plan that takes into account the patient's capacities for compliance with medical therapy. By providing ongoing education and supervision to the patient and caregivers, the case manager contributes substantially to compliance with the medical regimen. Patients who do not have family members available to assist in managing their care on a daily basis, such as patients who have long-distance caregivers, often benefit from case management services.

Patients who need services from different agencies can benefit from a case management approach. A frail elderly patient with mobility impairments and limited family support may require a case manager to arrange transportation for medical appointments, ensure that prescriptions are filled, and make arrangements for everyday needs such as grocery shopping, housekeeping, and laundry.

Even in the setting of substantial family support, patients and family members may be overwhelmed by the complexity of the systems providing health and community services. It is difficult for patients and their families to know which services are covered by insurance and for what duration of time. For example the cost of some medical needs may be covered by health insurance but only under specified circumstances for a limited period of time. Following the acute phase of a medical illness, previously independent elderly patients frequently require some level of continuing support. The case manager can be an important guide for obtaining the appropriate services in the most efficient and economic fashion.

Case management provides a rational coordinated approach to assess needs, identify appropriate community services that are available to meet those needs, and help patients and families coordinate, monitor, and evaluate the effectiveness of a comprehensive care plan that encompasses both medical and psychosocial needs.

Access to community resources

Most communities in the United States support a network of services designed especially for older people. The impetus for this aging services network was the passage

Table 8-1   Selected community services

Types of services	Description	Examples of problems	Typical payment sources†
Seniors' centers	Community sites that offer social activities, recreation, nutrition, and educational programs; professional services may also be available	Social isolation; depression	1
Nutrition sites	Sites that offer a midday meal and opportunities to socialize with peers	Poor nutrition; social isolation	1
Transportation	A variety of specialized programs that can include door-to-door pickup, wheelchair lifts, escorts, reduced-cost taxi and public transport service	Mobility impairment; inability to drive because of vision problems	1, 2, 3, 4, 6
Meals on Wheels	Meals delivered to homebound	Homebound; frail; poor nutrition; unable or unsafe to prepare meals	1, 2, 3, 4
Home health services	Nursing and other skilled medical services; can include home health aides to help with personal care needs	Ulcer care; monitoring of blood pressure; diabetes; compliance with medication; etc.	1, 2, 3, 4, 5, 6
Homemaker services	Nonskilled help in the home with personal care and home management needs	ADL and IADL* impairments; in need of help with bathing, meal preparation, shopping, etc.	1, 2, 3, 4, 6
Adult day care	Group settings for custodial care and social activities; may offer medical and rehabilitation services	Cognitive impairment; frail; in need of care for part of a day; caregiver stress; social isolation	1, 3, 4, 6

Service	Description	Indication	Payment sources†
Respite for caregivers	Short-term residential programs or in-home services to provide free time for primary caregivers	Caregiver stress	1, 2, 3, 4
Telephone reassurance	Daily telephone call from a volunteer; caller alerts agency if there is a problem	Social isolation	1
Friendly visiting	A volunteer visits on a regular basis	Homebound; loneliness; need for socialization	1
Emergency response systems	Electronic devices used as an alert system for emergencies	At risk for falls; lives alone	4
Retirement communities/life care communities	Apartments for independent older persons; some offer additional assistance as needs change, including 24-hour nursing care	Early stages of progressive illness; social isolation; IADL* impairment	4
Congregate housing for seniors	Apartments for independent and semi-independent older persons; some offer meals, housekeeping, and laundry services	Early stages of progressive illness; low income; social isolation; IADL* impairment	3
Case management	A designated worker is responsible for overall assessment of needs; arranges, coordinates, and monitors a comprehensive home care plan	Frail; complex problems; multiple service needs; long-distance family caregivers	1, 2, 3, 4, 5, 6
Legal assistance	Lawyers, paralegals, and trained/supervised volunteers offer a wide range of services for older people	Mobility impairment; disability affects family's financial health; cognitive impairment; unable to manage finances; need to plan for anticipated future disabilities associated with progressive illness	1, 2, 4

*ADL, activities of daily living; IADL, instrumental activities of daily living.
†Payment sources: 1, free or voluntary contribution; 2, subsidized, nominal fee; 3, subsidized, sliding-fee scale; 4, private pay for full cost of service; 5, Medicare reimbursement may be available on short-term basis for part of cost; 6, Medicaid payment may be available for low-income patients.

of The Older Americans Act of 1965. The Older Americans Act mandated each state to designate a single agency that serves as the state's office on aging and directed each state to plan services specifically for older people. Currently, this legislation continues to mandate that older people should not have to prove financial need for these services, but should be offered the opportunity to pay for these services on a voluntary basis. Some community services may be available to older persons free of charge or for a voluntary donation. Services available under The Older Americans Act vary greatly between states. The act allows for funding of programs that provide home care, transportation, meals, adult day care, seniors' centers, and other special services for older people.

In addition to programs funded by The Older Americans Act, private and public agencies offer a variety of home care and community services that vary considerably in quality and availability. The home care benefits include both skilled and unskilled services. Short-term skilled home health services may be reimbursed by Medicare or other insurance programs.

Table 8-1 depicts typical community services that may be available for older patients, as well as examples of the problems they potentially address. The array of services within different communities can be complex and difficult to understand. Similar services may be offered through government programs, private nonprofit agencies, and private for-profit agencies. Some states have obtained waivers under the Medicaid program to offer community-based services to low-income patients who might otherwise need more costly nursing home placements. The matrix of services and payment arrangements displayed in Table 8-1 can vary considerably between states and local communities.

Social workers are knowledgeable about all aspects of community-based services and payment sources. Social workers can inform patients, families, and clinicians about the options for services within the community that are relevant to each patient's needs and resources.

INCORPORATION OF SOCIAL WORKERS INTO MEDICAL PRACTICE

Social workers can make important contributions to the geriatric assessment process, treatment and planning conferences, decision making about goals of care, and for choosing and implementing services for coordinated care. When ambulatory geriatric clinics include social work as a component of an interdisciplinary team, an understanding of the levels of clinical social workers enables the selection of someone who meets the needs of the team and the patient population. Knowledge about the areas of specialization within the profession can be helpful in defining the role a social worker will perform in the ambulatory clinic.

Social work qualifications

The National Association of Social Workers recognizes three levels of clinical social work preparation: baccalaureate, graduate, and doctorate. Graduate level programs for education in social work provide for specialization within a field of practice. Most social workers who practice in geriatric clinics have specialized education in gerontology or medical social work. Social workers with a bachelor's degree usually practice in settings where they have access to supervision by social work practitioners at the master's degree level. Clinical social work practitioners at the master's level are generally prepared for independent practice, following two years of supervised practice where the second year of practice occurs within their areas of specialization. Therefore, geriatric social workers at the master's level will have at least 1 year of preprofessional experience in a general medicine or geriatric medicine setting. Advanced master's and doctoral levels of clinical social workers are licensed in most states and are eligible to participate as providers reimbursed by Medicare and other third-party payor programs.

Lower salaries for social work practitioners at the beginning level may appeal to a clinic's administrator. Lower salaries, however, should be weighed against the cost for supervision, the limited clinical skills of beginning-level practitioners, and the services that practitioners at this level provide, which are not reimbursed by third-party payors. On the other hand, the education of social workers at the bachelor's level includes training in individual and family interviewing, elementary psychosocial problem solving, and recommending community resources. These skills may be adequate for assisting with history taking, coordinating the clinic's services, and providing information about, and referrals to, community services if these are the roles assigned to the clinic's social worker. Many clinical settings benefit from a more highly trained clinical social worker who can function as an independent practitioner, deliver individual and group therapy, and command reimbursement for these services, in addition to the social worker's serving as a team member in performing comprehensive geriatric assessments.

REFERENCES

1. Cantor MH: Strain among caregivers: a study of experience in the United States, *Gerontologist* 23:597, 1983.
2. Capuzzi D, Gross D, Friel SE: Recent trends in group work with elders, *Generations* 14:43, 1990.
3. Colerick EJ, George LK: Predictors of institutionalization among caregivers of patients with Alzheimer's disease, *J Am Geriatr Soc* 34:493, 1986.
4. Lieberman MA, Bliwise NG: Comparisons among peer and professionally directed groups for the elderly: implications for the development of self-help groups, *Int J Group Psychother* 35:155, 1985.
5. Shanas E: The family as a support system in old age, *Gerontologist* 19:169, 1979.

CHAPTER 9

Advance directives and surrogate decision makers

JOAN TENO
JOANNE LYNN

KEY POINTS

- Collecting and documenting patients' preferences and values are essential in the care of older patients.
- Advance directives are especially important for elderly persons.
- The Patient Self-Determination Act mandates that health care institutions inform adult patients of their rights to accept or forego medical treatment and to formulate advance directives.
- A written directive giving instructions about the patient's future care, such as a living will, usually should focus on desirable and unacceptable outcomes.
- Elderly persons should initiate a written directive naming a proxy decision maker, ordinarily by choosing a durable power of attorney for health care decisions, if there is someone suitable to serve in that capacity.
- In assessing a patient's decision-making capacity, health care providers must consider both the patient's capabilities and the seriousness of the decision.

THE FRAMEWORK FOR ADVANCE DIRECTIVES

Health care providers for older persons have an important role in making decisions that profoundly impact their patients' lives. (The term *health care provider* acknowledges that, in addition to physicians, nurses, physicians' assistants, social workers, and others often have responsibilities for counseling patients and families and making important decisions.) These decisions involve a broad array of issues such as whether to provide or forgo life-sustaining care; whether to transfer a patient to a hospital or move the patient into a long-term care institution; whether an individual has the capacity to manage personal finances; and whether to treat systolic hypertension. Every one of these decisions requires knowledge of the patient's preferences and understanding of the relative burdens and benefits of the possible outcomes. Decisions regarding locus of care or life-sustaining treatment, for example, often could be resolved in more than one way, depending upon the patient's perspectives.

When the patient can participate in making choices, and good information and supportive counseling are provided to the patient, acceptable and appropriate decisions will ordinarily be made. However, when the patient cannot be involved, there still is a mandate to provide the best and most appropriate care within the context of the patient's values and preferences. One way to ensure this appropriate care is to document the patient's values and choices in advance.

The ambulatory care setting is the optimal environment for discussing advance directives and decision making. When compared with elderly patients in hospitals or nursing homes, older patients in an office setting generally will have a greater capacity functionally and cognitively to decide their preferences of care and outcomes. Moreover, information, preferences, and questions can be better communicated in a less stressful and urgent atmosphere such as a physician's office.

With the passage of the Patient Self-Determination Act in October 1990 as part of the Omnibus Budget Reconciliation Act,[4] each health care institution must notify adult patients, once they have been admitted to the facility, of their rights under state law to accept or forego medical treatment and to write formal advance directives (e.g., durable powers of attorney for health care, living wills, and health care proxies). This statute applies to acute care hospitals, nursing homes, home health agencies, hospices, and health maintenance organizations that accept Medicaid or Medicare payment. Increasingly, clinicians will need to counsel patients regarding advance directives and will encounter these documents in a variety of settings. They will need to know the relevant laws and regulations.

Over the past 3 decades, a fairly comprehensive model of health care decision making has evolved and been widely endorsed.[5,6,8] Since reasonable persons differ about the desirability of the likely outcomes associated with various treatment plans, including foregoing treatment, the health care provider must present information about patients' current health and explain possible outcomes (both beneficial and adverse) in the context of the probability that each will occur. The informed patient or proxy then should collaborate with the health care provider to make treatment choices that will achieve outcomes desired by the patient.

When a patient can assess the desirability of outcomes, decision making need not directly evaluate the merits of arguments for or against any course of care—the patient decides the course of care. When the patient lacks the decision-making capacity, someone else must take on the task of shaping the care plan to the patient's own preferences, a task that is always difficult and often falls short of ideal. One strategy to avoid the worst aspects of this situation is to have the patient give directions for future care, which might include designating a proxy, mandating or refusing certain treatment options, or giving advice about personal priorities.

THE VALUES DOMAIN OF COMPREHENSIVE GERIATRIC ASSESSMENT

Rationale for assessment of values

In comprehensive geriatric assessment, health care providers address the four dimensions of a biopsychosocial-functional model. One additional element is needed for health care providers to make good decisions in the course of caring for their elderly patients—the values domain. Without information about values, preferences, and formal advance directives, decision makers may not achieve their most important goals.

While information from the other four domains is needed to describe the possible future courses for a patient, this is not enough information to make decisions. The patient's evaluation of the desirability of the potential outcomes is essential. Problems arise if the patient cannot participate in the discussion at the time that decisions need to be made, as in the circumstance of severe cognitive impairment. To accommodate care plans to the patient's own values, health care providers must routinely collect information regarding the patient's values, preferred approach to care, and concerns about dying and other future prospects, and document it in the medical record.

The process of collecting and discussing the patient's values

Issues of survival and suffering must be discussed in a sensitive manner. Each health care provider should develop a style that is effective and comfortable. Each should also have these discussions as a routine part of providing comprehensive health care. Patients and families ordinarily welcome the opportunity to discuss and record the patients' preferences, especially when they realize that many treatment decisions involve compromises between different benefits and burdens.

Ideally, as mentioned above, discussions regarding advance directives should be held in an ambulatory setting when the patient is fairly stable and not facing urgent decisions. Discussions should occur preferably with a health care provider who has developed a rapport with the patient. The directives should be updated periodically because preferences may change over time, especially with changes in the patient's health status.

Specific elements of the values domain

Standardized forms have been developed to guide and record discussions about a patient's values.[3] With or without these forms, the patient needs to be encouraged to reflect on personal values and preferences. (See the accompanying box on page 75.)

Some clinicians worry that discussing these issues with patients will take a great deal of time and provoke troublesome anxiety. It is more likely that such discussions will save time and relieve anxiety. Countless hours might otherwise be spent in futile treatment pursued only because no one is certain that a decision to stop is justifiable.

THE VALUES DOMAIN

Current quality of life
Aspirations and fears
Religious beliefs
Outcomes that the patient would consider to be worse than an earlier death
Important personal values
Experience with end-of-life decision making with family members or friends
Preferences for surrogate decision maker
Preferences for treatments

More provider time and family satisfaction are lost when disputes erupt over the interpretation of the patient's values.

Most elderly patients are able to answer the question "If you became seriously ill and could not discuss health care decisions with your doctor, with whom should the doctor discuss these issues?" However, some patients may prefer to avoid envisioning and choosing future treatment. The clinician must individualize the content and timing of these discussions. Whenever possible, the natural history of the patient's diseases should be shared with the patient. For patients who are likely to die as a result of progression of their current illnesses, discussions should include consideration of the common situations encountered in the terminal care of such patients. For patients likely to face institutionalization, preferences about individual freedom, safety, remaining at home, and family burden need to be explored.

One procedure for generating advance directives is to determine the patient's preferences for various kinds of life-sustaining treatment under specified outcome states.[2] This task requires considerable thoughtfulness and perspective from the patients, but it may be reassuring and useful for some patients. A lengthy catalog of the patient's specific decisions may give a false sense that all has been resolved. This cannot ever quite be true, for the patient may face unexpected combinations of outcomes, unanticipated treatment options, or unavoidable ambiguity in the directives. These concerns are especially relevant with *the living will,* a frequently used treatment directive that is ordinarily stated in general terms and requires substantial interpretation.

Use of a proxy

These considerations (i.e., unavoidable ambiguity in directives) make it critically important for the patient to name a proxy to collaborate in decision making with health care providers should the patient be unable to participate. This proxy, whenever available, can interpret the patient's preferences in the context of the actual situation confronting the patient.

If there is a suitable proxy, there are only a few issues that would be advisable for the patient to determine in advance. The patient's perspectives about in which circumstances death would be preferred to life or the possibility to achieve a certain quality of life are of great importance. Likewise, at this time in the United States, litigation or adverse regulatory sanctions can largely be avoided by having the patients document their wishes to forego resuscitation, long-term tube feeding, and long-term life support during irreversible incompetence.

PREPARATION OF WRITTEN ADVANCE DIRECTIVES

Agreement between the health care provider and the patient usually provides sufficient authority for all likely health care decisions. The health care provider can enter the substance of the discussions and decisions in the medical record, and either the provider's recollection or record of the decisions will be sufficient to guide therapy. Nevertheless, the health care provider should encourage the patient to write formal advance directives. The aim of written advance directives is to allow patients' preferences and values to determine their health care choices at some future time, when the patients become unable to participate in these decisions. Written advance directives may reduce family strife, make the decision-making process more efficient, and decrease patients' anxiety about how their care will be managed, especially when the patients are dying.

Types of written advance directives

Advance directives can accomplish two functions: They specify care decisions and name the persons who should make care decisions. An *instruction directive* such as a living will is a written document that expresses the patient's preferences regarding future treatment. A *proxy* or *surrogate directive* is one that names another person to make health care decisions along with the responsible health care provider. The most common form of surrogate directive is the *durable power of attorney for health care*. The functions of both can usually be combined in a single document.

Instruction directives. If the patient has no one who is appropriate or willing to serve as a surrogate decision maker, then the patient must be encouraged to speak directly to as many issues as possible. While this instruction directive should focus on resuscitation and artificial feeding, it also should address likely complications of the known situation and any special concerns of the patient. It is hazardous for patients to write directives that completely bar or universally mandate the use of certain interventions. Some interventions might be used for a short time with full or significant recovery of the patient, instead of the patient's imagined scenario of long-term use with little recovery. Thus, the patient should avoid stating "no use of ventilator" and instead state "avoid long-term dependence upon ventilator" or "I would find it better to have died than to have survived in a mentally incompetent state and required long-term life support on a ventilator." It is generally better to be explicit about the patient's goals and values than to accept broad generalizations about specific treatments that might be at issue. For example, it is helpful to know that a patient is interested in living only with adequate cognitive function or without pain. It is not nearly so helpful, and can be hazardous, to have an unexplained document that purports the patient did not ever want a specific treatment. (e.g., hemodialysis).

Knowing whether the patient is committed to a religion with specific tenets about health care, such as Orthodox Judaism or Christian Science, can also be helpful. The health care provider also needs to know how seriously the patient adheres to the teachings of the religion.

Because it may have special importance, particularly after the Cruzan[1] case and other cases, a patient who has firm views that artificial feeding would be undesirable should have this conviction well documented. Similarly, a patient may believe that resuscitation should be foregone, and this viewpoint should be recorded. Otherwise, patients should speak to their own situations and concerns, focus on desirable and unacceptable outcomes, and leave final judgment to the proxy and the involved health care provider when the health care dilemma arises.

Surrogate directives. In general, formal advance directives should name a surrogate decision maker whom the patient trusts and with whom the patient has discussed treatment preferences. Naming one or more alternates is also wise. The surrogate has the authority to be a decision maker only when the patient becomes incapacitated to make decisions. If there is someone suitable, that person should be named durable power of attorney for health care and should be notified and given a copy of the document. The authority given to this person ordinarily should be quite broad, including making decisions about residence, treatment, life extension, and access to medical information. The patient should be encouraged to discuss preferences with the surrogate and include a written statement that advises the surrogate and others about the patient's most important preferences and values.

Legal considerations

Health care providers now must become familiar with state laws regarding advance directives in order to counsel patients about the best options for achieving their goals. Under the Patient Self-Determination Act, every state has been required to develop a statement of the local law governing health care decision making. This information should be available in every hospital and nursing home. In addition, most state and local hospital associations, medical societies, and other groups have developed educational materials for patients' and medical professionals' use. Potential resources for information include state offices on aging, state professional societies, and Choice In Dying, a national consumer-oriented organization with offices at 250 West 57th Street, New York, NY 10107 ([212]-246-6973). In becoming familiar with these issues, many clinicians will find that their state laws are unduly cumbersome or do not address certain important issues. Correcting these deficiencies requires the concerned involvement of health care providers as citizens.

Although each state requires certain formalities for advance directives, written documents that do not conform to these formats are ordinarily still respected and are not automatically disregarded.[7] In general, if the document seems to be a valid expression of the patient's intent while the patient was competent, the document will probably be quite important when a judge must make a ruling based on its content.[7] In fact, a long hand-written letter may be more important in decision making than a living will purchased at a stationery store and signed without counseling.

ASSESSMENT OF DECISION-MAKING CAPACITY IN OLDER PERSONS

Older persons with cognitive impairments pose complex dilemmas for clinicians. Often, a comprehensive assessment is undertaken to determine an impaired patient's ability to make decisions regarding finances or site of residence. These assessments must balance autonomy, dignity, safety, and patient and community well-being. The essence of such a determination lies in whether the patient should bear the responsibility for the decision that is proposed or be protected from bearing the responsibility for the outcome of the decision.

In addition, clinicians must frequently balance the concerns of the patient with those of the caregiving network. The well-being of a family caregiver may require that the patient be placed in a long-term care facility, even when the patient would have preferred otherwise. The clinician is often faced with important negotiations that ultimately benefit the patient but do cause serious adverse consequences for the caregiving network. Considerations such as these challenge the traditional view that the clinician serves solely as the patient's advocate.

Health care providers often must determine whether a patient has adequate capacity to make decisions and bear responsibility for those choices. However, only a court of law may determine a patient's *competence*. Competency determinations fall into two general areas: The patient's ability to manage personal finances and the ability to make decisions regarding health care and personal matters such as where to live. If the court finds the person unable to manage finances, a *conservator for the estate* is appointed. If the court determines the person is unable to manage personal and health decision making, a *guardian of the person* is appointed. Judging the patient's competency in court or decision-making capacity in the medical setting requires a determination of the patient's ability to understand alternatives and to choose a plan of action that is consistent with personal goals and preferences. This assessment of whether the patient has adequate decision-making capacity is complex and requires more than merely applying a predetermined threshold to a patient's cognitive screening test. The capabilities that the patient needs for decision making vary in different situations. The standard to be applied also relies on interpreting the community's understanding of the degree to which cognitively impaired individuals can continue to manage their own lives. The community has competing obligations to intervene to protect impaired persons from serious harm and to leave citizens alone to pursue their own ideas of what is good for them.

An assessment of decision-making capacity should include specific measurements of memory, attention, and judgment (at least regarding the skills needed to address the decisions at hand). The patient must be able to understand the important impact of the choices, to reason about the alternatives, and to make choices that are consistent with enduring personal values and preferences. The patient's decision-making capacity should be assessed in relation to the decision at hand. A patient may be unable to manage finances, yet participate in decisions regarding health care. Virtually any patient who can communicate at all can bear responsibility for certain trivial decisions like whether to eat now or in a few minutes. Many mildly demented patients should retain control over an array of ordinary decisions, while a surrogate should make more substantial or difficult decisions for them. Even when a guardian has been appointed by a court, health care decisions should be discussed with the patient and family. Similarly, when the health care provider has concluded that the patient's proxy should take on decision-making authority, the patient still should be consulted to the extent possible. Patients who might understand the issues should be informed that someone else is making decisions on their behalf, and they may protest if they wish. These ongoing attempts to guarantee due process are vital to protecting the patient's civil liberties and ensuring that health care providers generally will be allowed to manage decision making in health care issues without recourse to court for each case.

REFERENCES

1. *Cruzan v Director, Missouri Department of Health*, 110 Supreme Court 2841, 111 L. Ed. 2d 224, 1990.
2. Emanuel LL, Emanuel EJ: The medical directive: a new comprehensive advance care document, *JAMA* 61:3288, 1989.
3. Gibson J: National values history project, *Generations* 14(suppl):51, 1990.
4. Patient Self-Determination Act, in the Omnibus Budget Reconciliation Act of 1990, P.L. 101-508, sections 4206, 4751, enacted November 5, 1990.
5. President's Commission for the Study of Ethical Problems in Medicine and Biomedical and Behavioral Research: *Deciding to forego life-sustaining treatment*, Washington, DC, 1983, U S Government Printing Office.
6. Schneiderman LJ, Arras JD: Counseling patients to counsel physicians on future care in the event of patient incompetence, *Ann Intern Med* 102:693, 1985.
7. The Coordinating Council on Life-Sustaining Medical Treatment Decision Making by the Courts: *Guidelines for state court decision making in authorizing or withholding life-sustaining medical treatment: a project of the National Center for State Courts*, Williamsburg Va, 1991.
8. The Hastings Center: *Guidelines on the termination of life-sustaining treatment and the care of the dying*, Bloomington, 1987, Indiana University Press.

SUGGESTED READINGS

Annas GJ: The health care proxy and the living will, *N Engl J Med* 324:1210, 1991.
Brett AS: Limitations of listing specific medical interventions in advance directives, *JAMA* 266(6):825, 1991.
Buchanan AE, Brock DW: *Deciding for others: the ethics of surrogate decision making*, Cambridge, U.K., 1989, Cambridge University Press.

CHAPTER **10** _____

Managing dying at home

ZAIL S. BERRY

KEY POINTS

- Care for the dying patient should be individualized to meet the patient's goals, with the focus on increasing comfort and reducing suffering.
- Symptom management is an important skill for physicians who care for dying patients.
- Eliciting and validating the patient's and family's concerns about the dying process are important to the successful management of dying at home.
- Advance directives and planning for death are important components of end-of-life care.
- The use of a multidisciplinary team allows comprehensive care for dying patients.

Until the mid-twentieth century, dying at home was the norm for most older persons. With the development of life-sustaining technology, emphasis on life extension as the primary goal of medical care, demographic changes resulting in separation of extended families, and employment of traditional caregivers outside the home, hospitals and nursing homes became the locus of care for many older persons at the end of their lives.

An increasing number of persons are choosing to spend the last days and weeks of life in the comfort and familiarity of their own homes. The vast majority of medical needs of the dying patient can be met in the home setting by physicians skilled in symptom management who work with multidisciplinary teams of caregivers.

PALLIATION: SHIFTING THE FOCUS OF MEDICAL CARE

In the care of dying older persons, all aspects of the patients' well-being should be considered, and goals of care should be set that maximize the quality of life remaining for these patients.

80

The goals of care should be individualized to meet the needs and preferences of patients and their families, and potential interventions should be evaluated based on their benefits and burdens *relative to goals of care*. Living to see a granddaughter marry, preventing dyspnea from interfering with one's home routine, and keeping pain to a minimum are examples of individualized patient-centered goals. The patient's preferences as defined by the patient must determine the goals of medical care. The physician must be prepared to honor the patient's goals, which at times may not seem to be in the patient's best interest.

BIOMEDICAL ASPECTS

Symptom management

As symptoms appear in a dying patient, pathophysiological reasoning can help physicians assess the cause of the symptoms and support treatment decisions. Examples include pain caused by a space-occupying tumor, bowel obstruction as a result of tumor growth in the peritoneal cavity, or nausea as a side effect of medications. In the home setting where diagnostic resources may be less available, the clinician must rely heavily on physical examination skills and knowledge of pathophysiology to make accurate judgments about the causes of symptoms. General guidelines for symptom management in elderly patients are provided in the box below.

The treatment of one symptom with multiple psychoactive medications that promote delirium or sedation without producing greater comfort is to be avoided. However, the use of multiple psychoactive medications may be necessary to control pain or other symptoms, as in the treatment of both pain and anxiety. Occasionally medications can be selected so that their side effects are therapeutic. The use of amitriptyline for depressive symptoms or neuropathical pain, for instance, may have a beneficial effect on insomnia.

PRINCIPLES OF GERIATRIC SYMPTOM MANAGEMENT

Set goals of care through discussion with patient or surrogate decision makers; develop multidisciplinary therapeutic alliance

Anticipate greater sensitivity to medications; start with lower doses and increase gradually as needed

Avoid use of multiple psychoactive medications when increasing sedation does not yield greater comfort

Whenever possible, use nonpharmacological adjunctive treatments

Administer medications around the clock for symptoms that are constant and as needed for intermittent symptoms

Be aware of medications' side-effect profiles

Nonpharmacological therapy such as biofeedback, meditation, massage, music therapy, and relaxation techniques may help control pain, anxiety, and other symptoms in appropriately selected patients. Home hospice services are often helpful in providing guidance in this area to patients and physicians.

Pain. No biotechnical skill is used more in the care of the elderly dying patient than pain management.[1,2,3] A more complete discussion of pain management is presented in Chapter 39. This section provides practical information and guidelines.

Pain, as distinct from nociception (the neurological detection and signaling of a noxious event), is an inherently subjective phenomenon and is modulated by the patient's emotional and spiritual states, as well as socioeconomic circumstances. Pain can be significantly lessened by appropriate treatment of these factors.

The clinician's confidence that pain will be controlled has enormous value to the patient and family. Achieving that confidence requires knowledge of the medications, their properties, and their appropriate use. Medications to control pain should be used in the order of their increasing efficacy. For the treatment of mild to moderate pain, acetaminophen, (enteric-coated) aspirin, or nonsteroidal antiinflammatory medications can be initiated. When the effectiveness of these are not satisfactory, an opioid such as codeine or oxycodone can be added, typically administered as a fixed combination (e.g., acetaminophen with codeine [Tylenol #3, Tylenol #4], Percodan, Percocet). When these no longer provide sufficient comfort, morphine or hydromorphone (Dilaudid) should be substituted for the lower potency opioid.

The appropriate dosage of opioid medication is that dose which maintains the patient's comfort with a minimum of unwanted side effects. The appropriate interval for a medication can be determined from its duration of action, which varies among individuals because of differences in pharmacokinetics. Drug equivalencies, appropriate dosages, and typical starting doses in the geriatric patient are listed in Table 10-1. Side effects of opioids are listed in Table 10-2. Refer to Chapter 39 for a detailed discussion on use of opiate analgesics in elderly persons.

When a given dose is less effective than desired, or the desired effect disappears before the appropriate interval elapses, the dose should be increased from 30% to 50% at the next interval. In a situation where pain is severe, a small dose may be repeated frequently until the point of comfort is achieved (every 15 minutes for subcutaneously administered medication; every 30 to 60 minutes for oral medications). When comfort is achieved, a continuing dose of 50% to 75% of the total amount initially needed to achieve comfort can be initiated at the appropriate interval, with boluses (30% to 75% of the continuing dose) available between regular doses as needed.

Long-acting opioid preparations such as oral MS Contin (morphine) can be helpful in patients with relatively stable medication needs. Once the patient's requirement for pain medication has been ascertained with the use of shorter-acting compounds, the total amount of opioids administered within 24 hours is summed and the equivalent number of milligrams of morphine is administered as MS Contin, divided every 12

Table 10-1 Opioid analgesics for treatment of pain in dying patients

Drug	Equivalent doses*		Effective dosage	Typical starting dose†
	PO	SQ/IM		
Codeine	200 mg	130 mg	4-6 hr	30-60 mg
				Tylenol #3 = 30 mg
				Tylenol #4 = 60 mg
Oxycodone				
Percocet	30 mg	15 mg	3-5 hr	5-10 mg
				Percocet = 5 mg
Hydromorphone				
Dilaudid	7.5 mg	1.5 mg	3-4 hr	1-2 mg
Morphine				
Morphine sulfate	40-60 mg	10 mg	2-4 hr	5-10 mg
MS Contin	40-60 mg	10 mg	12-24 hr	30-60 mg
Fentanyl‡			72 hr	25 μg patch

*Equivalent to 10 mg intramuscular morphine sulfate.
†For opioid-naive patient.
‡Potency = 1:20 to 1:30; therefore, 25 μg patch = 8-12 mg morphine sulfate every 4 hr.

Table 10-2 Side effects of opioid analgesics

Side effect	Management of side effect
Constipation	Initiate stool softener and stimulant laxative when opiate started
Sedation	Some degree of tolerance usually occurs in 2-4 days; use adjunctive agents; if drowsiness is intolerable, adjust dose
Nausea/emesis	Treat symptomatically as for nausea due to other causes; if severe, use adjunctive agents or switch to another opioid
Myoclonus	Usually seen at higher doses; if intolerable, adjust dose
Urinary retention/spasm	If prolonged survival not expected, use indwelling catheter
Cardiovascular effects	Occasionally orthostatic hypotension develops; use support stockings, adjunctive agent with lower dose opioid, or switch to another opioid
Respiratory depression	Rarely a problem with gradually adjusted dose; if overdose occurs, administer naloxone in repeated small doses

hours. (See Table 10-1.) When changing from one opioid to another (i.e., morphine to hydromorphone), physicians should decrease the equivalent dosage by 30% to 50% because of incomplete cross-tolerance between opioids. Unlike morphine and hydromorphone, which are available in liquid or crushable tablets, long-acting morphine cannot be crushed without loss of the slow release property. Some brands of long-acting morphine are rather large pills. MS Contin by brand name may be preferable for those patients who have difficulty swallowing pills.

For patients who have difficulty swallowing, administration of their medications in the home setting can present a challenge. When a patient's expected length of life is short, caregivers can be taught to administer subcutaneous equivalents of oral medications by injection. For longer periods, a continuous subcutaneous infusion of medication can be administered by a small portable pump, available through home infusion companies, or rectal suppositories of hydromorphone (3 mg Dilaudid) may be used. There are clinical reports of successful transbuccal administration of oral opioids in hospice patients, but the degree of absorption is highly variable. Introduced in 1991, a new product that administers fentanyl by a transdermal patch (Duragesic) can be particularly useful in the home care setting for the patient who becomes unable to take oral medication for pain. Drawbacks of the fentanyl patch include a long period between dosage adjustments (3 days after initial application and 6 days thereafter) and the inability to regulate the dosage to the patients' needs because of variability in serum concentrations among patients and the limited dosages available (25, 50, 75, and 100 μg).

The use of meperidine (Demerol) in patients with chronic pain is *not* appropriate because of its short duration of action and the long half-life of its metabolite, which precipitates central nervous system dysfunction, including seizures. Other opiates *not* recommended for use are pentazocine, an opiate agonist-antagonist, which can precipitate withdrawal symptoms in patients with chronic pain, and methadone, whose duration of analgesia is shorter than the duration of its sedative effect, which results in excessive sedation for the degree of analgesia attained.

Dyspnea. Dyspnea, the sensation of shortness of breath, is effectively treated with opioids. Relief from the subjective sensation of dyspnea occurs at dosages much lower than those needed to depress respiratory drive significantly. When dyspnea is mild, treatment can begin with a low dose of a long-acting opiate, either MS Contin (15 to 30 mg every 12 hours) or a fentanyl patch (25 μg applied every 72 hours). More severe dyspnea can be treated as was previously described for acute pain. Although used widely in the past, benzodiazepines should be used to treat dyspnea only when there is a compelling reason to avoid opioids. Relief from dyspnea usually comes only with significantly sedating doses of benzodiazepines, and several studies of benzodiazepine treatment for dyspnea have failed to show objective benefits.[4]

Oral and respiratory secretions. As the dying patient's level of arousal declines, the inability to effectively handle respiratory and oral secretions develops. For the patient who is being cared for at home, this stage of illness is usually preceded by diminished ability to take in food and fluids, and the resulting mildly dehydrated state often prevents severe respiratory congestion. Respiratory congestion may be worsened by the administration of intravenous hydration. When oral and airway secretions are problematic, they can be managed with opioids that dry secretions and reduce associated dyspnea. Oral hygiene measures and home suction apparatus may be used to provide additional assistance.

Nausea and emesis. Phenothiazine antiemetics (prochlorperazine [Compazine] or promethazine [Phenergan]), metoclopromide (Reglan), lorazepam (Ativan), histamine (H_2) blockers, and antacids can be used to treat nausea and vomiting, just as they are used for other adult patients. Most physicians are accustomed to treating nausea and emesis arising from abdominal obstruction as a surgical emergency. A conservative palliative approach is a viable alternative for terminally ill patients who do not desire aggressive surgical intervention. In conjunction with the use of antiemetics, medications that diminish bowel activity can lessen pain and emesis. Opioids in usual dosages, and loperamide hydrochloride (Imodium) or diphenoxylate hydrochloride with atropine sulfate (Lomotil), can improve patients' comfort. For patients for whom these measures do not provide adequate relief, nasogastric suction can be managed at home with the use of a portable suction device. A week's trial of corticosteroids (40 mg prednisone per day) may diminish the degree of obstruction and reopen the intestinal lumen. Occasionally, bowel obstruction will reverse itself without specific therapy.

Oral discomfort. Efforts to prevent the drying of oral mucosa should begin as soon as oral intake decreases. Swabbing the inside of the mouth with glycerin solution or citric acid mouthwash can be done by using Toothette-type swabs. When oral mucosa becomes dry and uncomfortable, 2% viscous lidocaine can be applied topically or used as a mouthwash, although with frequent use tachyphylaxis will develop, diminishing its effectiveness.

Candidiasis of the oral muscoa (thrush) can contribute to oral discomfort. When mild, thrush can be treated with topical oral nystatin suspension or clotrimazole (Mycelex) troches 4 to 5 times daily. Patients with severe thrush or those with odynophagia usually require oral ketoconazole (Nizoral) 200 mg twice daily or oral fluconazole (Diflucan) 200 mg initially, then 100 mg daily to provide lasting relief.

Constipation. The prescription of opiates should routinely be accompanied by rigorous attention to maintaining patients' regular bowel movements. (See Chapter 49.) Stool softeners (docusate sodium [Colace]) and a stimulant laxative (senna [Senokot]) may suffice. If constipation occurs, motility stimulants such as bisacodyl (Dulcolax) or other contact laxatives (cascara sagrada) should be tried, followed by rectal suppositories (glycerin or bisacodyl [Dulcolax]), saline enemas (Fleet), and manual disimpaction.

Incontinence. Urinary and stool incontinence is to be anticipated at the end of a patient's life. Caregivers may wish to be prepared with commercial diaper-like products or, for men, a condom catheter. If the expected life span is short, the potential for infection associated with indwelling catheters is not significant.

Skin and wounds. Because of the diminished mobility, poor nutrition, and incontinence that are seen frequently in the dying patient, preventive measures to maintain the patient's skin integrity are essential. Adequate hygiene, pressure-distributing mattresses, and appropriate care of pressure sores should be ensured. (See Chapter 30.)

Patients with cancer may develop tumor masses that erode the skin. The disorganized structure of the tissue may lead to bleeding and necrosis, making such lesions painful, disfiguring, and malodorous. Pain control and proper hygiene and aesthetics should minimize the impact such lesions have on the patient. Bathing the lesions with water or saline can be soothing. Some practitioners recommend bathing solutions of herbal tea or buttermilk to diminish foul odors. Localized bleeding can be controlled with silver nitrate stick cautery or gauze pads soaked in 1:1000 epinephrine solution. Local irradiation should be considered when it can be expected to yield greater benefit than burden to the patient.

Anxiety. The source of the dying patient's anxiety should be sought and treated as specifically as possible. When pharmacological treatment is needed, the use of short-acting benzodiazepines such as lorazepam (Ativan) in low doses (0.5 to 1 mg orally, subcutaneously, or sublingually, every 6 hours as needed) can be initiated and increased as needed. Other medications with sedative effects such as antihistamines (hydroxyzine [Vistaril, Atarax] and diphenhydramine [Benadryl]) can also be used, especially for a second symptom such as pruritus or pain.

Agitation. As a component of delirium, agitation is often a result of metabolic abnormalities such as hypercalcemia, hypernatremia, hyponatremia, or uremia, or a manifestation of an underlying illness such as metastatic cancer or Alzheimer's dementia. Especially when accompanied by a hallucinatory component, agitation may be effectively treated by low doses of haloperidol ([Haldol] 0.5 to 2 mg every 6 to 8 hours).

Seizures. Central nervous system disease and metabolic abnormalities in the dying patient may result in seizures. With appropriate support, acute seizure activity can be managed at home with intramuscular lorazepam ([Ativan] 2 mg every 15 to 30 minutes as needed), which is better absorbed than diazepam (Valium). Oral phenytoin (Dilantin), oral or intramuscular phenobarbital, and other anticonvulsants are used to prevent further seizure activity.

Nutrition and hydration

At the end of their lives, patients usually reduce their oral intake and often cease eating and drinking shortly before death. Questions about nutrition, tube feedings, and intravenous hydration frequently arise from family, friends, and other caregivers.

People who regularly care for dying patients observe that as patients diminish their intake, they rarely complain of hunger or thirst. The more common associated discomfort is that of a dry mouth, which is easily prevented and treated with topical care. Dying patients who receive intravenous hydration frequently develop dyspnea and increased pain as extravasation of fluid leads to ascites, pulmonary edema, and peripheral edema. Feedings administered to dying patients by either nasogastric or gastrostomy routes can facilitate aspiration. Dying patients may have difficulty expectorating and swallowing a normal amount of respiratory and oral secretions, producing their frequent coughing, choking, and aspirating. The mild state of dehydration that accompanies the dying process is observed by those who care for the terminally ill to be a natural preparation for a peaceful death.

Symptoms immediately preceding death

Progressive weakness, declining level of consciousness, inability to swallow food and fluids, and the inability to expectorate and swallow respiratory secretions are extremely common developments in persons dying after prolonged illnesses, although the mechanisms of such changes are largely unstudied. Sudden demise can occur without these developments and usually results from an acute cardiac, pulmonary, or cerebrovascular event.

Rapid deep respirations reminiscent of those seen with ketoacidosis, slow shallow respirations, and Cheyne-Stokes respirations are common during the final hours of life. The sound of air being moved through an airway containing unexpectorated secretions is sometimes referred to as a *death rattle* and may indicate that death is close at hand. This condition usually causes far greater discomfort for caregivers and family members than for the patient.

Prognostication

Physicians are often asked to estimate the time remaining in the patient's life. A range of time can be provided so that the question does not go unanswered, but the degree of uncertainty should be communicated. The pace of change in a patient's condition is often more relevant to the amount of time remaining for that patient than the actual condition itself.

PSYCHOSOCIAL ASPECTS

Family concerns

If managing pain is the biotechnical skill most frequently called upon for the care of dying patients at home, then listening to patients and families is the most valuable interpersonal skill needed. Some issues commonly arise among dying patients and their families. In addition to questions about the length of life remaining, patients and their families frequently ask what signs and symptoms they should expect as the patients' conditions deteriorate.

Multidisciplinary home care

Successful care for patients dying at home requires a coordinated delivery of services. This coordination of services is usually accomplished by a formal or informal multidisciplinary team that may include physicians, nurses, home health aides, family members, friends, social workers, clergy, and others. In addition to serving the patient's medical and nursing needs, the home care team provides patient education, emotional support, and assistance with end-of-life planning.

If a home hospice program serves the patient's community, referral to that program may be all that is needed. A hospice team usually consists of a visiting nurse, social worker, and chaplain, as well as other professionals who are called upon as needed. The medical directors of such programs usually provide consultation on specific issues. Medicare provides a hospice benefit to fund home care services for persons who have a prognosis of 6 months or less, with the physicians' services billed separately. Where home hospice services are unavailable, social work staff can help to assemble a home care team that meets the patient's needs.

Advance directives

Advance directives for health care decisions are of great importance and ideally disclose the desirableness of the patient's possible outcomes and personal preferences for care. Issues that frequently arise are the use of antibiotics to treat conditions such as pneumonia and urinary tract infection, intravenous hydration and tube feedings when the patient is no longer able to consume foods and fluids, and cardiopulmonary resuscitation.

Funeral arrangements

Grieving family members may have difficulty making decisions about funeral arrangements at the time of the patient's death. Many families prefer to make arrangements in advance. Advance planning allows the patient to incorporate personal preferences into the funeral plans and may provide some comfort to both patient and family.

Pronouncement of death and death certification

Legal procedures and actual practices vary enormously between jurisdictions. The office of the local medical examiner and hospice or other health care professionals who are experienced with home deaths are good sources of information. Contacting the medical examiner in advance with information regarding the nature of the patient's illness and prognosis may facilitate arrangements for the certification of death and removal of the body. The death certificate is initiated and filed by the funeral director. The funeral director subsequently contacts the physician for information about the cause of death and the physician's signature. Advance contact with the funeral director is helpful for all involved.

Bereavement

Practices followed by physicians after a patient's death vary tremendously. A physician's actions will be determined by that physician's level of personal comfort with various practices and relationship with the deceased patient and surviving family members.

REFERENCES

1. Foley KM: Pharmacologic approaches to cancer pain management. In Fields HL, ed: *Advances in pain research and therapy*, New York, 1985, Raven Press.
2. Saunders CM: *The management of terminal illness*, ed 2, London, 1985, Edward Arnold.
3. Twycross RG, Lack SA: *Therapeutics in terminal cancer*, ed 2, London, 1990, Churchill Livingstone.
4. Tobin MJ: Dyspnea: pathologic basis, clinical presentation, and management, *Arch Intern Med* 150:1604, 1990.

SUGGESTED READINGS

Foley KM: The treatment of cancer pain, *N Engl J Med* 113:84, 1985.
Lynn J, ed: *By no extraordinary means: the choice to forgo life-sustaining food and water*, Bloomington, 1989, Indiana University Press.
Saunders CM: *The management of terminal illness*, ed 2, London, 1985, Edward Arnold.

CHAPTER 11

Financial concerns

JOHN J. DANNER

KEY POINTS

- A financial checklist should be used to assess the financial status of all older patients.
- Never assume that patients understand their health insurance coverage.
- Seniors often place medical concerns secondary to financial concerns.
- Medicare supplemental insurance policies vary greatly; the consumer must read the fine print.
- Many eligible seniors refuse government assistance as "charity" or are unaware of available programs.
- Seniors living alone are at particular financial risk.

Why does great-grandma save aluminum foil, plastic wrap, paper bags, and rubber bands? Can't she buy more? She has enough money, doesn't she? Why does she mumble about "saving for a rainy day" and "waste not want not"? The answer to all these questions was always: She lived through the Great Depression—it changed her life. The Depression influenced the older person's views about money perhaps more than any other event in American history.

Despite the variabilities among older persons, they do have some things in common with each other. Attitudes about saving and spending money, especially as they relate to medical care, are frequently similar in this age group. They, not unlike younger adults, tend to place financial security before health concerns. This behavior pattern, in part, may explain their reluctant use of preventive measures, inordinate delays in seeking acute services, problems with medication compliance, frequently missed appointments, and hesitation in seeking alternative medical care. It is important for health care professionals who work with older patients to understand their attitudes about finances as these views will determine the patients' use of health care services.

Like the Medicare system itself, older people tend to view medical care from an acute, hospital-oriented perspective. Preventive medicine or routine health maintenance examinations may be unusual concepts to many older persons (as well as clinicians). To them, most medical care comes about as a result of sudden illness and accidents and at the insistence of other family members who observe a functional decline. This may lead to a greater use of emergency room visits. Often the patients have no primary physicians to provide information about recent medical history or follow-up after the acute medical experience. As a result, care for many elderly persons is episodic and uncoordinated.

Added to these problems is the elderly patients' lack of information and awareness about how outpatient bills are paid. Many older patients have limited understanding about what services are covered by Medicare, whether they are eligible for some other kind of assistance, or what "assignment" means. In fact, they may understand their insurance coverage for the acute hospital experience better than their bills for doctor's office visits. Many of the elderly understand that Medicare does pay for most of an acute care hospital stay and 80% of office costs, if there is assignment. Because Medicare has only recently begun to emphasize preventive care and home care, it is not surprising that elderly persons lack knowledge about how these areas are financed.

COHORT BELIEF SYSTEM

The current population of those aged 65 to 85 years have a number of similar characteristics. Some of the most common characteristics are (1) the financial devastation of the Depression (1930s) and the resultant, ingrained, intense, financial wariness, (2) the view of the physician as all knowing, (3) the belief that increased need for medical care means death is near, (4) the belief that functional decline is to be expected at their age, (5) the lack of awareness about recent medical advances, and (6) the expectation that they cannot improve after a certain age.

Money and self-esteem are closely related. Money means freedom to make choices and provide for needs, and it serves as a marker for success in life. The not-so-subtle message is that if one has little or no money, one has no value. Even for those who have money, many are consumed with worries that they will lose it to financial disaster or illness. For instance, if illness intervenes, the ability to remain financially sound may provide the person with a sense of self-worth. Yet, in spite of these overriding concerns, many older persons have not made adequate financial plans (or do not have the funds) to cope with emergencies. Those who do not financially plan for medical emergencies may find that their entire "nest egg" is spent on catastrophic care and reap a self-esteem bankruptcy.[3]

When people retire, there is an average decrease by 50% of their income. This economic decline is expressed in survival terms. The seniors spend less because they may be frightened to spend any of the principal from their homes or are consumed by a fear of not having enough money for "a rainy day." As a consequence, many seniors neglect to spend for basic health maintenance or health insurance (Medicare supplements), tend to look for miracle cures, cut back on medication dosages, or are noncompliant with treatment regimens.

FINANCIAL CONCERNS AND INCOME LEVEL

Even when seniors are financially secure, these beliefs and realities strongly impact their doctor-patient relationships. Financially secure elderly persons may have saved and invested but hold even stronger views about their never having enough to be "safe" than do those of more moderate means or even the poor elderly population. Fortunately, higher incomes are associated with a lower prevalence of illness. However, the presence of wealth has no correlation to the ability to spend for health care.

The older adults with average income may have some savings and equity in their homes. The majority of married seniors own their own homes. Their self-esteem is connected to the preservation of these resources as well. This group is also reluctant to spend and, as a result, usually has enough money to be disqualified financially from public monies and programs. When retirement benefits and insurance coverage change as a result of corporate "adjustments," the already marginal financial balance for this group is tilted. If a spouse requires nursing home care, the average time it takes to spend to the poverty level is 13 weeks. This is especially true for widows on reduced benefits (widowhood results in reduced retirement income from a spouse's account) who rent, have $15,000 or less in the bank, and have no one else to pay for the costs of health care. If widows own their homes, that causes problems as well. Quick sales are difficult, and many wish to keep their homes in the hope that they will be able to return later. However, their homes prevent them from meeting Medicaid eligibility requirements. Eventually, poverty results.

About 10% of the elderly population are poor. The most vulnerable to poverty are widows and the very old. Thirty to 40% of this group are poor.[2] The poor have problems beyond their limited funds. This cohort may perceive public help as an admission of "moral weakness" and thus refuse it. The lingering negative stereotype of welfare from the 1930s inhibits this group from using public funds. Even when they apply for public assistance, the bureaucratic complexities and inadequate available resources of the system limit the fulfillment of the needs of older adults. Furthermore, poor elderly people often lack transportation for office visits, have a high rate of illiteracy, and have a higher rate of disability than the general older population.

APPROACH TO FINANCIAL ASSESSMENT

Physicians must be aware of older patients' beliefs and attitudes towards finances. A thorough knowledge of the financial issues that confront seniors will help physicians to understand the reasons behind some of their patients' attitudes, behaviors, and actions. Some physicians may feel uncomfortable discussing these issues with their patients and neglect to ask about financial resources. Often the physicians' office staff can be trained to perform sensitive inquiries that are necessary to obtain financial information. Such discussions should be a routine part of new patients' assessments,

---

FINANCIAL CHECKLIST

Insurance

Medicare Part A, Part B
Health maintenance organization (HMO)
Medicare supplement, parallel, carve-out policies
Medicaid

Monthly income

Social Security
Retirement benefits
Pensions
Annuities
Interest accounts
Work

Governmental assistance

Social Security Supplemental Income (SSI)
Section 8 Department of Housing and Urban Development (HUD)
In-Home Support Services (IHSS)

---

thereby allaying their fears that only those with limited means are assessed. A financial checklist can be used to obtain the needed facts. (See the box above.)

Many physicians assume that when seniors seek medical care, they are aware of the finances involved, payments expected, insurance policies' parameters and limits, copayments, deductions, as well as their financial responsibilities. However, many seniors are unaware of their health care finances. The physicians or office staff must educate patients about their financial obligations for health care. An up-front awareness prevents later misunderstandings that can result in nonpayment, collection procedures, abrupt termination of doctor-patient relationships, noncompliance, and poor medical care.

INSURANCE

Medicare

Medicare was developed in the 1960s and was the first program to focus on medical care for older Americans. It is financed at the federal level by deductions from the salaries of those presently working. Since the inception of the Medicare program, the number of older people who live below the poverty line has dropped. However, the percentage of income that elders pay for health care has risen (from 15% to 18%), primarily due to an increase in the use of hospitals and high technology interventions. Older persons pay about 29% of all their health care dollars out of pocket.

Medicare is available to those 65 years or older who contributed to Social Security. In 1972 benefits were extended to individuals of any age who had been disabled for 2 years and who were entitled to Supplemental Security Income (SSI). It was also made available to persons aged 65 or older who are citizens and had worked in jobs that did not pay into Social Security (migrant workers, domestics, some federal and state employees) and to individuals below age 65 who were not entitled to Social Security benefits but voluntarily enrolled and paid monthly premiums.

Part A. Hospitalization (Part A) covers most acute hospital expenses, limited skilled nursing facility care, and some home health and hospice care. A copayment of almost $652 per benefit period is required (as of 1992). There are also other copayments for those who have extended hospital stays. The older person automatically receives Medicare Part A once he or she becomes eligible for Social Security.

Part B. Participation in Part B of Medicare is voluntary. About 3% of the Medicare population elect not to purchase this insurance. A monthly fee is deducted from their Social Security payments (in 1992, $31.80). Physicians' charges for outpatient services, limited mental health services, laboratory services, radiological services, and some durable medical equipment are covered (Table 11-1). The coverage changes frequently, and information on the latest limits is available from the social security offices and the state's third-party processor for Medicare. Medicaid will pay the monthly fee for those who are eligible. Part B covers 80% of the local allowed charges; however, Medicare *does not* cover eyeglasses, medication prescriptions, routine examinations, immunizations (except for pneumococcal or hepatitis vaccine), cosmetic surgery, nonsurgical dentistry, dentures, foot care, or special shoes. Mammograms were recently added to the covered services list.

The physician must bill the Medicare processor for services rendered to the patient. The physician also must bill for Medicare supplements. If the physician accepts assignment, Medicare pays 80% of the local allowable charge. The patient is responsible for the remaining 20%.

Medicaid

Medicaid was established in 1965 to provide medical coverage to poor persons. It is funded by federal monies augmented by state and local funds. Unlike Medicare, this program is means tested (i.e., one must meet certain income and asset requirements to qualify). Generally, the asset requirement is fixed well *below* the poverty level. Fewer than 40% of those below the poverty level are covered by Medicaid. Each state has different eligibility requirements and coverage varies accordingly. Poor elderly persons use Medicaid as a supplement to Medicare. Medicaid is included when a person receives SSI benefits because of age, disability, or blindness.

Medicaid pays for (1) inpatient hospital coverage, (2) laboratory and x-ray services, (3) outpatient care from physicians, and (4) skilled nursing care. Some states have very liberal programs covering medications, rehabilitation, psychiatric services, routine screening, and diagnostic tests.[4] Others have only emergency care available.

Table 11-1 Services covered under Medicare Part B

Coverage	Physician services	Mental health services	Hospital outpatient services
Services included	Medical and surgical services; diagnostic procedures; radiology; pathology; drugs and biologicals that cannot be self-administered	Outpatient therapy for mental illness by physician, psychologist, or in comprehensive rehabilitation outpatient setting	Ambulatory surgery incident to services of physician; diagnostic tests (laboratory/x-ray); ER hospital-based medical supplies
Conditions that must be met	Care medically necessary for diagnosis and management of acute or chronic illness; care approved by Medicare carrier	SAPS*	Care approved by Medicare carrier
Deductible	$100 deductible covers all Part B series	SAPS	SAPS
Copayment	20% (100% for charges in excess of allowable charge by nonparticipating physicians)	50% (Maximum of $1,200)	SAPS
Reimbursement	Allowable charge lesser of actual charge, the physician's usual charge, or 75% of area prevailing charge, with annual increased limited by MEI†	SAPS	Varies by type of service; outpatient surgery in transition from facility, specific cost to national average cost; laboratory and x-ray are on fee schedule; ER‡ on facility-specific costs

Coverage	Independent laboratory services	Deductible medical equipment
Services included	Clinical diagnostic laboratory	Wheelchair; oxygen equipment but not oxygen
Conditions that must be met	Care ordered by physician	For use in home; to serve a medical purpose for people who are sick or injured
Deductible	None	SAPS
Copayment	None	SAPS
Reimbursement	Approved standard fee all laboratories must take assignment	Usually based on approved amount for rental fee

*SAPS, same as physician services. †MEI, Medicare economic index. ‡ER, emergency room.

Medicare supplements

If persons aged 65 years or older have Medicare Parts A and B, they probably will benefit from having a Medicare supplement (Medigap) when they do not qualify for Medicaid. Without the supplemental insurance policy, they must pay out of pocket all deductibles, copayments, and balances of their physicians' charges. Some people assume that they will never get ill or need a supplemental policy. About 70% of the Medicare population purchase such a policy.

There have been many problems with older people purchasing policies that were not true supplements. Some older persons believe that they have a good policy only to find that they have a "carve-out" or parallel policy. A *carve-out policy* is basically a Medicare duplicate offered by some retirement plans, which saves the company money. Some may purchase more than one policy, thinking that they are receiving added coverage. Only one Medicare supplement is needed. By law, Medigap policies must provide basically the same coverage. Several have added features such as coverage for private rooms, prescriptions, or up to 150% of local Medicare-approved amounts. These plans are considerably more expensive.

Health maintenance organization

A health maintenance organization (HMO) is a capitated program where the federal government contracts with an HMO to provide all care for the subscriber. The HMO is reimbursed at 95% of the adjusted average per capita costs (approximately $400 a month per enrollee). HMOs must provide both inpatient and outpatient care, as well as reduced-cost extra services (prescriptions, eyeglasses, etc.). About 5% of Medicare beneficiaries are enrolled in HMOs. The performance of HMOs has varied widely. Some provide benefits that are not available with the standard Medicare policy, while others cannot remain financially solvent because of the heavy caseload of patients requiring expensive services. A person may disenroll by going to the Social Security office and completing a minimal amount of paperwork. Disenrollment takes a maximum of 90 days and can be as short as 30 days. Many people belong to HMOs and do not know it. Some have actually "joined" when they thought they were requesting information through the mail. HMOs generally put warning stickers on the backs of the patients' Medicare cards. Always check for these stickers.

INCOME

Work-related income

Incomes of elderly persons are from a few basic sources. Most retired workers and their spouses receive Social Security Act (SSA) monthly payments. The amount is determined by the salary amount and the number of years that they contributed before retirement. This amount varies greatly. Spouses also receive Social Security;

however, widows receive smaller amounts than when their spouses were alive, even if they themselves did not work.

Others who worked for large corporations or were union employees may receive monthly retirement pensions. These plans also vary widely, depending on the plan and level of salary before retirement. Some seniors have saved and invested or receive income from properties and stocks they control.

Government assistance

For many older persons, financing their health care and living expenses becomes an impossible task. This is especially true for those aged 85 years or older. The median annual income of this group ($8,000) is only a few hundred dollars more than their annual health care expenditures. Such persons almost always will require some form of financial assistance.

However, many seniors who are eligible for assistance are unaware of the various programs designed to ease their financial burden. These programs include the Department of Housing and Urban Development's (HUD) housing projects, Social Security Supplemental Income (SSI), In-Home Support Services (IHSS), and, in some areas, case management through local departments of social services.

HUD has a federal partnership with local housing authorities that builds senior housing and supplements rentals for individuals who are financially eligible. People generally pay one fourth of their monthly income for rent, while the balance is covered by the HUD program.

SSI is a federal program through Social Security that augments Social Security payments up to the locally determined poverty level. Monthly payments range from about $400 for those living alone to $600 for couples. Some people are eligible even if they do not receive Social Security. Generally, such persons must be diagnosed as disabled. In most states, people who are eligible for SSI are also eligible for Medicaid; however, Social Security income is figured into the equation when their eligibility is determined. Also, some states pay for in-home workers who provide basic support for activities of daily living (ADL). The amount of coverage depends on the patients' level of need as determined by evaluators from the social services department and, secondarily, by a report from their physicians who verify that the patients are incapable of providing for themselves. It is very important that the physicians who fill out such forms accurately state the dependent functional levels of the patients.

In some communities, case management services are available to eligible seniors who are in need of coordination of care. These case managers can be of great assistance to physicians because they provide assessments, in-home services, placement assistance for community living, transportation, financial augmentation, and many more services that help to maintain community living and an increased quality of life for functionally impaired seniors. Local agencies on aging can provide options that are available in the community and will take referrals from physicians who have patients who are financially eligible and in need of case management.

FUTURE TRENDS

As the population continues to age, it is projected that community assessment systems should be developed to identify, in a timely manner, those who have functional decline so as to reduce the likelihood of costly institutionalization. Partnerships between local, state, and federal agencies are being formed to develop programs that will focus on educative and preventive measures to improve assistive community services. The program ideally will be rehabilitative and provide geriatric assessment to the general elderly population. A national health insurance program or service will remain on every political agenda for the foreseeable future. If modeled on programs of other countries, these programs would require interagency cooperation, a provision for preventive primary medical care, and mandatory case management to redistribute appropriately the limited funds that are available.

REFERENCES

1. Friedman E: Health care's changing face: the demographics of the 21st Century, *Hospitals* 65:36, 1991.
2. Kasper JD: Aging alone: profiles and projections: a report of the commonwealth fund commission on elderly people living alone, The Commonwealth Fund, 1988.
3. Larson R: Thirty years of research on the subjective well being of older Americans, *J Gerontol* 33:109, 1978.
4. US Dept of Health and Human Services: Social Security Administration, SSA Pub No HCFA 10050461250, Washington, DC, 1991, U.S. Government Printing Office.

SUGGESTED READINGS

Schneider EL, Guralnik JM: The aging of America: impact on health care costs, *JAMA* 263:2335, 1990.
Enthoven A, Kronick R: A consumer-choice health plan for the 1990s: universal health insurance in a system designed to promote quality and economy, *N Eng Med* 320:29, (Part 1), and 320:94 (Part 2), 1989.

APPROACHES TO ASSESSMENT

Overview to comprehensive assessment

KENNETH BRUMMEL-SMITH

KEY POINTS

- Comprehensive assessment is one of the most important tools that office-based physicians can use when caring for older persons.
- During assessment, physicians should attempt to understand how patients are functioning in their own homes.
- Physicians should become familiar with a few instruments for assessment and their applications, limits, and interpretations.
- Office personnel can be trained in the application of standardized assessment instruments.

Comprehensive assessment of the older patient has been termed the "technology of geriatrics." The term *comprehensive assessment* usually refers to a multifaceted examination that includes evaluations of the patient's physical, mental, social, economic, and functional health status. (See the box on p. 101.) Anticipatory discussion about the patient's ethical desires regarding intensity of care is also an appropriate component of the assessment. Unfortunately, the terms comprehensive assessment and functional assessment are often used interchangeably. In reality, functional assessment is but a part of the comprehensive assessment. Physicians providing care to elderly patients must be well versed in both types of assessment processes.

One of the basic aspects of geriatric care is its goal of maintaining the patient's function.[4] Standard medical care tends to be both disease and cure oriented. In a traditional approach, the patient may receive excellent care for a medical problem, such as diabetes mellitus that is out of control, but is left so functionally disabled due to weakness and excessive bed rest that the patient cannot continue to live at home independently.

_____ **COMPONENTS OF COMPREHENSIVE ASSESSMENT** _____

Medical health
Psychological health
Functional health
Social support system
Economic stability
Ethical decision making

Older persons, in general, are more concerned with functional outcomes than disease outcomes. Even when they have multiple problems, they tend to rate their health as good to excellent _if_ they can care for themselves. Their greatest fears are usually functionally based such as the fear of being dependent on their children, having to go to a nursing home, or falling.

The inability for patients to carry out their daily functions is usually not detected when practitioners use the traditional medical approach. For instance, a performance-based gait evaluation is far superior in detecting walking problems than a standard neurological examination.[11] Furthermore, there are often multiple reasons why patients may not be functioning at their highest possible levels. Biological, psychological, and social factors all interact to create one's ability to function. While any one factor may limit function, in common practice all the factors play a role to some degree.

For the frail older person in need of assistance, the influence of the caregiver is perhaps the greatest factor affecting function. In a study evaluating the various factors that determined use of formal health care services, the burden experienced by the caregiver was the most important factor found.[3] Both the use of home care services and nursing home placement were better predicted by measuring caregiver burden than by the patient's physical examination, diagnoses, or even activities of daily living (ADL).

GOALS OF COMPREHENSIVE ASSESSMENT

The National Institutes of Health convened a Health Consensus Development Conference in 1988 that elucidated the following goals for comprehensive assessment: (1) to improve diagnostic accuracy, (2) to guide the selection of interventions to restore or preserve health, (3) to recommend an optimal environment for care, (4) to predict outcomes, and (5) to monitor clinical change over time. (See the box on p. 102.) In office-based practice, assessment may meet one or more of these goals. The consensus panel also believed that targeting the assessment process to patients who are most in need was an important factor.[10]

_____ GOALS FOR COMPREHENSIVE ASSESSMENT* _____

Improve diagnostic accuracy
Guide the selection of intervention
Recommend an optimum environment for care
Predict outcome
Monitor change over time

---

*From National Institutes of Health, Health Consensus Development Conference, 1988.

EFFECTIVENESS OF COMPREHENSIVE ASSESSMENT

There have been a number of studies documenting the effectiveness of the comprehensive assessment approach in an outpatient setting.[9,12]

This multifaceted approach is generally provided by a team of health care providers in a hospital or institutional setting. However, in office practice it is usually the physician's role to perform the medical, psychological, and functional components. Naturally, this type of comprehensive assessment takes time and usually occurs over a number of visits. In some practices, an office assistant or nurse can be trained in the administration of assessment tools. Many physicians develop referral relationships with social workers in private practice or through their hospital affiliations.

LIMITS OF ASSESSMENT

There are limits to the process of comprehensive assessment. Some of these limits arise from the origins of the instruments, the inherent difficulties in obtaining functional, psychological, or social information, and the information gleaned from comprehensive assessment. Most assessment instruments (e.g., Barthel index, Lawton IADL scale[6]) were developed for research purposes but have not been studied specifically in office-based practice. Large multifaceted instruments, such as the Comprehensive Assessment and Referral Evaluation (CARE), have little application in office practice because of the training required to administer them and the time required to complete the evaluation. Many highly trained providers, such as physical therapists, rarely use standardized instruments and instead rely on a traditional set of evaluation measures. After all, virtually all experienced physicians rely on a non-standardized instrument—the physical examination. Standardized instruments do facilitate communication between providers by having a common language.

It has been suggested that there are five factors that must be evaluated when practitioners review an assessment instrument.[2] (See the box on p. 103.) Because it is difficult for the busy practitioner to evaluate each instrument personally, an excellent handbook has been written that reviews the various assessment instruments.[5]

EVALUATING AN ASSESSMENT INSTRUMENT

Does it have proven validity?

Does it have proven reliability?

Does it have sensitivity to detect changes over time?

Do summed scores hide important information (e.g., although a total score is within normal range, key items are responded to incorrectly)?

Does the design fit the target audience (e.g., men may score lower on instrumental activities of daily living (IADL) scales because such scales are often weighted toward activities carried out by women in their age cohort)?

Other problems arise that are related to the methods used by practitioners to obtain information during assessment. For instance, should the physician ask the patients if they are having any problems dressing, ask a family member to report any problems, or watch the patients attempt to dress themselves. Which source of information is the most reliable? Most standardized assessment instruments rely upon verbal reports by the patients or family members. Such reports are often fraught with problems.

One problem is the phenomenon of say do, can do, do do. Patients may have many reasons for "saying" they can do a particular activity. They may be able to do it, may fear the consequences of not being able to do it and hence exaggerate the truth, or may not be able to remember and make up an answer. Some patients are so fearful of being told they must move to a nursing home that they will try to design answers that overstate their capabilities. The same possibilities hold true for family members. There may be an overwhelming sense of burden felt by the caregivers which then limits their objectivity in every observation that they make.

What a person "can do" is best assessed by observing the patient's activity (Tinetti gait and mobility examination)[11] or a representative activity (Williams timed manual task test).[13] But this approach is also subject to misinterpretation. Some people may perform very poorly because of performance anxiety, while others may be so stimulated by the testing situation that they accomplish the task even though they rarely carry out such activities in the privacy of their own homes. Persons with severe depression may be physically and cognitively capable of performing activities of daily living but may have such severe psychomotor retardation that they fail to dress or feed themselves. Standardized instruments would rate them the same as severely demented persons. Therefore, the ideal piece of information would be what they "do do," those activities that they actually carry out in their own living environments. The most complete assessment would look at all three levels.

Talking with patients about their perceived capabilities and functional problems, corroborating information from friends and families, and administering appropriate performance-based tests when needed will most accurately define the patients' statuses. *The importance of an experienced clinical impression should not be forgotten.* No measurement instrument is sensitive enough to discern the subtle cues that are picked up during an in-depth interview or after years of continuous care and observation of a patient.

The best time to perform an assessment is another problem that arises. Obviously one would not like to use a procedure haphazardly that is both time consuming and expensive. Some have suggested performing a comprehensive assessment during the patient's major life changes, such as prior to discharge from a hospital or before admission to a nursing home, as is done in England. Guidelines from the Omnibus Reconciliation Act of 1987 (OBRA 1987) require such an assessment at these points, but then the problem arises as to who will do the assessment and where it will occur. Because of the advent of the prospective payment system (PPS) in 1983, there is not much time for an assessment to be done in an acute hospital setting. Even if an assessment was to be done there, who would perform it? If it is done soon after the patient's hospital discharge and admission to a nursing home, the patient may still be experiencing the effects of anesthesia, drugs, or sensory deprivation. Furthermore, it appears that targeting the assessment to those most in need of it has the highest yield in terms of detecting treatable conditions and effective positive functional outcomes.[10] It is not cost-effective to routinely perform comprehensive assessments for healthy elderly outpatients. In the office setting, it is probably wise to reserve the more comprehensive assessment procedures for those who have recent, significant, functional changes (especially after a recent hospitalization) or those who may be facing admission to a nursing home. Some type of periodic assessment of certain areas, in a much less extensive form, also is likely to benefit those who are without apparent functional losses at the time of routine health maintenance examinations.

Ideally, an assessment tool should detect changes over time. This is especially important for office-based practices because changes in patients' functional abilities usually occur insidiously and may escape the notice of patients and physicians. Most of the established tools have been evaluated for this feature and found to be acceptable. To document such changes, the use of a flow sheet to record performance and total scores is recommended.

DESIGNING INTERVENTIONS BASED ON ASSESSMENT

Those studies that failed to show positive benefits from comprehensive assessment did not include an intervention with the assessment process. In office practice, intervention is not likely to be a problem. The physician practicing geriatrics may need the services of a social worker and allied health providers (e.g., physical and occupational therapists, audiologists, etc.); hence, it is important to develop a list of resources who can be called upon to address the problems that are found during comprehensive assessment.

REIMBURSEMENT AND TIME MANAGEMENT FOR COMPREHENSIVE ASSESSMENT

Perhaps the most difficult topic is how to optimize appropriate reimbursement for this labor-intensive effort. The new Relative Value System, which places greater emphasis on primary care and cognitive-based assessments, may eliminate some of the problems.[7] Further efforts by physicians who care for older persons are necessary to: (1) demonstrate the effectiveness of comprehensive assessment, and (2) advocate appropriate reimbursement for those services.

Physicians in office practices can maximize their reimbursement for these services through a number of mechanisms. Programs for home assessment and care can be referred through a local chapter of the Visiting Nurse Association (VNA). These programs often provide case management services. A number of community hospitals are willing to fund a nurse-case manager who can serve as both a manager and case finder. This service improves patients' access to hospital facilities and promotes a positive image in the community.

In the office, assessments are often done during a number of visits. (See Chapter 2.) Most physicians will need at least 1 hour for the initial assessment. With training, other office personnel can administer standardized assessment instruments. If the patient requires ongoing case management services that only a physician can provide, it is possible to bill Medicare for these services as well.[1]

It is also wise to develop a summary sheet that enables the physician to quickly access needed information. This sheet should include the patient's medical, psychological, functional, and social problems. A list of current medications, especially if they are related to the medical diagnoses on the problem list, is also helpful. The problem list can be sent to VNAs or to a nursing home, should that become necessary. A flow sheet on which to record the dates of repeated assessments is also a useful tool.

REFERENCES

1. American Academy of Family Physicians: Medicare Part B information update, Kansas City, Mo, 1991, The Academy.
2. Applegate WB, Blass JP, Williams TF: Instruments for the functional assessment of older persons, *N Engl J Med* 322:1207, 1990.
3. Brown LJ, Potter JF, Foster BG: Caregiver burden should be evaluated during geriatric assessment, *J Am Geriatr Soc* 38:455, 1990.
4. Comprehensive geriatric assessment: AGS public policy committee, *J Am Geriatr Soc* 37:473, 1989.
5. Gallo JJ, Reichel W, Andersen L: *Handbook of geriatric assessment*, Rockville, Md, 1988, Aspen.

6. Lawton MP, Broady EM: Assessment of older people: self-maintaining and instrumental activities of daily living, *Gerontologist* 9:179–186, 1969.

7. Lee PR, Ginsburg PB, LeRoy LB, Hammons GT: The physician payment review commission report to Congress, *JAMA* 261:2382, 1989.

8. Natioinal Institutes of Health Consensus Development Conference Statement: Geriatric assessment methods for clinical decision making, *J. Am. Geriatr. Soc.* 36:342, 1988.

9. Rubenstein LZ: Geriatric assessment: an overview of its impacts, *Clin Geriatr Med* 3:1, 1987.

10. Solomon DH: Geriatric assessment: methods for clinical decision making, *JAMA* 259:2450, 1988.

11. Tinetti ME, Ginter SF: Identifying mobility dysfunctions in elderly patients, *JAMA* 259:1190, 1988.

12. Williams ME: Outpatient geriatric evaluation, *Clin Geriatr Med* 3:173, 1987.

13. Williams ME, Hadler NM, Earp JA: Manual ability as a marker for dependency in elderly women, *J Chron Dis* 35:115, 1982.

SUGGESTED READINGS

Applegate WB, Blass JP, Williams TF: Instruments for the functional assessment of older persons, *N Engl J Med* 322, 1990.

Gallo JJ, Reichel W, Andersen L: *Handbook of geriatric assessment*, Rockville, MD, 1988, Aspen.

Solomon DH: Geriatric assessment: methods for clinical decision making, *JAMA* 259:2450, 1988.

Williams ME: Outpatient geriatric evaluation, *Clin Geriatr Med* 3:173, 1987.

CHAPTER 13

Office assessment tools

LAURA MOSQUEDA

KEY POINTS

- Functional assessment more accurately predicts a patient's quality of life than a simple problem list.
- Functional assessment in the office setting provides information about the patient's self-care skills, neuromuscular function, and mental function.
- Assessment tools do not provide diagnosis but allow monitoring of the patient's responses to treatment and changes in function over time.

An older adult's quality of life is closely related to physical, psychological, and social function. Unfortunately, a simple examination of a patient's problem list does not accurately predict that patient's functional status. For example, a patient with six diagnoses on a problem list (diabetes mellitus, congestive heart failure, glaucoma, pulmonary disease, hypertension, and history of stroke) may be much more functional than a patient who has "only" one problem (osteoarthritis of the left hip). Thus, it is critically important to evaluate and document the geriatric patient's functional capacity in a systematic way. The tools described in this chapter are easily used in an office setting and assist the clinician with functional assessment of three general areas: (1) self-care skills, (2) neuromuscular function, and (3) mental function. However, these screening tools do *not* provide diagnoses. They do allow monitoring of the patient's responses to treatment and changes in function over time. They may also help family members understand their loved one's abilities and limitations.

SELF-CARE SKILLS ASSESSMENT

The activities of daily living (ADL) and instrumental activities of daily living (IADL) are formal assessment tools that outline functions which are necessary for day-to-day living. As will be described in detail, a person who requires assistance in any of these activities cannot function in a completely independent manner. It is

107

therefore critically important for the primary care physician to know how to ask about and document ADL and IADL. These tools provide insight about what patients *can do* for themselves. In addition, they provide the patient, family, support system, and physician with practical information that helps them decide what, if any, assistance is needed.

Activities of daily living

There are certain basic abilities a person must possess to remain at home independently. These abilities allow a person to accomplish basic self-care tasks which are referred to as activities of daily living. (See the accompanying box below.) ADL are typically divided into seven categories and may be easily recalled by the mnemonic *ABCDETT: Ambulation* or mobility describes a person's ability to move from place to place, with or without an assistive device; *Bathing* refers to sponge baths, traditional baths, and showers; *Continence* of bowel and bladder refers to sphincter control rather than ability to get to a commode; *Dressing* includes selecting and getting clothes, as well as the act of dressing; *Eating* does *not* include preparing meals but refers solely to the ability to feed oneself; *Toileting* involves going to the commode, undressing and dressing as needed, and cleaning oneself after voiding; and *Transferring* refers to getting in and out of a bed or a chair.

If a person is independent in all ADL, that individual is able to function inside a home without assistance. A disability in any one of these categories indicates that an in-home caregiver is required, at least on a part-time basis. It is crucial to remember that one's independence in ADL depends on the interaction of physical, psychological, and socioeconomic factors. The following example illustrates this interaction: An 83-year-old woman with osteoarthritis of both shoulders and hips is independent in all ADL, as long as her pain is well controlled. However, her pain gradually increases and she becomes unable to get in and out of the tub. An occupational therapist recommends that the physician prescribe a tub transfer bench and long-handled sponge. This simple intervention restores the woman's independence and obviates the need for a caregiver to assist with bathing. But if this same patient then becomes depressed following the death of her husband, or her socioeconomic status prevents

---

ACTIVITIES OF DAILY LIVING

Ambulation or mobility
Bathing
Continence
Dressing
Eating
Toileting
Transferring

her from getting the equipment she needs, a simple intervention may not be adequate. The combination of her biological, psychological, and social stressors may lead to a functional decline necessitating assistance for bathing, transferring, and toileting.

The Katz index of ADL allows the physician to assess six ADL: bathing, continence, dressing, feeding, toileting, and transfers.[4] (See the box below.) Each function is rated on a 3-point scale. For instance, continence is classified as (1) having complete

---

_____ KATZ INDEX OF ACTIVITIES OF DAILY LIVING* _____

1. **Bathing (either sponge bath, tub bath, or shower)**
   a. Receives no assistance (gets in and out of tub by self if tub is usual means of bathing)
   b. Receives assistance in bathing only one part of body such as the back or a leg
   c. Receives assistance in bathing more than one part of body or is not bathed

2. **Continence**
   a. Controls urination and bowel movement completely by self
   b. Has occasional "accidents"
   c. Needs supervision to keep urine or bowel control, uses catheter, or is incontinent

3. **Dressing (gets clothes from closets and drawers, including underclothes, outer garments; uses fasteners, including braces, if worn)**
   a. Gets clothes and gets completely dressed without assistance
   b. Gets clothes and gets dressed without assistance except in tieing shoes
   c. Receives assistance in getting clothes or getting dressed or stays partly or completely undressed

4. **Eating**
   a. Feeds self without assistance
   b. Feeds self except for assistance in cutting meat or buttering bread
   c. Receives assistance in feeding or is fed partly or completely by using tubes or intravenous fluids

5. **Toileting (going to the "toilet room" for bowel and urine elimination; cleaning self after elimination and arranging clothes)**
   a. Goes to "toilet room," cleans self, and arranges clothes without assistance (may use object for support such as cane, walker, or wheelchair and may manage night bedpan or commode and emptying same in morning)
   b. Receives assistance in going to "toilet room," cleaning self, or arranging clothes after elimination or receives assistance in using night bedpan or commode
   c. Does not go to room termed "toilet" for the elimination process

6. **Transferring**
   a. Moves in and out of bed or chair without assistance (may use object for support such as cane or walker)
   b. Moves in and out of bed or chair with assistance
   c. Does not get out of bed

---

*Response a., 3 points; b., 2 points; c., 1 point; maximum score, 18 points.

control of bowel and bladder (3 points), (2) having occasional "accidents" (2 points), or (3) requiring supervision to maintain control (1 point). Note that each task classification is based on what the patient is *actually* doing, not on what the patient is *capable* of doing. The Katz index of ADL is especially helpful in identifying patients who require minimal or moderate assistance with their basic abilities and functions. Physicians may not realize that these patients require help because their disabilities are not obvious without formal questioning. The index is an objective method for monitoring a patient's function over time and indicates when physicians should intercede (i.e., before a patient's functional decline becomes extreme).

Instrumental activities of daily living

IADL are the higher level abilities that allow a person to function independently in the home or community. (See the box below.) Early functional loss often occurs in the areas of transportation and housework. When patients or their families notice problems in these areas, this may serve as a harbinger of more significant functional decline.

The five-item questionnaire for the instrumental activities of daily living screening allows a practitioner to rate the patient's traveling, shopping, meal preparation, housekeeping, and money management skills.[2] (See the box on p. 111.) It is especially important for practitioners to be aware of the patient's psychosocial situation when they administer this questionnaire because it includes several tasks that are traditionally performed by women. For instance, an older man may say that he does not perform housework, shopping, or meal preparation simply because his spouse performs these tasks, not because of his functional limitations. Eventually he may have these functional deficits, but they will not become apparent until he is required to perform the tasks (e.g., after death of spouse).

INSTRUMENTAL ACTIVITIES OF DAILY LIVING*

Using the telephone
Shopping
Preparing meals
Doing laundry
Housekeeping
Taking medications
Managing money
Traveling

---

*Some clinicians also include reading, writing, climbing stairs, and paid employment.

FIVE-ITEM INSTRUMENTAL
ACTIVITIES OF DAILY LIVING SCREENING

1. **Can you get to places out of walking distance**
   a. Without help (can travel alone on bus, taxi, or drive own car)
   b. With some help (need someone to help or go with you when traveling)
   c. Or are you unable to travel unless emergency arrangements are made for a specialized vehicle such as an ambulance

2. **Can you go shopping for groceries or clothes (assuming that you have transportation)**
   a. Without help (can take care of all your shopping needs yourself)
   b. With some help (need someone to go with you on all shopping trips)
   c. Or are you completely unable to do any shopping

3. **Can you prepare your own meals**
   a. Without help (can plan and cook meals yourself)
   b. With some help (can prepare some things but unable to cook full meals yourself)
   c. Or are you unable to do any meal preparation

4. **Can you do your housework**
   a. Without help (can scrub floors, etc.)
   b. With some help (can do light housework but need help with heavy work)
   c. Or are you unable to do any housework

5. **Can you handle your own money**
   a. Without help (can write checks, pay bills, etc.)
   b. With some help (can manage day-to-day buying but need help with managing your checkbook and paying your bills)
   c. Or are you completely unable to handle money

*Scoring system has not been validated for interpretation.

NEUROMUSCULAR ASSESSMENT

The traditional neurological and musculoskeletal examinations are time-consuming processes. They yield detailed information about specific joints or muscle groups but give little information about a patient's overall function. A study by Tinetti and Ginter[8] revealed that the standard neuromuscular examination is poor at identifying a patient's mobility problems because it is the *interaction* of a person's strength, tone, mental status, sensation, and range of motion (to name but a few components) that determines a person's mobility. The following discussion describes two practical tools that assess a patient's neuromuscular function.

The performance-oriented mobility assessment (Table 13-1) is particularly useful for assessing a person's risk of falling.[8] This test is performed by first asking the patients to get up from their chairs without using their hands, walk to the end of the

Table 13-1   Performance-oriented mobility assessment

Position change or balance maneuver	Observations
Balance component	
Getting up from chair*	Potential risk of fall if patient does not get up with single movement; pushes up with arms or moves forward in chair first; unsteady on first standing
Sitting down in chair	Plops in chair; does not land in center
Withstanding nudge on sternum	Moves feet; grabs object for support
Romberg test (eyes closed)	Same as above; tests patient's reliance on visual input for balance
Neck turning	Moves feet; grabs object for support; complains of vertigo, dizziness, or unsteadiness
Reaching up	Unable to reach up to full shoulder flexion standing on tiptoes; unsteady; grabs object for support
Bending over	Unable to bend over to pick up small object (e.g., pen) from floor; grabs object to pull up on; requires multiple attempts to arise
Gait component	
Initiation	Hesitates; stumbles; grabs object for support
Step height	Does not clear floor consistently (scrapes or shuffles); raises foot too high (more than two inches)
Step continuity	After first few steps, does not consistently begin raising one foot as other foot touches floor
Step symmetry	Step length not equal; pathologic side usually has longer step length (problem may be in hip, knee, ankle, or surrounding muscles)
Path deviation	Does not walk in straight line; weaves side to side
Turning	Stops before initiating turn; staggers; sways; grabs object for support

*Use hard armless chair.

hallway, turn around, and walk back to the practitioner. The practitioner observes initiation of movement, gait pattern, turning, and ability to follow a verbal command. When patients return, the examiner nudges them lightly on the sternum three times, observes the patients with their eyes closed, and asks patients to turn their heads, to reach up, and to bend over. The patients are then asked to sit down without using their hands. The entire examination takes only a few minutes to perform but yields a wealth of information. This examination includes many provocative maneuvers that patients are likely to perform during a regular day.

The Rancho functional assessment screen (Table 13-2) focuses on the patient's upper extremity strength, range of motion, and ambulatory status.[1] Each test, such as having the patient put both hands behind the head, correlates with a function, for example, combing hair. Patients who can independently perform all of these tests

Table 13-2 Rancho functional assessment screen

Test	Functions tested	Normal	Limited	Unable
Put both hands together behind head	Combing hair; washing back, etc.			
Put both hands together in back of waist	Managing clothing; washing lower back			
Sitting, touch great toe with opposite hand	Lower extremity dressing; hygiene			
Squeeze examiner's two fingers with each hand	Grasp strength (approx. 20 lb of pressure needed for functional activities)			
Hold paper between thumb and lateral side of index finger while examiner tries to pull it out	Pinch strength (approx. 3 lb of pressure needed for functional activities)			
Stand from chair without using hand	Transfer ability; fall risk			
Walk 15-30 m	Velocity; household ambulatory status			

have a high level of physical function. The following example illustrates the utility of this assessment: An 82-year-old man has been living independently in an apartment. A functional assessment indicates that he is having increasing difficulty in touching his left great toe with his right hand. He tends to be off balance, and his left hip hurts because of the amount of flexion that is required for that maneuver. He is referred to an occupational therapist who provides him with adaptive equipment for lower body dressing, thus decreasing his pain and risk of falling.

MENTAL STATUS EXAMINATION

Cognitive assessment

The mini-mental state examination (MMSE) is a screening device for cognitive function.[3] It is a widely used, standardized tool that has good reliability and validity. A maximum score of 30 points is possible. It includes tests for orientation, registration, attention, recent recall, language (written and verbal, receptive and expressive), and visuospatial skills. (See the box on p. 114). Patients who score 25 or above are

───── MINI-MENTAL STATE EXAMINATION ─────

		Score	Total
1. Orientation			
What is the	day	——— 1	
	date	——— 1	
	month	——— 1	
	year	——— 1	
	season	——— 1	——— 5
What is the	city	——— 1	
	state	——— 1	
	county	——— 1	
	building	——— 1	
	floor	——— 1	——— 5

2. Registration

Name 3 objects and take 1 second to say each. Then ask the patient to repeat all 3 objects. (Give 1 point for each correct answer. Repeat until patient can get all 3 objects.)   ——— 3

3. Attention and calculation

Serial 7s: Ask the patient to count backward by 7s from 100. (Stop after 5 answers. Give 1 point for each correct answer.) Alternate: Spell *world* backward. (Give 1 point for each correctly placed letter.)   ——— 5

4. Recall

After 2 minutes, ask for the 3 objects' names in question 2. (Give 1 point for each correct answer.)   ——— 3

5. Language

Point to a pencil and a watch. Ask the patient to name each as you point. (Give 1 point for each correct answer.)   ——— 2

Ask the patient to repeat the following phrase: No *if*'s, *and*'s, or *but*'s. (Give 1 point for the correct answer.)   ——— 1

Ask the patient to perform the following three-stage command: Take this piece of paper in your left hand, fold it in half, and lay it on the table. (Give 1 point for each correct step.)   ——— 3

Ask the patient to read and carry out the following written command: Close your eyes. (Give 1 point for the correct response.)   ——— 1

Ask the patient to write a sentence. It must contain a noun and a verb and make sense. Ignore spelling errors. (Give 1 point for the correct answer.)   ——— 1

Ask the patient to draw 2 interlocking pentagons. There must be 5 sides to each pentagon and 4 interlocking sides. Example: (Give 1 point for the correct answer.)   ——— 1

TOTAL   ——— 30

considered normal; a score between 19 and 24 suggests mild impairment; a score between 16 and 19 suggests moderate impairment; and a score of less than 16 suggests a severe impairment.

Because of its widespread use and high interrater reliability, the MMSE is particularly useful when clinicians communicate with each other. However, this test must be used with caution because people who have fewer years of formal education tend to have lower scores. For example, a person with a third grade education always may have had difficulties with subtracting, reading, and writing. On the other hand, demented patients who are highly educated must have a fairly significant decline in cognitive abilities to be identified by the MMSE.

Prior to administering the examination, practitioners should put patients at ease by explaining to them that the various tests are routine parts of the examination (e.g., "In this part of the examination, I'm going to ask you a few questions that will test your memory. Some of the questions may seem easy and others may seem hard, so just do your best"). The first 10 points measure orientation. Incorrect answers can result for this part of the examination, for example, when new patients first come to the office but do not know the address or floor. The next 3 points are based on mental registration of 3 objects. Warn patients to keep these objects in mind because they will be asked to repeat them again in a few minutes. Patients with Alzheimer's disease may be able to register the words but cannot recall them a few minutes later. Asking patients to count backward from 100 by 7s can be an intimidating task, even for younger adults who are not demented. It is usually less threatening to ask patients to spell *world* backward; for every correctly placed letter they score 1 point. The patients are then asked to recall the 3 items that they mentally registered, and only those spontaneously remembered are credited. Patients who do poorly in the naming section generally have a moderately severe deficit. Patients who have early Alzheimer's disease will have difficulty naming *parts* of objects (pen clip, knuckle, watchband, etc.). The final question, which is worth 1 point, is the only test for patients' visuospatial abilities. Because the MMSE is heavily weighted toward orientation questions, it is just as important for practitioners to note what questions the patients missed as it is to note the total score. For example, a female patient who has a ninth grade education scores 22 on the MMSE. She has just moved to her son's home in a new state, does not know the county, town, hospital, day, or date, and spells *world* incorrectly backward. Another male patient, a retired astronomer, scores 24 on the MMSE, with points off for month, date, registering 2 of 3 objects, recalling 1 of 3 objects, and inability in copying the interlocking pentagons. Although the second patient has a higher score, the impairment is more global and severe than the first patient's impairment.

Depressed patients may have a low score on this examination, secondary to difficulty with concentration and low motivation to answer questions. These patients will usually show little effort and answer many questions with "I don't know." They are often aware of their memory problems and will complain about them to their physicians.

As with all other assessment tools, the MMSE neither provides a diagnosis nor differentiates dementia, delirium, amnesia, or aphasia. This tool assists clinicians in identifying the potentially demented patient so that they may further evaluate the cause of the cognitive impairment. (See Chapter 35.)

Depression

Many older adults were raised in a society that viewed depression as a sign of weakness. Thus it is not surprising that geriatric patients tend to underreport depression to their physicians. Depressed older adults are more likely to approach their primary care physicians with numerous somatic complaints than seek help from mental health specialists. Many of the illnesses that typically occur in older adults produce functional decline and predispose these patients to depression. It is, therefore, critically important for physicians to be vigilant for signs and symptoms of depression. (See Chapter 36.)

The older adult health and mood questionnaire (OAHMQ) was designed specifically as a brief screening tool for depression in geriatric patients.[5] Unlike other depression scales, OAHMQ includes criteria from the *Diagnostic and Statistical Manual of Mental Disorders* (DSM-III-R) along with age-associated differences for the reporting of depressive symptoms. The OAHMQ consists of 26 true or false statements. The 22 items are categorized into mood and non-mood questions. Odd-numbered statements reflect a patient's depressed mood by examining feelings such as anhedonia (I seem to have lost the ability to have any fun), irritation (I have been more easily irritated or frustrated lately), and hopelessness (I frequently feel like I don't care about anything anymore). Even-numbered statements reflect a patient's depressive symptoms that are related to behavior (It is hard for me to get started on my daily chores), cognition (My memory or thinking is not as good as usual), and somatic complaints (My appetite or digestion of food is worse than usual).

The OAHMQ is scored as follows: Patients who endorse (answer true) 0 to 5 items are not depressed; those who endorse 12 or more probably meet criteria for major depression. However, even those patients who score between 6 and 11 are likely to have enough depressive symptoms to interfere with their function. If a person has an intermediate score (i.e., 6 to 11) with more than 6 odd-numbered items endorsed, it is likely that a dysphoric mood is present.

MULTIDIMENSIONAL SCALES

Functional dementia scale

Many clinicians and family members who care for persons with dementia have noticed that the patients' functional abilities cannot be predicted by the amount of cognitive impairment present. The functional dementia scale (FDS) was designed as

_____ OLDER ADULT HEALTH AND MOOD QUESTIONNAIRE (OAHMQ)* _____

1. My daily life is not interesting .... T or F
2. It is hard for me to get started on my daily chores and activities .... T or F
3. I have been more unhappy than usual for at least a month................ T or F
4. I have been sleeping poorly for at least the last month .... T or F
5. I gain little pleasure from anything .... T or F
6. I feel listless, tired, or fatigued a lot of the time .... T or F
7. I have felt sad, down in the dumps, or blue much of the time during the last
   month ....T or F
8. My memory or thinking is not as good as usual......................... T or F
9. I have been more easily irritated or frustrated lately...................... T or F
10. I feel worse in the morning than in the afternoon........................ T or F
11. I have cried or felt like crying more than twice during the last month ...... T or F
12. I am definitely slowed down compared to my usual way of feeling......... T or F
13. The things that used to make me happy don't do so anymore............. T or F
14. My appetite or digestion of food is worse than usual .... T or F
15. I frequently feel like I don't care about anything anymore .... T or F
16. Life is really not worth living most of the time .... T or F
17. My outlook is more gloomy than usual .... T or F
18. I have stopped several of my usual activities............................ T or F
19. I cry or feel saddened more easily than a few months ago................ T or F
20. I feel pretty hopeless about improving my life........................... T or F
21. I seem to have lost the ability to have any fun........................... T or F
22. I have regrets about the past that I think about often .... T or F

*If patient has 0–5 true answers, no major depression; 6–11 true answers, intermediate or borderline; 12 or more true answers, probable major depression.

a fast, simple, and reliable method for clinicians to evaluate demented patients' functional abilities.[6] This scale is designed to be completed by the patients' caregivers and has a very practical orientation. (See the box on p. 118.) It includes questions about patients' self-care skills and disruptive behaviors. Each item is stated as a behavior (e.g., wanders at night or needs to be restrained to prevent wandering, hears things that are not there, cannot control bowel function). The caregivers rate each item on a scale from 1 (none or little of the time) to 4 (most or all of the time).

The FDS includes the caregivers' assessments in a systematic quantifiable fashion. This not only helps the physician to gather data, but it also helps validate the importance of the caregiver's role. The following example illustrates the use of the FDS: Mrs. H. is a 78-year-old woman who was diagnosed with Alzheimer's disease 1 year ago. She lives with her son and daughter-in-law. Her daughter-in-law takes her to the physician's office and says that Mrs. H. has been getting a lot worse, a lot faster, for the past few months. The daughter-in-law also mentions that Mrs. H. is confused and even violent at times. While examining the patient, the physician asks the daughter-in-law to complete the FDS. The physician's examination reveals mild congestive

---

FUNCTIONAL DEMENTIA SCALE

Circle one rating for each item:
1 = None or little of the time
2 = Some of the time
3 = Good part of the time
4 = Most or all of the time

Date: _____
Patient: _____
Observer: _____
Relation to patient: _____

1 2 3 4   1. Has difficulty in completing simple tasks on own (e.g., dressing, bathing, doing arithmetic)
1 2 3 4   2. Spends time either sitting or in apparently purposeless activity
1 2 3 4   3. Wanders at night or needs to be restrained to prevent wandering
1 2 3 4   4. Hears things that are not there
1 2 3 4   5. Requires supervision or assistance in eating
1 2 3 4   6. Loses things
1 2 3 4   7. Has disorderly appearance if left to own devices
1 2 3 4   8. Moans
1 2 3 4   9. Cannot control bowel function
1 2 3 4   10. Threatens to harm others
1 2 3 4   11. Cannot control bladder function
1 2 3 4   12. Needs to be watched so doesn't injure self (e.g., by careless smoking, leaving the stove on, falling)
1 2 3 4   13. Destroys materials around him or her (e.g., breaks furniture, throws food trays, tears up magazines)
1 2 3 4   14. Shouts or yells
1 2 3 4   15. Accuses others of doing him or her bodily harm or stealing his or her possessions when you are sure the accusations are not true
1 2 3 4   16. Is unaware of limitations imposed by illness
1 2 3 4   17. Becomes confused and does not know where he or she is
1 2 3 4   18. Has trouble remembering
1 2 3 4   19. Has sudden changes of mood (e.g., gets upset, angry, or cries easily)
1 2 3 4   20. Wanders aimlessly during the day or needs to be restrained to prevent wandering, if left alone

---

heart failure and a urinary tract infection, both of which are new findings for this patient. The physician notices that her score on the MMSE is only 2 points lower than it was 8 months ago. After reviewing the FDS, the physician has some specific functional information: Mrs. H. scores 3s and 4s on items such as moaning, controlling bladder function, shouting, and changing moods. The urinary tract infection and congestive heart failure are treated and the patient returns to the physician's office 3 months later. While Mrs. H. is waiting to be seen, the daughter-in-law is again asked to fill out the FDS. The same behaviors that were occurring "most of the time" (a score of 4) are now occurring "some of the time" (a score of 2). Although Mrs. H. still has a significant impairment, treatment of her medical problems optimizes her function, as is reflected in the FDS.

Hebrew rehabilitation center for the aged vulnerability index

The Hebrew Rehabilitation Center for the Aged (HRCA) developed an assessment tool that integrates self-care skills, neuromuscular function, and cognitive status. The HRCA vulnerability index was devised as a multidisciplinary screening instrument that identifies "high-need" elderly persons in the community.[7] (See the box below.) Unlike the other tools presented in this chapter, the HRCA vulnerability index provides little specific information; its goal is to identify those elderly persons who are at high risk of losing their independence. By administering this test periodically, the

---

THE HEBREW REHABILITATION CENTER FOR THE AGED VULNERABILITY INDEX

1. Now I will ask you about your meals. Do you prepare them yourself?
       _____ Yes   _____ No
   If Yes, ask: Do you have great difficulty doing it yourself?
   If No, ask: Do you need this help?
       _____ Yes   (P)   _____ No

2. Do you take out the garbage yourself?
       _____ Yes   _____ No
   If Yes, Ask: Do you have great difficulty doing it yourself?
   If No, ask: Do you need this help?
       _____ Yes   (P)   _____ No

3. Are you healthy enough to do the ordinary work around the house without help?
       _____ Yes   _____ No

4. Are you healthy enough to walk up and down stairs without help?
       _____ Yes   _____ No

5. Do you use a walker or four-pronged cane at least some of the time to get around?
       _____ Yes   (P)   _____ No

6. Do you use a wheelchair at least some of the time to get around?
       _____ Yes   _____ No

7. Could you please tell me what year it is?
       _____ Correct   _____ Incorrect (P)
   A. Record number of (P) boxes checked for questions 1. to 7.   A. ( )

8. In the last month, how many days a week have you usually gone out of the building in which you live?
       _____ 2 or more days a week
       _____ 1 day a week or less (P)

9. Are you able to dress yourself (including shoes and socks) without help?
       _____ Seldom, sometimes, or never
       _____ Frequently or most of the time (P)
   B. Record number of (P) boxes checked for questions 8. to 11.   B. ( )
   C. Person is functionally vulnerable if
       A. box is greater than 1 or
       A. box equals 1 and *B.* box is greater than 0.   C. ( )
       Check ( ) if vulnerable

primary care physician can detect problems for patients who may require an intervention or in-home assistance.

It is hoped that functional assessment tools will help the clinician identify treatable disabilities at an early stage. Just as we are vigilant in looking for early evidence of organ failure, we must attuned to looking for early evidence of "function failure."

REFERENCES

1. Brummel-Smith K: *The Rancho functional assessment screen*, Tech Rep, Downey, Calif, 1992, Rehabilitation Research and Training Center on Aging.
2. Fillenbaum GG: Screening the elderly: a brief instrumental ADL measure, *J Am Geriatr Soc* 33:698, 1985.
3. Folstein MF, Folstein S, McHuth PR: Mini-mental state: a practical method for grading the cognitive state of patients for the clinician, *J Psychiatr Res* 12:189, 1975.
4. Katz S et al: The index of activities of daily living: a standardized measure of biological and psychosocial function, *JAMA* 185:914, 1963.
5. Kemp B et al: The older adult health and mood questionnaire: a measure of depressive disorder, Tech Rep, Downey, Calif, 1991, Rehabilitation Research and Training Center on Aging.
6. Moore J et al: A functional dementia scale, *J Fam Pract* 16:499, 1983.
7. Morris JN et al: An assessment tool for use in identifying functionally vulnerable persons in the community, *Gerontologist* 24:373, 1984.
8. Tinetti ME, Ginter SF: Identifying mobility dysfunctions in elderly patients, *JAMA* 259:1190, 1988.

SUGGESTED READINGS

Folstein MF, Folstein S, McHuth PR: Mini-mental state: a practical method for grading the cognitive state of patients for the clinician, *J Psychiatr Res* 12:189, 1975.
Gallo JJ, Reichel W, Anderson L: *Handbook of geriatric assessment*, Rockville, Md, 1988, Aspen.
Goldsmith G, Brodwick M: Assessing the functional states of older patients with chronic illness, *Fam Med* 21:38, 1989.
Kane RA, Kane RL: *Assessing the elderly: a practical guide to management*, Lexington, Mass, 1981, DC Heath.

CHAPTER 14

Preoperative assessment and management

ELIZABETH L. COBBS

KEY POINTS

- Increasing numbers of elderly patients are safely undergoing diverse surgical interventions.
- Age in itself is not a contraindication to surgery.
- Comprehensive preoperative care provides the basis for the best possible outcomes for older patients.
- Assessment, goal setting, and decision making are important elements of the preoperative process.
- Coordination of the provider system is essential to ensuring the best possible outcome.
- Sufficient, pertinent, clinical documentation permits maximal coordination and continuity through a complex provider system.

CLINICAL RELEVANCE

The past two decades have produced significant advances in the safety and efficacy of surgical interventions for elderly patients. Careful preoperative assessment and management are the first steps to successful surgical interventions for older persons. To accomplish these important initial steps, health care professionals utilize the tools of geriatric medicine such as the comprehensive functional assessment and the biopsychosocial interdisciplinary team approach.

In recent years there has been a drastic shift from the hospital-centered preoperative care of the 1970s and early 1980s. Largely in response to the rising costs of health care, a large proportion of preoperative management now occurs in the outpatient arena. Many aspects of this ambulatory focus impact the elderly patient. The burden of orchestrating laboratory tests and complex evaluations may be substantial. Despite the proliferation of outpatient facilities that renders this task more easily accomplished, the planning and coordination continues to be time consuming and

121

labor intensive for patients and physicians. The preoperative management of an elderly patient in the ambulatory setting is ideally a *process* combining comprehensive assessment, individual goal setting, decision making, and coordination of medical, anesthetic, and surgical management. The responsibility for directing the preoperative management may fall on the primary care physician, the surgeon, or another member of the health care team, depending on the complexity of the patient's problems, the nature of concomitant problems, and the setting.

PREOPERATIVE ASSESSMENT

A comprehensive history and physical examination provide the foundation for a successful preoperative assessment. The scope of the assessment should be broad enough to identify any condition that deserves attention during the preoperative period or affects the patient's decision to have surgery. A functionally impaired elderly individual with complicated health problems is likely to require a detailed assessment to achieve optimal surgical results.

History

Elderly patients may be poor historians, unable to recall the details about past surgeries, drug allergies, or hospital stays. The physician is at a distinct advantage if the patient has been followed over time. In that event, the history is well established and needs only to be updated. It is worthwhile to obtain the patient's previous medical records to clarify sketchy historical data and avoid unwelcome surprises during the preoperative period.

A general review of systems should focus on recent changes in health status. An appreciation for the rate of change in function may be important to the decision for the patient to undergo surgery. Preoperative activity, ambulatory status, exercise tolerance, chest pain, and respiratory and neurological systems are particularly noteworthy. A history of falls is an important predictor of subsequent falls.

The patient's use of medications, including nonprescription remedies, must be carefully elicited. A history of frequent use of anxiolytics and sleep medications should be sought because the patient may exhibit signs of withdrawal when these medications are suddenly discontinued perioperatively. A history of substance abuse, especially alcohol, may not be suspected in older patients but should always be considered.

Physical examination

A comprehensive physical examination is essential to preoperative assessment and management and provides a baseline for the intraoperative and postoperative care. Vital signs should include weight and height. Orthostatic measurements of blood pressure and pulse serve as an assessment of volume status and as a predictor of postoperative falls. Blood pressure may fluctuate in elderly patients, thus a single measure that is mildly elevated need not cause undue concern. The patient's general appearance should be recorded, with reference to body habitus, affect, and behavior. Carotid bruits are often found in older persons, but in the absence of symptoms, they are not associated with significantly increased risk for subsequent stroke. Cardiac function merits careful attention. Signs of active congestive heart failure (such as a diastolic [S_3] gallop sound or jugular venous distention) heighten surgical risk of perioperative cardiac morbidity. Systolic murmurs, a common finding in elderly patients, are often associated with a sclerotic aortic valve but should be carefully characterized if there is a concern that aortic stenosis exists. Kyphoscoliosis may distort the apical impulse, making it an unreliable clue to cardiac size.

The pulmonary examination should assess respiratory function, including the patient's response to the exertion of rising from a chair or walking about the room. Basilar rales are not necessarily a sign of pathology in an elderly patient. Pedal edema is frequently associated with venous stasis and therefore is an unreliable sign of cardiac failure without associated findings. The neurological examination may uncover motor or sensory deficits that heighten the patient's risk for injury in the postoperative period. An assessment of visual and auditory acuities should be included because impairments of these senses may hinder the patient's ability to regain orientation immediately after anesthesia.

Mental status

The older patient with abnormal mental status should be characterized to the extent necessary so that the severity, likely cause, and potential for complications associated with surgery may be assessed. Further evaluation and treatment should be considered if new evidence of an affective or cognitive disorder is discovered. Delirium is a common postoperative occurrence in elderly patients undergoing major surgery. The presence of cognitive impairment, significant sensory impairment, and general frailty may increase the risk of acute confusional states postoperatively. (See Chapter 34.) A standard instrument for assessing the patient's cognitive function is helpful because it can be easily repeated by others in the hospital setting. (See Chapter 13.)

Functional assessment

Functional capacity is derived from the patient's combined biomedical, psychological, and social resources and is assessed through qualitative and quantitative data gathered from the history, physical, and mental status examination. (See Chapter 12.) Accurate assessment aids in predicting the older patient's response to the stresses associated with surgery and allows planning for the postoperative period. Comprehensive assessment of function should address mobility, cognition, medical condition, sensory impairment, use of aids, bowel and bladder continence. (See Chapter 13.)

Social assessment

Inquiry about social circumstances is always relevant in preparing elderly patients for surgery. Immediately following surgery, even the most independent individual needs assistance from others for transportation, meal preparation, general care, and supervision.

Laboratory

Most surgical centers require that a preoperative panel of laboratory data be obtained within a specified time interval. Generally, decisions about laboratory tests should be guided by the findings from the patient's history and physical examination. In the absence of diseases or medications that mandate particular tests, the minimum laboratory screening should include a complete blood count, blood or serum glucose, serum electrolytes, serum creatinine, urinalysis, electrocardiogram (ECG), and chest radiograph within a reasonable period of time. Shortly before surgery, patients coping with chronic medical problems should be measured for the appropriate parameters of their illnesses and their blood levels of medications. A test of thyroid function warrants consideration in a patient with vague symptoms and signs that may mimic those of normal aging.

Urinalysis is included in the preoperative screening because of the high incidence of urinary tract pathology in older patients. Asymptomatic bacteriuria is not uncommon in elderly patients and need not be treated (see Chapter 28); however, significant pyuria or hematuria should be identified prior to surgery. A urinary tract infection should be treated before elective surgery.

ECG is an important test for elderly surgical patients. The typical resting ECG of an elderly person reflects changes that are associated with atherosclerosis and degeneration of the conduction system. Sequential ECGs may be extremely helpful in determining whether nonspecific findings should raise concerns about cardiac ischemia or a silent myocardial infarction within the last 6 months. Elderly persons are much more likely to have silent myocardial infarctions. Echocardiograms have shown great utility for the noninvasive diagnosis of significant cardiac conditions in elderly patients. A murmur that suggests aortic stenosis warrants a preoperative echocardiogram.

Routine chest radiographs are unnecessary for most persons who have no pulmonary symptoms or signs. In healthy younger persons undergoing elective surgery, chest radiographs are unnecessary. However, preoperative chest radiographs in older patients will often reveal a significant finding relevant to postoperative management.[1] Heart size, for example, may be abnormal, and cardiomegaly may be a harbinger of postoperative complications. Pulmonary function tests are not usually necessary in the absence of significant chronic lung disease or if there is little concern about the patient's pulmonary reserve and ability to tolerate the proposed anesthesia and operation.

INTERVENTIONS

Goals of care

Elderly patients often face medical dilemmas that may not always have acceptable solutions. The goals of care should reflect each individual's medical situation in the context of the psychological, social, and economic circumstances. Cure of a disease process and subsequent prolongation of life are desirable goals whenever feasible in patients of any age. For example, cancer-directed operations or other surgical attempts at cure are highly efficacious in selected elderly patients. The importance of preserving function in elderly patients has been increasingly recognized. Older patients often face dilemmas of chronic symptom management for which surgical intervention may be appropriate. Total hip replacements have been shown to be well tolerated and to achieve excellent relief of pain in patients aged 80 years and older.[5] For chronically ill elderly patients, surgical interventions may be necessary to permit adequate nursing care for the patients. A gangrenous extremity in a nonambulatory, functionally disabled, chronically ill person who is dependent on others for wound care may be best managed by a conservative amputation, which leaves a more rapidly healing surgical site that can be safely and easily managed by the caregivers. Preservation of well-being and dignity is a compelling indication for surgery in any patient, old or young. For example, elderly persons may derive great psychological benefit from cosmetic surgery following disfiguring cancer surgery.

Goals of care are best established through collaboration with the patients, clinicians, families, caregivers, consultants, and significant others. For patients who cannot make their own medical decisions, it is often helpful to discuss the goals of care with a broad representation from the health care team. Nursing staff who know the patient well often contribute insightfully to such a discussion.

Calculation of risks and benefits

Accurate calculation of risks and benefits is essential to good medical decision making. At some time, most elderly patients will face a complex decision with implications for life span, function, or comfort, if not all of these. Choices frequently must be made between a number of imperfect options that carry relative risks. Patients and their surrogates make their choices based on assessments of the risks and benefits of various treatment options, in conjunction with their personal preferences.

In calculating patient-related risk, chronological age is associated with age-related, though variable, physiological decline and the increased likelihood that disease will be present. Attempts to quantitate the risks of surgery in older patients reflect the debate over how much risk should be attributed solely to age or to underlying disease processes. Assumptions about patient-derived risk cannot be assigned solely on the basis of chronological age.

One recent retrospective study of nonagenarian (ages 90 to 100) surgical patients asked these questions: (1) Does advanced age alone increase preoperative surgical risk?, and (2) What correctable causes of morbidity and mortality can be identified that might alter management and minimize surgical risk in the very old?[6] Specifically, the study sought to answer whether advanced age alone warranted invasive hemodynamic measures. Results suggested that many of these patients have outlived the period of peak risk for preventable cardiac disease and therefore did not warrant routine preoperative invasive hemodynamic monitoring. For these patients, the most important determinants of outcome appeared to be related to surgical technique, anesthesia, and preoperative care.

Cardiac risk has received considerable study because of the high probability for the presence of cardiovascular disease in elderly patients. In 1977 Goldman devised a risk factor index utilizing prospective analysis for patients over the age of 40 years who undergo non–cardiac surgery. (See Tables 14-1 and 14-2.) In 1987 Detsky et al.[2] elaborated the cardiac risk index by studying a group of higher risk patients who undergo preoperative evaluation. Gerson et al.[3] suggested that elderly individuals who are unable to complete exercise testing (2 minutes of bicycle exercise in the supine position to raise the heart rate above 99 beats/min) are at increased risk for cardiac complications during abdominal or non-cardiac thoracic surgery. Inability to exercise, however, is nonspecific and may be related to poor general medical condition, limited cardiovascular reserve, or cardiac disease.

Table 14-1 Goldman cardiac risk index

Criteria	Points
S$_3$ or jugular venous distention	11
Myocardial infarction during previous 6 mo	10
Rhythm other than sinus or premature atrial contractions	7
> 5 premature ventricular contractions/min anytime preoperatively	7
Age > 70 yr	5
Emergency operation	4
Significant aortic stenosis	3
Intraperitoneal, intrathoracic, or aortic surgery	3
Poor general medical status	3
PO$_2$ < 60 mm Hg	
PCO$_2$ > 50 mm Hg	
K < 3.0 mEq/L	
HCO$_3$ < 20 mEq/L	
BUN > 50 mg/dl	
Creat > 3.0 mg/dl	
Chronic liver disease	
Abnormal liver function tests	
Chronically bedridden from noncardiac causes	
TOTAL POSSIBLE POINTS	53

Modified from Goldman L et al: Multifactorial index of cardiac risk in noncardiac surgical procedures, *N Engl J Med* 297:845, 1977.

Table 14-2 Postoperative morbidity and mortality according to Goldman cardiac risk index

Class	Point total	No/minor complications	Life threatening	Cardiac deaths
I	0-5	99%	0.7%	0.2%
II	6-12	93%	5.0%	2.0%
III	13-25	86%	11.0%	2.0%
IV	> 25	22%	22.0%	56.0%

Adapted from Goldman L et al: Multifactorial index of cardiac risk in noncardiac surgical procedures, *N Engl J Med* 297:845, 1977.

Medical knowledge of cardiac risk factors is evolving. Significant ventricular ectopy is a risk factor for sudden death in patients who have either postmyocardial infarction or severe left ventricular dysfunction. However, in the absence of these factors or evidence of structural heart disease, the healthy older patient probably does not have an increased risk of cardiac complications during the preoperative period. For active patients who have angina pectoris provoked by exertion only, chronic stable angina has not been a risk factor for preoperative cardiac complications.

Significant aortic stenosis is best detected and quantified by Doppler echocardiography and should be identified prior to surgery. Some research shows that elderly patients who have severe aortic stenosis can safely undergo surgery when they are carefully managed through cardiac monitoring and meticulous anesthesia techniques.[4] Active congestive heart failure (as evidenced by an early diastolic gallop [S_3] or jugular venous distention) is an important potentially reversible risk factor and should be vigorously treated prior to surgery.

Pulmonary risks are enhanced in older patients because of changes associated with aging such as decreased compliance of the lungs and thoracic cage, increased residual volume and dead space, increased alveolar-arterial oxygen gradient, and decreased forced expiratory volume in the first second (FEV1). This enhanced vulnerability to hypoxemia is exacerbated by pain, sedation, and infection. Pulmonary risks are further heightened by the patient's history of smoking, along with a productive cough, obstructive lung disease, and obesity.

The risk of postoperative renal failure is increased by a glomerular filtration rate (GFR) of less than 50 ml/min. It is not possible to uniformly predict the creatinine clearance (a measure of GFR) based on the age, weight, and serum creatinine of an older patient. While many individuals will manifest a marked decrease in GFR as they age, some older persons who are free of renal and cardiovascular diseases will have a well-preserved GFR. An actual measurement of creatinine clearance is necessary if accurate determination of renal function is needed.

Patients who have suffered recent strokes are at a relative risk for another stroke, which diminishes over time. The greatest risk for recurrent strokes occurs in the first few months. Poor medical conditions of the patients, reflected through organ failures and substantial acute or chronic illnesses, confer increased risks for elderly patients.

Malnutrition, as evidenced by a serum albumin of less than 3.0 g/dl, has been associated with a high incidence of postoperative complications.

Surgical risk may derive from the patient, surgeon, procedure, timing of the procedure, and system of care. Frail elderly patients are vulnerable in all of these domains and benefit from aggressive attempts to minimize the risks in each area.

Procedure-related risks derive from multiple factors, including site of the incision, length of the operation, and anesthesia time. Pulmonary risks are increased by upper abdominal and thoracic incisions. The risk of postoperative renal failure is increased by procedures that are longer than 3 hours and operations that involve clamping of the aorta above the origin of the renal arteries.

The characteristics of the health care providers themselves are important determinants of risk, particularly the experience and expertise of the surgeon and anesthesiologist. The more delicate the patient and proposed surgery, the more important become the judgment and operative finesse of the surgical team. Though difficult to measure, the quality of the health care system contributes significantly to the outcomes of surgical interventions for elderly patients. Medical records, pharmacy, laboratory, housekeeping, and other departments contribute services that are essential to high-quality perioperative care for elderly persons. Teamwork and continuity is essential to producing good surgical outcomes. Communication and cooperation become absolutely necessary, especially when health professionals care for elderly patients who have cognitive impairments and must rely to a great extent on support from their environment. As in all age groups, emergency surgery confers increased risks to elderly patients through a variety of mechanisms.

Decision to have surgery

The circumstances of each elderly patient are unique, and decisions about surgery may be complex. Good decision making is based on individual goals of care, risk-benefit assessments of the various treatment options, and ethical principles such as autonomy, beneficence (acting in the patient's best interest), and nonmaleficence (doing no harm to the patient). Though the patient's age may be one factor in the decision, considerations of coexistent disease, individual preferences, timing of surgery, and anticipated functional outcomes are likely to weigh more heavily.

A surgeon who demonstrates experience and capability should be selected. A second surgical opinion is frequently advisable and often required by insurers. Patients should view second opinions as opportunities for greater education and quality assurance. Consultants should be sought who appreciate the special qualities of the elderly population and who participate in collaborative decision making, which are necessary to achieve the best possible outcomes. The clinician should seek the best results with the least invasive procedures such as interventional radiology, endoscopy, and laparoscopy. Finally, when clinicians have a choice of sites where surgery may be performed, "site friendliness" to elderly patients should be considered.

Optimizing the patient's status

The preoperative period is the time to pursue any maneuvers that minimize the detrimental effects of coexistent diseases and age-related physiological decline.

Preoperative conditions, such as congestive heart failure, bronchospasm, or hypothyroidism, that can be ameliorated by medical treatment should be vigorously sought during the preoperative assessment. Other conditions, such as renal failure, also increase the patient's operative risks but are immutable. Avoiding treatments or diagnostic maneuvers that aggravate these conditions is paramount in planning the preoperative care.

Polypharmacy should be aggressively addressed. The preoperative period presents an ideal opportunity to discontinue any medications that are not absolutely necessary. Current practice allows most medications that are truly necessary to be continued with careful monitoring throughout the postoperative period. Estrogen replacement in postmenopausal women does not increase the risk of their developing deep venous thrombosis and therefore should not be discontinued in anticipation of surgery.

Cardiac status and blood pressure are best controlled over time through gradual titration of medication, which prevents volume depletion or wide fluctuations in the blood pressure. Pulmonary optimization can be achieved in elderly patients who have chronic lung disease by exhorting the patient to quit smoking and instituting deep breathing maneuvers, chest physiotherapy, bronchodilators, and antibiotics when indicated.

Patients who have histories of stroke are at risk for recurrent strokes, and elective surgery probably should be delayed at least 2 weeks after the event to minimize further complications. It is not often possible to achieve substantial amelioration of the patient's nutritional status in advance of surgery, but it is worthwhile to address the options.

Blood transfusions may be required in elective surgery (e.g., total hip replacement, prostatectomy). Optimally, the patient's own blood, donated in advance of surgery, should be utilized. This usually can be arranged through the Red Cross or the hospital's blood bank.

The perioperative plan

Planning for the postoperative period should begin in the preoperative phase, and the patient's needs for transportation and appropriate care following the surgery should be anticipated. Functional impairments should be expected. Pain, confusion, and decreased vision and mobility place the patient at risk for injury. Special consideration is necessary for cognitively impaired patients and their caregivers. Falls frequently occur postoperatively, especially when the patient is in the hospital or other unfamiliar environment. A social worker can identify community resources and arrange for supplemental services for an elderly person who has few social supports. Single elderly women who live alone are likely to need these kinds of services.

Designation of a surrogate decision maker

Before surgery, each patient should designate a surrogate who would make health care decisions if the patient becomes unable to make decisions. Documents attesting to that designation and to the patient's advance directives should be included in the preoperative packet.

Communication and documentation

Sufficient sharing of information enables a team of caregivers to deliver well-coordinated perioperative care. The preoperative note, summarizing the key elements of the assessment, is collated with all the relevant documentation, including laboratory data, advance directives, and caregiver information, into a complete preoperative packet for use by the surgical and anesthetic team.

REFERENCES

1. Boghosian SG, Mooradian AD: Usefulness of routine preoperative chest roentgenograms in the elderly patient, *J Am Geriatr Soc* 35:142, 1987.
2. Detsky AS et al: Predicting cardiac complications in patients undergoing non-cardiac surgery, *J Gen Intern Med* 1:211, 1986.
3. Gerson M et al: Cardiac prognosis in noncardiac geriatric surgery, *Ann Intern Med* 103:832, 1985.
4. O'Keefe JH, Shub C, Rettke SR: Risk of noncardiac surgical procedures in patients with aortic stenosis, *Mayo Clin Proc* 64:300, 1989.
5. Petersen VS, Solgaard S, Simonsen B: Total hip replacement in patients aged 80 years and older, *J Am Geriatr Soc* 37:219, 1989.
6. Schrader LL et al: Is routine preoperative hemodynamic evaluation of nonagenarians necessary?, *J Am Geriatr Soc* 39:1, 1991.

SUGGESTED READING

Keating JH, ed: *Clinics in geriatric medicine: perioperative care of the older patient*, W.B. Saunders, Philadelphia, PA, August, 1990.

CHAPTER 15

Evaluation for driving

SUSAN M. LILLIE

KEY POINTS
- Age alone does not predict skill in driving.
- Older drivers compensate for age-related changes by altering their driving patterns.
- An objective evaluation is needed for determining older drivers' needs for independence versus the potential danger of their continued driving.
- Education and rehabilitation can improve many drivers' skills.
- Care documentation offers the best legal protection.
- Functional performance in driving takes precedence over medical diagnoses alone.

A PROFILE OF OLDER DRIVERS

While accurate statistics are not available on the numbers of drivers aged 55 and older, drivers aged 65 and older constituted 12.5% of the driving population in 1989.[7] Malfetti and Winter[8] project that 1 of every 3 drivers will be over 55 years old by the year 2000. Those persons over the age of 65 who are eligible to drive will increase to 50 million in the year 2020, and of that group over half will be 75 or older.[7] Growing concern over the safety risk of older drivers, however, is often exaggerated. Identifying the skills that result in a good or bad driver is an arduous task and current research is inconclusive. Even simple data gathering is complicated by enormous discrepancies in licensing procedures among the 50 states and the lack of a centralized data base on older drivers.

Driving patterns and performance

As a group, older drivers compensate for age-related changes by minimizing driving on freeways, during rush hour, in inclement weather, and at night. They drive less frequently and fewer miles. Older drivers prefer familiar routes and vehicles; familiar tasks enable drivers to fully attend to the demands of driving. Modifications

131

COMMON DRIVING ERRORS IN OLDER DRIVERS

Difficulty backing up and making turns
Not seeing traffic signs or other cars quickly enough
Difficulty in locating and retrieving information from dashboard displays and traffic
   signs
Delayed glare recovery when driving at night
Not checking rearview mirrors and blind spots
Bumping into curbs and objects
Not yielding to oncoming traffic or right-of-way vehicles
Irregular or slow vehicle speeds
Difficulty with situations requiring quick decision making

---

in driving behavior partially compensate for decreased skills. However, compensation techniques for driving only manage the activity of driving and enhance safety rather than "remediate" the drivers' declining functional skills.

The largest segment of new or novice drivers is older women. An increase of 120% in the numbers of women drivers is expected within 5 years.[1] Because many older women presumably depend on their spouses for transportation, the infirmity or death of their partners forces these women to depend more on others for their transportation needs or learn how to drive at a later age. Women also drive less and stop driving, altogether, much sooner than do older men, which frequently curtails their independence prematurely.[6] Hence every effort should be made to encourage a qualified older patient to continue driving.

Moving violations sharply increase for older drivers. The accompanying box summarizes common driving errors of older drivers. Some of these errors can be attributed to the fact that most experienced older drivers never had the benefits of formalized driver education and training.

Accidents among older drivers generally occur as low-speed, two-car, intersection collisions during daylight hours in fair weather. While older drivers are more likely to have serious injuries or fatalities from accidents than younger drivers, automobile fatalities constitute only one half of 1% of deaths for persons over the age of 60.[4]

THE EVALUATION PROCESS

Primary care physicians will often be the first professionals to identify deficits in skills that are essential for driving. Physicians have four purposes for evaluating the driving skills of their patients: (1) to establish a baseline of data to determine future changes in performance, (2) to monitor medications or medical conditions that could affect safe driving, (3) to recommend rehabilitative interventions necessary to maintain or prolong independence in driving, and (4) to identify those patients whose driving clearly poses a threat to the safety of themselves or others. Physicians are entrusted with the very difficult task of balancing the independence of older people with the public safety. Physicians can help their older patients to recognize changes in their driving skills through therapeutic use of their established relationships and trust.

Table 15-1 Resources for older drivers

Resource	Service
The Handicapped Driver's Mobility Guide American Automobile Association Traffic Safety Department 1000 AAA Drive Heathrow, FL 32746 Approximately $3.00	State by state listing of driver evaluation programs, including those with an occupational therapist, driver instructors, vehicle modification vendors, and basic guidelines for vehicle modification
A Flexibility Fitness Training Package for Improving *Older Driver Performance* (pamphlet) American Automobile Association Foundation for Traffic Safety 1730 M Street, N.W., Suite 401 Washington, DC 20036	Provides written directions and diagrams for flexibility exercises for the neck, shoulder, trunk, and back specific to driving
Reporting Alzheimer's Disease and Related Disorders *Guidelines for Physicians* State of California Health and Welfare Agency Department of Health Services PO Box 942732 Sacramento, CA 94234	Provides reporting guidelines and legal information for patients with dementia; while specific to California law, it is generally useful for determining interventions
Perceptual Motor Evaluation for Head Injured and *Other Neurological Impaired Adults* Santa Clara Valley Medical Center Occupational Therapy Department 751 South Bascom Avenue San Jose, CA 95128 Approximately $15.00	Provides directions for administering gross visual screenings and other perceptual motor tests and includes an established scoring system
Drivers 55 Plus: Test Your Own Performance (booklet) *55 Alive/Mature Driving 1991* (pamphlet) Publication No. PF3798(791).D934 American Association for Retired Persons 601 E Street, N.W. Washington, DC 20049	Provides self-test booklet for older drivers, materials on the 55 Alive/Mature Driving Program for both participants and prospective instructors, and other miscellaneous materials
U.S. Department of Transportation National Highway Traffic Safety Administration 400 Seventh Street, N.W. Washington, DC 20590	Provides consumer information in brochures or newsletters about traffic safety for older drivers; gathers data; conducts research; institutes plans for national highway traffic safety of older drivers
Older Driver Resource Directory Circular #385 National Research Council 2101 Constitution Ave., N.W. Washington, DC 20418	Provides domestic and international listing of persons and agencies involved with older drivers.

Motor vehicles department

The motor vehicles department (MVD) in each state is the sole legal licensing authority for driving privileges. An evaluation of older people's driving skills by physicians or driving evaluation programs results in data upon which subsequent recommendations are made. Recommendations by physicians or driving programs are encouraged by more MVDs because they provide additional information that the MVDs are unable to obtain. It is rare when a state has the time, evaluation tools, and medically trained evaluators to fully assess drivers who have physical or cognitive deficits. Frequently, the only clinical evaluation that an MVD can offer are an interview, a visual acuity test, and occasionally a visual fields or depth perception test. Functional performance testing by an on-the-road test is generally of such a short duration that it does not adequately place drivers in situations requiring rapid judgments or problem solving.

Physicians should cultivate a contact within their local MVD office. Physicians should ask for the names of staff who conduct tests of people who have medical conditions. Physicians also should ask what information the MVDs find helpful when they evaluate drivers and if they have any graduated licensing that would benefit the patients. This relationship will prove useful to physicians and MVDs for developing driver evaluation materials, assisting patients with paperwork, and understanding how the licensing, reporting law, or reevaluation procedures affect the patients.

Examination schedule and evaluation components

A set of assessments can be developed to screen patients in the office for evaluation of their driving skills. Educating older patients about the need for periodic examinations as a part of their overall medical treatment plans can reduce stress during the assessments. The Canadian Medical Association[3] in 1991 recommended that evaluations be performed every 3 years from ages 45 to 70, every 2 years from ages 70 to 80, and annually for those drivers aged 81 years or older.

A clinical evaluation should always include vision assessment, medication review, physical examination, cognitive and psychosocial status assessments, and driving history. Odenheimer[9] provides useful guidelines in the evaluation of the older patient, while Reuben, Sullivan, and Trainer[10] examine specific age-related diseases of driving and the ethics of legal requirements and interventions with older drivers. Both studies are valuable resources in the evaluation of an older patient's driving skills.

EVALUATION TOOLS AND PROCEDURES

Vision

It is well established that driving requires good vision. Patients often do not recognize visual impairments because of their gradual onset, which can cause serious repercussions while these patients drive. All states except for Alabama and Kansas require initial vision tests before drivers secure their licenses, but subsequent vision tests are required only every 4 years in 66% of states and much longer in others, particularly those with renewal-by-mail systems.[9,10] In California's renewal-by-mail system, for example, good drivers can go as long as 12 years without vision examinations. The primary care physicians can incorporate simple vision tests into their patients' visits. If their vision appears impaired, the patients can be referred to the appropriate specialist for diagnosis and treatment long before their vision tests are due at the MVDs.

Visual acuity and visual field requirements vary from state to state. Most states require a minimum of 20/40 corrected vision; this does not mean that one cannot drive if these requirements are exceeded, but more thorough examinations through the MVD and possibly vision specialists are required. Visual field requirements are less generalizable because there is tremendous variance among the states. The Canadian Medical Association[3] recommends that patients who are diagnosed with homonymous or bitemporal hemianopia should not be allowed to drive under any circumstances.

Visual testing should include visual acuity and visual fields. (See Chapter 55.) While a link between acuity and driving performance has not been found, visual acuity is the hallmark vision test for driving both in the United States and abroad and thus should be included. Testing of acuity can be accomplished through a Snellen eye chart; other vision testing equipment is more accurate (and expensive), but the Snellen test is used solely as a screening for gross visual impairments and the standard eye chart suffices.

The occupational therapy department at Santa Clara Valley Medical Center in San Jose, California, publishes an inexpensive manual for perceptual motor evaluations (Table 15-1) that includes tests for gross visual skills, ocular pursuits, visual fields, and visuospatial neglect. The tests can be quickly administered (about 5 minutes for all those mentioned). Designed for neurologically impaired patients, the tests are easily applied to the older population for the specific purpose of gross visual screening.

Medications

Research is scarce concerning the use of medications and driving. Despite the lack of research, common sense and personal experience tells most people that medications affect driving skills and must be evaluated.

Careful review of medications, their side effects, and how they interact is essential. Laux and Brelsford[6] found that the more medications patients took, the higher the rate of near misses because patients did not observe other cars and perceive traffic signals quickly, which required emergency braking to stop in time. The rate of near misses increased for those drivers taking medications with known central nervous system (CNS) effects.

Physicians have two primary responsibilities regarding medications and older drivers: They must manage their patients' medications and warn them of potential side effects. A history of alcohol use should also be considered, and patients should be warned against combining alcohol and drugs. Documentation of conversations would be prudent.

Physical assessment. Most physicians do not have adequate time to examine all tasks that are necessary for driving, including a patient's ability to enter and exit the vehicle, fasten and unfasten the seat belt, reach the dashboard controls, turn the steering wheel, use the transmission gearshift, and lift the foot on and off the gas and brake pedals. With this in the mind, the physician should administer the following tests on all of the patient's extremities: range of motion, muscle strength, sensation, coordination, and balance. If significant impairments in strength or other functions are found, referral to an occupational or physical therapist is advisable for the patient's rehabilitation, as well as to determine adaptations and modifications. Table 15-2 lists common physical limitations of elderly drivers.

Cognition and perception. Judgment, information processing speed, decision making, and visuospatial function are critical skills for safe driving. The impact that cognition and perception have on patients' driving skills is much greater than that of their physical conditions. Evaluation of the patients in these areas is complex. Minimal score criteria for safe driving is still being evaluated. However, the literature does list four tests that assist physicians. These include the mini-mental state examination (MMSE), activities of daily living (ADL), instrumental activities of daily living (IADL), and symbol digit test.

Studies indicate that scores on MMSE for drivers were higher than non-drivers.[9] The same study also showed that (1) driving skills and the ability to perform ADL and IADL are linked, possibly because they both require high-level cognitive functioning for success, and (2) the need for assistance with ADL is not equated with an inability to drive.

The symbol digit test from the Wechsler adult intelligence scales was the most revealing test for age-related information processing speed.[6] The symbol digit test serves as an indicator of the speed at which information is perceived, processed, and a reaction generated, which are requisite skills for safe driving. The test is quickly administered and involves the verbal and written transcription of symbols into digits; age-specific scores and standard deviations provide quantitative scores and norms.

Driving history

Driving history and knowledge of rules of the road are basic parts of a driving evaluation. One should never assume that a driver is experienced. A questionnaire can be used to assess the age at which older adults began driving, whether there are any restrictions on their licenses, and the types of training they obtained for driving.

Table 15-2 Common physical limitations of elderly drivers*

Problem	Impact on driving	Options
Limited neck range of motion (ROM)	Decreased ability to turn head for visual checks; impairments in seeing cars, traffic signs, and pedestrians	OTR/RPT† to increase ROM and strength; driving program or vendor for special mirrors
Limited shoulder ROM	Difficulty or inability to fasten seat belt; difficulty turning the steering wheel	OTR/RPT to increase ROM and strength; OTR to modify seat belt for independent use
Arthritic changes in hand	Difficulty opening car door and grasping/turning keys	OTR key holder, door opener devices; driving program or vendor for steering device, built-up steering wheel, modified dashboard knobs
Impaired or nonfunctional upper limb	Unsafe steering with one hand, especially in turns or emergencies; unsafe operation of transmission shift lever or turn signals	Driving program or vendor for steering device, cross-over transmission, or turn signal lever
Lower back syndrome or orthopedic changes	Impaired visual checks; limited driving; decreased concentration	OTR/RPT to increase strength, flexibility, and positioning; driving program or vendor for lumbar supports, rear view mirror
Lower extremity impairment	Difficulty lifting legs in and out of car; difficulty lifting foot up from low accelerator pedal to high brake pedal	OTR/RPT to increase ROM and strength, modify transfer technique; driving program or vendor for foot pedal extensions, left foot accelerator
Cognitive	Slow information processing and delayed or impaired judgments; impaired recognition of unsafe driving practices	OTR for cognitive evaluation and training; driving program or motor vehicles department to road test for a minimum of 30 min

*The vehicle of choice for all older drivers is a two-door car with automatic transmission, power steering, and power brakes.
†OTR, occupational therapist, registered; RPT, registered physical therapist.

Information about driving errors such as the number and circumstances of traffic violations or vehicular accidents that have occurred within the last 3 years is also needed. However, patients may be reluctant to write this information down, especially if they feel that their licenses are in jeopardy.

Dementia

Debate continues on whether or not patients who are diagnosed with senile dementia of the Alzheimer type (SDAT) should drive. Studies of actual on-the-road performance are exceedingly rare. The University of Washington Medical Center is currently conducting a study that road tests drivers who have questionable dementia and those who have mild dementia.[5] A third category of drivers who do not have dementia is used as the control group. Preliminary evaluation of 40 subjects revealed that 56% of those drivers who were diagnosed with mild dementia did not pass, yet all the remaining drivers, those who do not have dementia and those who have questionable dementia, passed the 60-minute driving test. While this study suggests that the degree of the dementia and the functional performance is more significant than the diagnosis alone, additional research is needed.

The Canadian Medical Association[3] also believes that the patient's functional ability to drive is more significant than the diagnosis alone. Nevertheless, close monitoring is required for those who have diagnoses of dementia because changes can be rapid. Family members may provide first reports of aberrant behavior that may affect a patient's driving ability.

INTERPRETATION AND RECOMMENDATIONS

Physicians must determine actions to be taken based on the patients' test scores and physical, medical, and functional statuses. Interventions should be timely, meaningful to the patients, and within their financial means if at all possible. Recommendations must clearly state the physicians' judgments about their patients' abilities to drive. Examples of these are as follows:

1. No deficits noted; the patient appears to have the capacity to drive
2. Mild physical and/or cognitive deficits noted; patient appears to have capacity for continued driving upon completion of the recommended actions (new corrective lenses, range of motion or exercise program, etc.)
3. Moderate to severe physical and/or cognitive deficits noted; patient advised to stop driving until the recommended actions are accomplished (adaptive driving equipment installed, road test by MVD to assess driving performance, referral to therapist, etc.)

The recommendation for a patient to stop driving may be temporary, as in the case of a mild to moderate stroke, or permanent, as in the case of severe dementia. Physicians who discover cognitive deficits in their patients should request, when state law permits, that the MVDs test the patients for a minimum of 20 to 30 minutes on the road in traffic conditions that are similar to those in which the patients drive.

EDUCATION AND REHABILITATION

Interventions for older drivers often involve education and rehabilitation.

Education is an important tool for the older driver to become aware of and compensate for age-related changes. Because some driving errors can be attributed to outdated or "rusty" knowledge of rules of the road or to age-related changes, a review course can aid many drivers in minimizing their risks of driving. The most immediate education that physicians can provide to their patients is information about their strengths and weaknesses in driving skills, which is obtained through the evaluation process. Immediate discussion of the potential problems and required coping mechanisms is valuable to older drivers. Frequently, a more formalized education process is desirable.[1]

Attempts should be made to restore function, as well as provide adaptive devices or techniques, to older persons who appear capable of driving safely. Referral to an occupational and/or physical therapists is essential.

Cognitive and perceptual rehabilitation should not be overlooked. Some cognitive impairments may be treated through occupational therapy. Speech therapists and psychologists also provide cognitive training.

Driver evaluation programs

Patients who have moderate to severe physical or cognitive impairments, multiple medical conditions, neuromuscular or neurological impairments, and progressive diseases may require a referral to a formal driver evaluation program. Patients who have mild impairments require referrals only if there is specific cause to question their driving safety. Most third-party payors do not cover driving evaluations. However, there will be times when the question of safety overrides any concern over ability to pay. On occasion, a free or low-cost driver evaluation program can be located, which is usually supported by private funding and grants. Another low-cost alternative is vendors who install adaptive driving equipment. Vendors lack medical training but are able to provide vehicle modifications for patients who have mild to moderate impairments. Vendors only charge for parts and labor, making this choice financially attractive. *The Handicapped Driver's Mobility Guide* provides listings for evaluation programs, drivers' training, and vendors for all 50 states (Table 15-1).

Legal considerations

Testing procedures for older drivers should be consistent for legal purposes. If physicians perform frequent evaluations of driving skills for older patients, development of an evaluation form is advantageous. The best legal protection is documentation. No legal precedent for damages against a physician who allows an older person to drive has yet been established. There have been judgments against physicians when injuries and accidents have occurred because the drivers were taking medications or emotionally distraught and did not receive adequate warning against driving, and because a physician failed to follow reporting law procedures exactly as recommended.[2] Reporting laws will vary from state to state—only six states have mandatory reporting laws. Familiarity with state laws is imperative, and when a physician does report a patient to the MVD, it should be based on the potential danger rather than the "actual" danger that a patient poses to themselves and the public, since actual danger cannot be determined or projected by clinical testing.[10]

Recommendations should be made to patients in writing. These recommendations should document all communications regarding medications, an action plan, what written materials were provided and to whom, and whether or not the patient agrees to follow the physician's instructions. A form that lists frequently prescribed actions is advisable. A copy can be given to the patient and the original can be placed in the patient's medical record.

REFERENCES

1. American Association of Retired Persons: *55 alive/mature driving 1991, Pub* No PF3798(791).D934, Washington, DC, 1991, The Association.
2. Antrim JM, Engum ES: The driving dilemma and the law: patients' striving for independence vs public safety, *Cognit Rehabil* 7(2):16, 1989.
3. Canadian Medical Association Council on Health Care's Subcommittee on Emergency Medical Services: *Physician's guide to driver examination,* ed 5, 1991, The Association.
4. Cerrilli E: *Older drivers: the age factor in traffic safety,* Pub No DOT HS 807 402, Washington, DC, 1989, US Department of Transportation, National Highway Traffic Safety Administration.
5. Hunt L: *Dementia and road test performance: summary of proceedings of the conference on driver competency assessment,* Sacramento, Calif, 1990, State of California Department of Motor Vehicles, Program and Policy Administration, Research and Development Section.
6. Laux LF, Brelsford J: *Age-related changes in sensory, cognitive, psychomotor and physical functioning and driving performance in drivers aged 40 to 92,* Houston, 1990, Rice University, The Human Factors Laboratory, Department of Psychology and American Automobile Association Foundation for Traffic Safety.
7. Malfetti JL: *Older driver graduated licensing: summary of proceedings of the conference on driver competency assessment,* Sacramento, Calif, 1990, State of California Department of Motor Vehicles, Program and Policy Administration, Research and Development Section.
8. Malfetti JL, Winter DJ: *Drivers 55 plus: test your own performance: a self-rating form of questions, factors and suggestions for safe driving,* Falls Church, Va, 1986, Safety Research and Education Project and American Automobile Association Foundation for Traffic Safety.
9. Odenheimer GL: Cognitive dysfunction and driving abilities. Presented at the Annual Meeting of the American Geriatrics Society, Atlanta, May 18, 1990.
10. Reuben D, Silliman RA, Trainer M: Aging drivers: medicine, policy, and ethics, *J Am Geriatr Soc* 36:1135, 1988.

SUGGESTED READING

Eberhardt JW: *National Highway Traffic Safety Administration prospective: summary of proceedings of the conference on driver competency assessment*, Sacramento, Calif, 1990, State of California Department of Motor Vehicles, Program and Policy Administration, Research and Development Section.

McPherson K, Ostrow A, Shaffron P: *Physical fitness and the aging driver*, 1989, West Virginia University, Department of Safety Studies and Department of Sport and Exercise Studies and American Automobile Association Foundation for Traffic Safety.

Reuben D, Silliman RA, Trainer M: Aging drivers: medicine, policy, and ethics, *J Am Geriatr Soc* 36:1135, 1988.

CHAPTER 16

Outpatient evaluation for nursing home admission

REBECCA ELON

KEY POINTS

- A physician's written approval is required for a patient to be admitted as a resident to a nursing home.
- The comprehensive assessment of a patient for possible admission to a nursing facility should include a thorough evaluation of the patient's functional and cognitive statuses in addition to the medical assessment.
- Utilization of community resources may delay or prevent nursing home admission.
- When evaluating an individual for possible nursing home admission, the caregiving network, which may be helping to sustain the patient within the community, should be assessed.
- While residing in the nursing facility, each resident must be under the care of a physician.
- A nursing home component of a primary care practice can be a rewarding and satisfying endeavor, but it is important for the physician to affiliate with carefully selected facilities.
- Serving effectively as an attending physician in a nursing home requires a relationship not only with the patient and the family but with the facility's staff as well.
- Knowledge of the current regulatory requirements for medical practice in the nursing home is necessary for attending physicians who care for patients in nursing homes.

COMMUNITY RESOURCES THAT HELP
LONG-TERM CARE PATIENTS TO REMAIN AT HOME

Meals on Wheels
Home health aides
In-home physical or occupational therapists
Domestic workers or chore aides
Adult day care centers
Psychiatric day hospitals
Friendly visitors
Respite care
Caregiver support networks
Case management services

When older people become physically or cognitively impaired to such a degree that their abilities to function independently are compromised, they typically need long-term care services to help them carry out activities of daily life that most healthy people perform without effort. Gerontologists have classified these endeavors of daily life into two categories: activities of daily living (ADL) and instrumental activities of daily living (IADL). (See Chapter 13.) Older persons who have difficulties in performing ADL and IADL tasks may benefit from long-term care services to help sustain them in the community. The long-term care services that are usually required to support community-dwelling, functionally impaired, older patients include personal care, social, and health care services. The majority of long-term care that is provided to older people comes from family members.[1] In addition to family support, many community-based services are available to help sustain older people while they live at home. (See the box above.)

If an elderly, functionally impaired patient's requirements for long-term care and supportive services exceed or exhaust the available resources of the family and the community, the patient may be brought to the physician's office for evaluation for possible nursing home admission.

LONG-TERM CARE SERVICES: THE PHYSICIAN'S ROLE

Physicians are the gatekeepers for many long-term care services. Their signatures are usually required to authorize in-home services, day care centers, and nursing home admissions. However, few physicians receive formal training regarding their roles within long-term care. Among physicians who serve as attending physicians within long-term care, the degree of involvement varies. The minimal level of involvement is fulfilled by physicians who merely review and sign the medical orders from a home health agency or nursing home. Historical examples exist of attending physicians at nursing homes who signed orders that were sent to their offices, mailed them back to the nursing homes throughout the years, and never entered the nursing homes or examined the patients. Whether the authorizing signature represents the culmination of a professional medical evaluation and recommendation or is merely a perfunctory administrative act depends upon the knowledge and commitment of the attending physician.

ASSESSMENT FOR NURSING HOME ADMISSION

The physician in the ambulatory practice of geriatric medicine is frequently confronted by family members who have decided that their elderly parents need to enter a nursing home and have selected a facility. The physician is asked to sign the paperwork authorizing the admission.

In a busy outpatient practice where a 10- to 15-minute appointment is scheduled for an office visit, the physician may be tempted, after hearing the family's rationale for the decision, to comply with the request and sign the paperwork.

If the patient is to receive an appropriate assessment for nursing home admission, the patient and family should be scheduled to return to the physician's office when adequate time can be devoted to performing a comprehensive geriatric assessment. The purpose of this assessment is to determine whether alternatives other than institutionalization exist, which would allow appropriate long-term care to be delivered to the patient. Typically, the physician uses the biopsychosocial model to define ways in which a patient's overall function could be enhanced. Components of this assessment should include the following:

1. A complete history and physical examination
2. A mental status examination
3. A functional assessment
4. A detailed social history that identifies unmet needs of the patient or caregivers, which can lead to nursing home placement
5. An assessment of the potential for rehabilitation or functional improvement
6. A values history to determine the preferences of the patient (e.g., does the patient wish to enter a nursing home)
7. A determination of the patient's capacity to make financial or health care decisions
8. A determination of whether advance directives or a designated surrogate decision maker (such as durable power of attorney for health care decisions) exist
9. A determination about legal guardianship should be made if the patient lacks the capacity to make health care decisions and a designated surrogate does

not exist (e.g., there are differing opinions among family members about what should be done for the patient, decisions are being made by the family that do not appear to be in the patient's best interest, the patient's wishes are strongly divergent from the family's decisions)

10. An evaluation of whether options other than nursing home admission exist for the patient

11. A determination of whether the facility under consideration has the appropriate level of care, staff who are skilled and knowledgeable about the patient's particular problem, and accessibility for family and significant others.

During the course of the assessment it is important for the physician to remain cognizant of the fact that it is generally the patient, and not the family, who is the "client." There is a strong tendency when a cognitively impaired older patient is brought to the physician's office by the family for the physician to speak to the family, referring to the patient in the third person as though the individual were absent when he or she is sitting in the same room. In order to avoid this situation which can be embarrassing and humiliating to people even in the presence of cognitive impairment, the physician should make conscious efforts to direct the conversation toward involving the patient. When this is not possible, efforts should be made to speak to the family in private without the patient being present.

Precipitants of nursing home admission

The older person who is at risk for nursing home admission may be brought to the physician's office by family members, case managers, friends, neighbors, or perhaps workers from adult protective services. Events that prompt such an office visit are frequently related to the patient's progressive decline in cognitive capabilities, which results in functional impairments. Sometimes precipitating events have placed the elderly patient in crisis, for example, a landlord who terminates a rental agreement because the patient no longer fulfills the obligations of tenancy. Concerns about the patient's safety may be paramount. Common circumstances that precipitate nursing home admission include the following:

1. Difficulty handling financial affairs (sometimes evidenced by having utilities discontinued when bills are unpaid).
2. History of fires at home from an unattended stove.
3. Reports of grossly inappropriate behavior.
4. Repeated inappropriate telephone calls to relatives in the middle of the night.
5. Weight loss as a result of forgetting to eat or inability to obtain food.
6. Inattention to personal hygiene.
7. Nocturnal wakefulness that disrupts the patterns of the rest of the household.
8. Wandering outdoors and becoming lost.
9. Incontinence of bowel.
10. Recurring falls.

Strategies to prolong community-dwelling capacity

The comprehensive geriatric assessment may uncover medical or psychological conditions that are potentially remediable. Additionally, deficits in the social support of an older functionally impaired individual may be identified that are amenable to support from long-term care services in the community. A social worker who is knowledgeable about community resources and decision making for long-term care can make important contributions to the comprehensive geriatric assessment. (See Chapter 8.) In addition, social workers often serve as case managers for frail elderly persons who do not have adequate family support and can no longer manage the burden of coordinating the long-term care services that are necessary to continue living in the community. Such social workers are often members of the interdisciplinary team in a geriatric medicine practice, or they may be available as consultants through a community's senior citizen centers and other agencies that provide services for elderly persons.

Additionally, an evaluation by an occupational therapist and/or a physical therapist may contribute important information about the patient's functional capacity and potential for rehabilitation. (See Chapter 4.) A course of occupational or physical therapy may bolster the patient's function to such an extent that the transfer of the patient to a nursing home can be delayed or averted.

CONSIDERATIONS IN CHOOSING A NURSING HOME

Since the family, in most circumstances, will be visiting the patient with greater frequency than will the physician, the geographic *location* of the nursing home should facilitate the family's participation in the life of the patient. If the patient has lived in a particular neighborhood for many years and has a strong network of social support there, a nursing home in that geographic location is highly desirable to maintain longtime friendships and the patient's participation in the life of the community.

The *quality* of the nursing home is an important consideration that may override the desirability of the geographic location. If the only nursing home located near the patient's family or neighborhood is one of poor quality, then perhaps the patient would be better served in a high-quality nursing home at another location.

PHYSICIANS' INVOLVEMENT FOLLOWING NURSING HOME ADMISSION

Continuity is valued by physicians and patients as an important component of high-quality medical care. Nursing home admission is an event that may disrupt a long-established doctor-patient relationship. While physicians may be deeply committed to the principle of providing continuity of care, they should consider several factors before making a commitment to be a nursing home attending physician.

The geographic proximity of the nursing home to the physician's own home or office may be a key factor in the physician's decision to serve as attending physician. Nursing homes that are distant to the physician's usual practice sites will be visited less often, despite the best intentions of the physician.

Serving as the attending physician for one or two patients in a community nursing home is often an unsatisfactory arrangement for the patient, physician, and staff of the nursing home. By serving only one or two patients, a physician is likely to visit the nursing home infrequently, making it difficult for the physician to gain adequate familiarity with the facility and staff or make visits on short notice. An office-based practitioner may find that such a small nursing home practice is not financially viable because of current reimbursement constraints.

If the physician serves as an attending physician in a particular facility, it is advisable to follow a sufficient number of patients to make a minimum of one regularly scheduled visit to the nursing home each week. This allows the physician to develop a working relationship with the nursing home staff, and places the physician in a better position to assess the quality of care that the patients are receiving. Regularly scheduled physician's visits and telephone contact times prevent excessive urgent telephone calls from nursing home staff to the physician. When nursing staff knows that the physician visits or calls the nursing home on a regular schedule, many questions and routine matters can be resolved during those times.

Office-based physicians who decide that it is not feasible to serve as the attending physicians for their patients who have been admitted to nursing homes still can contribute significantly to continuity of care for these patients. Simple measures such as telephoning the physician who will be caring for the patients in the nursing home is helpful and appreciated by the attending physician. Providing key elements of information about the patients' histories is an effective method to ensure smooth transitions in the patients' care. Maintaining contact with the patients and/or families during the period following admissions to nursing homes may ease feelings of loss and abandonment that some patients experience when their care is transferred to another physician.

If a physician decides to care for patients in a nursing home, it is helpful to call the medical director of the facility to determine the requirements for attending physicians. Federal regulations for nursing homes include specific standards of practice for the delivery of primary care in such facilities.[2] To meet the requirements of nursing home practice, a physician must be familiar with the relevant federal and state regulations.

If a physician who serves as an attending physician in a nursing home later discovers that it is not feasible to continue in that capacity, the matter should be discussed with the nursing home's medical director who may transfer the patients to a new attending physician. Most nursing homes maintain a group of physicians who are willing to accept additional patients within the facility. Prompt transfer of a patient to another physician is preferable to a situation in which the attending physician cannot meet the requirements of the role and delays transferring the patient.

Serving as primary care physician for a cohort of nursing home patients can be a deeply rewarding and satisfying endeavor. However, the physician must be affiliated only with carefully selected facilities. Particular attention must be paid to the organization and management of the nursing home practice to provide primary care services that are appropriate for long-term care settings and to ensure appropriate reimbursement for the work.

REFERENCES

1. Kane RA, Kane RL: *Long-term care: principles, programs and policies*, New York, 1987, Springer.
2. Conditions of participation, *The Federal Register*, p 48865, Sept 26, 1991.

SUGGESTED READINGS

How to Choose a Nursing Home, Health Care Financing Administration's Beneficiary Education Program, Washington, DC, 1991, Government Printing Office.
Lanspery S: Nursing homes. In Doress PB, Siegal DL, eds: *Our bodies growing older*, New York, 1987, Simon & Schuster.
Ouslander J, Osterweil D, Morley J: *Medical care in the nursing home*, New York, 1991, McGraw-Hill.

CHAPTER 17

Hearing assessment

GREGG WARSHAW
ANGELA WALTHER

<u>**KEY POINTS**</u>

- Hearing loss should be addressed for each elderly patient through history, physical examination, and screening.
- A practical screening method for hearing impairment is the pure tone otoscope with or without the hearing handicap inventory for the elderly.
- The audiogram identifies the extent and type of hearing loss while the evaluation for speech discrimination tests the patient's understanding of speech.
- Along with proper rehabilitation, a hearing aid can greatly improve a patient's sensorineural hearing loss.

Hearing impairments are extremely common among the aged. Approximately 8 million senior citizens have hearing impairments, the third leading chronic problem of the aged. Twenty-five percent of the population aged 65 years and older report hearing impairments, and 30% show hearing impairments through audiological testing.

Hearing impairments adversely affect quality of life for elderly persons.[1] Hearing impairment has been linked to decreased cognitive functioning in elderly persons. Through proper education, treatment, sensory aids, and rehabilitation, elderly patients who have sensory impairments can experience increased independence and quality of life.

AGE-RELATED CHANGES

Hearing depends upon the integration of three systems: (1) the peripheral sensorineural component (external, middle, and inner ear; eighth cranial nerve), (2) central auditory system (auditory brain stem and cortex), and (3) central nervous system. Several physiological changes in these systems are associated with aging.[3] These changes include atrophy of Corti in the basal turn (area responsible for high-frequency sound), loss of hair cells, and loss of cells in auditory centers of the cortex

149

_____ **CRITERIA FOR DIAGNOSING PRESBYCUSIS** _____

Onset after age 60
Hearing loss equal for bone and air conduction
Progressive
Bilateral high-frequency sensorineural hearing loss
No past or present ear disease
No use of ototoxic medications

From Mader S: Hearing impairment in elderly persons, *J Am Geriatr Soc* 32(7):548, 1986.

and brain stem. Perhaps more important are functional changes associated with aging. Decreased speech discrimination, distortion of signals, and increased interference from outside noise can decrease an individual's understanding of speech. Difficulty in localizing sound, slowing of cognitive processes, and changes in memory also occur with age. These changes can interact to decrease hearing and communication skills.

PRESBYCUSIS

Diagnostic criteria and history

Presbycusis is a slowly progressive sensorineural hearing loss that is most predominant at high frequencies. The criteria for diagnosing this condition are shown in the box above.

The first step in diagnosing presbycusis is obtaining a good history. Difficulties understanding speech in a noisy room, hearing someone whisper, and hearing the telephone or radio all suggest hearing impairments. Diagnosis of presbycusis can be facilitated by the hearing handicap inventory for the elderly person—screening version (HHIE–S). (See box on p. 151.) The HHIE–S has an overall accuracy of 75%. When the fail cutoff is 24, the HHIE–S sensitivity and specificity are 41% and 92%, respectively, with positive and negative predictive values of 67% and 78%, respectively. The HHIE–S can be combined with the pure tone audioscope (see discussion on screening audiometry below) and the overall accuracy increases to 83%.

The second step in diagnosing presbycusis is the physical examination. The otoscopic examination should routinely be done to remove occluding cerumen and check for otitis media. The most widely recommended test for the physical examination is the whispered voice test. The clinician whispers *three to six words* at a set distance (6 to 24 inches) behind the patient. Reported sensitivities and specificities range from 75% to 100%. Inability to repeat 50% of the words constitutes failure. The whispered voice test as a screening tool is limited by inconsistent word choice and decibel level. Other tests for the physical examination include the ticking watch, finger rub (index finger and thumb), and the Rinne and Weber tests.

HEARING HANDICAP INVENTORY
FOR THE ELDERLY–SCREENING VERSION (HHIE–S)*

	Yes (4)	Sometimes (2)	No (0)
1. Does a hearing problem cause you to feel embarrassed when meeting new people?	_____	_____	_____
2. Does a hearing problem cause you to feel frustrated when talking to members of your family?	_____	_____	_____
3. Do you have difficulty hearing when someone speaks in a whisper?	_____	_____	_____
4. Do you feel handicapped by a hearing problem?	_____	_____	_____
5. Does a hearing problem cause you difficulty when visiting friends, relatives, or neighbors?	_____	_____	_____
6. Does a hearing problem cause you to attend religious services less often than you would like?	_____	_____	_____
7. Does a hearing problem cause you to have arguments with family members?	_____	_____	_____
8. Does a hearing problem cause you difficulty when listening to TV or radio?	_____	_____	_____
9. Do you feel that any difficulty with your hearing limits or hampers your personal or social life?	_____	_____	_____
10. Does a hearing problem cause you difficulty when in a restaurant with relatives or friends?	_____	_____	_____

From Ventry IM, Weinstein BE: Identification of elderly people with hearing problems, *American Speech-Language-Hearing Association* 25:37, 1983.
*Range of total points, 0–40; 0–8, no self-perceived handicap; 10–22, mild to moderate handicap; 24–40, significant handicap.

Screening audiometry

Audiologists recommend audiograms when patients' hearing impairments are clinically suspected following their screening tests (i.e., hearing handicap inventory for the elderly–screening version [HHIE-S], whispered voice test, and pure tone otoscope). Studies of the pure tone otoscope have shown sensitivities of 87% to 96% (depending on failure criteria) and specificities of 70 to 90% in aged persons.[2] Screening of asymptomatic patients is not yet recommended by the U.S. Preventive Task Force Service due to lack of evidence for cost-effectiveness; however, recent studies support

Table 17-1 Hearing loss and related speech difficulty

Decibel loss	Grade	Speech difficulty
<25	Normal	No difficulty
26–40	Mild	Difficulty with faint speech
41–60	Moderate	Difficulty with normal speech
61–80	Severe	Difficulty with loud speech
>81	Profound	Cannot understand speech

testing ambulatory older patients in the office with a pure tone otoscope. The audioscope also can be used to detect pure tone deficits when significant history, physical examination, or assessment indicates a possible communication or hearing disorder for the patient.

Before the audioscope is used, ear pathology and occluding cerumen should be extracted. Forty decibels (dB) is tested in both ears at the following frequencies: 500 Hz, 1000 Hz, 2000 Hz, and 4000 Hz, which are usually preceded by a tone at 60 dB and 1000 Hz to be certain that the patient understands the directions and can hear at a greater decibel level. If the patient misses any frequency, the test should be repeated after directions are given again. Failure criteria are (1) failing to hear one frequency in each ear, or (2) failing to hear two frequencies in one ear.

Table 17-1 shows the grading for hearing loss at various frequencies and the predicted speech difficulty. Losses greater than 40 dB are considered clinically significant and are graded moderate to severe. Decibel level is averaged over 500, 1000, and 2000 Hz.

AUDIOLOGY: INTERPRETING AN AUDIOGRAM

An audiogram is a useful tool for evaluating hearing impairment. Pure tone audiograms answer the following three questions: (1) What kind of hearing loss is present (i.e., sensorineural, conductive, or mixed)?, (2) Is the loss unilateral or bilateral?, and (3) At what frequencies does the loss occur?

Sensorineural hearing loss is characterized by abnormal and equal decreases in air and bone conduction. Disorders of the inner ear, cochlea, and vestibular and auditory centers often show sensorineural hearing loss. Conductive hearing loss shows a reduction for air- but not bone-conducted tones. The audiogram for a conductive hearing loss will show an air-bone gap. Conductive hearing loss is characteristic of disorders that impede normal transmission of sound waves through the external canal and tympanic membrane or that interfere with the functioning of the ossicles. Mixed hearing loss shows a reduction of both air and bone conduction, but *loss of air conduction is greater.* A typical audiogram is shown in Fig. 17-1. The hearing loss ranges from 40 to 80 dB, corresponding to a frequency range of 250 to 8000 Hz. Normal decibel level is 0 to 20. The frequencies are essentially equal for both air and bone conduction, indicating sensorineural hearing loss. It is also a bilateral loss, greatest in the high frequencies. The pure tone audiogram in Fig. 17-1 is consistent with presbycusis.

Speech audiometry is also done by the audiologist (Fig. 17-1). First, the average of pure tones (PTA) from 500 to 2000 Hz is calculated for both right and left ears. This is then compared to the speech reception threshold (SRT), the lowest decibel level that the patient can respond to correctly for 50% of the speech stimuli presented. The PTA and SRT should be within 5 to 10 dB. Speech discrimination, which is the percentage of words that the patient can repeat correctly when those words are presented at a sufficiently loud level, is listed for each ear. Speech discrimination is generally recorded at a sensation level (SL) of 40 dB above the PTA and is a good functional indicator of a patient's communication ability. The relationship between a sensorineural hearing loss that shows on the audiogram and speech discrimination is variable. An elderly person may have only a small sensorineural hearing loss but

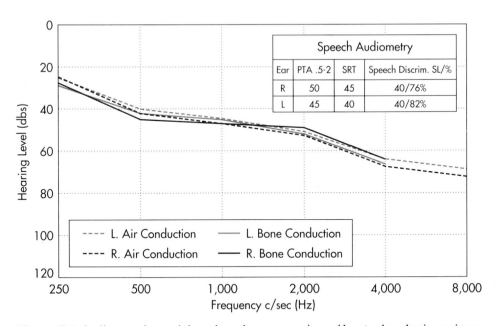

Speech Audiometry			
Ear	PTA .5-2	SRT	Speech Discrim. SL/%
R	50	45	40/76%
L	45	40	40/82%

Figure 17-1 Audiogram shows a bilateral, moderate, sensorineural hearing loss that is consistent with presbycusis. Speech discrimination is consistent with presbycusis. (*See text for explanation.*) *L*, left; *R*, right; *PTA*, pure tones average; *SRT*, speech reception threshold; *SL*, sensation level (decibels above PTA).

a low speech discrimination, which results either from the type of presbycusis or other aging processes in the brain stem, auditory centers, or central nervous system. It also could be due to a retrocochlear lesion or a pathological condition involving the brain stem or cortex. With cochlear lesions, a good correlation usually exists between sensorineural hearing loss that shows on the audiogram (i.e., sensory presbycusis) and speech discrimination. Also, speech discrimination may worsen as one travels more medially through the auditory system. Testing for speech discrimination is important in presbycusis since values less than 50% suggest poor results with a hearing aid.

OTHER CAUSES OF HEARING LOSS

Table 17-2 lists other causes of hearing impairments in elderly persons. The most common and easily remedied is cerumen impaction, which can cause a 40 dB conductive hearing loss. Other causes of conductive hearing loss are otosclerosis and tympanosclerosis. Tympanosclerosis consists of sclerotic changes in the tympanic membrane and middle ear mucosa caused by past middle ear infections. On otoscopic examination, chalky white plaque in the tympanic membrane may be seen. If plaque extends to the ossicular chain, conductive hearing loss may occur later in life; this can be corrected through surgery. Otosclerosis consists of a focus of new bone growth on the medial wall of the middle ear. A stapedectomy may be required if fixation of the footplate of the stapes occurs. If otosclerosis occurs in a patient with presbycusis, mixed hearing loss will be found.

Paget's disease of the bone causes hearing loss in 30% to 50% of patients who have skull involvement. It is usually bilateral and most commonly causes conductive hearing loss. However, sensorineural hearing loss can be caused by changes around the foramina of the acoustic nerve. Conductive hearing loss may result from stenosis of the external auditory meatus or ossification of the stapedial tendon. Hearing loss is one of the indications for medical treatment of Paget's disease.

Table 17-2   Other causes of hearing loss in elderly persons

Conductive	Sensorineural
Cerumen	Ototoxic medications
Otosclerosis	Noise trauma
Paget's disease	Vascular disease
Tympanosclerosis	Paget's disease
	Ménière's disease
	Tumors

Other possible causes of sensorineural hearing loss in elderly persons include ototoxic medications, noise trauma, vascular causes, and Ménière's disease. The accompanying box lists ototoxic medications. Diuretics and antibiotics, especially aminoglycosides, can cause sensorineural hearing loss. The hearing loss that is associated with diuretics usually occurs in patients who have coexisting renal failure. Aspirin causes tinnitus that can be associated with hearing loss; this is reversible once the aspirin is discontinued. Noise-induced hearing loss is generally a high-frequency sensorineural loss like presbycusis. However, noise-induced loss is characterized on the audiogram by a positive deflection (hearing gain) at frequencies of 6000 to 8000 Hz. Ménière's disease causes a sensorineural hearing loss that is usually greater in the low frequencies, which are associated with severe vertigo, and patients usually develop symptoms before they are 65 years old. Vascular disease can cause a sensorineural loss that occurs suddenly.

Losses of sensorineural hearing and speech discrimination that do not fit the criteria for presbycusis, noise trauma, or ototoxic medications can be further evaluated by acoustic immittance and auditory brain stem response to determine if lesions are cochlear, retrocochlear, or central. As mentioned previously, cochlear lesions usually show some correlation between the degree of sensorineural hearing loss and speech discrimination. The battery for acoustic immittance includes tympanometry and acoustic reflex testing. Tympanometry evaluates the flow of acoustic energy through the middle ear with variation of the air pressure. High-impedance abnormalities such as otitis media can be differentiated from low-impedance abnormalities such as interruption of ossicles. Testing the patient's acoustic reflex also measures the stapedius

---

OTOTOXIC MEDICATIONS

Antibiotics
- Aminoglycosides
- Erythromycin
- Vancomycin

Antimalarials

Antineoplastics
- Cisplatin
- Nitrogen mustard

Antiinflammatory agents
- Aspirin (reversible)

Diuretics
- Furosemide
- Ethycrynic acid

muscle reflex. In some cases, middle ear pathology that is not detected by an audiogram can be identified by an immittance battery. Reflex testing of the stapedius muscle also helps differentiate retrocochlear lesions from cochlear lesions. Examples of retrocochlear lesions are acoustic neurinoma, hemorrhage, and meningioma. Acoustic neurinoma causes a unilateral sensorineural hearing loss. Central lesions are rare causes of deafness, but this can occur if auditory areas in both hemispheres are compromised by a vascular lesion.

REFERRAL INDICATIONS

A patient who has a history that is consistent with presbycusis, complains or has difficulty hearing, or fails a pure tone otoscope examination should be referred to an audiologist. When a patient complains of sudden or unilateral hearing loss, has an audiogram that is consistent with presbycusis, or has a significant difference in hearing loss and speech discrimination, a prompt referral to an otolaryngologist is recommended.

HEARING AIDS

The five types of hearing aids are (1) behind-the-ear (BTE), which houses the components in a case behind the ear and sound travels to an ear mold in the ear canal; (2) in-the-ear (ITE), which fits entirely into the external ear; (3) in-the-canal (ITC), which is housed entirely in the canal; (4) body-worn, which is physically the largest; and (5) eyeglass, which is not usually recommended because it combines two sensory aids. The first three types are most popular with patients. With technological improvements, the ITC hearing aid is gaining popularity. In the older population, lack of dexterity can limit use of ITC and ITE hearing aids. For some, the BTE hearing aid also can be difficult to adjust. Hearing aids work best at a 50 to 80 dB hearing loss; however, if the hearing loss is greater than 80 dB, improvement is generally small.

The success of a hearing aid depends on the patient's education and aural rehabilitation. First, the patient must realize that it takes a period of time to adapt to the hearing aid. Second, good communication must exist between patient and audiologist, and the patient must be motivated to use the hearing aid. Third, the patient must be aware that the hearing aid is to be used in conjunction with speech reading and, at times, other assistive listening devices. Fourth, hearing aid training and communication with others who use hearing aids enable the patient to become comfortable with the device.

Audiology evaluations and hearing aids are not paid for by Medicare. Medicaid, in many states, will pay for hearing aids. Cost, which varies from $500 to $1000 for the evaluation and hearing aid presents a problem for many older patients. Before hearing aids are purchased, they can generally be used on a trial basis for 30 days. Many patients try a hearing aid for 30 days in one ear and 30 days in the other to determine which gives the best results. For patients who have difficulty with internal distortion and localization, binaural hearing aids (hearing aids for each ear) are often recommended since they increase the signal-to-noise ratio. These binaural aids should also be tried on a 30-day basis. If a patient cannot afford a hearing aid or does not want one, certain assistive listening devices can be used to increase day-to-day functioning.

Even with a hearing aid, many hearing-impaired individuals require assistive listening devices in certain surroundings.[5] Because of increased external noise in public places, assistive listening devices are being used in concert halls and theaters. A microphone is placed near the speaker or stage, and the sound is amplified to the listener through one of several transmission modes, including audio loops, infrared devices, or FM radio. This increases the signal-to-noise ratio that is delivered to the listener.

In addition, there are several inexpensive amplifiers for use on the television or telephone for the hearing impaired. Many public telephones are equipped with an amplifier. Closed-captioned entertainment is growing in popularity. Other assistive listening devices include vibrating alarm clocks, accessory headsets for television or radio, and telephone and doorbell signaling devices. An audiologist can provide more information about the various devices that are available (Table 17-3).

The box on p. 158 lists suggestions for improving communication with hearing impaired patients. Additionally, an amplifier can be used by the physician during office visits.

Table 17-3 Listening aids and approximate prices

Listening aid	Cost* ($)
Portable telephone amplifier that fits on any receiver	15–25
Amplifier that fits in pocket with earphone and microphone	100–140
Telecommunication devices for the deaf, includes typing messages and intermediate relay system	400
Telephone adapters for use on telephone	15–25
Light and strobe telephone signal systems	20–30
Amplifiers for general use	20–30
Hard-wire amplification systems for interview purposes	25–70

*Cost may vary depending on model, company, location sold, etc.

IMPROVING COMMUNICATION SKILLS
FOR HEARING-IMPAIRED ELDERLY PERSONS

Be certain to have the person's attention
Speak face to face
Repeat by paraphrasing
Speak at normal level or slightly louder
Speak a little more slowly
Stand within 2 to 3 feet
Reduce background noise
Pause at end of sentences
Avoid appearing frustrated
Write down key words if person can read
Have person repeat to be certain message was understood

REFERENCES

1. Kane R, Ouslander J, Abrass I: *Essentials of clinical geriatrics*, ed 2, New York, 1989, McGraw-Hill.
2. Mulrow C, Lichtenstein M: Screening for hearing impairment in the elderly, *J Gen Intern Med* 6(May-June):249, 1991.
3. Rees T, Duckert L: Auditory and vestibular dysfunction in aging. In Hazzard W, Andres R, eds: *Principles of geriatric medicine and gerontology*, New York, 1990, McGraw-Hill.
4. Ventry IM, Weinstein BE: Identification of elderly people with hearing problems, *American Speech-Language-Hearing Assoc* 25:37, 1983.
5. Weinstein B: Geriatric hearing loss: myths, realities, resources for physicians, *Geriatrics* 44(4):42, 1989.

SUGGESTED READINGS

Kane R, Ouslander J, Abrass I: *Essentials of clinical geriatrics*, ed 2, New York, 1989, McGraw-Hill.
Mader S: Hearing impairment in elderly persons, *J Am Geriatr Soc* 32(7):548, 1986.
Rees T, Duckert L: Auditory and vestibular dysfunction in aging. In Hazzard W, Andres R, eds: *Principles of geriatric medicine and gerontology*, New York, 1990, McGraw-Hill.

CHAPTER 18

Safety in the home

PETER A. BOLING

KEY POINTS
- Home safety assessment may prevent many catastrophic events for the older patient.
- Office-based home safety assessment may miss key findings.
- Assessment can be performed by a non-physician health care provider.
- Assess the home in relation to the patient's unique needs.
- Review the patient's daily routines to assess home safety.
- Avoid cultural bias and consider the patient's alternatives.
- Learn about and use community resources to correct problems.

The busy clinician making a house call often encounters a spectrum of issues that variably affects the patient's health. However, a wise clinician seeking to prevent catastrophic events will find the time to perform home safety assessment when the clinical issues have less urgency. Overall, accidents are the fifth most common cause of deaths among elderly persons; the high prevalence of accidental death makes this an important area for the geriatric clinician.[6] Burns result in 41 annual hospitalizations per 100,000 adults aged 85 years and older, a rate that is 50% higher than the rate in the general population.[3] Residential fires killed 1278 senior citizens in 1984[4], nearly one tenth as many as the 13,500 who died from renal failure.[2] Falls cause two thirds of accidental deaths, with an annual death rate of 57 per 100,000 persons aged 75 years and older.[5] This compares with a death rate of 183 per 100,000 resulting from pneumonia and influenza.[2] Ramsdell et al[11] found that after a thorough clinical evaluation of 154 patients, in-home assessment exposed 55 new problems related to safety (22% of 255 new problems).[11] Twenty of these problems involving wandering (9), driving (9), and household risks (2), appeared to be a threat for immediate death or serious morbidity.

Beyond preventing catastrophes, home safety assessment by an alert clinician or other health care provider may generate adaptive strategies that will enhance quality of life for the older patient. For example, a wheelchair ramp can foster independence; a long-armed grabber can improve daily functioning; and a telephone with oversized numbers may facilitate communication. Such in-home assessment and management yield immediate benefits and often engender positive relationships between physician, patient, and caregiver.

The following discussions focus on specific recommendations for home safety assessment and management. Somewhat arbitrary distinctions are made between physical or structural hazards and "medical" hazards. The special concerns of households with cognitively impaired elderly persons are also considered separately.

The importance of a clinician's entering the home as a respectful guest, with an unbiased perspective and a watchful eye, should be stressed. Home safety assessment calls for common sense and for examining each patient's environment in the context of that patient's unique medical status and functional capacity.

The accompanying box summarizes guidelines for home safety assessment.

PHYSICAL OR STRUCTURAL HAZARDS FOR ANY ELDERLY ADULT

Although physical and structural hazards are widespread, they are most prevalent in older homes and economically disadvantaged areas.

Beyond the basics (i.e., a house with structurally adequate roof, floors, and stairs, as well as functional toilet), adequate cooling (preferably an air conditioner but minimally a fan and good ventilation) should be provided for patients at high risk for heat stroke who live in those regions where sustained temperatures above 90° are common. High-risk patients include those who have severe immobility, moderate dementia, advanced cardiorespiratory diseases, and those who take anticholinergic or diuretic drugs. Access to fluids and reliable caregiver support are also critical for many of these patients. There are well-documented epidemics of heat stroke among older patients in southern cities.[8] These studies probably underestimate heat-related morbidity and mortality since they do not identify patients who suffer deterioration in cardiac, respiratory, or other physiological functions because of heat-induced stress. Evidence supporting this theory may be found by epidemiologic studies.[12]

The danger of freezing is less often overlooked by patients and families. Still, referrals for timely preventive intervention by social services (e.g., fuel purchase assistance) can be very helpful.

Residential fires are likely to be fatal for frail, less mobile, geriatric patients. Ill-advised or hazardous use of kerosene heaters, open burners on a gas stove, and loose or poorly insulated wiring, as well as smoking in bed and placing oxygen tanks near flames of any type should be addressed. Heat injury is also frequently caused by hot tap water when the water heater thermostat is set too high or by heating pads that are used at high settings by sleeping patients or the cognitively impaired.[7]

Potential causes of falls often can be spotted when the clinician examines the usual pathways that the patient uses in the house. Verbal accounts may suffice, but often one must watch the patient move around the home to assess risk. Chapter 31 should be reviewed for further recommendations about preventing falls in the patient's home.

A quick look in the kitchen may disclose absence or unavailability of suitable nutrients or fluids, which prompts further appropriate evaluation. Occult malnutrition is becoming common in the elderly population. Similarly, evidence of grossly unsanitary areas for food preparation or florid infestation with insects or rodents should be noted. Occult alcoholism may also be evidenced by the cans or bottles in the home.

Finally, security precautions are important in high-crime areas, especially if older patients are living alone. Violent crimes against older persons are common and can be emotionally and financially devastating when they are not fatal.

COMMON "MEDICAL" HAZARDS

Medication-related misadventures may contribute to as many as one quarter of hospitalizations for older persons and are considered directly causal in nearly 8% of admissions.[10] Factors involved in these medication-related incidents include poor communication between doctor and patient, unwise prescribing practices, and intentional noncompliance. (See Chapter 3.) Adherence to medical regimens (drug and diet) is vital for some frail geriatric patients, while other patients are far less dependent on their medications than their physicians believe them to be. At times, failure to comply may even be lifesaving.

Every safety assessment should include a careful review of the patient's medication. How are medicines handled and delivered to the patient in the home? Are the bottles labeled correctly? Are any outdated? Is the person who organizes and administers the medication responsible and well informed about the medication's use? These and other medical issues need to be assessed. (See the box on p. 162.)

Evaluation for the patient's access to fluids or undesirable foods may be noteworthy. Availability of telephone communications may be important, especially if the patient lives alone. Certain types of adaptive equipment may be medically vital such as inflatable mattresses for patients at risk of bedsores or walkers for patients at high risk for falls.

Patients with severe psychiatric or cognitive impairments

Patients who have severe psychiatric or cognitive impairments require special consideration. Wandering behaviors, impulsive actions, and impaired judgment increase the chance of misadventures. Most important is the reliable availability of a

---
GUIDELINES FOR HOME SAFETY ASSESSMENT

Basic structure
- Intact roof
- Solid floors and stairs
- Functioning toilet (or outhouse)
- Source of fresh water

Temperature control
- Fan/air conditioner
- Proper use of heating pads
- Proper hot water heater temperature
- Adequate heat/insulation

Nutrition
- Types of foods in cabinets
- Evidence of alcohol use
- Kitchen condition
- Pests

Fire prevention and response
- Use of kerosene heaters
- Use of open gas burners on stove for heat
- Smoking in bed
- Use of oxygen
- Dangerous electrical wiring
- Smoke alarms
- Exit plans in case of fire

Crime prevention
- Locks
- Method of calling for help

- Proximity of neighbors
- Surrounding criminal activity

Preventing self-injury, suicide, accidental homicide
- Loaded guns
- Knives
- Household toxins
- Car keys
- Swimming pool
- Power tools

Medication management
- Duplicate medicines, outdated drugs, pill box
- Correct labeling
- Storage safety, accessibility, refrigeration if needed
- Caregiver familiar with medications

Wandering control (demented patients)
- Doortop latches, special locks
- Fenced yards with latches hidden
- Identification bracelets
- Electronic wandering alarms
- Caregiver supervision

Miscellaneous
- Emergency phone numbers by telephone
- Wheelchair ramp

---

*See Chapter 31 for fall prevention.

capable well-informed caregiver; some patients require 24-hour supervision. Accurate assessment of caregiver support often requires serial home visits.

Attention to the potential for falls is even more critical for a cognitively dysfunctional patient who is able to rise unassisted than for a cognitively intact frail elder. Stairs pose a great hazard. The patient's wandering alone outside can also be very dangerous. Likewise, unsupervised access to medications, firearms, sharp instruments, toxins (e.g., cleaning agents or pesticides), and stoves or other materials (e.g., cigarettes) that might cause fires is undesirable.

RECOMMENDATIONS AND INTERVENTIONS

Home safety assessment may be time consuming, but it can be reasonably accomplished by an experienced community health nurse, office-based nurse, nurse practitioner with geriatric expertise, or physician. Although it is not always feasible for an office-based practice, a team approach in which each member makes a unique contribution often is best. Sometimes the assessment can be accomplished by conversations with a reliable patient or caregiver in the office. In most cases, the assessment is more accurate when performed in the home. Supplying the patient or caregiver with a self-help form may also be a useful strategy.

In seeking an optimal home situation, all providers should avoid being overly judgmental or critical when evaluating home safety and should rely instead on reasonable minimal standards. Suggestions should be tempered with awareness of the patient's financial and social situation, prognosis, availability and acceptability of alternative caregiving situations, as well as the preferences of the patient and family. Providers should become familiar with and enlist the aid of the extended family, friends, neighbors, religious groups, social service departments, area agencies on aging, and other sources of support.

Clear-cut or probable neglect or abuse must be reported to appropriate authorities (adult protective services, local ombudsman, etc.). On occasion, the simple act of investigation by an external authority can change a caregiver's behavior. Reporting neglect or abuse may also jeopardize the physician's relationship with the caregiver, sometimes without improving the patient's situation; therefore, reporting should be done selectively.

A number of home safety checklists and interventional strategies are available.[1,5,9] One approach is to conduct the evaluation room by room.[5,9] Alternatively, organizing the evaluation around the patient's daily routine is appropriate.

PROVIDER SAFETY: RECOGNIZING DANGER

Medical professionals are rarely endangered during home visits, even in economically disadvantaged neighborhoods. However, some areas are potentially dangerous, particularly in larger cities, and providers should be aware of these danger signs. Intoxicated patients or caregivers who exhibit aggressive behaviors are of concern, as is the presence of persons in the home who are not related to the family and who may be involved in illegal activities (e.g., drug sales). Providers should be aware when they enter an area known for high crime rates or extreme poverty and alert when there are possible risks related to race and sex differences between providers, care recipients, and members of the household. Safety recommendations for providers are summarized in the box on p. 164.

In high-crime areas, it is advisable to make visits early in the day because people who are involved in criminal activities and substance abuse often are asleep. Visits to such areas after dark should be avoided. In the high-crime neighborhoods, it is sometimes best to send two providers. Calling ahead is wise because the patient or family can decline a visit if they know it is unsafe for the provider or want to prevent

```
————————— PROVIDER SAFETY DURING HOME VISITS —————————
```

Recognize potential risk factors and danger signs
- Location of home in a high-crime area
- Race or sex differences between provider and household
- Intoxicated patient/caregiver exhibiting aggressive behavior
- Presence of people who may be criminals

Interventions
- Visit dangerous areas early in the day
- Do not visit dangerous areas after dark
- Call ahead (household can determine if environment is safe)

- Use alternate provider (male in place of female)
- Do not carry medicines and advertise that policy
- Visit in groups of two or more when in very dangerous areas
- Communicate with other professionals regarding unsafe homes
- Give patient alternative sources for care if safety reasons force withdrawal
- Report unsafe homes to agencies for adult protective services

confrontations between medical professionals and those involved in criminal activity. Occasionally, families and neighbors also will keep an informal watch over the provider's car in certain neighborhoods.

It is also important to communicate with visiting nurses and other professionals about safety concerns that have been identified. When a situation is deemed unsafe, inform the patient (e.g., by telephone, certified letter, or in person) about other possible sources for medical care and discontinue services in the home; however, this should rarely be necessary.

REFERENCES

1. Blodgett HE, Deno E, Hathaway V: For the caregivers: caring for someone with loss of brain function, *Clinical Report on Aging* 1(2):16, 1987.
2. Brody JA, Borck DB, Williams TF: Trends in the health of the elderly population, *Annu Rev Public Health* 8:211, 1987.
3. Gulaid JA, Sacks JJ, Sattin RW: Deaths from residential fires among older people: United States 1984, *J Am Geriatr Soc* 37:331, 1989.
4. Gulaid JA, Sattin RW, Waxweiler RJ: Deaths from residential fires 1978-1984 in Public Health Surveillance of 1990 Injury Control Objectives for the Nation. CDC Surveillance Summaries MMWR No. SS-1 37:39, 1988.
5. Hindmarsh JJ, Estes EH: Falls in older persons: causes and interventions, *Arch Intern Med* 149:2217, 1989.
6. Hogue C: Injury in late life: Part I. Epidemiology, *J Am Geriatr Soc* 30:183, 1982.
7. Hogue C: Injury in late life: Part II. Prevention; *J Am Geriatr Soc* 30:276, 1982.
8. Hope W et al: Illness and death due to environmental heat: Georgia and St Louis 1983, *JAMA* 252:209, 1984.
9. Josephson KR, Fabacher DA, Rubenstein LZ: Home safety and fall prevention, *Clin Geriatr Med* 7(4):707, 1991.

10. Nolan L, O'Malley K, Prescribing for the elderly: part 1: sensitivity of the elderly to adverse drug reactions, *J Am Geriatr Soc* 36:142, 1988.
11. Ramsdell JW et al: The yield of a home visit in the assessment of geriatric patients, *J Am Geriatr Soc* 37:17, 1989.
12. Schuman SH: Patterns of Urban Heat-Wave Deaths and Implications for Prevention: Data from New York and St. Louis during July, 1966. *Environmental Research* 5:59, 1972.

SUGGESTED READINGS

Josephson KR, Fabacher DA, Rubenstein LZ: Home safety and fall prevention, *Clin Geriatr Med* 7(4):707, 1991.
Ramsdell JW et al: The yield of a home visit in the assessment of geriatric patients, *J Am Geriatr Soc* 37:17, 1989.

PART THREE

PREVENTION AND HEALTH MAINTENANCE

CHAPTER 19

Successful aging

JOHN WALSH

KEY POINTS

- Individuals age very differently (heterogeneity of aging)
- With age there is reduced functional reserve capacity.
- Successful aging is an adaptive process involving *selection, optimization,* and *compensation* of motivational, physical and cognitive capabilities and skills.
- There is no unanimity on the criteria and predictors of successful aging.

Aging can be viewed from a positive or negative vantage point. Americans live longer, but do they live healthier lives? Aging is considered to be synonymous with significant losses and, therefore, is usually perceived negatively. A common universal assumption is that older people have substantial declines in their physical and mental functions. A considerable amount of literature dwells on losses that are associated with the aging process, including loss of work, income, friends, family, and self-esteem. Old age is often stigmatized by decremental disease, dementia, depression, and death. On the other hand, there are vigorous, happy, and productive older people who are aging well and living longer, and others wish to know the formula that will help them to age optimally. Obviously, middle-aged people today are more preoccupied with healthy lifestyles in preparation for their productive, healthy, and problem-free old age.

VARIABILITY OF AGING

Nonetheless, many physiological functions begin to decline progressively after age 30.[5] The rate of decline in organ function is not uniform, and individuals age at different rates (interindividual variability). Thus, physiological age is not always synonymous with chronological age. Functional decline not only varies substantially between individuals, but organ losses within each individual also occur at different rates (intraindividual plasticity). Like younger people, most older people have considerable functional reserve. But with the passage of time, these reserves progressively dwindle, an inevitable accompaniment to aging. While healthy older people usually maintain normal organ function in the resting state, their reduced reserve capacities often prevent optimal function under stressful conditions.

Aging itself cannot be held responsible for all losses occurring after middle age. The variability in the rate of decline among older people, usually attributed to genetic control, is generally due to several additional factors (i.e., personal habits, environmental conditions, and psychosocial factors[14]). Genetic and medical considerations both influence the rate of functional decline among older people, along with social and economic factors such as sanitation, nutrition, and working or living conditions. In addition, adequate income and education are predictors of better quality of life, whereas poverty, ignorance, and social isolation are associated with more illness and disability.

Lifestyle factors such as lack of exercise, poor diet, obesity, smoking, and alcohol affect the functional decline of older people, but they are also risk factors for diseases such as hypertension, heart disease, stroke, chronic obstructive lung disease, lung cancer, and diabetes mellitus, all of which have deleterious effects on functional ability.[2,7,8,10] Social and behavioral factors cannot be ignored when smoking, unhealthy diets, lack of exercise, and poor stress management are blamed as risk factors for poor health. These risk factors are socially learned and reinforced by behavior. Not only disease but also medications have imposing effects on the aging process. In clinical evaluation it is often difficult to separate the effects of diseases, medications, personal habits, and dietary and environmental influences from the effects of the aging process. This dilemma influences the management of health care for older people. Clinicians can alter the lifestyle and environmental factors for older patients and treat diseases that influence morbidity and mortality, such as hypertension and diabetes mellitus, even though clinicians are unable to alter progressive losses that result from the aging process itself. In essence, modification of the extrinsic factors of aging fosters a better quality of life, which is as important as its influence on longevity itself.

Already, there has been a dramatic decline in some diseases, such as coronary artery disease, stroke, and lung cancer, because of changes in health behaviors. Strokes have waned largely because hypertension is diagnosed and treated more effectively, cigarette smoking has ceased and better dietary control is practiced, aspirin is used for prophylaxis, and anticoagulants are used for atrial fibrillation. Similarly, the decline in mortality from ischemic heart disease has been related to changes in lifestyle and treatment of hypertension, and recently the lower rate of coronary artery disease in women was reported to result from estrogen replacement therapy.[17] Furthermore, there is convincing evidence that seat belts and refraining from driving while under the influence of alcohol prevent accidental injury and death. Lung cancer and chronic obstructive pulmonary disease can be prevented by the cessation of cigarette smoking and are further examples of positive effects from risk modification. Similarly, a number of nonfatal chronic diseases such as urinary incontinence, osteoporosis, and fractures, as well as falls, are preventable or potentially modifiable.

IMPACT OF CHRONIC DISEASE

An attractive hypothesis (compression of morbidity) espoused by Fries and Crapo argues that successful aging is attained by people who optimize their lifestyle factors for the goal of delaying the onset of chronic disease until later in life.[8,9] Thus, chronic illness will occur only during the final years of a longer life, thereby increasing the length of a healthier life. Similar conclusions are advanced by Bortz[3] who supports the idea that lifestyle factors influence the aging process and blames many of the physiological losses that are ascribed to aging on physical inactivity or disuse. Alternatively, a pessimistic view argues that chronically ill people are unquestionably kept alive longer but with an increasing number of diseases. Those investigators who disagree with these hypotheses and concepts maintain that Alzheimer's disease, osteoarthritis, fractures, Parkinson's disease and other chronic afflictions that are associated with older people will become an increasing health burden.[15,16]

There is a paucity of data on the impact that chronic disease morbidity has on active life expectancy. The concept of "active life expectancy" is that fraction of the remaining lifetime that will be spent in a functionally independent state; it is an estimate of the quality years of life remaining for older people. Clearly one's recovery from disability and dependency resulting from chronic illness, as it influences active life expectancy and therefore quality of life, must be considered. Studies show that 19% to 24% of the dependent population return to independence within 2 years.[12,13] While a compression of morbidity would add years of active life, so would recovery from a disability. There are several approaches to one's attaining improved health, maintaining health, recovering from poor health, or delaying the onset of illness.

NORMAL AGING: SUCCESSFUL OR USUAL

In the study of the aging process, it has become increasingly important for clinicians to differentiate normal aging, with its variable physiological losses, from the changes produced by disease (sick or pathologic aging). Rowe and Kahn[14] have suggested that with normal aging there are variable physiological losses that can be subdivided into two groups, successful and usual (Figure 19-1). *Successful aging* describes individuals who demonstrate few or minimal physiological decrements that are due to aging alone and for which there is less need for further modifications in personal habits or environments. In *usual aging*, the more common mode of aging, there are significant physiological losses along with substantial reduced reserve capacity. For example, with usual aging there are influential impairments to a patient's

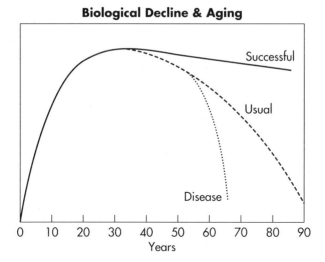

Figure 19-1 Successful and usual patterns of normal aging. Incremental growth (physiological, functional, or reserve capacities) peaks at age 30; thereafter, there is a variable decline with successful aging showing minimal decrements.

glucose metabolism, which are shown by abnormal glucose tolerance tests, systolic hypertension, atherosclerosis, declining renal and immune function, decreased bone density, decreased sensory input (visual/hearing loss), declining crystalized (verbal) and fluid (inductive) reasoning, and progressive slowness of movement. These changes can be substantially modified to mitigate their effects on the patient's functional reserve capacity and to reduce the risks of superimposed disease.

Baltes and Baltes[1] have used the terms *normal* and *optimal* aging, which correspond to the terms *usual* and *successful* aging used by Rowe and Kahn.[14] Other terms for successful aging that is uncomplicated by disease include *aging well* and *optimal, productive,* and *healthy aging. Healthy aging* implies an absence of disease, and the terms *successful* or *optimal aging* additionally emphasize the absence of significant physiological decline. These catchwords shift attention away from the belief that old age is always associated with decline and loss to a positive viewpoint that encourages optimism about aging. This perspective focuses attention on extrinsic factors that modify aging, thereby fostering health promotion and prevention. The concept of successful aging promotes healthful strategies such as exercise, modification of diet, cessation of smoking, and social and intellectual stimulation. The aggregate of these strategies potentially enhances a patient's quality of life and prevents the shrinkage of physiological reserves or postpones the onset of chronic disorders. From a research point of view, the concept of successful aging isolates aging itself as a process that is uncomplicated by significant physiological decline or disease.

INDICATORS FOR SUCCESSFUL AGING

The concept of successful aging is complex, with different meanings for different disciplines. Thus there is no specific prescription for successful aging. In many respects it is intensely subjective, with individuals themselves playing major roles in coping with life's problems. Length of life alone is not a sufficient criterion; longevity must be accompanied by other measures that enhance quality of life. These are the lifestyle and behavioral measures that challenge individuals' plasticity to maximize their reserve capabilities. Multiple criteria have been suggested as indicators for successful aging, although there is no consensus on their relative importance.[1,18]

One's physical and mental health coupled with longevity are characteristics of aging well. Mental health reflects one's ability to cope with grief, failures, and conflicts. Adaptive competence is a major criterion for successful aging. It draws upon the individual's capacity to respond with resilience to physical, mental, psychosocial, or environmental challenges of later life. Adaptability measures one's behavioral ability to deal with a variety of life's demands. In general, one's adaptive responses to environmental challenges become less sensitive and slower with age.[6] Furthermore, psychosocial adjustment is considered to be a dimension of successful aging. These attributes emphasize job satisfaction and relationships with people and circumstances that lead to life satisfaction and self-esteem.

Personal control or autonomy is another yardstick for successful aging.[6,11] Autonomy fosters the ability to set and follow one's own rules, an important component to the health of the older person. Older individuals perform better when they have a sense of purpose and control over their activities. In contrast, those who are denied this prerogative perform less well and may be at increased risk for illness or injury. A common example is relocation or moving and its attendant loss of friends, family, and neighbors. Autonomy-enhancing environments enable older individuals to cope with problems, while environments where condescending and overly concerned attitudes prevail only encourage older people's helplessness. The latter is seen in some nursing homes or at the patient's home, where there is an overly solicitous spouse.

As a consequence of interindividual variability and intraindividual plasticity, successful aging is considered to be an adaptive process to experience social, physical and cognitive losses involving selection, optimization, and compensation.[1] As people grow older and their biological, mental, and social reserves decline, they use these adaptive processes. Older people focus on areas (selection) that permit self-satisfaction and are manageable. Older people enhance their behaviors to optimize their capabilities. When behavioral capacities are lost or reduced, older people compensate by altering their behaviors. An example of someone who used these strategies to facilitate successful aging is Rubenstein. He conquered the weaknesses of aging that affected his piano playing by (1) reducing his repertoire and playing fewer pieces (selection), (2) practicing these more often (optimization), and (3) slowing the speed of his playing prior to any fast movements, thereby enhancing the impression of speed in the fast movements (compensation).[1]

Only a small percentage of people aged 65 years and older, and even a much smaller number over age 80, do not have chronic diseases or disabilities combined with minimal physiological changes to qualify as candidates for the pure model of successful aging as proposed by Rowe and Kahn.[14] Successful aging used in this context suggests that the oldest old who have any chronic disease are unsuccessful and have failed to age well. This message and all that it implies may be demoralizing to those older people who are vigorous and maintain high levels of physical and social functioning, despite their underlying chronic diseases. Many older people effectively compensate for physiological changes and diseases by adapting to their disabilities or restoring functional capacities by rehabilitation. Recently the term *effective aging* has been used to recognize these patients.[5] Many older people fit this definition, having adapted to physical, psychological, and social challenges. Comfort's book *A Good Age*[4] is replete with examples of positive strategies used by older people to remain energetic and active. Among his many examples is Anna Mary Moses who farmed until her late 70s. She stopped embroidering on canvas when she was 78 because of arthritis in her fingers and began to paint pictures in oils of rural America. In 1960 at age 100 she illustrated an edition of *The Night Before Christmas*. This painter was "Grandma Moses."

The concept of successful aging has variable meanings for individuals, society, and even among various disciplines of the health care profession. To some, successful aging indicates one's ability to adapt effectively and optimally to change, disease, and environmental imbalance. Perhaps the term *optimal aging* more clearly defines the concept of one's minimal physiological losses that are uncomplicated by disease. Optimal aging has a less objectionable connotation than do other terms that imply some older are aging unsuccessfully. The concept of *successful aging* needs to be better understood, including its criteria, predictors, and variables. More data on the impact that lifestyle, behavioral, and environmental influences have on active life expectancy, morbidity, and mortality are likely to contribute to a better idea of successful aging. Meanwhile, the study of aging individuals who are free of disease as a "standard" for health facilitates better research on aging and provides better insight about risk factors for chronic disease and its prevention or postponement.

REFERENCES

1. Baltes PB, Baltes MM, eds: Psychological perspectives on successful aging: the model of selective optimization with compensation. In *Successful aging: perspectives from the behavioral sciences*, Cambridge, Canada, 1990, Cambridge University Press.
2. Benfante R, Reed D, Brody J: Biological predictors of health in an aging cohort, *J Chron Dis* 38:385, 1985.
3. Bortz WM: Redefining human aging, *J Am Geriatr Soc* 37:1092, 1989.
4. Comfort A: *A good age*, New York, 1976, Crown.
5. Curb JD et al: Effective aging: meeting the challenge of growing older, *J Am Geriatr Soc* 38:827, 1990.
6. Evans JG: Prevention of age-associated loss of autonomy: epidemiological approaches, *J Chron Dis* 37:353, 1984.
7. Fried LB, Bush TL: Morbidity as a focus of preventive health care in the elderly, *Epidemiol Rev* 10:48, 1988.

8. Fries JF: Aging, natural death, and the compression of morbidity, *N Engl J Med* 303:130, 1980.
9. Fries JF, Crapo LM: *Vitality and aging: implication of the rectangular curve*, San Francisco, 1981, W.H. Freeman.
10. Guralnik JM, Kaplan GA: Predictors of healthy aging: prospective evidence from the Alameda County Study, *Am J Public Health* 79:703, 1989.
11. Rodin J: Aging and health: effects of the sense of control, *Science* 233:1271, 1986.
12. Rogers RG, Rogers A, Belanger A: Active life among the elderly in the United States: multistate life-table estimates and population projections, *Milbank Q* 67:370, 1989.
13. Rogers A, Rogers RG, Belanger A: Longer life but worse health?: measurement and dynamics, *Gerontologist* 30:640, 1990.
14. Rowe JW, Kahn RL: Human aging: usual and successful, *Science* 237:143, 1987.
15. Schneider EL, Brody JA: Aging, natural death, and the compression of morbidity: another view, *N Engl J Med* 309:854, 1983.
16. Schneider EL, Buralnik JM: The aging of America: impact on health care costs, *JAMA* 263:2335, 1990.
17. Stampfer MJ et al: Postmenopausal estrogen therapy and cardiovascular disease, *N Engl J Med* 325:756, 1991.
18. Valliant GE: Avoiding negative life outcomes: evidence from a forty-five year study. In Baltes PB, Baltes MM, eds: *Successful aging: perspectives from the behavioral sciences*, Cambridge, Canada, 1990, Cambridge University Press.

SUGGESTED READINGS

Baltes PB, Baltes MM, eds: Psychological perspectives on successful aging: the model of selective optimization with compensation. In *Successful aging: perspectives from the behavioral sciences*, Cambridge, Canada, 1990, Cambridge University Press.
Rowe JW, Kahn RL: Human aging: usual and successful, *Science* 237:143, 1987.
Valliant GE: Avoiding negative life outcomes: evidence from a forty-five year study. Baltes PB, Baltes MM, eds: *Successful aging: perspectives from the behavioral sciences*, Cambridge, Canada, 1990, Cambridge University Press.

CHAPTER 20

Nutritional assessment and dietary recommendations

JAMES W. MOLD

KEY POINTS

- Older persons who are poor, physically frail, or live alone are at particular risk for malnutrition.
- The diagnosis of nutritional deficiencies for older patients depends primarily upon their dietary histories and assessment of their risk factors, supplemented by physical examinations, including height and weight, and selected laboratory tests.
- Older people in the United States often consume too little water, dietary fiber, calcium, potassium, magnesium, iron, zinc, selenium, chromium, and B vitamins.
- Significant health problems can result from the ingestion of excessive amounts of zinc and vitamins A, B_6, and D.
- Dieticians can be of great help to older patients and should therefore be consulted regularly.

Adequate nutrition is essential for good health. If too little attention has been paid by physicians to nutrition in the past, it may be because most adults in this country consume adequate amounts of the essential nutrients. In fact, nutritional excesses are much more common than deficiencies. In contrast to younger adults, older persons are at substantial risk for nutritional deficiencies. For example, it has been estimated that approximately 30% of older Americans ingest less than the required amounts of one or more essential nutrients. Among those aged 75 years and older, 40% of men and 30% of women are at least 10% underweight.[1] Such estimates, while probably accurate, are made difficult by the lack of well-established guidelines for optimal weight and height and recommended daily allowances (RDAs) for essential nutrients for people aged 75 years and older. In addition to inadequacies of dietary intake, older persons are more likely to have increased requirements for certain nutrients as a result of problems with absorption, acute and chronic metabolic stressors (infections, trauma, etc.), and medication-nutrient and disease-nutrient interactions.

Despite the frequency of documented dietary deficiencies among older persons, the biochemical evidence of nutritional deficiencies is relatively scant. This should not be interpreted as evidence that malnutrition among older people is uncommon. In fact, a substantial percentage of older individuals have inadequate nutritional reserves, a problem that manifests itself during illnesses, injuries, and surgical stress. Nearly 50% of persons aged 65 years and older are clinically malnourished at the time of admission to the hospital. (See also Chapter 45.)

NUTRITIONAL ASSESSMENT

Nutritional assessment must be a routine part of ambulatory geriatric care. The four basic components of nutritional assessment are (1) dietary history, (2) assessment of risk factors for malnutrition, (3) routine physical examination, and (4) selected laboratory tests.[6]

In an ambulatory setting, the most commonly used dietary history consists of the patient's recall of foods that were consumed during the previous 24 hours. It is important to recognize that the older patient's ability to recall information is often impaired for a variety of reasons, so corroborative information from family members or friends is also important. Occasionally it may be necessary to request a 3-day diet diary.

Questionnaires can be particularly useful for gathering the large amount of information that is required for geriatric assessment. If a screening questionnaire is used, general dietary questions can be included on it, or these same questions can be asked during the clinical interview. (See the box on p. 177.)

More important than the collection of older patients' dietary information is the recognition of their risk factors for malnutrition. (See the box on p. 178.) This information, which routinely should be obtained as part of the general evaluation process (functional assessment, cognitive assessment, social support, financial assessment, etc.), must be assimilated for purposes of nutritional assessment. Computerized record systems can facilitate this kind of analysis.

The most critical elements of the physical examination are the patient's general appearance and vital signs. In particular it is important to notice affect, body build, muscle bulk, subcutaneous fat, skin pigmentation and texture, and overall vitality. Accurate measurements of height and weight should be obtained regularly and charted in such a way as to document trends. More sophisticated anthropometric measurements such as biceps circumference and skinfold thickness are not usually necessary in an ambulatory setting.

_____ **NUTRITION SCREENING QUESTIONS** _____

1. Do you have a good appetite?
2. Has your weight changed recently?
3. Have you noticed any problems with taste or smell?
4. Do you have problems with chewing or swallowing?
5. Do you wear dentures? Are you having any problems with them?
6. What problems have you had in shopping for food?
7. What problems have you had in preparing meals?
8. Are you following a special diet of any kind?
9. Are there any foods that you cannot eat?
10. How much milk do you drink in a typical day? How much cheese, yogurt, and ice cream do you eat?
11. How many 10-ounce glasses of water or other liquid do you drink in a typical day?
12. Do you generally eat several portions of meat, fruits and vegetables, and breads and cereals daily?
13. Have you experienced nausea, vomiting, or diarrhea recently?
14. Have you ever had an operation on your stomach?
15. How much alcohol do you drink during an average day or week?

Several routine laboratory tests are particularly important. These include serum albumin (normal is 3.5 g/dl or greater), total lymphocyte count (normal is 1500 cells/ mm^3 or greater), hemoglobin and/or hematocrit, blood urea nitrogen (BUN), serum creatinine, and the BUN/creatinine ratio. In addition, under certain circumstances, serum B_{12}, serum folate, serum 25-hydroxycholecalciferol (25-OH vitamin D), and serum transferrin levels can be very helpful.

INCREASED RISK FOR MALNUTRITION

Some of the factors that put older people at increased risk for malnutrition are listed in the box on p. 178. (See also Chapter 45.) It is important to recognize that as a result of decreased activity levels and possibly decreased basal energy expenditures, older people tend to consume less food. Despite decreased energy requirements, there is no reduction in the need for fluids, proteins, vitamins, or minerals. A diet containing 1000 to 1500 kilocalories per day therefore must be particularly rich in these essential nutrients if it is to supply the required amounts. For this reason, food selection is critical. Individuals who have limited incomes may select or purchase suboptimal foods. Present-day elders were raised in a very different environment than exists today. Convenience foods and microwave ovens are a recent phenomenon. Some need to completely relearn how to cook; some men may never have learned.

Probably because of their constant struggle with health problems, older persons seem to be particularly susceptible to dietary fads. Media attention directed at lowering

RISK FACTORS FOR MALNUTRITION

Social isolation
Homebound
Low income
Inadequate transportation
Impaired taste or smell
Impaired vision
Cognitive deficits
Masticatory problems
Dysphagia
Gastric or esophageal pathology
History of gastrointestinal surgery
Impairments of manual dexterity
Mobility problems
Recent and/or frequent hospitalizations
Depression or bereavement
Alcohol abuse
Multiple medications

fats and cholesterol, for example, has caused many older people to unwisely restrict essential dietary components. Vitamins, minerals, and herbal remedies are frequently taken in excessive amounts.

Social isolation is another major risk factor for malnutrition.[2] Eating is a social event. Individuals who live alone may find meal preparation for one to be more trouble than it is worth and dining alone to be unenjoyable. Loneliness and bereavement can diminish the desire for food.

A variety of health-related problems can cause anorexia, food aversion, or poor food selection. The aging process seems to be associated with some diminution in the abilities to taste and smell.[5] When compounded by diminished salivary flow (commonly the result of anticholinergic medications), dentures, or poor oral hygiene, the taste and smell of food may further be altered. Classically, salty and sweet tastes are the first to be lost. For this reason, low-salt diets may be particularly unpalatable, and foods such as bell peppers, which have both sweet and bitter tastes, simply taste bitter.

Oral pathology can result in substantial problems that are associated with appetite, mastication, and swallowing. Older people are less likely to visit a dentist regularly and more likely to be edentulous or to have significant gingival diseases than younger adults. Among edentulous individuals, nonuse or unavailability of dentures is an important risk factor for the development of malnutrition, despite the fact that edentulous individuals are able to chew and swallow most foods even without their dentures.

Certain medications are particularly likely to interfere with a patient's adequate nutrition. Digoxin is a leading offender since it may cause anorexia, even when the patient's serum level is within the therapeutic range. Several commonly prescribed antidepressants including trazodone and fluoxetine can suppress appetite. Sedative and hypnotic agents may cause apathy and decreased food intake. Centrally acting antihypertensive drugs may adversely affect appetite by depressing the patient's mood.

COMMON SPECIFIC NUTRITIONAL DEFICIENCIES

Several specific nutritional deficiencies are particularly important in ambulatory geriatric care, including (1) underhydration, (2) protein-calorie malnutrition, (3) calcium deficiency, (4) zinc deficiency, and (5) inadequate intake of dietary fiber. In addition, community surveys have found that a substantial percentage of older people consume less than 60% of the RDAs for iron, riboflavin, nicotinic acid, vitamins C and D, folate, potassium, and magnesium. Table 20-1 summarizes the RDAs for various nutrients for elderly persons and lists common dietary sources of each.

Hydration

Water is perhaps the most essential ingredient of life because it is the solution in which nearly all biochemical reactions take place. Relatively minor changes in the concentrations of certain solutes can significantly affect metabolic processes. Acute water losses of as little as 2% can reduce the patient's work capacity by as much as 20% and performance on cognitive tests by as much as 10%. In addition to its function as a solute, water serves as a thermal buffer (sweat), cleansing agent (tears, saliva, sputum, urine), and transport substance (urine, feces, saliva). Adequate salivary flow is necessary to transport chemicals in food to the taste buds of the tongue, for example.

It has been well documented that total body water as a percentage of body mass decreases with increasing age. There are reasons to believe that decreased water intake may be at least partly responsible. With increasing age, both renal water conservation mechanisms and thirst perception are consistently impaired. While older people often require more water, they tend to consume less. Self-imposed water restriction is sometimes seen in those who have urinary incontinence.

Despite suboptimal fluid intake, most older people are not clinically dehydrated. However, older people are at increased risk for significant dehydration when they are faced with acute fluid losses or even further decreased intake. There is almost no reliable information available regarding the health effects of chronic subclinical underhydration. However, most geriatricians routinely urge their patients to consume at least 1500 to 1800 ml of liquid daily. This prescription translates to about one 10-ounce glass of water or other liquid with each meal and one between meals, for a total of five to six glasses daily.

Table 20-1 Aging and various nutrients

Nutrient	RDA	Causes of deficiency	Primary food sources
Calories	30 kcal/kg	Decreased intake; multiple	All
Protein	1.0 g/kg	Decreased intake; multiple	Many
Water (free)	1500 ml	Decreased thirst; urinary frequency; incontinence	Liquids
Calcium	male: 1000 mg female: 1500 mg	Decreased intake; decreased absorption; lactose intolerance; loop diuretics; noncalcium antacids; soft drinks	Dairy products; broccoli; cauliflower
Zinc	15 mg	Decreased intake; alcohol; diuretics; digoxin; renal disease; cancer	Meat; eggs; seafood; milk; whole grains
Selenium	50-200 µg	Decreased intake	Fish; shellfish; grains; onions
Chromium	50-200 µg	Decreased intake	Meat; cheese; grains; condiments
Copper	2-3 mg	Decreased intake; excess zinc	Shellfish; nuts; raisins; legumes; organ meats
Iron	10 mg	Vegetarian diet; decreased intake vitamin C; blood loss; clay or starch ingestion	Meat; green vegetables
Magnesium	male: 350 mg female: 300 mg	Decreased intake; diuretics; digoxin; alcohol	Green vegetables; grains; seafood
Vitamin C	60 mg	Decreased intake; high dose salicylates	Citrus fruits; melons; tomatoes; potatoes; grains; green leafy vegetables
Vitamin D	400 IU + sunlight	Homebound; mineral oil; anticonvulsants; isoniazid	Milk; egg yolks; salmon
Vitamin B_1 (thiamine)	0.5 mg/1000 kcal	Decreased intake; alcohol; antacids; gastric cancer; dialysis	Whole grains; potatoes; pork; fortified cereals
Vitamin B_6 (pyridoxine)	male: 2.2 mg female: 2.0 mg	Decreased intake; alcohol; isoniazid; L-dopa; penicillamine	Milk; oatmeal; legumes; beef; pork; glandular meats
Folic acid	400 µg	Decreased intake; antacids; triamterene; phenobarbital; methotrexate; sulfa drugs; H_2 blockers	Green leafy vegetables; beef; fish; eggs; asparagus; broccoli; fortified cereals

Table 20-1 Aging and various nutrients—cont'd

Nutrient	RDA	Causes of deficiency	Primary food sources
Vitamin B$_{12}$	3.0 μg	Pernicious anemia; vegetarian diet; colchicine	Dairy products; eggs; liver; meat
Vitamin A	male: 3000 IU female: 2500 IU	Decreased intake; alcohol; mineral oil; cholestyramine; cigarettes	Yellow and green leafy vegetables; fortified margarine; milk; liver; cantaloupe
Vitamin E	male: 10 mg female: 8 mg	Decreased intake	Green leafy vegetables; egg yolks; nuts; wheat germ
Vitamin K	70-140 μg	Warfarin; mineral oil; tetracycline; cholestyramine	Cabbage; peas; turnips
Vitamin B$_2$	0.6 mg/1000 kcal	Decreased intake; alcohol; laxatives; malabsorption	Dairy products; green leafy vegetables; eggs; enriched cereals
Vitamin B$_3$ (niacin)	male: 16 mg female: 13 mg	Decreased intake	Fish; meat; poultry; grains

Protein-Calorie

Protein-calorie malnutrition is also generally subclinical in the ambulatory elderly person and is more a problem of reserve capacity than overt malnutrition. However, physicians caring for older patients will encounter marasmus (both protein and calorie deficiencies) or kwashiorkor (isolated protein deficiency). Individuals at greatest risk for these syndromes are those who are very old, physically frail, chronically ill, poor, and/or socially isolated. Marasmus is associated with weight loss and therefore should be easily detectable. Kwashiorkor, on the other hand, may not be accompanied by weight loss and is more often discovered by laboratory testing. Both conditions are associated with low serum albumin and transferrin levels and low total lymphocyte counts.

Protein-calorie malnutrition is a life-threatening problem that should be managed aggressively. Resistance to infection, wound healing, muscle strength and mobility, and cognition are significantly impaired. Mortality rates are substantially higher for these individuals particularly if they become acutely ill. Most also will have vitamin and mineral deficiencies, which need to be corrected.

Calcium

Older people require, on average, more dietary calcium than younger people. Despite an increased need for calcium, older persons tend to consume less calcium than younger adults. This is probably the result of both an overall decreased food intake and changes in food selection.

The primary source of calcium in the average American diet is dairy products. (See Table 20-2.) Unfortunately, many older people are unable to tolerate dairy

Table 20-2   Sources of dietary calcium

Source	Quantity	Amount of calcium (mg)
Milk	1 cup	300
Ice cream	½ cup	100
Yogurt	8 oz	400
Cheese	1 oz	175-275
Broccoli	½ cup	100
Collards	½ cup	150
Spinach	½ cup	100
Chick-peas	¼ cup	75
Cereal (whole grain)	¾ cup	150
Shrimp	3 oz	100
Tofu	4 oz	100
Almonds	1 oz	75

products because of acquired lactase deficiency. These individuals must either use exogenous lactase with their ingestion of dairy products or take calcium supplements to meet their calcium requirements and prevent the chronic wasting of calcium from bone. Yogurt is often better tolerated than other dairy products. If lactase is used, its effect is maximal when added to milk at least 12 hours before ingestion. Milk that has been pretreated with lactase is now available in many supermarkets. A 500-mg tablet of calcium carbonate contains 200 mg of elemental calcium. Calcium carbonate is almost always well absorbed when taken with a meal. Calcium citrate is more predictably absorbed by those persons with achlorhydria. Calcium supplementation is relatively safe and well tolerated by most individuals. However, caution should be used when clinicians prescribe calcium to individuals who have a history of calcium-containing renal stones and those who take thiazide diuretics. In contrast, patients who take loop diuretics such as furosemide, which enhance calcium excretion, have increased calcium requirements.

Vitamin D

Up to 35% of hospitalized geriatric patients in the United States have low or borderline serum levels of 25-OH vitamin D. Individuals who consume very little milk or who rarely go outside are at particularly high risk for vitamin D deficiency.[3] Those with significant hepatic or renal disease may have difficulty converting vitamin D to its active form and may require supplementation with vitamin D_2 or vitamin D_3. The RDA for vitamin D is only 400 international units (IU). Higher doses can be associated with significant toxicity.

Zinc

Zinc, which is most commonly obtained from meat, eggs, seafood, milk, and whole grains, is present in inadequate amounts in the diets of many older people.

Diuretics, digoxin, renal disease, cancer, and alcoholism can all contribute to zinc deficiency as well. The manifestations of zinc deficiency include impaired taste and smell, immunological deficits, hypogonadism, and dry flaky dermatitis, all of which closely resemble changes that are commonly attributed to aging.

The RDA for zinc is 15 mg. This amount can be found in many multivitamin-mineral preparations. Treatment with larger doses of zinc (80 mg twice daily) has been shown in at least one study to increase the rate of healing of pressure ulcers. There is so far no evidence that zinc supplementation will improve taste or smell in the majority of individuals who have these sensory deficits.

Fiber

Dietary fiber is important for proper bowel function. It probably plays a role in the prevention of diverticulosis and colon cancer. It may help to ameliorate diabetes mellitus and hypercholesterolemia. Because there are so many types of dietary fiber, it is practically impossible to make simple recommendations regarding daily requirements. Patients should be advised to choose whole grain breads and cereals and increase their consumption of fresh fruits and vegetables rather than canned and prepared foods. Psyllium and methylcellulose are probably acceptable alternatives. Oat bran and other primarily soluble fibers may not be as effective at improving bowel function. Increases in the patient's dietary fiber consumption should be instituted gradually and accompanied by increases in fluid intake to avoid constipation and bloating.

POTENTIAL ADVERSE EFFECTS OF DIETARY COMPONENTS

Most vitamins and minerals are surprisingly nontoxic and can be taken in large amounts with very little hazard. However, several of them can cause serious health problems if taken in higher than recommended doses over long periods of time.[4]

Vitamin A

Many vitamin supplements contain as much as 10,000 IU per tablet. Individuals who are consuming several different preparations containing these quantities of vitamin A are at risk for significant toxic effects including hepatic injury, leukopenia, hypercalcemia, impaired wound healing, headaches, and malaise.

Vitamin B$_6$

Chronic consumption of vitamin B$_6$ in excess of 75 to 100 mg daily can cause peripheral neuritis and neuropathy. Most ordinary multivitamin preparations contain from 2 to 5 mg of vitamin B$_6$. However, vitamin B complex and pure vitamin B$_6$ preparations containing from 50 to 150 mg can be purchased in most pharmacies and health food stores.

Vitamin D

The manifestations of vitamin D toxicity include bone resorption, hypercalcemia, hyperphosphatemia, heterotopic calcification (e.g., in kidneys and heart), weakness, nausea, and vomiting. It is now difficult to take excessive amounts of vitamin D without help from a physician since the most potent over-the-counter preparations contain only 1000 IU.

Vitamin C

Vitamin C is often consumed in large amounts in hopes that it will enhance one's resistance to infections and cancer, improve wound healing, prevent blood clots, and improve bowel function. The official daily requirement is only 60 mg, but many people regularly consume 2000 mg or more each day in supplements. Abrupt discontinuation of large doses of vitamin C can precipitate a syndrome called rebound

Table 20-3   Effects of selected medications on nutrients

Drug	Effect
Calcium carbonate	Decreases iron absorption
Cholestyramine	Decreases absorption of vitamins A, D, E, and K, iron, folic acid, and fats
Colchicine	Decreases absorption of vitamin B_{12}
Corticosteroids	Reduce levels of vitamin D thereby decreasing calcium absorption; can cause a negative nitrogen balance by increasing gluconeogenesis
Diphenylhydantoin	Accelerates metabolism of vitamin D; increases rate of utilization of folic acid
H_2 blockers	Decrease vitamin B_{12}, iron, and calcium absorption
Isoniazid	Directly antagonizes the activities of vitamin B_6, niacin, and tryptophan
Loop diuretics	Increase urinary excretion of sodium, potassium, magnesium, and calcium
Methotrexate	Folic acid antagonist
Mineral oil	Decreases absorption of vitamins A, D, E, and K, carotene, calcium, and phosphorus
Mysoline	Accelerates metabolism of vitamin D; increases rate of utilization of folic acid
Nitrofurantoin	Folic acid antagonist
Omeprazole	Decreases absorption of iron, calcium, and vitamin B_{12}
Phenobarbital	Accelerates metabolism of vitamin D; increases rate of utilization of folic acid
Phenolphthalein	Decreases absorption of vitamin D and calcium
Psyllium	Decreases absorption of riboflavin
Salicylates	In high doses, increase vitamin C and potassium excretion; causes chronic blood loss and iron deficiency
Sulfasalazine	Decreases absorption of folic acid
Thiazides	Increase urinary excretion of sodium, potassium, and magnesium
Triamterene	Folic acid antagonist
Trimethoprim	Can cause folic acid depletion

scurvy, which is manifested by perifollicular, gingival, and gastrointestinal hemor-rhages, and mental status changes. Megadoses of vitamin C can also cause deficiencies of vitamin B_{12} and folic acid.

MEDICATION-NUTRIENT INTERACTIONS

Table 20-3 lists some of the more relevant effects of commonly used drugs on specific nutrients.

Several medications can impair the absorption of specific nutrients.[7] Cholestyra-mine binds with fat soluble vitamins and folic acid. Histamine (H_2) receptor blockers, antacids, anticholinergic agents, and omeprazole—by reducing gastric pH—interfere to some degree with the absorption of calcium, iron, and vitamin B_{12}. Aluminum-containing antacids decrease the absorption of vitamin B_{12}.

Medications can also interfere with the metabolism or biochemical activity of nutrients. Diphenylhydantoin inhibits the 25-hydroxylation of vitamin D. Isoniazid inhibits the activities of vitamin B_6, niacin, and tryptophan. Methotrexate, triamter-ene, and trimethoprim all interfere with the actions of folic acid.

Some nutrients can affect the pharmacokinetics or physiological effects of certain medications. For example, the clinical effects of lithium are highly dependent upon the sodium content of the patient's diet; low-salt diets increase lithium's toxicity, while high-salt diets increase its therapeutic effectiveness. Quinidine toxicity may be precipitated by a high intake of fruit juices. The risk of kidney stones is increased when probenecid is taken with a diet that is high in purines and proteins. Calcium supplements may to some degree decrease the effectiveness of calcium chan-nel blockers.

USE OF CONSULTANTS

Printed handouts listing foods that are high in sodium or calcium may be useful, but for more complex issues, particularly when significant behavioral changes are required of patients, physicians should consult a registered dietician. Dieticians can be found most easily in hospitals but also may be in private practice where they are affiliated with large medical clinics, nursing homes, or home health care agencies.

Individuals who have multiple risk factors for malnutrition probably should be evaluated by a case manager who can determine whether services such as mobile meals or assistance with shopping or meal preparation are needed and available. The case manager then arranges those services that are to be provided. Areawide agencies on aging, which administer the Older Americans Act and other senior programs throughout the United States, maintain comprehensive listings of services such as mobile meals, congregate meal sites, senior centers, and other services for older people. Physicians or their office staff should be aware of these and other community services.

REFERENCES

1. Beattie BL, Louie VY: Nutrition and health in the elderly. In Reichel W, ed: *Clinical aspects of aging,* Baltimore, 1989, Williams & Wilkins.
2. Davis MA et al: Living arrangements and dietary patterns of older adults in the United States, *J Gerontol* 40:434, 1985.
3. Dawson-Hughes B et al: Effect of vitamin D supplementation on wintertime and overall bone loss in healthy postmenopausal women, *Ann Intern Med* 115:505, 1991.
4. Dipalma JR, Ritchie DM: Vitamin toxicity, *Annu Rev Pharmacol Toxicol* 17:133, 1977.
5. Massler M: Geriatric nutrition: the role of taste and smell in appetite, *J Prosthet Dent* 43(3):247, 1980.
6. Roe DA: Nutritional assessment of the elderly, *World Rev Nutr Diet* 48:85, 1986.
7. Trovato A, Nuhlicek DN, Midtling JE: Drug-nutrient interactions, *Am Fam Physician* 44(5):1651, 1991.

SUGGESTED READINGS

Roe D: *Handbook on drug and nutrient interactions: a problem-oriented reference guide,* ed 4, Chicago, 1989, American Dietetic Association.
Watkin DM, ed: *Nutrition in older persons, Clin Geriatr Med* 3(3):253-412, 1987.

CHAPTER 21

Physical Activity and Exercise

ROBERT M. SCHMIDT

<u>KEY POINTS</u>

- Assessment of exercise and physical activity of older patients should include four domains: aerobic fitness, strength, flexibility and balance.
- Before prescribing a comprehensive exercise regimen, clinicians should evaluate the health status of older patients while they are clinically stable.
- Patients should be reevaluated at the time of major changes in physical activity or health.
- Exercise stress tests are usually normal for healthy individuals and need not be repeated at regular intervals unless there are major changes in health status.
- Consider less traditional physical activity (e.g., gardening, housework) as exercise, especially for the oldest old (85 + years) and persons who have symptoms of chronic disease.
- Patients should be told that it is never too late to start exercising and increasing their physical activity.

An exercise regimen for an older patient should not be limited to the usual aerobic (isotonic or oxygen-utilizing) activities that are recommended for younger adults. Many older persons obtain most of their exercise through physical activities that are not generally included in exercise advice provided by clinicians. Furthermore, most assessment tools are *not* designed to evaluate ambulatory geriatric outpatients or healthy older persons. Alternative forms of exercise such as housework, yardwork, and gardening need to receive more attention. Exercise assessment and subsequent prescriptions for older patients should include activities that enhance flexibility, strength (isometric or non–oxygen-utilizing exercise), and balance, in addition to aerobic benefit.

For older persons it is never too late to begin a physical activity and exercise regimen, and numerous healthy outcomes can be achieved. The primary care physician has an excellent opportunity to offer exercise advice and an exercise prescription during each office visit. Results of recent studies demonstrate high patient compliance rates, enthusiasm (of patients and physicians alike), and commitment by older patients to work on physical activities that are recommended by their primary care physician.[8,9]

EXERCISE PHYSIOLOGY AND AGING

Maximal physiological function and performance of many physical activities are thought to decline with one's chronological age, usually beginning in the third or fourth decade. Some of the more important aging-related changes are summarized in the accompanying box. There are significant person-specific differences in the onset and rate of these physiological changes. A major challenge for the primary care physician is to differentiate between individual rates of aging and development of signs and symptoms of disease. Often, the combination of a patient's declining physiological function and development of acute and chronic diseases contributes to a general loss of ability to perform physical exercise and recover from its effects.[3]

Maximum oxygen consumption and cardiovascular function

Exercise capacity (for overall aerobic fitness) is assessed by measuring the patient's maximum oxygen consumption (Vo_2 max), which is the product of cardiac output and systemic arteriovenous oxygen difference. This determination represents the maximal ability of the cardiovascular system to deliver oxygenated blood to the periphery and the capacity for muscle and other tissues that are exercised to extract oxygen from the blood. Although a 5% to 10% per decade decline in Vo_2 max has

---

**PHYSIOLOGICAL
PARAMETERS THAT CHANGE WITH NORMAL AGING**

Decrease in maximal cardiorespiratory performance
Decline in Vo_2 max*
Loss of muscle mass and strength
Decrease in bone density
Decline in glucose tolerance
Deterioration in lipid metabolism
Increase in percent body fat
Loss of height
Decrease in nerve conduction velocity

Vo_2 max, maximum oxygen consumption (or maximum aerobic capacity).

been reported in persons aged 25 to 75 years, this decrease is no longer thought to be secondary to age alone. Unrecognized coronary artery disease and physical deconditioning could account for such a decline in the study's subjects. Furthermore, healthy older persons may compensate for age-related decline in maximal heart rate by an increase in stroke volume; those who have more muscle mass may also ameliorate the decline in Vo_2 max.

Isometric exercise (strength)

In addition to isotonic (aerobic) forms of exercise in which muscle length changes (walking, running, swimming), isometric (anaerobic, static work, strength) exercise represents the common tasks and activities of daily living (lifting, pushing, or pulling against a fixed resistance). With isometric exercise, muscle length does not change and tension develops within the muscle to accommodate the load. Isometric activities are measured as strength (i.e., quantity of weight that can be lifted, pushed, or pulled).

The isometric contraction increases venous return and heart rate, resulting in increased cardiac output and elevation in both arterial and diastolic pressures. Many studies have demonstrated the gradual loss of one's maximal isometric strength between the ages of 30 and 80, which presumably results from a loss in the number of muscle fibers rather than size. In one's seventh decade, fibers that are primarily involved in isometric work decline by 5% to 10%. The number of functioning motor units in both upper and lower extremities also declines with one's age.

Increasingly, the accelerated loss of strength in older individuals appears to result from inactivity or nonuse of their muscles. If individuals perform the correct type and amount of exercise throughout their lives, strength can be maintained even among the oldest age groups. It is very important for older people to work on increasing their strength. Strength training can prevent accelerated muscle atrophy that occurs with years of inactivity. Activities of daily living are easier for persons who have greater strength, and more difficult work can be accomplished without fatigue. Stronger muscles are less likely to be injured. Exercise that increases patients' muscular strength also may be important for stimulating bone growth and retarding osteoporosis and fractures among the oldest age groups.

Flexibility

Flexibility is the range of motion around any particular joint. Flexibility is limited by the elasticity (or lack thereof) of the tendons, ligaments, and muscles that hold a joint together. Although flexibility is generally thought to decrease as one ages, this is not due to aging per se but to inactivity. Anyone (old or young) who is inactive loses flexibility. Flexibility exercises increase the blood flow to the muscles, making them an effective warm-up before other types of exercise. Additionally, a more flexible body may be less likely to sustain injury during activity.

Balance

Balance is one's ability to maintain equilibrium or to maintain the center of the body mass over the base of support. Studies of older adults indicate that small but significant disruptions in the temporal organization of postural muscle responses occur when subjects are given external threats. Older adults also have more difficulty with their balance when sensory inputs contributing to balance such as proprioception and vision are reduced.

ASSESSMENT OF EXERCISE AND PHYSICAL ACTIVITY IN OLDER PATIENTS

There are no valid assessment tools that measure or predict overall "healthy" life expectancy. Many instruments that assess the physical activity of older adults have been developed to exclude disease or decreased function. The following discussion reviews a primary care physician's assessment of physical activity for an ambulatory older patient during a routine office visit and emphasizes how to enhance the patient's healthy aging.

Exercise testing for older patients primarily assesses their safety to participate in exercise programs and helps physicians to formulate exercise prescriptions. Individualizing the patient's exercise goals is important for patients to achieve maximal benefit, compliance, enjoyment, and long-term participation.

Since cardiovascular, pulmonary, musculoskeletal and neurological dysfunctions are common in older patients, their primary care physicians must perform comprehensive health assessments, including medical history, physical examination, review of laboratory tests (especially serum cholesterol and HDL), physiological tests (weight, height, blood pressure, heart rate and percent body fat), and psychosocial and behavioral parameters. Based on these health status outcomes, the physicians should selectively order exercise tests that will help them to write appropriate exercise prescriptions. Some patients self-select for exercise testing, regardless of their preliminary health status outcomes or risk factors.

Exercise (stress) tests for aerobic exercise (endurance)

The most common instruments for evaluating a patients' aerobic capacity are the treadmill and the stationary bicycle ergometer. A bicycle test has several advantages: A patient's work rate can be easily varied and accurately quantified, thus V_{O_2} can be approximated in a patient for whom it is not possible to measure gas exchange. This is not the case for treadmill exercise where the work performed depends in part on the patient's weight. Bicycle ergometers are also less expensive, less bulky, and less noisy than treadmills. With upright bicycle ergometry, the patient's upper body remains stationary, which allows blood pressure to be measured easily and reduces motion artifact on the electrocardiogram.

However, the majority of exercise tests are performed on the treadmill. Many patients have leg muscle or knee joint pain, feel awkward riding a bicycle, or find the seat uncomfortable. (For further details about treadmill and bicycle ergometry testing, see the work by Weber and Janicki.[11])

A graded exercise test is indicated for any older person who is beginning a vigorous exercise program. Testing protocols use a constant treadmill speed with work increments that can be changed by adjusting the treadmill's incline. Speeds of 1.7 to 3.5 mph are often used for healthy adults, but testing of frail or severely deconditioned patients requires reduced intensity. The duration of each stage should be long enough for the subject to reach a steady state (at least 2 to 3 minutes). Grade increments should be chosen with the goal of expressing the patient's full range of exercise performance over a reasonable period of time.

If oxygen consumption can be measured during the stress test, functional capacity can be expressed in milliliters of oxygen consumed/kilogram/minute (ml/kg/min) and related to heart rate. The energy expenditure for most physical activities is calculated in METs (1 MET = resting oxygen consumption = 3.5 ml/kg/min or 1 kcal/kg/h) and can be extrapolated to a safe range of exercise intensity, usually 4 to 7 METs for most older individuals who display no cardiovascular limitations during maximal exercise testing. Physical activities suitable for ambulatory older patients are summarized from data published by Amundsen,[1] Birrer,[2] and Weber and Janicki.[11] (See the box on p. 192.)

For aerobic exercise to enhance a patient's cardiopulmonary capacity and metabolic function, large muscle groups (legs, back, shoulders) must be used repetitively in activities such as walking, swimming, stationary bicycling, and jogging. For older patients, aerobic exercises 3 to 4 times per week are recommended. Each session should include 5 to 10 minutes of warm-up stretches, 20 to 30 minutes of aerobic exercise, and 5 to 10 minutes of cool-down. The physician and patient together should review all health status outcomes and agree to a program that is likely to meet the patient's expectations and ensure compliance. A frequently recommended method for determining a target heart rate for aerobic exercise is summarized in Table 21-1. It should be remembered that the maximum heart rate for older patients should be recommended only after an appropriate exercise assessment and prescription have been individualized for the patient.

Assessment of strength

Isometric testing can be performed in a number of ways and on a variety of muscles. The hand dynamometer is a device that indicates the isometric effort of a patient's handgrip in pounds or kilograms and measures length of time that an isometric contraction can be maintained. Routine assessment of a patient's ankle and knee strength could prove helpful to the physician prescribing strengthening exercises.

PHYSICAL ACTIVITIES
SUITABLE FOR AMBULATORY OLDER PATIENTS

Very light (<3 METs; Vo_2 3.5-11 ml/kg/min)*

Activities of daily living
Driving an automobile
Shuffleboard, horseshoes, archery
Walking (level at 2 mph)
Playing golf (using a cart)
Stationary bicycling (very low resistance)

Light (3-5 METs; Vo_2 11-18 ml/kg/min)

Doing housework
Dancing (social)
Playing golf (walking)
Sailing
Playing tennis (doubles)
Walking (3-4 mph)
Level bicycling (6-8 mph)
Doing light calisthenics

Moderate (5-7 METs; Vo_2 18-25 ml/kg/min)

Gardening
Climbing stairs (slowly)
Carrying objects (30-60 lb)
Playing tennis (singles)
Walking (4.5-5 mph)
Bicycling (9-10 mph)
Swimming (breast stroke)
Snow skiiing (downhill)

Heavy (7-10 METs; Vo_2 25-32 ml/kg/min)

Swimming (fast)
Walking (6-7) mph
Playing squash
Cycling (12-14 mph)
Playing handball

From Amundsen LR: Cardiac considerations and physical training. In Jackson OL, ed: *Physical therapy of the geriatric patient*, ed 2, New York, 1989, Churchill Livingstone; Birrer RB: Prescribing physical activity for the elderly. In Harris R, Harris S, eds: *Physical activity, aging, and sports*, vol 1, Albany, NY, 1989, Scientific and Medical Research; Weber KT, Janicki JS: *Cardiopulmonary exercise testing: physiologic principles and clinical applications*, Philadelphia, 1986, WB Saunders.
*See text for explanation of METs and Vo_2.

Table 21-1 Determination of target heart rate for exercise

1. Take your pulse for 60 sec when you first wake up in the morning, 3 days in a row.
2. Add up the numbers and divide by 3 to get your average. Use the table below to determine your target heart rate. (The example is for a person age 70 years who is just starting a walking program.)
3. Beginners should exercise at about 60% of their maximum heart rate, intermediates at 70%, and advanced at 80%.

	You	Example
	220	220
Subtract your age	− _____	_____ 70
Your maximum heart rate		150
Subtract your resting rate	− _____	− _____ 72
		78
Your target heart zone (60%)	× _____ .60	× _____ .60
		47*
Add your resting rate	+ _____	+ _____ 72
Your target heart rate	_____	_____ 119

*46.8 rounded to 47.

Functional ankle movement becomes limited as one ages and could be improved by strengthening weak dorsiflexor muscles.

Exercises for strength are performed as repetitions of movements, with the total work done being the product of the resistance (e.g., a 5-lb weight) and the number of repetitions. As an individual becomes stronger over a period of weeks, total work should increase so that the patient continues to improve strength. Total work may be increased either by increasing the resistance or by increasing the number of repetitions. For older patients, the best formula for strength training is low resistance, high repetition.

Assessment of flexibility

Because flexibility is not a general measurement but rather specific to each joint or group of joints, commonly performed assessments like the sit-and-reach test provide limited information, except for flexibility of the trunk and hips while the patient bends forward. More accurate methods to determine the flexibility of a joint include the goniometer, Leighton flexometer, or Elgan electrogoniometer, the most accurate method.

Until agreement is reached about an adequate assessment for a patient's flexibility, the primary care physician may limit testing to the patient's activities of normal daily living where flexibility is necessary (e.g., tieing one's shoes). Besides inactivity, flexibility may be limited by the patient's age, arthritis, obesity, injuries, and congenital abnormalities.

The only way to increase one's flexibility is by regularly performing stretching exercises. Stretching should be done slowly and under control, since muscles tend to resist stretching if it is done too quickly. Patients should focus on stretching large muscle groups, especially the lower back and the hamstring muscles. Stretching should be done for a minimum of 20 to 30 min/day before and after other forms of exercise, and anytime a person feels the need.

Assessment of balance

There are currently no standardized methods of assessment for balance. Until standardized instruments for assessment are available, the physician must rely upon traditional evaluations of balance, including the patient's history, physical examination, and performance-based tests. (See Chapter 13.)

PRESCRIPTION FOR EXERCISE AND OTHER HEALTH BEHAVIORS

Evidence is accumulating from both cross-sectional and longitudinal studies, and recently from controlled intervention studies, that interventions for healthy behaviors play major roles in reducing morbidity and improving quality of life for the patient at any age.

Investigators also have demonstrated the benefits of increasing physical activity and exercise for older men and women (e.g., psychological functioning, physical performance, skeletal muscle mass and function, aerobic endurance, strength, balance, and flexibility[2,4,5,7]). Conditions and function decrements that are associated with aging but ameliorated or enhanced by physical activity are listed in Table 21-2.

Table 21-2 Aging-associated conditions and function decrements ameliorated or improved with exercise and physical activity

Conditions	Function decrements	
Arthritis	Balance	Lung reserve
Atherosclerosis	Bone density	Metabolic function
Back pain	Control	Mobility
Depression	Energy	Muscle mass
Diabetes mellitus	Enthusiasm	Reaction time
Falls and fractures	Flexibility	Self-esteem
Heart disease	Heart reserve	Self-efficiency
Hypertension	Independence	Sleep quality
Memory loss	Individuality	Strength
Obesity	(self-expression)	Weight control
Osteoporosis		Well-being
Stress		
Thrombophlebitis		
Varicose veins		

These studies and others provide strong evidence that a primary care physician who treats a patient of any chronological age and baseline health status can implement a person-specific health assessment to evaluate outcomes of interventions for healthy aging, promotion of health, and preventive medicine for that patient.[6,10]

REFERENCES

1. Amundsen LR: Cardiac considerations and physical training. In Jackson OL, ed: *Physical therapy of the geriatric patient*, ed 2, New York, 1989, Churchill Livingstone.
2. Birrer RB: Prescribing physical activity for the elderly. In Harris R, Harris S, eds: *Physical activity, aging, and sports*, vol 1, Albany, NY, 1989, Scientific and Medical Research.
3. Blumenthal JA et al: Long-term effects of exercise on psychological functioning in older men and women, *J Gerontol* 46:353, 1991.
4. Brown M, Holloszy JO: Effects of a low-intensity exercise program on selected physical performance characteristics of 60- to 71-year-olds, *Aging* 3:129, 1991.
5. Fiaterone MA et al: High-intensity strength training in nonagenarians: effects on skeletal muscle, *JAMA* 263:3029, 1990.
6. Morey MC et al: Two year trends in physical performance following supervised exercise among community-dwelling older veterans, *J Am Geriatr Soc* 39:986, 1991.
7. Posner JD et al: Low- to moderate-intensity endurance training in healthy older adults: physiological responses after fou. months, *J Am Geriatr Soc* 40:1, 1992.
8. Schmidt RM: Healthy aging research: application to primary health care in a retired cohort of men and women age 65 to 89, *Gerontologist* 31:359, 1991.
9. Schmidt RM et al: Evaluating outcomes of healthy aging interventions: the health watch or Arizona study in the Sun Cities, *Gerontologist* 30:8, 1990.
10. Schmidt RM, Wu M: Health watch: a person-specific assessment system to evaluate outcomes of healthy aging interventions, health promotion, and preventive medicine in an aging America. In Felitti VJ, ed: *Health evaluation: searching for the hidden defect*, Rockville, Md, 1991, International Health Evaluation Association.
11. Weber KT, Janicki JS: *Cardiopulmonary exercise testing: physiologic principles and clinical applications*, Philadelphia, 1986, WB Saunders.

SUGGESTED READINGS

Schmidt RM, Kligman EW, Lutz MA: *Health and wellness resource guide: health watch of Arizona*, Sun City, Ariz, 1989, Allied University Research in Aging/Sun Health Corporation.
U.S. Preventive Services Task Force: *Guide to clinical preventive services: an assessment of the effectiveness of 169 interventions*, Baltimore, 1989, Williams & Wilkins.
Shepart RJ: The scientific bases of exercise prescribing for the very old, *J Am Geriatr Soc* 3:62, 1990.

CHAPTER 22

Preventive interventions

RICHARD REED

KEY POINTS

- Preventive services should be incorporated into daily office practice.
- Preventive activities occur at three levels: primary prevention (preventing development of disease), secondary prevention (detecting asymptomatic disease), and tertiary prevention (reducing complications and disabilities from existing disease).
- Although several preventive interventions are beneficial and cost effective for older persons, there is a lack of data on potential benefits of many preventive services for this population.

The care of the older patient in the ambulatory setting increasingly requires a preventive orientation. However, data specifically demonstrating the value of several preventive procedures are limited for older persons. This is particularly true for the very old (e.g., 75 years and older) for whom extrapolating data from middle-aged populations may not be appropriate. For example, elevated blood pressure in the very old actually appears to be protective for survival in men in one study.[5] The goal of this chapter is to highlight what is and is not known in this rapidly evolving area. Current recommendations made by the U.S. Preventive Services Task Force (USPSTF)[10,11] and the Canadian Task Force (CTF),[3] two advisory groups that provide comprehensive recommendations for screening and counseling activities, will be reviewed.

Preventive activities are typically divided into three levels, including primary, secondary, and tertiary prevention. *Primary prevention* involves preventing the development of disease in individuals. Typical interventions include modifying high-risk health behaviors (e.g., smoking or high-fat diet) or chemoprophylaxis of disease (e.g., use of agents to prevent cancer or osteoporosis). *Secondary prevention* or screening involves detecting disease while it is asymptomatic or in an early stage of development. Screening is most effective if an intervention cures or significantly ameliorates further development of complications that are associated with the disease state. *Tertiary prevention* involves preventing subsequent disability from a disease that has already manifested itself. Much of the rehabilitation process can be labeled tertiary prevention. Comprehensive geriatric assessment and treatment, a systematic process for identifying causes of functional disabilities in older subjects who have clinical diseases, is increasingly important for tertiary prevention.

PRIMARY PREVENTION

A variety of primary preventive services that promote health should be available for older patients. These services include counseling, immunizations, and chemoprophylaxis.

Counseling to change health behaviors

Smoking cessation. The decision to quit smoking is the most important health-related change in behavior that an individual can make, regardless of age. There is a high prevalence of smoking among older age groups, with 19% of older persons aged 65 to 74 who are current cigarette smokers and 9% of those aged 75 and older who are smokers.[4] In addition, nearly 8% of men aged 75 and older report their using snuff or chewing tobacco. Although trials of techniques for smoking cessation have not been specifically studied for older adults, studies for younger populations indicate that direct face-to-face advice is preferred where a brief unambiguous statement about the need to stop smoking is made. Data on quitting and reassurance that smokers require several attempts prior to successful long-term cessation can also aid in patients' adherence to their physician's recommendations. Scheduled support visits or telephone calls can enhance compliance. Use of nicotine gum has not been studied for elderly persons and therefore cannot be recommended.

Physical activity. The USPSTF recommends that physicians provide information about the role exercise has in disease prevention as well as select the appropriate exercises. The use of preexercise evaluation is often indicated. A more complete discussion of exercise is described in Chapter 21.

Nutrition. Individuals below the poverty level and those who have multiple chronic diseases are most in need of specific nutritional interventions. Overnutrition (obesity) is also a significant concern; however, mild obesity may be somewhat protective for mortality, particularly for the very old who may benefit from the additional energy stores during periods of acute illness. (See Chapter 45.) Components of the diet are a special concern, and physicians' counseling concerning dietary intake of calories, fat and cholesterol, complex carbohydrates, calcium, sodium, and fiber is recommended by the USPSTF. (See Chapter 20.)

Injury prevention. Injuries are the fifth most common cause of deaths for individuals aged 65 years and older. Approximately two thirds of these deaths are attributed to falls. Several risk factors have been associated with falling, but no study has demonstrated that reversing these risk factors results in a lower incidence of falls or fall-related morbidity or mortality for older individuals. (See Chapter 31.) Several trials are currently in progress. The USPSTF recommends that physicians counsel older patients or their caregivers about home inspection and modification, as well as test patients' vision and monitor their use of drugs that are associated with increased risk of falling. (See Chapter 18.) Exercise programs are also recommended to improve mobility and flexibility for patients who have no contraindications.

Other preventive recommendations such as not driving while intoxicated, crossing streets safely, using seat belts, handling firearms with care, not smoking in bed, and decreasing hot water temperature also should be considered for discussion.

Oral health. Daily brushing and flossing of teeth and regular dental checkups on a yearly or biannual basis are recommended for older patients. Physicians should routinely perform oral examinations and look for decayed teeth or oral lesions. (See Chapter 47.)

Immunizations

Influenza vaccine. Few preventive services have had as substantial a documented efficacy as the influenza vaccine, which should be given annually to all those persons aged 65 years and older. During an influenza A outbreak among persons who are at especially high risk, such as those living in retirement centers or nursing homes, amantadine prophylaxis also should be given daily immediately for 2 weeks after immunization or if immunization is contraindicated, for the duration of influenza activity in the community.

Pneumococcal vaccine. Pneumococcal vaccine is recommended for all persons aged 65 years and older. This is based on convincing clinical trials in younger populations. The cumulative weight of evidence from several case-control studies suggests an efficacy of approximately 60% for the vaccine's preventing bacteremic disease in immunocompetent persons.[2] Pneumococcal vaccine is underutilized by primary care physicians.

Tetanus vaccine. The efficacy of tetanus vaccine in preventing tetanus is well documented. In addition, tetanus more commonly leads to death for older persons than for younger adults. Therefore, there is almost universal agreement that a primary series of immunizations should be given in older adults who have not previously been vaccinated, and previously immunized patients should receive a booster every 10 years.

Chemoprophylaxis

Aspirin. Aspirin decreases the risk of strokes for patients who have transient ischemic attacks (TIAs) or histories of stroke, prevents recurrent myocardial infarctions (MIs) for survivors of MI, reduces mortality for patients who have acute MIs, and prevents MI and death for individuals who have unstable angina.[6,9] The USPSTF recommends discussion of the risks and benefits of aspirin for primary prevention of MI for individuals who have high cholesterol or other risk factors and do not have contraindications for therapy. These contraindications include uncontrolled hypertension, peptic ulcer disease, a history of any type of bleeding or bleeding disorders, risk factors for bleeding or cerebral hemorrhage, and liver or kidney disease. Some controversy still exists because an increased incidence of cerebral hemorrhages was noted in some studies.

Estrogen replacement. The USPSTF recommends that physicians consider estrogen treatment for women who have risk factors for osteoporosis, including low mineral content of bone, white or Asian race, slender body build, and history of bilateral oophorectomy before menopause or history of early menopause. Contraindications include thromboembolic disorders, history of hormone-dependent cancer, undiagnosed vaginal bleeding, or active liver disease.

Vitamin and mineral supplements. Use of vitamin and mineral supplements is a very common practice by older individuals. Oversupplementation is frequent, although toxicity is rarely reported. Supplementation appears to be prudent for individuals who consume less than 1000 kilo-calories per day, which may be up to 16% of white and 18% of black individuals aged 60 to 74.[1] However, for the remainder of older individuals who consume adequate calories and a full range of foods, these supplements are probably not necessary, with the exception of calcium, which is generally lacking in the diets of both women and men. (See Chapter 20.)

SECONDARY PREVENTION
Cancer

Several screening services should be provided routinely to geriatric patients. Table 22-1 lists cancer screening guidelines that are recommended by the USPSTF, CTF, and American Cancer Society (ACS).[7]

Breast cancer. Screening techniques for breast cancer include self-examination, examination by a physician, and mammography. Both examination by a physician and mammography are additive in the detection of breast carcinomas. A negative mammogram in the presence of a palpable mass still should be considered suspicious. Thus, the examination and mammogram should be viewed as complementary procedures. The frequency of physical examination and mammography is somewhat controversial and varies among different organizations.

Colorectal cancer. Colorectal cancer is the leading cause of death from cancer in the United States. For those who are over the age of 50, current screening recommendations for colon cancer vary widely among medical advisory groups. Several clinical trials of fecal occult blood testing (FOBT) and flexible sigmoidoscopy are currently being tested or planned. It may be prudent for physicians to screen those

Table 22-1 Cancer screening for persons 65 years and older

Cancer screening modality	Recommendations		
	U.S. Preventive Services Task Force	American Cancer Society	Canadian Task Force
Breast cancer			
Self-examination	No evidence	No evidence	No evidence
Clinical examination	Every 1-2 years until 75	Yearly	Yearly
Mammogram	Every 1-2 years until 75	Yearly	Yearly
Colon cancer			
Fecal occult blood	No evidence*	Yearly	No evidence*
Sigmoidoscopy	No evidence*	Every 3-5 years according to physician	No evidence*
Cervical cancer			
Pap smear	NR† if consistently normal up to age 65	Yearly; less frequently if consistently normal 3 times or more	Every 5 years; more or less depending on clinical judgement
Prostate cancer			
Digital rectal examination	No evidence	Yearly	No evidence
Prostate specific antigen	NR	No evidence	NE‡
Skin cancer			
Self-examination	No evidence	NE	NE
Clinical examination	If high risk	Yearly	If high risk
Ovarian cancer			
Pelvic examination	NR	Yearly above 40	NE
Oral cancer			
Clinical examination	NR except if high risk	Yearly	No evidence

*No evidence; there is insufficient evidence for or against the use of a test in asymptomatic persons aged 65 and older without risk factors; further data are needed (*for low risk groups only).
†NE, not recommended.
‡NR, not evaluated.

Table 22-1 Cancer screening for persons 65 years and older—cont'd

Cancer screening modality	Recommendations		
	U.S. Preventive Services Task Force	American Cancer Society	Canadian Task Force
Thyroid cancer			
Clinical examination	Regularly if exposed to upper body radiation	Yearly	NE
Testicular cancer			
Clinical examination	NE	Yearly	No evidence

who have a previous diagnosis of inflammatory bowel disease, adenomatous polyps or colorectal cancer, a previous history of endometrial, ovarian or breast cancer, and those with first-degree relatives with colorectal cancer.[11] Colonoscopy is recommended for those with familial polyposis or family cancer syndromes.[11]

Cervical cancer. Approximately three fourths of women who are aged 65 years and older have not received Papanicolaou smears on a regular basis. Currently, the USPSTF recommends that screenings for women may stop when they are 65 years old if regular screenings have been negative. If screening has not been done or has been erratic, regular examinations including Papanicolaou smears should be undertaken at an interval of once every 1 to 3 years.

Prostate cancer. Prostate cancer is currently the most common cancer in American men, and is predominantly manifested in elderly men. (See Chapter 25.) However, there is no definitive evidence that early intervention in the treatment of prostate cancer significantly alters the course of the disease. Although screening tests such as digital rectal examination, transrectal ultrasound, and prostate-specific antigen exist, the ability of screening programs to alter morbidity or mortality rates from this disease has not been demonstrated. The ACS currently recommends routine digital rectal examinations in asymptomatic men while the CTF and USPSTF do not recommend this procedure. Other tests are being evaluated.

Skin cancer. Skin cancer is increasing at epidemic proportions and particularly afflicts older individuals. (See Chapter 29.) A clinical evaluation of individuals who have increased exposure to the sun should occur on a regular basis, and regular evaluation of older individuals who have normal exposure may be clinically prudent. Data concerning self-examination is insufficient to make a recommendation.

Other carcinomas. Currently, it is not recommended by the USPSTF that screenings should be performed for lung cancer, oral cancer, pancreatic cancer, or ovarian cancer. With the exception of lung cancer, these are not universal recommendations. Current recommendations are listed in Table 22-1.

Coronary artery disease and stroke

Coronary artery disease. Over 80% of deaths from coronary artery disease (CAD) occur in people aged 65 years and older, making CAD the most common cause of death in the elderly population. The only primary screening mechanism for CAD is electrocardiography. Routine electrocardiography (ECG) is not recommended for screening of asymptomatic individuals. The USPSTF states that it may be clinically prudent for physicians to perform screening ECGs on asymptomatic men who have two or more cardiac risk factors. (See Table 22-2.)

Table 22-2   Screening examination for vascular disease among asymptomatic people 65 years or older

Vascular disease	U.S. task force	Canadian task force
Asymptomatic CAD		
Resting ECG	May be clinically prudent for asymptomatic men who have two or more risk factors or those who would endanger public safety because of sudden cardiac events	Poor evidence regarding inclusion of asymptomatic patients; recommendations made on other factors
Exercise ECG	May be prudent in sedentary or high-risk males who are beginning vigorous exercise	Poor evidence regarding inclusion of asymptomatic patients; recommendations made on other factors
Cerebrovascular disease		
Carotid bruit	No recommendations; may be prudent if CAD or risk factors for cerebrovascular disease are present	Poor evidence regarding inclusion of asymptomatic patients; recommendations made on other factors
Noninvasive testing	No recommendations; may be prudent if CAD or risk factors for cerebrovascular disease are present	Not evaluated
TIA symptoms	Should ask about history of symptoms	Not evaluated
Peripheral artery disease		
Noninvasive testing	Not recommended	Not evaluated

Cerebrovascular disease (stroke). Cerebrovascular disease is the third leading cause of death in the United States, with the majority of deaths (55%) occurring among those who are 65 and older. The USPSTF concludes that there is insufficient evidence for auscultation of carotid bruits or other noninvasive testing to support recommendations in this area. The task force notes that it may be clinically prudent for physicians to screen by carotid auscultation those patients who have established risk factors for stroke, including advanced age, smoking, hypertension, CAD, atrial fibrillation, diabetes mellitus, neurological symptoms of transient ischemic attacks (TIA), or previous stroke. (See Table 22-2.)

Risk factors associated with coronary artery disease and stroke (Table 22-3)

Hypertension. Both diastolic and systolic blood pressure appear to be important risk factors for CAD among older persons. (See Chapter 53.) Blood pressure should be evaluated every 1 to 2 years for individuals who are normotensive. The diagnosis of hypertension requires abnormal pressure readings on at least three separate occasions. Nonpharmacological therapy should be tried initially, unless the patient's blood pressure is substantially elevated, and should include an exercise prescription, weight loss for the obese, and a limitation on sodium and alcohol consumption.

Table 22-3 Risk factors for coronary artery disease and stroke and recommendations for screening

Risk factor and screening measurement	U.S. task force	Canadian task force
Hypertension		
Blood pressure measurements	Screen every 2 years	At least every 2 years; should be done at all visits to physician
Obesity		
Anthropometric measurements	Height and weight should be measured routinely	Not evaluated
Diabetes mellitus		
Fasting glucose	Not recommended for asymptomatic adults; may be prudent for high-risk adults (obese, family history of diabetes, history of gestational diabetes)	Not recommended for general population; some evidence for inclusion in high-risk group
Lipids		
Cholesterol	Should be done at intervals at discretion of physician	Not evaluated
Lipid profile	For those who are receiving or may receive drug therapy	Not evaluated

Smoking. Smoking cessation always should be recommended.

Obesity. Obesity is a risk factor for a patient's developing coronary artery disease, diabetes mellitus, elevated blood pressure, and increased serum cholesterol. (See Chapter 45.) The USPSTF currently recommends that weight and height measurements should be made, and either a table of desirable weights should be used or body mass index (weight/height^2) should be calculated. A body mass index that is higher than 27.8 for men or 27.3 for women or 20% above desirable weight measurements should serve as a threshold for dietary and exercise recommendations.

Diabetes mellitus. There is no evidence that early diagnosis of diabetes mellitus decreases a patient's risk for CAD or other complications. Screenings for asymptomatic patients are therefore not recommended. (See Chapter 43.)

Cholesterol and lipid profile. Serum cholesterol is still positively correlated with CADs for elderly persons, but the degree of correlation is one third lower than that for younger cohorts. Currently, the National Cholesterol Education Program[8] recommends that all adults who have high blood cholesterol (240 mg/dl or above) and those who have borderline high cholesterol (200 to 239 mg/dl) with known CAD or two or more risk factors (male gender, premature CAD in first-degree relative, smoking, hypertension, high-density lipoprotein cholesterol below 35 mg/dl, diabetes mellitus, stroke, peripheral vascular disease, or severe obesity) should receive counseling on dietary modifications.

SCREENING FOR OTHER CONDITIONS
Functional status

Monitoring an individual's functional abilities over time is an important component of all geriatric care. Instrumental activities of daily living (IADL) and activities of daily living (ADL) are predictive of a patient's mortality, health care needs and cost, as well as quality of life. Mechanisms to evaluate these abilities on a routine basis are strongly recommended. Physicians can do these evaluations informally through clinical histories or by formal questionnaires and performance-based testing. (See Chapter 13.)

Both the USPSTF and CTF recommend hearing screenings with follow-up otoscopic examinations and audiometric tests for individuals who have evidence of hearing loss, which may identify treatable causes. (See Chapter 17.)

The USPSTF recommends that physicians routinely test elderly patients' visual acuity and make follow-up referrals to eye specialists. The task force does not recommend routine tonometry by primary care physicians but believes that it may be clinically prudent to advise elderly persons about glaucoma testing by their eye specialists. (See Chapter 55.)

Psychological and social issues

Depression and bereavement. The USPSTF currently does not recommend screening for depression in asymptomatic older adults but does recommend questioning patients concerning their emotional well-being when histories reveal risk factors for suicide such as recent divorce or separation, depression, alcohol or other drug abuse, serious medical illness, or recent bereavement.

Alcohol and other drug use. Alcoholism continues to be an important problem throughout a patient's life span. Estimates suggest that approximately 10% of persons aged 65 years and older have a drinking problem, while 8% are alcohol dependent.[3] The USPSTF recommends that physicians should routinely ask patients about their use of alcohol or other drugs. Alcohol screening questionnaires are also useful.

Metabolic and nutritional problems

Thyroid disease. Thyroid disease is common among older populations.[11] The USPSTF recommends that routine screening may be clinically prudent for older persons, especially women. A specific screening test was not recommended. (See Chapter 44.)

Osteoporosis. Osteoporosis is a common concomitant of aging, particularly for women. (See Chapter 42.) Although early detection and treatment may potentially result in better outcomes, there is no evidence of clear-cut improvements in outcomes. Currently, measurement of bone-mass density is not recommended for asymptomatic women. All older female patients should receive counseling about the risks and benefits of calcium supplementation, exercise, and estrogen replacement, particularly those who have risk factors for osteoporosis (e.g., smoking history or white race).

Other screening techniques

Urinalysis. Currently there is no consensus about the optimal methodology for urinary screening or whether the urinalysis has a significant sensitivity and specificity for routine screening. The USPSTF believes that it is clinically prudent for periodic testing for asymptomatic bacteriuria, hematuria, and proteinuria in elderly patients.

Anemia. Because the morbidity and mortality associated with anemia are usually caused by coexisting disorders, routine screening for anemia in asymptomatic individuals is not recommended. (See Chapter 46.)

Tuberculosis. Tuberculosis rates are highest for elderly persons, and the majority of these cases occur among those living in the community. Individuals who are thought to be at higher risk (e.g., minority populations, low body weight, and those living in enclosed high-density settings) should be routinely screened by tuberculin skin tests and appropriate follow-ups. Testing for the booster phenomenon is indicated for frail older populations.

TERTIARY PREVENTION

All health care should include an effort to prevent subsequent disability. For instance, the astute primary care physician caring for a patient who had a stroke can do much to prevent further sequelae of this devastating illness. Recognition and treatment of depression, reduction of medications, prevention of hypotension, and specific rehabilitation interventions are tertiary preventive measures for the stroke patient. Similarly, excess disability in the patient who has dementia can also be prevented. Associated depression can be treated, the patient's medical condition can be optimized, and drug side effects can be limited.

MAINTAINING A PREVENTIVE EMPHASIS IN AMBULATORY PRACTICE

Important preventive services can be incorporated into the physician's daily office practice. An annual examination can be scheduled for systematic review of an individual's preventive services needs, in addition to the physician's addressing these issues during routine visits. Another useful adjunct is the development of an age-specific checklist that addresses relevant preventive issues. These checklists need to be dynamic as new data become available for the patient and require individual decision making after the physician carefully reviews the relevant literature.

REFERENCES

1. Abrahams S et al: Dietary intake of persons 1-74 years of age in the United States: advance data from vital and health statistics of the National Center for Health Statistics, Pub No 6, Rockville, Md, March 1979, Health Resources Administration, Public Health Service.
2. Broome CV, Breiman RF: Pneumococcal vaccine: past, present and future, *N Engl J Med* 324:1500, 1991.
3. Canadian Task Force on the Periodic Health Examination: The periodic health examination. II. 1989 update, *Can Med Assoc J* 142:955, 1990.
4. Centers for Disease Control: Tobacco use by adults: United States, *MMWR* 38:685, 1989.
5. Langer RD, Ganits TG, Barrett-Connor E: Paradoxical survival of elderly men with high blood pressure, *Br Med J* 298:1356, 1989.
6. Manson JE et al: A prospective study of aspirin use and primary prevention of cardiovascular disease in women, *JAMA* 266:521, 1991.
7. Mettlin C, Dodd G: The American Cancer Society guidelines for the cancer-related checkup: an update, *CA* 41:279, 1991.
8. Report by the National Cholesterol Education Program Expert Panel on detection, evaluation, and treatment of high blood cholesterol in adults, *Arch Intern Med* 148:36, 1988.
9. Steering Committee of the Physician's Health Study Research Group: Final report on the aspirin component of the ongoing physicians' health study, *N Engl J Med* 321:129, 1989.
10. Woolf SH et al: The periodic health examination of older adults: the recommendations of the U.S. Preventive Services Task Force. I. counseling, immunizations and chemoprophylaxis, *J Am Geriatr Soc* 38:817, 1990.
11. Woolf SH et al: The periodic health examination of older adults: the recommendations of the U.S. Preventive Services Task Force. II. screening tests, *J Am Geriatr Soc* 38:93, 1990.

SUGGESTED READINGS

Woolf SH et al: The periodic health examination of older adults: The recommendations of the U.S. Preventive Services Task Force. I. counseling, immunizations and chemoprophylaxis, *J Am Geriatr Soc* 38:817, 1990.

Woolf SH et al: The periodic health examination of older adults: The recommendations of the U.S. Preventive Services Task Force. II. screening tests, *J Am Geriatr Soc* 38:933, 1990.

CHAPTER 23

Social and spiritual contributors to independence

LEAH ELLENHORN STROMBERG

KEY POINTS

- Social function and spirituality of elderly patients impact their overall health and the utilization of health services.
- Social and spiritual supports can enhance life satisfaction for the elderly persons, even in the face of declining health.
- Interventions involving informal and formal social and spiritual resources can help prevent depression, disease and an unnecessary decline in function for the elderly persons.
- Psychosocial and spiritual interventions can assist elderly people in developing and maintaining social and spiritual reserves (or credits) for future use.
- Special populations must be approached thoughtfully; the recognition and acceptance of cultural diversity by clinicians can lead to the effective selection of specialized resources and treatment modalities.

SOCIAL FUNCTION IN THE CONTEXT OF OVERALL FUNCTION

The assessment of social function involves an investigation of the patient's interactions with others and with the environment. Kinship ties, friendships, and group affiliations are important aspects of the patient's social function as are activities such as work, hobbies, and interests. Cultural and religious connections provide a framework for living and link individuals with others who hold common values. The availability and quality of social resources such as family support, housing, and income are key ingredients of social function as are the patient's inner resources, expectations, motivation, and adaptability. These key components all determine, to a large extent, the degree to which aging becomes a process that is filled with enrichment and meaning or despair and disappointment.

The relationship between social function and health becomes evident when one examines the use of health services by elderly people. Older persons who are depressed, alone (and lonely), or have difficulty adapting to change are more likely to appear in their physicians' offices than those who have good social support systems and histories of creative adaptations to life's transitions. Studies have shown that, regardless of marital status, elderly persons who live with others are less likely to use health services than elderly persons who live alone.[3] However, elderly spouses who are caregivers report impaired social function and more physical ailments, depression, and fatigue than age-matched populations.

The physical symptoms that elderly patients have may often be in part the expression of underlying psychosocial dysfunction. Elderly patients, especially those in the current cohort groups, may be reluctant to reveal social or emotional problems because of their fear of embarrassment or ridicule. In some cultures it is unacceptable to share personal matters with outsiders; it is far more acceptable to complain of sleeplessness or pain, for example. While poor nutrition may have its origins in an organic malfunction, it may also be symptomatic of a psychosocial problem such as poor adaptation to widowhood, inability to budget limited finances, or a reaction to the loss of an important social support.

The challenge to persons in medical and human service professions is to assess health and treat illness by considering the interaction between the patient's physical, emotional, and social characteristics. A change in physical health can have profound effects upon an individual's ability to maintain independence and well-being. Conversely, a change in one's social resources can begin a chain of events leading to a decline in physical health and overall function. Social function like other functional domains (physical, cognitive, emotional, environmental) impacts the overall function of an elderly person.[5]

This concept that social function impacts the overall function of the elderly is meaningful for several reasons. First, it demonstrates the interdependence of the various elements that comprise overall function including physical, cognitive, emotional, spiritual, and social factors. An individual's physical health is affected by such factors as heredity, diet, and exercise; social factors such as environment and family support can greatly influence the overall equation for functional capacity. Important clues to the diagnosis and treatment of health problems can be detected through careful exploration of the patient's social function. Second, and of great significance to the clinician, there are areas of social function that are amenable to intervention. Often the most beneficial and easily accomplished treatments are those that incorporate psychosocial, environmental, and spiritual interventions. Dial-a-ride transportation, friendly visitor programs, telephone reassurance, congregate meals, and case management are examples of community-based social services that can prevent the chain of events leading to disease, depression, and unnecessary institutionalization of elderly persons.

PERSONS AT RISK FOR PSYCHOSOCIAL DYSFUNCTION

It is difficult to characterize elderly people as a group because enormous diversity exists regarding their health, social and environmental supports, financial security, and cultural and personal philosophies. However, elderly persons are distinctive for two reasons: (1) certain developmental milestones impact large numbers of older persons (e.g., retirement, widowhood), and (2) large numbers of elderly persons lack the resources and resourcefulness (i.e., the social reserves) to cope effectively with aging-related phenomena. Many situations require elderly persons to draw upon their accumulated social reserves to adapt to change and restore well-being.

Elderly persons seem to be most vulnerable to psychosocial dysfunction when they experience change. (See the box below.) Events such as retirement, widowhood, deaths of close friends, and changes in household composition may be the impetus for physical and mental health problems. Relocation, immigration, and financial difficulties also may signal the need for elderly persons to mobilize their inner strengths and social reserves. When these resources are either insufficient or maladaptive, elderly people develop a high risk for psychosocial and medical problems. The following is a discussion of the most common areas of risk.

Retirement and role loss

For some elderly persons retirement is a long awaited and celebrated occasion to enjoy freedom from regimentation and accountability. Studies have shown that retirement will be a stressful event for a minority of elders for whom retirement has negative implications.[2] Many older persons, especially those who are in good health, take on new more satisfying activities—even second careers. However, for others retirement may mean the loss of prestige, status, or sense of accomplishment that accompanied their jobs, as well as the loss of a network of social relationships throughout the work place. Many elderly persons, especially those whose retirement has come about involuntarily, find themselves feeling isolated, displaced, and uncomfortable without the structured activity of the office or factory. Often retirees mourn the loss

---

_____ **RISK FACTORS FOR PSYCHOSOCIAL DYSFUNCTION** _____

Retirement/role loss
Widowhood
Deaths of close friends
Family problems
Relocation
Financial problems

of their feeling productive, which was provided by their work, and experience emptiness after retirement. Married retirees are commonly affected by a phenomenon called *impingement*, which is characterized by complaints about a general lack of privacy and an inequitable division of labor in the home.[9]

As older people live longer and healthier lives, many seek greater flexibility in the work place. In many settings, the mandatory retirement age has increased or has been abolished. Opportunities for part-time work, consulting, volunteering, and second careers have increased as well. Many corporations offer extensive preretirement planning services to help prepare employees for the future. Unfortunately, many older workers must face early retirement, often involuntarily, because of plant closings and layoffs. The Social Security system provides some benefits to those who wish to retire earlier than age 65.

Many older persons retire to care for their aged parents or spouses. The substitution of one set of responsibilities for another, without the benefit of pay or social contact, can be depressing and stressful. Caregiver burden may manifest itself in many different ways, including physical symptoms, fatigue, isolation, depression, domestic violence, substance abuse, and noncompliance with medical advice.

Death of a spouse

Approximately one half of all women aged 65 years and older are widows. Among males, 13% of those aged 65 years and older are widowers.[4] A bereaved person usually receives a large amount of community and family support immediately after experiencing a loss. This support diminishes considerably over time as family and friends return to their own responsibilities, while the older person begins to adjust to the loss of a spouse.

Most widows and widowers initially choose to live alone. Some move in with adult children or siblings. There may be drawbacks to either decision. While living alone offers older people the opportunity to maintain their independence, it may be lonely and frightening for those who are unskilled at finding substitute sources of friendship and support. Alternatively, many elderly persons and their families regret the decision to live together. Older persons often feel rejected, scrutinized, and uncomfortably dependent. The families may feel burdened by parent-child role confusion and expenses and may feel intruded upon by their older relatives.

Losing a spouse may be the event that signals an abrupt change in financial status for an older person. Many older people find their incomes drastically reduced by the loss of benefits at a time when they are unlikely to earn additional income. Some widows and widowers are completely unprepared for the task of managing money. The death of a spouse frequently is preceded by months or years of illness. In addition to the grief and exhaustion experienced after the loss of a partner who had been ill, the bereaved spouse may face the unfortunate task of sorting through thousands of dollars of unpaid medical bills.

While much has been written about the problems of elderly widows, attention also must be given to the needs of elderly widowers. In the current cohort groups, men are often inexperienced in household activities.

It must be noted that one's grief and sadness following the death of a spouse may be accompanied by feelings of relief and even gladness. All marriages are not universally blissful, and many elderly persons remain unhappily married for personal, religious, and cultural reasons. Others may express feelings of liberation after the deaths of spouses who had been ill and in need of a great amount of caregiving.

Single and childless elderly persons

The single and childless elderly population is important for several reasons. First, the number of persons in this category is increasing as divorce rates are increasing and fertility rates are decreasing. This category also includes many homosexual elderly persons whose special needs are often overlooked. Second, single and childless elderly persons are more likely to find themselves in residential care or institutions than elderly people who are married or have children.

The popular conception that older people are alienated from their families is a myth. Even when there are no children, older people often strengthen their relationships with other kin, particularly siblings.[8] In times of stress most unmarried older persons or those who have lost their spouses turn to family for support, even when close ties with friends and neighbors exist. Because friendships are by definition voluntary associations, there may be great reluctance for elderly people to burden friends about psychosocial needs. When families are not available or do not exist, older people are vulnerable to problems if they cannot solicit support from resources that are available through friends or formal organizations.

Family problems and changes in household composition

Many types of family scenarios can create high-risk situations for elderly people such as divorce (their own or that of a child) or adult children who move back home, often with grandchildren. In addition, the adult children may resist moving out. If the adult children are financially dependent, many elderly persons find themselves supporting their adult children by Social Security retirement benefits or SSI (Supplemental Security Income for low-income persons) when they cannot afford to do so. Older adults may have to provide care for disabled spouses, children, or grandchildren. There may be a substance abuse problem (their own or that of a close relative). Elderly persons may experience personal void resulting from "empty nests" as their children leave home. Finally, there may be well-meaning but overprotective relatives who restrict elderly people's autonomy by taking away their responsibilities and rights to make decisions and take risks.

SPIRITUALITY AND HEALTH

Numerous studies have confirmed the importance of faith and religious belief to older persons. Older persons are more involved in church activities than the general population; 97% of persons aged 65 years and older report their having religious affiliations.[6,7] Among those aged 75 years and older, participation in religious activities outside the home diminishes, but prayer and religious expression remain critical forces in maintaining life satisfaction and mental health.

The significance of spirituality in helping older people to cope with the changes that are brought on by aging cannot be underestimated. Research has shown that elderly persons who are involved in religious activities, as well as those who express their spiritual feelings in more personal and informal ways, are less prone to depression and have an easier time adjusting to the variety of losses that may accompany aging.

Many physicians feel uncomfortable about discussing spiritual matters with their patients, just as patients may be guarded about their spiritual beliefs and practices. This discomfort may result from physicians' lack of understanding, or physicians may feel that their patients use religion to deny reality rather than confront it.

As elderly persons live longer lives with more chronic conditions, many change their perspectives about medicine and technology. While most older people have witnessed incredible advances in medical treatment, the limitations of medicine also have become apparent. The experiences of living with one or more chronic illnesses and of losing loved ones to conditions for which treatment has been unsuccessful reinforce their beliefs and spiritual commitments.

Openness by physicians about their patients' spirituality can lead to a greater sense of trust and teamwork. Physicians can encourage patients to discuss spiritual matters, if the patients desire. Religious institutions also provide concrete support for older persons. Research on elderly black communities reveals that the church is the single most important and trusted source of psychosocial and spiritual support for great numbers of black elderly persons. Members of the clergy increasingly receive credentials in psychology, social work, and pastoral counseling and render their services in hospitals and social service agencies.

PSYCHOSOCIAL AND SPIRITUAL INTERVENTIONS FOR ELDERLY PERSONS

The goal of all medical treatment for elderly patients is "the management of physical and mental problems in a way that compromises social functioning as little as possible."[2] The impact of medical treatment on the ability of older persons to maintain what they define as quality of life should always be a primary consideration. Many elderly persons are willing to tolerate great discomfort, expense, or risk to maintain lifestyles that are meaningful and satisfying. Personal fulfillment in old age

AIMS OF COMPREHENSIVE
INTERDISCIPLINARY INTERVENTIONS FOR ELDERLY PERSONS

The prevention of disease, depression, and other events that can lead to a disastrous outcome

The enhancement of life satisfaction through available linkages and social supports

The preservation of the critical balance between simply reacting to change and having personal autonomy

The development and protection of social and spiritual reserves for future use

The prevention of social iatrogensesis (e.g., prescription for an inappropriate social resource)

comes not only from one's reacting successfully to the challenges of loss, illness, and change, but also from continuing to direct one's life and initiate worthwhile activity.

Medical, psychological, social, and spiritual interventions for older persons should incorporate the aims outlined in the accompanying box.

Techniques for integrating social and spiritual interventions into medical practice

The first objective for clinicians is to know and evaluate the social and spiritual supports that are currently available to their patients. One way to obtain this information is to ask patients to complete a diagram for mapping social support networks (Figure 23-1).[1] Patients are asked to look at the diagram of three concentric circles surrounding a smaller circle containing the word "YOU." The patients must then write into the circle the names of persons who are most important in their lives, placing their closest friends' or relatives' names within the innermost circle. Patients also may indicate organizations to which they belong. Once this is accomplished, it is possible to visualize the supports that are available to older people in their time of need and to examine further the nature of the relationships in the various concentric circles, including the following:

1. Are they reciprocal?
2. Are they dependent upon payment?
3. What is the frequency of contact with the patient?
4. What is the availability during the patient's time of need?
5. Who was left out of the diagram (e.g., estranged children) and why?
6. Who was surprisingly included (e.g., ex-spouses) and why?

Efforts can be directed at strengthening the supportiveness of families and close friends or at filling in social support gaps with community-based social services.

Often families and friends are unaware of or misinformed about the needs of patients until the physicians discuss them openly. Family conferences that include

Diagram for Mapping a Social Support Network

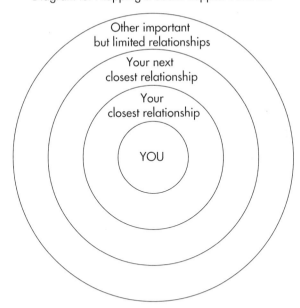

Figure 23-1 Diagram for mapping a social support network. *(See text for explanation.) (Reproduced with permission from Antonucci TC: Hierarchal mapping technique,* Generations *10:11, 1986.)*

patients and significant others chosen by the patients are valuable in validating needs and in generating solutions to social support problems. Family conferences also enable physicians to detect family dysfunction that may prevent adequate family support. Unrealistic expectations by the patients, families, or physicians also become visible during family conferences.

There also is a wide array of formal social supports available in the community. However, many elderly people feel uncomfortable about seeking help in the community. When encouraging older people to utilize community resources, physicians often encounter the patients' resistance, fear, and ignorance. It is not enough simply to recommend a senior center, for example; the patients may need encouragement to try something new and often frightening. The following are important points for referring for psychosocial support:

1. If patients have ethnic or religious preferences, seek resources offered by those groups. Physicians should respect cultural preferences and tolerate some prejudices with which they may not agree. Try to overcome unreasonable objections but respect differences. A non–English-speaking patient may require services that are provided in a foreign language.

2. Keep a list of the telephone numbers of community resources and initiate referrals by telephone calls to introduce the patients. Give patients a social prescription form or other printed material that lists types of available resources and telephone numbers (e.g., case management, home health care, residential care, financial eligibility, legal planning, skilled nursing facilities). Patients should inform their physicians about the outcome of the referrals.

3. Attempt to match the outside resources with the personality style of the patient. Some elderly persons feel quite comfortable in large groups (e.g., senior centers); others may be more comfortable with individual, private services that can be rendered in the home.

4. Acknowledge hardships. Patients feel supported and are more likely to follow through on recommendations when plans are personalized and hardships such as transportation problems and finances are understood by their physicians. The level of caregiver burden should always be a consideration when treatment options are considered.

REFERENCES

1. Antonucci TC: Hierarchal mapping technique, *Generations* 10:11, 1986.
2. Bosse R et al: How stressful is retirement?: findings from the normative aging study, *J Gerontol* 46:13, 1991.
3. Cafferata GL: Marital status, living arrangements, and use of health services by elderly persons, *Gerontology* 42:613, 1987.
4. Huttman ED: *Social services for the elderly*, New York, 1985, Free Press.
5. Kane RA: Assessing social function in the elderly, *Clin Geriatr Med* 3:87, 1987.
6. Koenig HG, George LK, Siegler IC: The use of religion and other emotion-regulating coping strategies among older adults, *Gerontologist* 28:303, 1988.
7. Moberg D: Social indicators of spiritual well-being. In Thorson J, Cork L, eds: *Spiritual well-being in the elderly*, Springfield, Ill, 1980, Charles C Thomas.
8. Shanas E: Social myth as hypothesis: The care of the family relative of old people, *Gerontologist* 19:6, 1979.
9. Vinnick BH, Ekherdt DJ: Retirement and the family, *Generations* 13:54, 1989.

SUGGESTED READINGS

Kane RA: Assessing social function in the elderly, *Clin Geriatr Med* 3:87, 1987.
Moberg D: Social indicators of spiritual well-being. In Thorson J, Cork L, eds: *Spiritual well-being in the elderly*, Springfield, Ill, 1980, Charles C Thomas.

COMMON GERIATRIC SYNDROMES AND PROBLEMS

CHAPTER 24

Urinary incontinence

HERBERT C. SIER

KEY POINTS

- Urinary incontinence is underreported by patients.
- In addition to the genitourinary tract, there are multiple factors, including neurological and functional disabilities of the patients, that can lead to incontinence.
- The four major patterns of persistent incontinence are urge, stress, overflow, and functional.
- Behavioral therapies are an important component in treatment of urge and stress incontinence.
- Anticholinergic medications are helpful in urge incontinence.
- Estrogens and alpha-adrenergic agonists are useful in stress incontinence.
- Surgery can be helpful in stress incontinence and in outlet obstruction.

CLINICAL RELEVANCE

Prevalence, epidemiology, complications

Urinary incontinence may be defined as an involuntary loss of urine that is objectively demonstrable and leads to a social or hygienic problem. Its prevalence among elderly persons residing in the community is between 10% and 20%. Recent studies in the United States have found that the prevalence of urinary incontinence among elderly persons is as high as 30%. In one study, the prevalence of incontinence was 37.7% and 18.8% in elderly women and men, respectively.[2]

Incontinence is associated with impaired cognitive statuses of the patients and with their dependency on others for activities of daily living. An incontinence study among community-dwelling patients who have dementia demonstrated that those with incontinence had greater impairments to their cognitive functions and more frequent behavioral problems. Visuospatial difficulties in finding the bathroom were observed among the dementia patients who had incontinence.[6]

In the study by Diokono et al,[2] several epidemiological findings were observed. Women who had incontinent episodes during pregnancy were more likely to be incontinent later in life. For men, cardiovascular disease was correlated with incontinence. In both sexes, mobility problems, lower urinary tract problems, pulmonary diseases, neurological diseases, constipation, and prior genital surgeries were more common in the incontinent elderly population.[2] Ouslander et al[7] found that with the exception of diuretics, medications were not more prevalent among incontinent versus continent patients.

The complications for urinary incontinence among elderly persons who dwell in the community include medical and psychosocial issues, as well as significant economic costs.[10] In 1987, the direct cost of urinary incontinence among community dwellers was $7 billion, of which $4.8 billion was spent on care for older adults.[12]

Urinary incontinence is frequently underreported by patients for various reasons. Often individuals are embarrassed or believe that incontinence is a normal process of aging, or they are afraid of the therapies used to manage this problem. Consequently, many older adults are never evaluated by their physicians for this problem. They often purchase pads or undergarments or use tissue paper to manage the leakage.[5] Physicians underreport urinary leakage for their elderly patients. It is essential that physicians ask their older patients if urinary leakage is a problem.

Physiology

As people age, physiological changes occur that predispose individuals to urinary incontinence. However, in most older adults urinary leakage does not develop. Incontinence should not be thought of as a normal accompaniment to aging. In men, the prostate enlarges and this can lead to an outlet obstruction or unstable bladder contractions (detrusor motor instability). In postmenopausal women, estrogen decreases and this can lead to atrophic vaginitis and urethritis, as well as to a poor mucosal seal. In older women, maximal pressure for urethral closure and urethral length decrease. Pelvic laxity may develop and contribute to stress incontinence.[10,11]

In both sexes, the rate for urine flow decreases, bladder capacity declines, uninhibited bladder contractions increase, and postvoid residual volumes increase. The postvoid residual volume should not increase to more than 50 ml.[11] Unstable bladder contractions can be observed on cystometrograms for 10% to 20% of continent individuals who have minimal urinary symptoms.[7] For men and women, there appears to be increases in nocturia.

The structures involved in micturition include the brain, spinal cord, autonomic nervous system, bladder outlet (internal and external sphincters), and pelvic floor muscles.[14] The sympathetic nervous system promotes storage of urine in three ways.

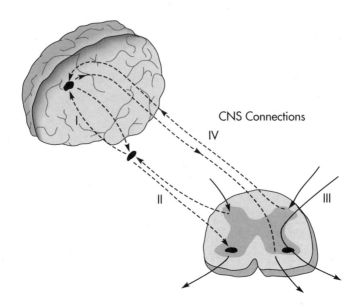

Figure 24-1 Central nervous system (CNS) control of voiding. Loop I, voluntary control over reflex arc of voiding (loop I). Loop II, reflex arc of voiding. Loop III, involuntary control of pelvic floor musculature. Loop IV, voluntary control of external urethra and pelvic floor musculature. *(Reproduced with permission from Williams ME, Pannill FC: Urinary incontinence in the elderly: physiology, pathophysiology, diagnosis and treatment,* Ann Intern Med, *97[6]:895, 1982.)*

First, the dome of the bladder contains beta-adrenergic agonist receptors, and during storage the bladder can expand to accept more urine. Second, the sympathetic nervous system can inhibit the parasympathetic nervous system. Third, the sympathetic nervous system contracts the smooth muscle fibers of the internal sphincter in which lie alpha-adrenergic agonist receptors. The parasympathetic nervous system controls voiding because it contracts the detrusor muscle. The somatic nervous system via the pudendal nerve controls the pelvic floor musculature.[10]

The process of voiding may be considered as a series of loops (Figure 24-1).[15] Loop II is the reflex arc of voiding. The bladder's sensory nerves course up the spinal cord to the brain stem detrusor nucleus, and efferent fibers descend to the spinal detrusor motor nucleus. Axons then synapse in the pelvic ganglia leading to contraction of the bladder.

Sensory information from the brain stem detrusor nucleus ascends to the frontal lobes and thalamus. Efferent fibers descend to the brain stem nucleus and modulate an inhibitory control over loop II. Thus, loop I gives voluntary control over the reflex arc of voiding. This central control allows individuals to hold back their urine, even when they feel it is time to void.[15]

Loop III allows involuntary control of the pelvic floor musculature. Loop IV allows volitional control over the external urethra and the pelvic floor musculature. When the bladder is full and voiding occurs, loop II activity predominates as loop I releases its inhibition. Loops III and IV allow the external sphincter and pelvic floor musculature to relax as the detrusor muscle contracts.[15]

The major neurotransmitter in loop II-mediated contraction of the bladder is acetylcholine. Prostaglandins also may cause bladder contraction. Enkephalins and vasoactive intestinal peptide are proposed inhibitory neurotransmitters.[13]

CLINICAL MANIFESTATIONS

Acute incontinence

The causes of acute incontinence are highlighted by the mnemonic DRIP:[10] delirium, (urinary) retention, restricted (mobility) infection, (fecal) impaction, polyuria, and pharmaceuticals. Pharmaceuticals that can cause or exacerbate incontinence are anticholinergics (antihistamines, narcotics), psychotropics (antidepressants, sedative hypnotics, antipsychotics), diuretics, alcohol, calcium channel blockers, and alpha-adrenergic agonists and antagonists.

Persistent incontinence

The various types of persistent incontinence are urge, reflex, detrusor hyperactivity with impaired contractility, stress, overflow, functional, and iatrogenic. Ouslander et al[7] found that within a geriatric outpatient population the most common presentation of symptoms among the incontinent were mixed. Diokono et al[2] observed that in women and men, 55% and 29%, respectively, had mixed urge and stress symptoms. Pure obstructive symptoms are more common for men, while stress symptoms are more common for women. Urge symptoms alone can be found among both sexes.

Urge incontinence is the most frequent cause of persistent incontinence among men and women.[7] Urge incontinence is characterized by a frequent desire to void, involuntary voiding, and leakage of moderate to large amounts of urine. Detrusor motor instability occurs when the bladder contracts spastically, and during a cystometrogram a rise in pressure of 15 cm of water or greater cannot be inhibited at low bladder volumes. A second type of urge incontinence is sensory urge incontinence in which there are urge symptoms, but the bladder does not contract unstably. This may be related to atrophic urethritis and a poorly compliant bladder.[10]

The causes of urge incontinence are better understood by examining the loops described previously. Disorders in the central nervous system that interfere with the functions of loop I may be associated with the loss of cortical inhibition. If the cause of urge incontinence is a problem of the central nervous system, it is called detrusor hyperreflexia.[11] Loop II fires without any modulation and frequent urination occurs. A second cause would be a hyperactive stimulus to loop II, which could be related to disorders in the lower genitourinary tract. If a central nervous system disorder is identified after the patient is examined, focal neurological findings may be present. Perineal sensation probably is normal and postvoid residual urine is low.

Reflex incontinence is characterized by a patient's involuntary leakage of urine without warning and is due to detrusor hyperreflexia, an impaired sensation of bladder filling, and the absence of bladder symptoms. It is caused by a lesion of the suprasacral spinal cord that interferes with loop I function. Coordination between bladder contraction and bladder outlet relaxation is also interrupted, leading to bladder dyssynergia and a large amount of postvoid residual urine.[11]

Detrusor hyperreflexia with impaired bladder contractility causes frequent voiding but incomplete emptying. Findings are similar to urge incontinence, except the postvoid residual urine may be high. There is no bladder dyssynergia or outlet obstruction in this condition.[11,12]

Stress incontinence refers to weakness of the urethral sphincter and results in small to moderate amounts of urine loss when there is an increase in intraabdominal pressure such as a cough or sneeze. Pure stress incontinence is accompanied by normal perineal sensation and sacral reflexes and a low amount of postvoid residual urine.[10]

Overflow incontinence is characterized by hesitancy, dribbling, poor urinary stream, leakage of small amounts of urine and high postvoid residual.[10,11] If a patient has an acontractile bladder from a diabetic neuropathy, sensation will be impaired. However, if a male patient has prostatic hypertrophy or a female patient has large cystocele that causes an obstruction, perineal sensation and sacral reflexes are usually intact.

Functional incontinence implies that normally continent persons leak urine because of impairments primarily to their functional abilities. It may result from physical or psychological barriers to appropriate voiding. Cognitive or mobility deficits may be found when the patient is examined. An example might be the older adult who lives in the community, develops a major depression, and commences to leak urine.[13]

Iatrogenic incontinence develops after a physician's interaction. A good example would be an older adult who has hypertension, takes a diuretic to control blood pressure, and develops urge incontinence. This patient would be better treated with another class of antihypertensives such as a calcium channel blocker or an angiotensin-converting enzyme inhibitor.[13]

DIAGNOSTIC APPROACH

It is important to take the patients' histories carefully. The onset, timing, duration, frequency, and amount of leakage are key questions to ask the patients about their incontinence.[10,11,12] Physicians should suggest that their patients keep a bladder record. Patients record the times when they void and whether they were wet or dry with the episodes. The presence of obstruction, stress, frequency, constipation, fecal incontinence, straining, and dysuria should be determined. However, of these symptoms, only stress complaints have a high predictive value. For example, if an older man describes frequency, it is possible that he has urge or overflow incontinence or both. It is necessary to record any medical conditions of the patients that could interfere with the functions of the various loops such as diabetes mellitus or various neurological disorders. If there is peripheral edema, this could lead to an increased frequency of nocturia. The medications that patients take should be assessed. Past genitourinary history, including previous surgery, radiation, or dilatations should be recorded. For example, it is important for a physician to question carefully a female patient who has a history of urine leakage during pregnancy. A careful assessment of the functional statuses of patients, especially their mobility, also should be determined.

The mental status and neurological examination of the patient are essential.[10] Examinations of the abdomen to find bladder distention and rectum to assess sphincter tone, prostate, fecal impaction or mass, and perineal sensation should be performed. Finally, for a female patient, a pelvic examination for atrophic vaginitis, pelvic mass, uterine prolapse, cystocele, or rectocele is necessary.

A urinalysis and urine culture should be done to evaluate a urinary tract infection. An assessment of the patient's postvoid residual urine is helpful, and if it is greater than 100 ml, acontractile bladder, bladder outlet obstruction, bladder dyssynergia, or detrusor hyperactivity with impaired contractile function may be present.[11]

Ouslander et al[9] designed an algorithm that includes simplified bedside testing. A catheter is introduced into patients after they void normally, and their postvoid residual urine is measured. Sterile water is introduced at 50 ml aliquots through a syringe held at 15 cm above the symphysis pubis, with the plunger removed. A simple bedside cystometrogram is performed, and bladder capacity, first urge to void, and unstable contractions are observed if the water rises in the syringe. Stress maneuvers are done before the postvoid residual urine is determined and after bedside bladder filling. If there is immediate leakage of urine when the physician performs a stress maneuver, then the patient has stress incontinence. If it takes a few seconds for urine leakage to occur after the patient coughs and there is a large amount of urine lost, there is probably a stress-induced detrusor contraction. When these conditions occur, both urge and stress incontinence are present.[10]

In this algorithm, the following criteria mandate urological referral: inability to pass the catheter, postvoid residual urine greater than 100 ml, hematuria, marked pelvic prolapse, severe obstructive symptoms, suspicion of prostate cancer, recurrent urinary tract infections, recent pelvic surgery or irradiation, or an uncertain diagnosis.[9] For patients who did not require referrals to urologists, diagnostic and therapeutic accuracy were both 88%. Approximately one-half of the patients met at least one criterion for formal urologic referral.[3]

The algorithmic approach to incontinence is helpful for the majority of elderly persons in the community as an initial step in their evaluation. The Agency for Health

Care Policy Research has recently promulgated clinical practice guidelines for urinary incontinence that recommend as a basic evaluation a focused history, physical examination, urinalysis, and postvoid residual. Simple cystometry as described above, as well as more complex urodynamic tests, are recommended only for those patients whose management cannot be determined by the basic evaluation.[14] More prospective studies should be done in the community setting to ascertain the appropriateness of a shortened evaluation. One of the major pitfalls in this algorithm is the risk of precipitating urinary retention for a patient who has bladder emptying problems.

INTERVENTION

The various modalities for treating persistent incontinence are shown in Table 24-1. Table 24-2 summarizes drugs that are used for treating urinary incontinence.[8] The three reasons to use an indwelling catheter are (1) management of severe pressure ulcers, (2) overflow incontinence associated with obstruction or an acontractile bladder that cannot be treated by another means, and (3) patients who are frail, severely dysfunctional, and bedridden, which makes it difficult to change them because of agitation or pain.[10] External catheters for men are associated with skin breakdown, *Candida* infections, and urinary tract infections. Those patients who have external catheters show a moderate incidence of bacteriuria in comparison to individuals who wear indwelling catheters and those who do not use any catheters.[12] External catheters for women are available, but more studies are necessary to assess their efficacy and complications for frail, community-residing, elderly persons.[12] Intermittent catheterization is a viable means for managing incontinence among elderly persons, and it

Table 24-1 Treatment of Persistent Incontinence

Type	Treatment
Urge	Behavioral: biofeedback; drugs: anticholinergics; antidepressants; estrogens; surgery in selected cases; electrical stimulation
Reflex	Treat like urge but need to decompress bladder with alpha antagonist or intermittent catheterization
Detrusor hyperactivity with impaired contractility	Behavioral; drugs: anticholinergics but prevent urinary retention
Stress	Behavioral: Kegel exercises; biofeedback; drugs: estrogens and alpha agonists; surgery: bladder neck suspension; artificial sphincter pessary; collagen or Teflon injection; electrical stimulation
Overflow	Remove offending drug; surgery: transurethral resection of prostate; intermittent or indwelling catheter; drugs: alpha antagonists
Functional	Improve function
Iatrogenic	Prevent precipitating factors

Table 24-2   Medications for the Treatment of Urinary Incontinence

Drug	Pharmacological changes with age/adverse effects	Precautions and recommendations
Anticholinergic/ antispasmodic	Decreased bladder capacity with age	Use primarily when urge incontinence is present
Oxybutynin	Dry mouth; blurry vision; delir-	2.5-5 mg tid
Propantheline	ium; constipation; elevated in-	15-30 mg tid
Flavoxate	traocular pressure	100-200 mg tid
Imipramine		25-50 mg tid
Alpha-adrenergic agonists	Sphincter weakness	Use with stress incontinence; avoid tri- cyclics with significant heart block
Pseudo- ephedrine	Hypertension; tachycardia;	30-60 mg tid
Imipramine	Orthostasis; anticholinergic	25-50 mg tid
Conjugated es- trogens	Decreased estrogen in post- menopausal women	Use with stress and sensory urge inconti- nence; consider adding progesterone
Oral, Topical	Endometrial cancer; elevated blood pressure; gallstones when used long term	0.625 mg/day 0.5-1 g/application
Cholinergic ago- nists	Bradycardia; hypotension; bron- choconstriction; gastric acid secretion	Short-term use only; overflow inconti- nence with atonic bladder due to anti- cholinergic agents
Bethanechol		10-30 mg tid
Alpha-adrenergic antagonist	Orthostatic hypotension	Use in overflow incontinence
Prazosin		1-2 mg tid

Adapted from Ouslander, JG, Sier HC: Drug therapy for geriatric urinary incontinence, *Clin Geriatr Med* 2(4):790, 1986.

appears that the incidence of symptomatic disease is lower than that of continuous catheterization but more studies are required.[11]

Behavioral interventions are important such as restricting fluids at night for individuals who have profound nocturia. Kegel exercises are conditioning exercises that help patients who have stress incontinence. During Kegel exercises, a woman practices stopping her flow of urine. Once the woman learns how to tighten her outlet, she practices 15 contractions 3 times a day.[1]

Cognitive function is a key determinant of the success of these behavioral therapies. For individuals who have cognitive deficits, a regimen for toileting or prompted voiding is applicable.[1] With scheduled toileting, caregivers toilet individuals at a set interval of time. With prompted voiding, caregivers ask patients if they need to urinate, and if they answer affirmatively, they are taken to the bathroom and given positive reinforcement at a fixed interval of time. In bladder retraining, the patient uses the bladder record and learns to lengthen gradually the intervals between voiding episodes. Fantl et al[4] found that by using a bladder retraining protocol for women who have pure urge incontinence, pure stress incontinence, and a combination of urge and stress incontinence, incontinence episodes decreased by 57%. With biofeedback, pressure in the rectum, vagina, or bladder is recorded for the patient. The patient is instructed to tighten the outlet by squeezing the rectum while relaxing the bladder and abdominal musculature.[1]

Disposable diapers and pads are used by approximately half of the elderly persons who live in the community and are incontinent.[5] These devices should not supplement a careful diagnostic evaluation because therapies often exist that may preclude the use of these undergarments.

REFERENCES

1. Burgio KL: Behavioral training for stress and urge incontinence in the community, *Gerontology* 36 (suppl 2):27, 1990.
2. Diokno AC et al: Medical correlates of urinary incontinence in the elderly, *Urology* 36(2):129–138, 1990.
3. Dubeau CE, Resnick NM: Evaluation of the causes and severity of geriatric incontinence: a critical appraisal, *Urol Clin North Am* 18(2):243, 1991.
4. Fantl JA et al: Efficacy of bladder training in older women with urinary incontinence, *JAMA* 265(5):609, 1991.
5. Herzog AR et al: Methods used to manage urinary incontinence by older adults in the community, *J Am Geriatr Soc* 37(4):339, 1989.
6. Ouslander JG et al: Incontinence among elderly community-dwelling dementia patients: characteristics, management, and impact on caregivers, *J Am Geriatr Soc* 38(4):440, 1990.
7. Ouslander JG et al: Genitourinary dysfunction in a geriatric outpatient population, *J Am Geriatr Soc* 34(7):507, 1986.
8. Ouslander JG, Sier HC: Drug therapy for geriatric urinary incontinence, *Clin Geriatr Med* 2(4):789, 1986.
9. Ouslander JG et al: Prospective evaluation of an assessment strategy for geriatric urinary incontinence, *J Am Geriatr Soc* 37(8):715, 1989.
10. Ouslander JG: Incontinence. In Kane RL, Ouslander JG, Abrass IB, eds: *Essentials of clinical geriatrics*, ed 2, New York, 1989, McGraw-Hill.
11. Resnick NM: Voiding dysfunction and urinary incontinence. In Cassel CK, Riesenberg DE, Sorensen LB et al, eds: *Geriatric medicine*, ed 2, New York, 1990, Springer-Verlag.
12. Resnick NM, Ouslander JG, eds: Urinary incontinence in adults: National Institutes of Health consensus development conference, *J Am Geriatr Soc* 38(3):263, 1990.
13. Solomon DH et al: New issues in geriatric care, *Ann Intern Med* 108(5):718, 1988.
14. U.S. Department of Health and Human Services: Clinical Practice Guideline: Urinary Incontinence in Adults, March, 1992.
15. Williams MW, Pannill FC: Urinary incontinence in the elderly: physiology, pathophysiology, diagnosis and treatment, *Ann Intern Med* 97(6):895, 1982.

SUGGESTED READINGS

Ouslander JG: Incontinence. In Kane RL, Ouslander JG, Abrass IB, eds: *Essentials of clinical geriatrics*, ed 2, New York, 1989, McGraw-Hill.
Resnick NM: Voiding dysfunction and urinary incontinence. In Cassel CK, Riesenberg DE, Sorensen LB et al, eds: *Geriatric medicine*, ed 2, New York, 1990, Springer-Verlag.
Resnick NM, Ouslander JG, eds: Urinary incontinence in adults: National Institutes of Health consensus development conference, *J Am Geriatr Soc* 38(3):263, 1990.
Williams MW, Pannill FC: Urinary incontinence in the elderly: physiology, pathophysiology, diagnosis and treatment, *Ann Intern Med* 97(6):895, 1982.

CHAPTER 25

Prostatism and prostate cancer

EILA C. SKINNER

KEY POINTS

- The natural history of obstruction to the bladder outlet due to benign prostate hypertrophy (BPH) is variable and often unpredictable.
- The actual size of the prostate in BPH does not correlate with the patient's degree of symptoms or response to treatment.
- The most common indication for medical or surgical intervention of BPH is the patient's degree of symptoms.
- Prostate cancer is the most commonly diagnosed cancer for men and its prevalence is increasing.
- Curable prostate cancer is almost always asymptomatic and is detected on routine screening examinations.
- Prostate-specific antigen (PSA) is a sensitive but somewhat nonspecific marker for prostate cancer, which is useful in early detection, staging, and follow-up.
- Choice of treatment depends on the stage of the disease and an estimation of the patient's general health and longevity.

Benign prostate or prostatic hypertrophy (BPH) and carcinoma of the prostate are both extremely common problems among elderly men. The two problems together are estimated to affect up to 50% of men aged 65 years and older. Because both problems increase dramatically with age, their prevalence is expected to rise significantly as the population ages.

BENIGN PROSTATIC HYPERTROPHY

Clinical relevance

Autopsy studies suggest that histological BPH occurs in more than 70% of men aged 60 years and older, and approximately 25% have clinically significant symptoms. In the past, adenomatous growth was thought to be an unremitting process, which would eventually result in obstruction to the bladder outlet for all patients. This belief was the basis for the recommendation of "prophylactic" treatment for asymptomatic or mildly symptomatic men who have enlarged glands. Although few prospective cohort studies have been done, it is now recognized that the natural history of BPH is extremely variable. While many patients develop progressive symptoms, others remain asymptomatic, have symptoms that spontaneously wax and wane, or have stable mild symptoms for many years without treatment.[1]

Clinical manifestations

The typical symptoms of obstruction to the bladder outlet due to BPH are a constellation of complaints, including urinary hesitancy, decreased force of stream, postvoid dribbling, double voiding, nocturia, and sensation of incomplete emptying of the bladder. Patients also may complain of more irritative symptoms such as dysuria, daytime frequency, urgency, and urge incontinence. In the absence of urinary infection or another process that irritates the bladder (e.g., bladder stone or carcinoma), these latter symptoms result from hypertrophy of the detrusor muscle and loss of normal cortical inhibition of detrusor contractions.

BPH is the most common cause of microscopic hematuria among elderly men and is believed to result from dilated friable veins on the surface of the adenomatous tissue. A full evaluation is required to exclude other causes of the hematuria such as bladder or renal carcinoma. Significant gross hematuria also can result from BPH and may require a transurethral resection of the prostate (TURP) to control the bleeding.

Approximately 10% of patients have an episode of acute urinary retention. Acute urinary retention is often brought about by a diuretic load, bladder overdistention, or over-the-counter cold medications that contain alpha-adrenergic agents (e.g., pseudoephedrine or phenylephrine). Often, patients who have retention can recover the ability to void after draining the bladder with a catheter for a few days. However, most patients who have retention eventually require treatment of the BPH, usually within a few months of the episode.

BPH is also the most common cause of acute urinary tract infections among elderly men. The first episode of such an infection in the absence of genitourinary manipulation warrants an evaluation for BPH, even for the patient who has a normal voiding pattern. Recurrent infections place the patient at significant risk for developing urosepsis with all of its potential complications.

A few patients have so-called silent prostatism with renal insufficiency due to bilateral hydronephrosis but have no complaints about voiding. This continues to occur occasionally today, even among patients receiving regular medical care.

Concomitant medical problems that are complicated by abnormal bladder function (e.g., diabetes mellitus, neurological disease) can cause diagnostic confusion for patients who have complaints about urinary patterns. Formal urodynamic evaluation may be necessary to differentiate these problems from BPH and determine which patients will benefit from surgical treatment of the prostate.[10]

Physical examination may reveal a palpably distended bladder, and during rectal examination the prostate is enlarged, smooth, and rubbery. The shape of the prostate can vary widely, and it is well known that the degree of symptoms correlates poorly with the actual size of the prostate. Most importantly, the prostate should be neither boggy and tender, which indicates infection, nor rock hard, which indicates carcinoma. The patient also should be examined for evidence of an intact sacral reflex arc (anal sphincter tone and bulbocavernosus reflex).

Diagnostic approach

When a patient has obstructive symptoms, the initial evaluation should include a general physical and rectal examination, urinalysis, and urine culture if indicated. Blood work should include renal function studies, complete blood count, and serum prostate-specific antigen (PSA). If possible the PSA should be drawn before a digital rectal examination is performed to decrease the chance of a falsely elevated result. If kidney function is impaired a renal ultrasound is indicated. Hydronephrosis that resolves with catheter drainage is one of the absolute indications for prostatectomy. When patients do not have elevated serum creatinine or hematuria, most studies suggest that there is no value to routine examinations of the upper genitourinary tract for patients being treated for BPH. However, many urologists routinely perform either an intravenous pyelogram or a renal ultrasound as a screening test before considering surgery.

Prostate-specific antigen is a protein secreted by the prostate epithelium and is a sensitive but nonspecific marker for prostate cancer. The normal range is 0 to 4.0 ng/ml (Hybritech assay) or 0 to 2.5 ng/ml (Yang assay). The probability of finding prostate cancer increases proportionately with the absolute level of PSA.[6,13,14] (See Table 25-1). However, approximately 25% of all patients who have only BPH also have an elevated PSA, with 5% having a PSA greater than 10.0 ng/ml. Other conditions that may elevate PSA transiently include acute prostatitis or prostatic abscess, urinary retention, prostatic massage, and prostatic biopsy. Elevation of PSA may persist for several weeks after such events.[13] Following the above initial evaluation, the patient should be referred to a urologist for cystoscopy. Cystoscopy is mandatory for patients who have microscopic or gross hematuria so that urologists may discover bladder tumors.

Table 25-1   Probability of detecting prostate cancer by abnormal digital rectal examination and PSA

	Percent positive* at PSA (ng/ml) level		
Rectal examination	**0-4.0**	**4.1-10.0**	**>10.0**
Normal	9%	20%	31%
Abnormal	17%	45%	77%

From Cooner WH et al: Prostate cancer detection in a clinical urological practice by ultrasonography, digital rectal examination and prostate-specific antigen, *J Urol* 143:1146, 1990.
*Percent positive, number of positive biopsies divided by total number of biopsies.

Other studies for BPH that are often done by urologists include abdominal ultrasound (to measure the volume of postvoid residual urine and to assess prostate size and kidney integrity) and measurement of urine flow (to document outlet obstruction and its response to therapy).[6]

Intervention

The indications for treatment are listed in the accompanying box.

There is little argument about the appropriateness of treatment for patients who have the absolute indications, but these patients make up a small percentage of the 400,000 prostatectomies that are performed annually. Most patients receive treatment because of the severity of symptoms. Severe obstructive symptoms can be very disturbing to patients, especially frequent nocturia, which disrupts sleep. The size of the prostate is *never in itself* an indication for treatment.

There has been an increase during the past 5 years in treatment options for patients who have BPH, and the specific indications and contraindications for each have not yet been worked out. Many treatment options still must be considered experimental

---

**INDICATIONS
FOR INTERVENTION IN BENIGN PROSTATE HYPERTROPHY**

Absolute indications
- Hydronephrosis that resolves with catheter drainage
- Persistent urinary retention
- Recurrent urinary tract infections

Relative indications
- Obstructive symptoms
- Bladder calculi
- Gross hematuria emanating from the hypertrophied prostate

┌───┐

TREATMENT OPTIONS FOR BENIGN PROSTATE HYPERTROPHY

Medical

- Alpha-adrenergic blockers (terazosin, prazosin)
- Androgen blockers (luteinizing hormone-releasing hormone agonists, flutamide)
- 5-alpha-reductase inhibitor (finasteride)

Surgical

- Open prostatectomy (suprapubic, retropubic)
- Transurethral prostatectomy (TURP)
- Transurethral incision of the prostate (TUIP)
- Transurethral laser ablation of the prostate
- Transurethral balloon dilation
- Microwave hyperthermia

└───┘

and should be offered only in the setting of an ongoing study. The treatments can be divided into medical and surgical options, with surgical options that include several minimally invasive approaches. (See the box above.)

The alpha blockers have been the most important new approach to BPH, and their increased use has dramatically reduced the number of patients undergoing surgery. Alpha blockers act by decreasing the tone in the smooth muscle component of the prostate and the bladder neck. Terazosin (Hytrin) is the most commonly used drug because of its once-per-day dosage. It is started at 1 mg at bedtime and titrated up to 5 to 10 mg in a single nightly dose. Prazosin has similar actions to terazosin but requires doses every 6 hours. Although postural hypotension is a possible side effect of all alpha blockers, it is rarely seen at these doses and the drug is well tolerated by elderly patients. Several weeks may be required to achieve a patient's response to the drug since the dose must be increased gradually. This limits the usefulness of these drugs for acute retention or hydronephrosis. Patients who have moderate symptoms and low residual urine (less than 200 ml) respond the best. Many urologists do not give most patients a trial of alpha blockers before considering surgical treatment.[4] (See Table 25-2 for recommendations for dosage.)

Androgen blockers are effective for achieving a decrease of prostate volume and improving symptoms and urine flow rates in about one third to one half of patients who have significant BPH.[12] The standard approaches such as oral estrogen and luteinizing hormone-releasing hormone (LHRH) agonists (Lupron, Zoladex) all cause impotence and hot flashes as possible side effects, making them unacceptable to most patients. Flutamide causes less impotence but diarrhea is a common side effect. The costs of both LHRH agonists and flutamide, currently more than $300 per month for each, may be prohibitive for many patients. A promising new drug is finasteride (Proscar), which blocks the action of the 5-alpha-reductase in converting testosterone

Table 25-2 Precautions and recommendations for drug prescribing in ambulatory elderly patients

Drug	Pharmacological changes with age/adverse effects	Precautions and recommendations
Terazosin (Hytrin)	Postural hypotension(rare); GI upset	Begin at 1 mg/day at bedtime; increase every 4-5 days to 5-10 mg daily
Prazosin (Minipress)	Postural hypotension; GI upset	Begin at 1 mg at bedtime; increase every 4-5 days to 1 mg bid to tid
Diethylstilbestrol (DES)	Thrombotic events; contraindicated for any patient who has significant cardiac or vascular disease; impotence; hot flashes	2-3 mg daily
Leuprolide (Lupron)	Hot flashes; impotence	7.5 mg SQ q 28 days
Goserelin (Zoladex)	Hot flashes; impotence	3.6 mg SQ q 28 days
Flutamide (Eulexin)	Diarrhea; occasional impotence	250 mg tid
Finasteride (Proscar)	Rare impotence	5 mg q day

to dihydrotestosterone in the prostate. This drug has minimal side effects and recently has received FDA approval.

The standard surgical approaches (i.e., transurethral resection of the prostate [TURP] and open prostatectomy) remain the mainstay of treatment for patients who do not respond to medical therapy. Transurethral resection is routinely performed on patients who are well into their 80s and beyond and often have multiple medical problems. The procedure can be performed while the patient is under spinal anesthesia and usually requires only 3 days' hospitalization, with minimal recovery at home. The most common complications include early or delayed bleeding, infection, and occasional incontinence. Strictures of the urethra or bladder neck also can develop late and can be a significant problem.

Open prostatectomy is required for patients who have prostatic enlargement greater than 50 or 60 g, which cannot safely be resected transurethrally. This procedure also can be performed while the patient is under spinal anesthesia but requires 4 to 7 days' hospitalization and 4 to 6 weeks' recovery at home.

Other less commonly used procedures include transurethral incision of the prostate, which has been used extensively in Europe and appears to be effective for some patients, especially those who have small prostates; balloon dilation of the prostate, which has been investigated recently and is well tolerated by patients under local anesthesia; and microwave hyperthermia, which is applied either transurethrally with a specially adapted catheter or transrectally via a probe and actually causes necrosis of the periurethral adenomatous tissue.[2]

Follow-up after any treatment of BPH consists primarily of periodic assessments of the patient's symptoms and renal function. It is important to recognize that treatment for BPH, including open surgical prostatectomy, does not decrease a patient's risk of developing prostate cancer.[7] The *surgical capsule,* consisting of a normal peripheral zone of prostate tissue, is always left intact after such procedures. Therefore, digital rectal examination and perhaps serum PSA should be performed on a yearly basis.

PROSTATE CANCER

Clinical relevance

Prostate cancer is currently the most common malignancy diagnosed among men and causes over 30,000 deaths per year. More than 80% of prostate cancer occurs in men aged 65 years and older. The age-adjusted incidence has been increasing steadily at about 2% per year over the past 2 decades. The exact etiology of prostate cancer is unknown, but it clearly depends on the presence of testosterone. Other known risk factors include family history (approximately twofold higher risk for patients with a father or brother who has prostate cancer) and race (approximately twice the risk for American blacks compared with whites). High dietary fat intake also may play a role.

It has been known for years that many men die of other causes, with clinically unsuspected prostate cancers detectable at their autopsies. This fact led to the concept of "latent" prostate cancer, which does not require treatment. Studies now suggest that the only difference between these autopsy cancers and clinically significant cancers is the volume of disease. Prostate cancer is clearly a very slow-growing malignancy, with the doubling time of well-differentiated tumors estimated at 2 years or more. Yet the morbidity from advanced prostate cancer should not be underestimated, with urinary retention, renal failure, hemorrhage, severe bone pain, anemia, and inanition causing a slow and very painful death. Because patients who have prostate cancer are often in their 70s or beyond, the challenge is to predict which patients will develop symptomatic local or metastatic disease before they succumb to another illness.

There currently is considerable controversy over the routine use of PSA as a screening test for prostate cancer in completely asymptomatic patients. It is not an ideal test by itself, since up to 40% of patients who have organ-confined cancer have normal PSAs, and 25% of patients who have BPH have elevated PSAs. Many of the former would be detected by an abnormal digital rectal examination. However, the addition of PSA to the yearly rectal examination clearly has allowed clinicians to detect early prostate cancers that are not palpable.[5]

The controversy about screening tests involves cost. Although the blood test is relatively inexpensive, prostate ultrasound and biopsy must be done to diagnose the cancer definitively, at the cost of several hundred dollars per patient. Some experts have recommended biopsies only for patients who have PSAs of more than 10 ng/ ml or those who have abnormal rectal examinations because these groups have the highest likelihood of cancer. Others, including myself, perform biopsies for any patients who have PSAs greater than 4.0 ng/ml, recognizing that many negative biopsies will be performed for each cancer detected. The key question of whether early detection and treatment will translate into improved survival rates remains to be definitively answered.

Clinical manifestations

Localized, curable, prostate cancer is by definition asymptomatic. When obstructive symptoms are caused by prostate cancer, they are indistinguishable from those caused by BPH, and generally at that point the cancer has already spread outside the capsule of the prostate. (See Table 25-3 for the clinical staging system). Patients who have metastatic disease most often have symptoms of bone pain or anemia. The axial skeleton is most often involved, especially the lumbar spine, sacrum, and iliac wings; however, any bone may be involved. Vertebral involvement may impinge on the spinal cord, and the presenting symptom is an acute lower extremity paralysis, which is a surgical emergency. Finally, extension into the bladder trigone or pelvic lymph nodes can cause ureteral obstruction, and often the presenting symptom is acute renal failure. Other sites of metastases such as the lung, liver, or brain are very rare, even with widespread disease.

Diagnostic approach

Digital rectal examination and serum PSA, followed by transrectal ultrasound and prostate biopsy are the keys to diagnosis of prostate cancer. Transrectal ultrasound has become the standard approach for physicians to obtain biopsies, which can be done in the office without anesthesia and with minimal risk. In addition to diagnosing the cancer, the ultrasound provides information regarding the extent of disease, and the pathology indicates the degree of differentiation of the tumor. These are both strong prognostic indicators and helpful in planning the patient's treatment.

The mean level of PSA relates directly to the stage of disease in every large study

Table 25-3 Clinical staging system for prostate cancer

Stage	Findings
A	Detected in specimen from simple prostatectomy (TURP or open)
A1	Less than 5% of prostate tissue involved
A2	More than 5% of prostate tissue involved
B	Palpable lesion confined to the prostate
B1	Nodule less than 1.5 cm diameter confined to one lobe
B2	Nodule greater than 1.5 cm diameter confined to one lobe, or both lobes involved
C	Palpable extension outside confines of prostate to pelvic sidewalls, bladder neck, or seminal vesicles
D1	Extension to pelvic lymph nodes
D2	Extension to bones or nodes outside pelvis

of patients undergoing radical prostatectomy. However, there is a wide range of PSA levels within any one stage such that it becomes a much less useful predictor of the stage of disease on an individual basis. Nevertheless, most studies show that a patient who has a PSA of greater than 15.0 ng/ml is unlikely to have a pathologically confined tumor at radical prostatectomy.[8]

Once the cancer has been detected, other blood tests should include blood urea nitrogen and serum creatinine, serum alkaline phosphatase, and serum prostate acid phosphatase. A bone scan still is ordered routinely by most urologists, although it is unlikely to be positive for the patient who has a PSA less than 10.0 ng/ml. Many surgeons also perform computerized tomography and magnetic resonance imaging of the pelvis to find pelvic adenopathy. Unfortunately, the false positive and false negative rates of both these tests are very high (20% to 40%), which limits their usefulness. Finally, an evaluation of the upper genitourinary tract and cystoscopy are often performed routinely before physicians decide on the patient's treatment.

Intervention

There are basically four possible treatment options for patients who have prostate cancer, which are listed in the box below. The best treatment for any one patient depends on a variety of factors, many of which may be difficult to quantify.

One of the most difficult problems in prostate cancer therapy is estimating an individual's life expectancy. Because prostate cancer often afflicts patients at age 70 and beyond and because it is a slow growing tumor that is asymptomatic until it reaches an advanced stage, the clinician must determine whether an individual patient will become symptomatic before he dies from another disease. This issue is ideally considered *before* the asymptomatic patient undergoes biopsy because there is little justification for early diagnosis if active treatment is not a reasonable option.

TREATMENT OPTIONS FOR PROSTATE CANCER

No treatment
Radical prostatectomy
Radiation therapy
• External beam
• Interstitial implants
• Combined (beam plus implants)
Hormone therapy
• Orchiectomy
• Diethylstilbestrol
• LHRH agonists (Lupron, Zoladex)
• Flutamide (Eulexin)
Chemotherapy

Stage A1 disease (less than 5% of tissue removed at TURP or open prostatectomy contains well-differentiated cancer) in the past was not treated because the risk of progression was considered to be very small. Recent data suggests that at least 15% of patients who survive 8 years or more will develop progressive disease, and the majority of patients will have more cancer found in the prostate if they receive radical prostatectomy. Therefore, urologists now recommend prostatectomy for many patients in their 60s who have A1 disease and are thought to have a good 15-year life expectancy.

Stage A2 disease (greater than 5% of tissue is involved) represents diffuse disease and actually has a worse prognosis than stage B1 tumors. Current studies suggest that the best long-term cure rates in stage A2 and B disease are achieved by radical prostatectomy. For patients who are not surgical candidates, radiation therapy offers a reasonable alternative.

In the past, radical prostatectomy was a much-feared surgery, with serious blood loss and frequent, debilitating, long-term complications such as impotence and incontinence. However, with current surgical and anesthetic techniques average blood loss should be less than 1000 ml and operative mortality less than 1%. Impotence often can be prevented in the early stages of disease, and significant incontinence rates are less than 5% to 10% in most recent studies. Much of this improvement is due to a clearer understanding about the anatomy of the prostate and urethra, which facilitates the development of the nerve-sparing surgical approach.[15]

Radiation therapy for prostate cancer has gone through a continual evolution of techniques and agents, with the ideal form of treatment still unclear. Current options include external beam therapy and/or interstitial implants using radioactive gold seeds, iridium wires, iodine, or palladium. Although patients may remain clinically free of disease for many years after radiation, studies using PSA or routine biopsies for follow-up have demonstrated residual tumor in the vast majority of patients.[9] Thus, the suggestion has been made that radiation slows the natural course of prostate cancer without actually affording a cure. However, for elderly patients, this difference may not be as significant as it appears. At this point radiation therapy is reserved for patients who either refuse surgery or are not considered reasonable candidates for prostatectomy.

Clinical stage C disease represents an area of considerable controversy. Both radical prostatectomy and radiation therapy can achieve good local control for these patients, but many will develop metastatic disease. Combined treatment modalities (surgery, radiation, and hormonal therapy) are being studied to increase the true cure rate in this group.[3]

Similarly, controversy exists regarding the proper treatment for the patients who have lymph nodes that are positive for cancer, which are discovered at the time of radical prostatectomy. Studies from the 1970s suggested that there was no survival advantage afforded by the patients' proceeding with radical prostatectomies in these cases, so most urologists now obtain frozen sections at the time of surgery and abandon prostatectomies if the nodes are positive for cancer. However, the surgery can be completed with much lower complication rates now than previously, and recent studies have shown improved survival for patients who proceed with the prostatectomies and receive early hormonal therapy.[6]

Metastatic prostate cancer can be significantly palliated with hormonal manipulation. Blockage of serum testosterone can be achieved equally well with orchiectomy, oral diethylstilbestrol (DES), and LHRH agonists. DES is very inexpensive but carries unacceptable risks for cardiovascular complications, especially among elderly patients. LHRH agonists are given in a depot form once every 4 weeks. They are very expensive but prevent the emotional trauma of orchiectomy. All three of these treatments cause impotence in the majority of patients, often with a loss of libido. Gynecomastia and hot flashes are other potential side effects.

There currently is much debate over the usefulness of adding flutamide (Eulexin) to orchiectomy or LHRH agonists for stage D2 disease. At least two randomized trials have shown an increase in survival of a few months for patients who received combined therapy.[4] However, several other randomized trials have not demonstrated any difference related to recurrence of the disease or survival for patients. Again cost is a significant factor, with flutamide currently costing more than $300 per month. Ultimately clinicians may identify a subgroup of patients who clearly will benefit from the combined therapy. For now, however, physicians must be cautious before they recommend flutamide for every patient who has metastatic disease.

REFERENCES

1. Begun FP: Benign prostatic hyperplasia: subjective and objective criteria for transurethral resection of the prostate, *Problems in Urology* 5:397, 1991.
2. Boyd SD, Sapozink MD, Astrahan MA: Microwave hyperthermia for the treatment of benign prostatic hyperplasia, *Problems in Urology* 5:441, 1991.
3. Carter GE et al: Results of local and/or systemic adjuvant therapy in the management of pathological stage C or D1 prostate cancer following radical prostatectomy, *J Urol* 142:1266, 1989.
4. Crawford ED et al: A controlled trial of leuprolide with and without flutamide in prostatic carcinoma, *N Engl J Med* 321:419, 1989.
5. Cooner WH et al: Prostate cancer detection in a clinical urological practice by ultrasonography, digital rectal examination and prostate-specific antigen, *J Urol* 143:1146, 1990.
6. De Kernion JB et al: Prognosis of patients with stage D1 prostate carcinoma following radical prostatectomy with and without early endocrine therapy, *J Urol* 144:700, 1990.
7. Gerber GS, Chodak GW: Detection of clinically occult prostate cancer in men with benign prostatic hyperplasia, *Problems in Urology* 5:380, 1991.
8. Hudson MA, Bahnson RR, Catalona WJ: Clinical use of prostate-specific antigen in patients with prostate cancer, *J Urol* 142:1011, 1989.
9. Kabalin JN et al: Identification of residual cancer in the prostate following radiation therapy: role of transrectal ultrasound guided biopsy and prostate-specific antigen, *J Urol* 142:326, 1989.
10. Kreder KJ, Webster GD: Urodynamic assessment of bladder outlet obstruction, *Problems in Urology* 5:386, 1991.
11. Lepor H, Henry D, Laddu AR: The efficacy and safety of terazosin in the treatment of BPH, *Prostate* 18:345, 1991.

12. Matzkin H et al: Treatment of benign prostatic hypertrophy by a long-acting gonadotropin-releasing hormone analogue: 1-year experience, *J Urol* 145:309, 1991.

13. Oesterling JE: Prostate-specific antigen: a critical assessment of the most useful tumor marker for adenocarcinoma of the prostate, *J Urol* 125:907, 1991 (review).

14. Stamey TA, Kabalin JN: Prostate-specific antigen in the diagnosis and treatment of adenocarcinoma of the prostate. I. Untreated patients, *J Urol* 142:1070, 1989.

15. Walsh PC: Radical retropubic prostatectomy with reduced morbidity: an anatomic approach, *NCI Monogr* 7:133, 1988.

SUGGESTED READINGS

Begun FP: Benign prostatic hyperplasia: subjective and objective criteria for transurethral resection of the prostate, *Problems in Urology* 5:397, 1991.

Cooner WH et al: Prostate cancer detection in a clinical urological practice by ultrasonography, digital rectal examination and prostate-specific antigen, *J Urol* 143:1146, 1990.

Gittes RF: Carcinoma of the prostate, *N Engl J Med* 324:236, 1991.

Oesterling JE: Prostate-specific antigen: a critical assessment of the most useful tumor marker for adenocarcinoma of the prostate, *J Urol* 125:907, 1991 (review).

CHAPTER 26

Gynecological disorders

AMANDA CLARK

KEY POINTS
- Annual gynecological assessment offers many opportunities to physicians for primary, secondary, and tertiary prevention of disease.
- Hormone replacement therapy provides relief of the patient's uncomfortable symptoms of menopause.
- Hormone replacement therapy contributes to the health and longevity of older women by reducing cardiovascular disease and osteoporosis.
- Vulvovaginal disorders, genital prolapse, and incontinence are common conditions affecting older women.

CLINICAL RELEVANCE

Women in the geriatric age group are well into the postmenopausal years because menopause occurs on the average at age 50. With exogenous estrogen replacement, clinicians can treat the uncomfortable symptoms that are associated with menopause and prevent some of the adverse health effects of menopause such as osteoporosis. Physicians also have learned how to prevent endometrial cancer that is associated with the use of estrogen. But the ability to provide hormone replacement therapy (HRT) also has created new therapeutic dilemmas regarding cardiovascular disease, breast cancer, and unwanted vaginal bleeding. There remains much to be learned about ideal HRT.

Cancers

The prevalence of many female genital cancers continues to increase among the geriatric population. Although screening programs exist only for breast and cervical cancer, an awareness of the common presenting symptoms of uterine, ovarian, and vulvar cancer are important to the early diagnosis of these lesions.

239

There are few data to guide screening programs for breast and cervical cancer among the geriatric population. There is no general consensus about how frequently mammograms should be performed for older women; however, many clinicians recommend that mammograms should be given annually to patients between ages 50 and 70. (See Chapter 22.) Because the prevalence of breast cancer continues to rise as the population ages, it seems prudent to continue mammography every 1 or 2 years for patients beyond age 70.

The incidence of cervical cancer declines in the geriatric years, but 40% of all deaths due to cervical cancer occur in women aged 65 years and older.[4] There are no firm guidelines for proper screening intervals of Papanicolaou (Pap) smears. The American College of Obstetrics and Gynecology and the American Cancer Society recommend that screening intervals be based on the patients' risk factors for cervical cancer and adequacy of their past screenings. Women who are at higher risk should continue to have annual screenings—women who have histories of cervical dysplasia, condyloma, multiple sexual partners, or whose partners have multiple partners. Women at low risk who have had consistent screenings may decrease frequency to every 3 years. Some have advocated stopping Pap smears after age 60 for low-risk women. I disagree with this recommendation because of the difficulty in clearly assessing a patient's risk status. An additional value of the Pap smear is that it encourages women to visit their physicians for preventive health care. Pap smears should be continued after hysterectomy because cervical tissue left behind at the vaginal vault closure can place patients at risk for cancer. The frequency of Pap smears after hysterectomy should again be determined according to the patients' risk factors. In addition, many women among the geriatric age group have had a subtotal hysterectomy with the cervix left in place. These women are still at risk for developing cervical cancer and endometrial carcinoma from residual endometrial tissue.

The incidence of endometrial cancer is highest around the time of menopause, which is probably related to the patient's increased unopposed estrogen stimulation at this time. Women who receive estrogen replacement therapy without progestins remain at increased risk for endometrial cancer. Obese women who do not receive HRT may be at increased risk for cancer from endogenous estrogen that is produced by peripheral conversion of androgens in fat tissue. As vaginal bleeding is the most common presenting symptom of this cancer, any vaginal bleeding in postmenopausal women requires careful evaluation.

The incidence of ovarian cancer increases until women reach age 70, then declines. Most ovarian cancers are diagnosed as palpable ovarian masses, but the disease is usually advanced at time of detection. Screening programs using vaginal ultrasound and tumor markers such as CA 125 are being investigated but are not recommended at this time.

Vulvar cancer peaks in incidence at age 85. It is very curable in its early stages but very difficult to treat as the disease advances. Unfortunately when vulvar cancer is diagnosed for most patients, symptoms of vulvar pruritus, as well as the lesion, have been present for 1 to 2 years. Both patients and their physicians tend to neglect the symptoms, attributing them to common benign causes. Also, many older women are too embarrassed to discuss vulvar symptoms. Annual query and vulvar inspection are simple measures to ensure early diagnosis for this skin cancer.

Other disorders

Vulvovaginal problems are common in this population. Vulvovaginal atrophic changes—vaginal dryness and dyspareunia—increase in severity beyond menopause. Vulvar dystrophies are common. Genital prolapse, urinary incontinence, urgency, frequency, and fecal incontinence increase in incidence and severity.

CLINICAL MANIFESTATIONS AND DIAGNOSTIC EVALUATION

History

A gynecological history and examination should be included in the annual evaluation of the patient. The clinician should recognize the normal changes of aging and the common gynecological disorders that are experienced by elderly women. Women should be asked about breast changes, lumps, pain, or nipple discharge. They should be encouraged to practice breast self-examination. Women who are not taking HRT should be asked about menopausal symptoms. Hot flushes are not common in the geriatric age group because they usually resolve within 2 years after menopause; however, they persist indefinitely in some women. Vaginal dryness, dyspareunia from atrophy, and urinary symptoms related to estrogen deficiency—frequency, urgency and incontinence—tend to worsen after menopause. Any vaginal bleeding is *abnormal* in a postmenopausal woman who is not taking HRT. If a woman is taking hormone replacement, vaginal bleeding must be evaluated considering the HRT schedule.

Decreased lubrication and resultant dyspareunia are common, secondary to vaginal atrophy or other vulvovaginal pathology. Although most clinicians agree that questions about sexual function should routinely be asked, these questions often get lost in the patients' myriad problems. Health professionals often feel anxious about initiating a sexual history. A helpful approach is simply to ask "Do you have any sexual concerns to discuss?" This lets the patient know that the caregiver thinks these issues are important and are appropriate to be discussed. If the patient has concerns, more detailed history and dialogue naturally follow. If not, the patient then knows that she can express her concerns at a later time.

Certain symptoms need to be specifically elicited because patients tend not to report them spontaneously. Patients should be asked about vulvar itching because this is the primary presenting symptom of vulvar cancer. To remember to do this, routinely ask this question at the time of vulvar inspection during the pelvic examination. Then inspection can be directed exactly to the area of symptoms.

Other symptoms that need to be specifically elicited are those of urinary and fecal incontinence and genital prolapse. Woman are often more embarrassed to address these issues than sexuality questions. Symptoms of genital prolapse are often reported as a sensation of pelvic or introital pressure, a mass at the vaginal introitus, or lower abdominal and back pain.

Examination

Routine examination should include a systematic evaluation of the breast tissue, expression of the breast for nipple discharge, and assessment of axillary lymph nodes. The breast tissue becomes easier to examine with aging, as parenchymal tissue is replaced with fat and fibrocystic changes recede. Cyclical changes may persist if a woman is on a cyclical regimen of HRT.

Vulvovaginal atrophic changes occur both from normal aging and estrogen deficiency, with the latter having a more pronounced effect. The labia majora lose their fat pads, tha labia minora shrink, and the introitus may shrink if the patient is not sexually active. When inspecting the vulva, physicians should pay particular attention to changes associated with irritative symptoms. Biopsies of any suspicious lesions should be done because precise diagnoses for vulvar lesions are difficult to obtain from inspection alone. Any discrete lesion that is raised, ulcerated, white, red, brown, or associated with irritative symptoms is suspicious.

The vaginal mucosae lose their rugae and become shiny, dry, and paler pink in color. The introitus may be narrowed but the vaginal length is usually normal. Therefore, the best speculum to use for older women is a small Pederson speculum (long and narrow) instead of the small Graves speculum (short and narrow). The cervix protrudes less into the vaginal vault and sometimes becomes flush with the vaginal mucosa. The endocervical mucosa and transition zone move upward into the cervical canal and are rarely visible on the ectocervix. Thus, it is important to go 1 to 2 cm into the patient's endocervical canal if possible to obtain a Pap smear. An endocervical specimen is best obtained with a small brush that is inserted into the cervix (Cytobrush). An ectocervical specimen should be taken with the spatula.

Pelvic prolapse cannot be assessed with the speculum in place because the blades of the speculum support the patient's vaginal walls and uterus. The patient should be asked to strain downward after the speculum has been removed. The vaginal walls or cervix may appear at the vaginal introitus. To determine which structure is descending, the physician may need to examine the patient by using a single blade of the speculum (Figures 26-1 and 26-2).

During bimanual examination of the patient, any vaginal stenosis that may cause dyspareunia should be noted. If the patient has urinary retention, the bladder may be palpable. If the patient has incontinence, the patient's ability to perform Kegel exercises can be assessed by asking her to squeeze the pelvic floor muscles. The uterus shrinks to about 6 cm in length after menopause. Fibroid tumors tend to regress even

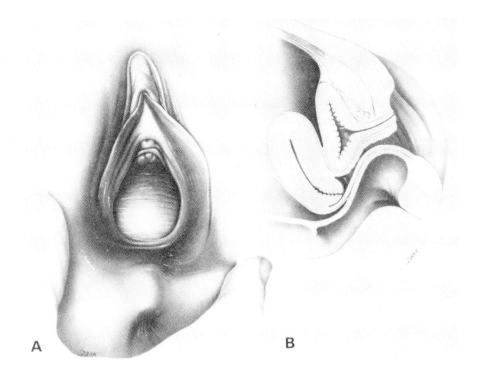

Figure 26-1 Cystocele (**A**) Exposed by a Sims speculum. (**B**) Sagittal view. The patient has been asked to bear down and cough. *(Reproduced with permission from Danforth DN, Scott J: Obstetrics and gynecology, ed 5, Philadelphia, 1986, Lippincott.)*

with estrogen replacement therapy. The ovaries shrink to $1 \times 1 \times 2$ cm and should not be palpable, regardless of HRT status. Should the ovaries be palpable, ovarian cancer must be considered. Rectovaginal examination may allow easier palpation of the uterus and adnexal region. At the same time, the rectum can be assessed for masses and stool obtained for occult blood testing.

INTERVENTION

Indications for hormone replacement therapy

The decision to initiate hormone replacement therapy is complex. The potential benefits and risks must be carefully presented and thoughtfully discussed with the patient. The decision of whether or not to receive HRT ultimately rests with the patient.

The most obvious benefit to the patient is relief of menopausal symptoms. Relief of hot flushes occurs promptly with estrogen replacement, but flushes may recur if estrogen is withdrawn. Improvement of vulvovaginal and urinary symptoms is much

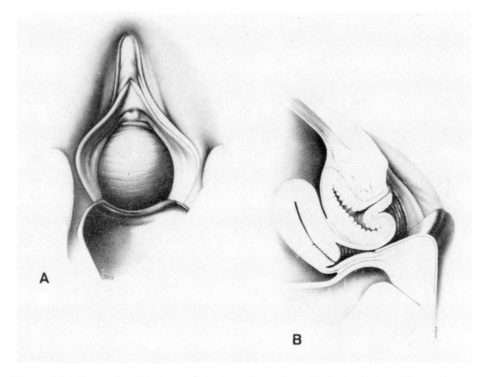

Figure 26-2 Rectocele. (**A**) Exposed by lateral traction. (**B**) Sagittal view. The patient is straining as if passing stool. *(Reproduced with permission from Danforth DN, Scott J:* Obstetrics and gynecology, *ed 5, Philadelphia, 1986, Lippincott.)*

slower. Patients may expect some improvement after 1 to 2 months, but full benefits of estrogen therapy may not be achieved for 6 to 12 months. The beneficial effect of estrogen in preventing osteoporosis has been shown clearly. (See Chapter 42.) At the time of menopause, there is accelerated loss of the mineral content of bone at approximately 1% to 2% per year. HRT arrests this loss but only as long as therapy continues. HRT cannot restore the mineral content of bone to prior levels but helps maintain bone density at its current level. For maximum benefit, HRT must be started at the time of menopause and continued indefinitely. Benefits still may be gained by patients who start HRT several years after menopause. It has been shown for women aged 65 to 74 that addition of estrogen remote from menopause is effective in preventing hip fractures.[3]

Estrogen clearly has been shown to reduce the patient's risk for cardiovascular disease. Because cardiovascular disease is so prevalent, the greatest benefit of estrogen is that it reduces the number of deaths from cardiovascular diseases. This protective effect is achieved in part by a positive impact on the patient's lipoprotein levels, but there are unknown protective mechanisms that do not involve lipoproteins. The effect of progestin on patients who are at risk for cardiovascular diseases is not yet known, but there is minimal impact to lipid profiles of those patients who currently take progestin.

The greatest potential risks of estrogen are estrogen-dependent neoplasia, endometrial carcinoma, and breast cancer. The patient's risk for endometrial carcinoma is increased by the use of estrogen that is unopposed by progestin. Addition of progestin reduces the patient's risk of endometrial carcinoma to levels below that of a postmenopausal woman who is not taking HRT.[1]

Although the risk of breast cancer is associated with factors that are influenced by estrogen—early menarche, late menopause, delayed childbearing—the bulk of evidence shows no increase in breast cancer associated with *postmenopausal* HRT.[5]

Women who need estrogen for treatment of menopausal symptoms should be reassured that HRT is safe. Unless contraindicated, HRT is recommended for women who are asymptomatic because of its overall health benefits. Because of estrogens, the reduction in the number of deaths from cardiovascular diseases and osteoporosis is significant, and it is greater than the potential increase in deaths from estrogen-related breast cancer. Studies confirm that there is an overall reduction in mortality from all causes among those who use estrogen.[2]

Contraindications for hormone replacement therapy

Estrogen replacement therapy is contraindicated for older women who have histories of advanced endometrial or breast cancer. If patients had stage I, grade I, endometrial cancer, surgery alone is curative and women may be placed safely on regimens of HRT with progestational agents. It is generally accepted that women who have breast cancer should not receive estrogen replacement, but the actual risk is unknown.

Clinicians are reluctant to give HRT to women who have histories of cardiovascular diseases largely because of the association of thrombosis with the use of oral contraceptives, which contain estrogen. But the positive impact that HRT has on the prevention of cardiovascular disease supports the use of HRT for these patients. Early data about HRT show a 50% reduction in the number of deaths from cardiovascular diseases among women who had experienced previous myocardial infarctions or strokes.

Treatment regimens

There are multiple treatment regimens. The most commonly used dose of estrogen is 0.625 mg of conjugated estrogen or 1 mg of micronized estradiol. This is the minimum dose that has been shown to prevent loss of bone density. This dose provides relief of menopausal symptoms for most women. The ideal dose for the prevention of cardiovascular disease is not known. Initially it was thought that a period of estrogen withdrawal was important for the prevention of uterine cancer; hence, the estrogen was given for 1 to 25 days. It is now apparent that the addition of progestin is critical to the prevention of endometrial cancer. Daily estrogen therapy simplifies HRT, enhances compliance, and prevents symptoms of estrogen withdrawal on the days that the hormone is not taken. Estrogen in vaginal cream is well absorbed and has all the systemic effects of oral estrogen. Oral administration produces more consistent absorption and is easier for patients to do, though vaginal administration may give quicker and better relief of vulvovaginal symptoms.

There are two schedules for progestin therapy—sequential and continuous. Ten days of medroxyprogesterone at a daily dose of 10 mg is effective in preventing endometrial hyperplasia. Medroxyprogesterone is usually given the first 10 days of the month with continuous estrogen or on days 16 through 25 with the interrupted estrogen schedule. On this regimen, 90% of women have enough endometrial stimulation to have normal estrogen-progestin withdrawal bleeding. If the bleeding occurs regularly 1 to 2 days after cessation of the progestion, the patients can be counseled that this is normal and no evaluation is necessary. Many women do not like the continued cyclical bleeding; the continuous progestin regimen may be offered to address this concern. Endometrial hyperplasia can be prevented with 2.5 mg of medroxyprogesterone given daily; thus, cyclical vaginal bleeding is prevented. Many patients experience irregular breakthrough bleeding during the first 3 to 4 months on this regimen. After 1 year on this regimen, 90% of patients have no further vaginal bleeding.

Obese women who are not taking estrogen may need progestin therapy for prophylaxis against endometrial hyperplasia and cancer from increased endogenous estrogen. Ten days of medroxyprogesterone at 10 mg a day should be administered; if withdrawal bleeding occurs, the patients should continue progestin therapy. Women who have had hysterectomies do not need progestin therapy, unless they have previous histories of endometrial cancer or endometriosis or have had supracervical hysterectomies.

Postmenopausal bleeding

The most common cause of postmenopausal bleeding is vulvovaginal atrophy. However, the most serious cause is carcinoma of the genital tract; bleeding from atrophy must be a diagnosis of exclusion. For women who do not take HRT, any vaginal bleeding must be investigated. For those who take sequential HRT, regular withdrawal bleeding should be anticipated and does not require evaluation unless the bleeding begins before the tenth day of progestin therapy. Any irregular bleeding must be evaluated. Since women who receive continuous HRT normally have irregular bleeding initially, the decision of when to evaluate them is more difficult. The decision must be made based on the patients' risk factors and levels of concern. Evaluation of postmenopausal bleeding should consist of a careful inspection of the vulva, vagina, and cervix for obvious lesions. A Pap smear should be done, followed by an endo-cervical curettage and endometrial biopsy.

SPECIFIC GYNECOLOGICAL DISORDERS

Vulvovaginal atrophy

Estrogen provides the best relief of symptoms. Vaginal dryness resulting in dys-pareunia can be alleviated with artificial lubricants. Water-based products such as Astroglide, Lubrin, and K-Y jelly are superior to oil-based lubricants such as petroleum jelly. Vaginal stenosis secondary to atrophy can be corrected by vaginal dilators, used with estrogen and lubrication, to gradually stretch the vaginal introitus. Plastic syringe covers are an inexpensive and readily available source for vaginal dilators.

Lichen sclerosus

Lichen sclerosus, a form of vulvar dystrophy, is a dermatological condition of the vulva of unknown etiology. Primary symptoms are vulvar pruritus and dyspareunia. Its presenting symptom is a symmetrical lesion affecting all or part of the vulva. Most commonly, the affected vulvar mucosa becomes thin and white and develops a "parchment paper" appearance. The labia minora appear to fuse into the labia majora and disappear. Areas that are erythematous or hyperkeratotic may be difficult to distinguish visually from carcinoma in situ, but lichen sclerosus is not considered to be premalignant. Diagnosis is made by biopsy; simple dermal punch biopsy in the office will suffice. The condition is incurable and treatment is directed toward controlling the patient's symptoms. Topical testosterone is most effective in reversing the patient's skin changes. Topical corticosteroids are effective in reducing pruritus, but they aggravate the atrophic changes and therefore should be used sparingly.

Squamous hyperplasia of the vulva

The presenting symptoms of squamous hyperplasia (formerly hypertrophic dystrophy) most often include raised white or red plaque, but the patient also may have atrophic changes. The lesions may be well demarcated or poorly defined. The labia minora do not fuse and disappear. Biopsy is required for diagnosis. Histologically there is hyperplasia of the epithelium. If atypia is present in the hyperplastic epithelium, the lesion may be premalignant. Treatment consists of topical corticosteroids for up to 6 months. Squamous hyperplasia with atypia should be observed closely for its progression to carcinoma in situ.

Carcinoma in situ and invasive squamous carcinoma

The appearance of carcinoma in situ is similar to other vulvar lesions. It may be a velvety-red patch or a raised, white, hyperkeratotic lesion. It also may be a brownish-pigmented lesion or a combination of these appearances. Any areas of ulceration, induration, or granularity are suggestive of invasion. Again, biopsy is necessary for diagnosis. Treatment for carcinoma in situ is primarily local excision of the lesion to provide a specimen that can be carefully examined by the physician for signs of invasion. Invasive disease often requires radical vulvectomy.

Genital prolapse and incontinence

The uterus, vagina, bladder, and rectum are held in place by the levator muscles and ligamentous supports of the pelvis. With aging and parturition, these attachments may become weakened and the pelvic organs descend out of their normal locations. All or part of the pelvic organs may be affected and each to various degrees, which results in various presenting symptoms. For all types of prolapse, patients may sense pressure on the pelvis or introitus, a mass protruding from the vagina, or low back pain.

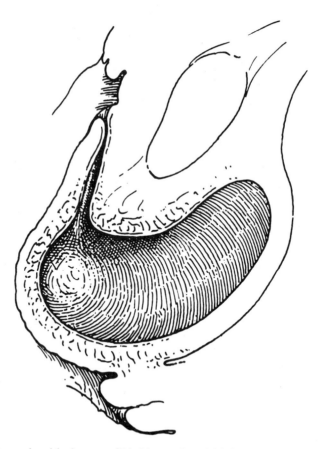

Figure 26-3 Cystocele with descent of bladder neck and bladder base. (*Reproduced with permission from Nichols DH, Randall CL:* Vaginal surgery, *ed 3, Baltimore, 1989, Williams & Wilkins.*)

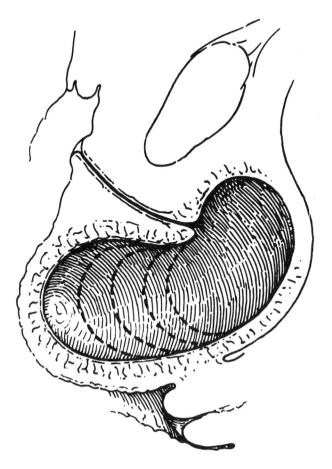

Figure 26-4 Cystocele with descent of bladder base. *(Reproduced with permission from Nichols DH, Randall DL: Vaginal surgery, ed 3, Baltimore, 1989, Williams & Wilkins.)*

A cystocele results from downward displacement of the bladder and anterior vaginal wall. If the urethra and bladder neck are displaced, the patient is prone to incontinence (Figure 26-3). If the cystocele involves only the upper vaginal wall and bladder base, the urethra may be kinked, sometimes improving continence and producing voiding difficulties for the patient (Figure 26-4). Genuine stress incontinence is highly associated with anterior vaginal wall prolapse, but the presence of a cystocele does not predict the presence of incontinence or its cause. When patients have urinary incontinence, they should be given a full evaluation that explores all possible causes, and their incontinence should not be attributed merely to the prolapse. (See Chapter 24.)

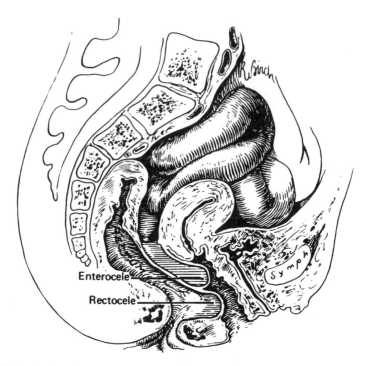

Figure 26-5 Sagittal section demonstrating the relative positions of a cystocele and rectocele. (*Reproduced with permission from Te Linde RW, Mattingly RF:* Operative gynecology, *ed 4, Philadelphia, 1970, Lippincott.*)

A rectocele results from downward displacement of the rectum and posterior vaginal wall (Figure 26-5). Symptoms of a rectocele include the patient's difficulty in evacuating the rectum and need for placing digital pressure in the vagina to empty the rectum. Rectoceles probably contribute to fecal impaction.

An enterocele results from the elongation and descent of the cul-de-sac or pouch of Douglas (Figure 26-5). Primary symptoms are a bulging sensation in the vagina and lower back pain. Enteroceles occur most commonly with uterine prolapse and with post-hysterectomy vaginal vault prolapse. With extreme uterine or vaginal vault prolapse, the patient's vagina may become completely inverted outside the body. With massive eversion, the ureters may become kinked, leading to obstructive uropathy. Obstructive uropathy is the only serious medical consequence of prolapse.

Prolapse may severely limit a patient's ability to be physically and sexually active. Treatment of prolapse is directed toward alleviating the patient's symptoms. Reducing a chronic cough, avoiding heavy lifting, and losing excess weight and constipation are measures that may help the patient.

A vaginal pessary can support prolapsed pelvic structures. The type of pessary used depends on the size of the vagina, type and degree of prolapse, and maintenance plan for the pessary. Ideally, the patient learns how to insert and remove the pessary herself. Some patients are unwilling to do this or are limited by lack of manual dexterity and cannot manage the pessary. They then must make regular visits to a health provider to remove and clean the pessary. Pessaries should be changed no less frequently than once a month—more often if a foul-smelling vaginal discharge develops. HRT is recommended to help the patients maintain vaginal mucosal integrity. Patients should be examined frequently for development of vaginal ulcers. A neglected pessary can result in a vesicovaginal or rectovaginal fistula from pressure necrosis.

Surgical repair offers correction of the prolapse and allows better function. A vaginal approach is preferred particularly for elderly patients to avoid abdominal incisions and facilitate the patients' recoveries. The type of surgery depends on which organs are affected and the types of symptoms that patients have, the details of which are beyond the scope of this chapter.

Fecal incontinence is associated with genital prolapse, but its etiology and treatment are poorly understood. Strengthening of the pelvic floor muscles may help patients to regain control. If stool consistency is loose, antidiarrheal agents may improve patients' stool consistency and bowel control.

REFERENCES

1. Gambrell RD Jr, Babgnell CA, Greenblatt RB: Role of estrogens and progesterone in the etiology and prevention of endometrial cancer: a review, *Am J Obstet Gynecol* 146:696, 1983.
2. Henderson BE, Paganini-Hill A, Ross RK: Estrogen replacement therapy and protection from acute myocardial infarction, *Am J Obstet Gynecol* 159:312, 1988.
3. Kiel DP et al: Hip fracture and the use of estrogens in postmenopausal women: the Framingham study, *N Engl J Med* 317:1169, 1987.
4. Mandelblatt JS, Fahs MC: The cost-effectiveness of cervical cancer screening for low-income elderly women, *JAMA* 259:2409, 1988.
5. Sillero-Arenas M et al: Menopausal hormone replacement therapy and breast cancer: a metaanalysis, *Obstet Gynecol* 79:286, 1992.

SUGGESTED READINGS

Byyny RL, Speroff L: *A clinical guide for the care of older women*, Baltimore, 1990, Williams & Wilkins.
Mishell DR Jr: *Menopause: physiology and pharmacology*, Chicago, 1987, Year Book.
Friedreich, EG Jr: *Vulvar disease*, ed 2, Philadelphia, 1983, WB Saunders.

CHAPTER 27

Sexual dysfunction

THOMAS MULLIGAN

KEY POINTS

- The most common reason for declining rates of sexual activity among the elderly population is male sexual dysfunction.
- Male dysfunction most often includes erectile failure and is frequently due to neurovascular diseases.
- Female sexual dysfunction most often includes dyspareunia due to hypoestrogenic vaginal atrophy.
- Successful treatment of sexual dysfunction requires a sensitive clinician who knows when medical, surgical, or psychological therapies are appropriate.

CLINICAL RELEVANCE

With aging, individuals' sexual interest (libido) declines to a mild degree, while sexual activity declines dramatically. However, when health status is factored into any analysis of age-related changes pertaining to sexuality, it becomes apparent that healthy elderly individuals demonstrate fewer changes in sexual interest, ability, or activity as they age, while those who develop age-associated diseases (e.g., diabetes mellitus, hypertension) lose their ability and are less active but retain sexual interest. Declining sexual ability is more often present in the aged man than in the woman and usually includes erectile failure.

The focus of sexual activity also changes during adult development. In young adulthood, sexual contact is directed toward orgasm. In contrast, during middle age, the individual looks for pleasure rather than just release. Although the sexual interaction often ends in orgasm, other pleasurable sensations are as highly rated as orgasm itself. During old age, there is a strong desire for tenderness and intimacy, even in the absence of penile-vaginal intercourse with orgasm. Thus sexual needs change but do not usually cease.

SEXUAL DYSFUNCTION IN MALES

Clinical manifestations

The first step in evaluating sexual dysfunction of the elderly male is to identify the problem. Although sexual dysfunction is common, patients often do not complain. Patients may be influenced by their own or their practitioners' ageist biases and may be fearful of discussing the problem. Therefore a sexual history should be part of every comprehensive geriatric assessment.

Diagnostic approach

The box lists the common causes of erectile failures among elderly men.

History. The sexual history includes three basic components: (1) sexual interest, (2) sexual ability, and (3) sexual activity. The clinician must be aware that sexual interest declines to a modest degree with aging.[1] Sexual ability, on the other hand, declines dramatically; the vast majority of aged men report inadequate erections for vaginal intercourse.[6] Sexual activity also declines dramatically among aged men, primarily because of their declining erectile function or other manifestations of declining health.

Determining the onset and course of the erectile dysfunction can be particularly helpful in the evaluation of the patient. Erectile failure that has an acute onset and a temporal association with the initiation of a new drug therapy suggests drug-induced impotence. Those drugs that are associated with erectile failure include diuretics, centrally acting antihypertensives, beta blockers, and virtually any agent with anticholinergic effects. Psychogenic erectile failure is similarly acute in its onset but temporally related to an emotionally stressful event. However, psychogenic impotence is variable in its course, with the patients' having normal erections during masturbation or with different partners. In addition, patients who have psychogenic erectile failure often report firm, long-lasting, morning erections. Psychogenic impotence is relatively uncommon in elderly men.

Erectile failure that has a gradual onset is most common among aged men and is usually associated with neurological or vascular disease. The course is typically in-

---

COMMON CAUSES OF ERECTILE FAILURE AMONG AGED MEN

Combined neurovascular disease	30%
Vascular	21%
Diabetic neuropathy	17%
Nondiabetic neuropathy	11%
Psychogenic	9%
Drug effects	4%
Hypogonadism	3%

sidious and unremitting. Older men usually first report difficulties in maintaining erections, followed months or years later by difficulties in initiating erections. Their problems of obtaining firm erections through masturbation mirror problems that they have during sexual activity with their partners. Upon awakening, the men's erections are either absent or of limited duration and rigidity.

Physical examination. The physical examination is helpful in establishing vascular, neurological, endocrinological, or genital disorders that may be related to the patient's erectile failure. Specifically, the clinician should look for visual field defects, gynecomastia, abdominal or femoral bruits, testicular atrophy, penile plaques, diminished peripheral pulses, and peripheral neuropathy. The assessment of the bulbocavernosus reflex, which assesses the reflex arc of the pudendal nerve and sacral spinal cord, is easily administered to determine the patient's penile-somatic innervation. The absence of this reflex suggests penile neuropathy. With the information provided by the history and physical examination, the clinician can make one of the following presumptive diagnoses:

1. normal age-related change
2. adverse drug reaction
3. psychogenic impotence
4. hypogonadism
5. penile neuropathy, or
6. penile vascular disease.[5]

However, distinguishing between patients who have penile neuropathy, arterial insufficiency, venous insufficiency, or multifactorial causes often requires laboratory-based assessment.

Laboratory assessment. Blood tests usually include a fasting blood glucose and serum free testosterone. The fasting glucose (or alternatively, hemoglobin A_{1c}) may be measured to determine whether diabetes mellitus, with associated autonomic neuropathy, might be the underlying cause of erectile failure. The testosterone level is obtained to diagnose hypogonadism. However, the clinician should be aware that hypogonadism is associated more clearly with the patient's low sexual interest rather than impaired erectile function. Nevertheless, when free testosterone levels are low or marginal, a trial of testosterone supplementation may prove beneficial.

Assessment of the patient's nocturnal erectile function is helpful when psychogenic impotence is suspected. The presence of sleep-associated erections confirms the clinician's suspicion that the erectile mechanisms are intact, despite the patient's complaints to the contrary. A simple measure of nocturnal erectile function can be obtained by the outdated "stamp test" or the snap gauge (Dacomed). Radial pressure that is adequate to break the snap gauge correlates with penile rigidity. The snap gauge may be helpful as a screening test, but it has limitations in sensitivity and specificity.

The penile arterial supply can be noninvasively assessed by comparing the penile systolic pressure to the brachial systolic pressure using a Doppler probe (penile brachial index). However, injection of papaverine into the penis may be more sensitive for diagnosing penile vascular insufficiency. Arterial inflow and the restriction of venous outflow are probably adequate among those patients who develop rigid erections in response to papaverine that is injected intracavernosally.

Penile somatic innervation can be evaluated by nerve conduction velocity studies (electromyogram) of the pudendal nerve. Delayed nerve conduction velocity confirms a neuropathic diagnosis for diabetics and other patients who may have peripheral neuropathy. Unfortunately, assessment for the autonomic innervation of the erectile mechanism is not available.

Interventions

Table 27-1 summarizes treatment options for patients who have erectile failure. For patients who have hypogonadism, 200 mg of testosterone intramuscularly every 3 weeks may be effective. Newer transdermal delivery systems are being tested and may mimic the usual diurnal variations in testosterone levels. Oral testosterone undecanoate is hepatotoxic and should be avoided. Yohimbine and vitamin E are frequently used but have not been adequately evaluated to support their being recommended.

A variety of external devices (penile orthoses, vacuum entrapment devices) are currently available. Initial studies of vacuum-induced erections reported a good response rate from patients and few adverse effects other than ecchymoses. However, devices for vacuum-induced erections require a degree of manual dexterity that may preclude their use by elderly males who have arthritic or otherwise dysfunctional hands. One of the external devices (Erection System by Synergist) uses suction to draw the penis into a condomlike device but relies on the innate stiffness of the device to facilitate vaginal penetration. Although penile orthoses are appealing because of their reversible and noninvasive nature, they also have not been adequately studied.

Table 27-1   Treatment options for geriatric erectile failure

Treatment	Advantages	Disadvantages
Testosterone	Noninvasive	Rarely effective
Erecaid (Osbon)	Noninvasive	Cumbersome; not effective for arteriogenic dysfunction
Erection System (Synergist)	Noninvasive; effective regardless of causes	Decreases sensitivity; unaesthetic
Papaverine	Erection looks normal	Cavernosal fibrosis
Prostaglandin E_1	Erection looks normal	Burning sensation
Malleable prosthesis	No mechanical parts to malfunction	Permanent erection
Inflatable prosthesis	Erection looks normal	Often requires reoperation

Intracorporeal pharmacotherapy is an area under active investigation. Injection of papaverine, either alone or in combination with phentolamine, or prostaglandin E_1 will produce penile erections for men who do not have severe vascular disease. Self-injection has been used by thousands of patients worldwide and is accepted as a nonexperimental only slightly invasive option. Short-term complications include prolonged erections that need to be reversed if they last more than 4 hours. Long-term studies are only nearly complete; however, papaverine likely results in penile fibrosis in a small percentage of cases. In contrast, prostaglandin E_1 causes a painful burning sensation for some patients but is thought to be safer for long-term use because of the lower incidence of penile fibrosis.[2]

When noninvasive or slightly invasive options are not satisfactory, the implantation of a penile prosthesis may be successful. Prosthesis implantation should be considered after other less invasive options because a penile implant can be performed when other therapies have failed; however, less invasive therapies are of limited benefit after an implant fails. Depending on the type of prosthesis, costs are approximately $5,000 to $8,000. Available prostheses include rigid, malleable, multicomponent inflatable, and self-contained inflatable devices. The choice of prosthesis depends upon the patient's and spouse's preferences. Satisfaction of patients and partners immediately following prosthesis implantation has been good, although long-term studies have not been adequate.

Penile arterial revascularization potentially corrects the underlying problem but has met with limited success. The high prevalence of distal vessel disease among elderly men usually precludes successful revascularization. Penile venous ligation in patients who have abnormal venous drainage also has met with a disappointing success rate of less than 50%.

SEXUAL DYSFUNCTION IN FEMALES

Clinical manifestations

A sexual history should be part of the comprehensive geriatric assessment. Like the sexual history for males, the sexual history for females includes three basic components: (1) sexual interest, (2) sexual ability, and (3) sexual activity. Sexual interest declines to a greater degree among aging women than among aging men. However, sexual ability does not decline as dramatically for women compared with men's sexual ability. Sexual activity declines because of the loss of erectile function in the male partner or the death of the male partner.

Sexual dysfunction among older women is often related to menopause.[7] However, there is controversy as to which changes occur as a result of estrogen deficiency alone or other age-related changes. The decrease in estrogen is responsible for the increased alkalinity of vaginal secretions (contributing to increased frequency of vaginitis), decreased vaginal lubrication during sexual stimulation, and reduced labial and clitoral engorgement during stimulation. (Atherosclerosis is also contributory.) Other age-related changes include loss of subcutaneous fat in the mons pubis and labia majora and thinning of labia minora resulting in exposure of the clitoris and urinary meatus. These may result in irritation to the clitoris or urethra. Furthermore, the vaginal wall gradually atrophies. Any of the above changes can result in dyspareunia with secondary vaginismus. However, sexual activity does not necessarily decrease as a result of these changes. In fact, some women report an increase in sexual activity and enjoyment, which is attributed to their loss of the fear of unplanned pregnancies.[3]

Diagnostic approach

The most important aspect of diagnosis is a sensitive clinician who can create an environment where the woman feels comfortable to share intimate feelings. Questions that explore past and present sexual problems are important. Does the patient have a sexually functional partner? What is her present living situation (independence versus dependence)? Are her religious beliefs in conflict with her sex life? What are her concerns regarding menopause?

If dyspareunia is the main sexual complaint, the clinician should explore its severity and whether vaginismus is also present. Symptoms of uterine cramping should be evaluated as well. The patient should be queried about adverse drug reactions (e.g., vaginal dryness due to anticholinergics).

The history should be followed by a gentle and careful physical examination of breasts and genitalia. (See Chapter 26.) Some women prefer having a mirror during the examination of the genitalia to better understand some of the changes that have occurred. The genitalia should be examined for loss of subcutaneous fat of the labia majora and thinning of the labia minora. Gently place a finger in the vaginal introitus and observe for involuntary muscle contraction, which may suggest vaginismus. Insertion of a warm moist speculum (correctly sized) allows inspection of the vaginal wall. The well-corrugated, thickened, reddish-purple vagina of youth may be replaced by a less corrugated, thin, light-pink vaginal wall due to hypoestrogenemia. The examiner should observe for signs of irritation or bleeding.

Few laboratory tests are required to diagnose sexual dysfunction in the female. Serum estradiol levels are occasionally helpful.

Interventions

Education related to aging is an important aid in dispelling myths. Discussion of topics such as romance, privacy, and self-esteem can facilitate exploration of the psychosocial aspect of sexuality. Medical conditions such as vaginitis obviously need attention. For iatrogenic sexual dysfunction, discontinuing the drug may resolve the problem.

If dyspareunia is the result of menopause, treatment options are multiple. Estrogen replacement relieves dryness of the vagina, a major cause of dyspareunia, and may increase orgasmic frequency and sexual enjoyment. (See Chapter 26.) The less common uterine cramping that follows orgasm also can be eliminated by estrogen replacement. However, hormonal therapy is not free of side effects and should not be used indiscriminately. Nevertheless, estrogen replacement for properly selected patients (i.e., those who have no estrogen-sensitive cancers) is safe and effective in relieving many of the symptoms that contribute to sexual dysfunction.[4] If estrogen replacement is contraindicated, other methods for alleviating dyspareunia are available. For delayed or diminished vaginal lubrication, the woman and her partner can prolong foreplay. If this is still not sufficient, artificial lubricants (K-Y jelly) can be quite successful. The tube of lubricant should be warmed to body temperature for best results.

Vaginismus can be treated by gently inserting a finger with a slightly downward pressure into the vagina; a vaginal dilator also may be used. The number of fingers inserted into the vagina should be increased gradually until adequate relaxation of the vaginal muscles has occurred. Depending on the severity of the patient's vaginismus, this procedure may continue for days or weeks but is usually successful if the partner is supportive and patient.

Guidelines for successful sexual activity also should be discussed. Physical rest and a warm bath relax the musculoskeletal system and may enhance sexual activity. Awareness and improvement of physical appearance, nutrition, and atmosphere are also important. Slow and gentle love making, avoiding heavy thrusting, and varying the positions all may contribute to successful sexual activity.

Finally, all must realize that there is more to sexuality than penile-vaginal intercourse. Intimacy, including sharing, hugging, kissing, and holding each other, offers immense satisfaction. Why must the warm sensual experience of simply holding and being held be viewed as a failed sexual experience because one or both partners didn't attain orgasmic release?

REFERENCES

1. Davidson JM et al: Hormonal changes and sexual function in aging men, *J Clin Endocrinol Metab* 57:71, 1983.
2. Krane RJ, Goldstein I, De Tejada IS: Impotence, *N Engl J Med* 321:1648, 1989.
3. Gupta K: Sexual dysfunction in elderly women, *Clin Geriatr Med* 6:197, 1990.
4. Mooradian AD, Greiff V: Sexuality in older women, *Arch Intern Med* 150:1033, 1990.
5. Mulligan T, Katz PG: Erectile failure in the aged: evaluation and treatment, *J Am Geriatr Soc* 36:54, 1988.
6. Pfeiffer E, Verwoerdt A, Wang H: Sexual behavior in aged men and women, *Arch Gen Psychiatry* 19:753, 1968.
7. Sarrel P: Sexuality and Menopause, *Obstet Gynecol* 75:26s, 1990.

SUGGESTED READINGS

Bretschneider JG, McCoy NL: Sexual interest and behavior in healthy 80- to 102-year olds, *Arch Sex Behav* 17:109, 1988.
Vermeulen A: Androgens in the aging male, *J Clin Endocrinol Metab* 73:221, 1991.

CHAPTER 28

Urinary tract infection

THOMAS T. YOSHIKAWA

<u>KEY POINTS</u>

- Urinary tract infection is the most frequent bacterial infection found among older persons.
- Symptoms may be atypical or absent; acute confusion or functional changes may be the presenting clinical manifestations.
- Urine culture is necessary for diagnosis.
- Expect gram-negative bacteria other than *Escherichia coli*.
- Treat patients with oral trimethoprim-sulfamethoxazole, first generation cephalosporin, or quinolone.
- Follow up with patients in 24 to 48 hours.

CLINICAL RELEVANCE

Urinary tract infection (UTI) is the most frequent bacterial infection found among the geriatric population. Bacteriuria is defined as the presence of a uropathogen, at least 100,000 colonies/ml urine, on the patient's culture (UTI is *symptomatic* bacteriuria) and occurs in 5 to 15% of aging men and 10 to 30% of aging women who live in the community.[1] Most cases of bacteriuria among older adults are asymptomatic (i.e., there are no associated genitourinary or systemic complaints with the infection). An unknown but significant number of elderly persons who have asymptomatic bacteriuria experience symptomatic infection or urosepsis. Some individuals have persistent asymptomatic bacteriuria, and other older adults have bacteriuria that resolves spontaneously.

CLINICAL MANIFESTATIONS

Urinary tract infection should be suspected for any elderly person who has an acute change in health status, functional capacity, or feeling of well-being. This

259

information is especially important for older adults who have histories of genitourinary instrumentation, obstructive uropathy, urinary incontinence, genitourinary stones, other functional or anatomical abnormalities of the genitourinary tract, urosepsis, diabetes mellitus, or immunocompromised state.

As previously stated, bacteriuria is most often asymptomatic among aging adults. Nevertheless, symptomatic infection does occur and patients may manifest classic symptoms of dysuria, frequency, urgency (triad of the dysuric syndrome), flank or abdominal pain, fever, or chills. Alternatively, symptoms may be quite nonspecific and the patient only may exhibit decline in functional capacities, poor appetite, listlessness, weakness, confusion, falls, or occasionally urinary incontinence; fever also may be absent.

DIAGNOSTIC APPROACH

The diagnosis of UTI is confirmed by culturing at least 100,000 colonies of a uropathogen/ml urine. A preliminary *presumptive* diagnosis of UTI may be made from a patient's urinalysis. However, since the causes of UTI among aging persons may be more diverse and less predictable than for younger adults, a urine culture with antibiotic susceptibility data is essential for proper management of this infection. Whereas *Escherichia coli* causes 80% to 90% of uncomplicated UTI for young adults, *E. coli* may be isolated in 50% to 70% of older patients who have bacteriuria or UTI. The accompanying box lists uropathogens found among elderly patients who have UTI or asymptomatic bacteriuria. Older persons who have urinary catheters often have multiple microorganisms, including enterococci (25% of patients who are catheterized have enterococci), in their urine.

Urine collection

Proper collection of urine, which is essential for accurate microbiological data, may be more difficult for less functionally independent older persons. For elderly men who are circumcised, first-voided urine specimens are adequate for urinalysis

---

UROPATHOGENS IN ELDERLY PERSONS WITH BACTERIURIA

Citrobacter diversus	*Klebsiella pneumoniae* (indole-negative)
Citrobacter freundii	*Morganella morganii*
Enterobacter aerogenes	*Proteus mirabilis* (indole-negative)
Enterobacter cloacae	*Proteus vulgaris* (indole-positive)
Enterococcus faecalis	*Providencia rettgeri*
Enterococcus faecium	*Providencia stuartii*
Escherichia coli	*Pseudomonas aeruginosa*
Klebsiella oxytoca (indole-positive)	*Serratia marcescens*

and culture; careful cleansing of the glans penis and obtaining a midstream specimen are unnecessary.[4] However, for uncircumcised men, cleansing of the glans penis is recommended, which should then be followed by collection of a first-voided sample.

For many elderly women, assistance by a nurse or nursing assistant is necessary for proper collection of urine, since the risk of contamination of the urine specimen with perineal, vaginal, and skin microflora is significant. A sitting reversed position on the toilet facilitates abduction of the lower extremities and thus reduces the risk of perineal and skin contamination during voiding and collection of urine.[2]

Aging patients who are unable to provide a voided urine sample may require catheterization of the bladder in order to obtain a specimen. Although catheterization of women is relatively easy, the procedure is much more difficult and traumatic for elderly men. The risk of bacteriuria following a single catheterization of the bladder may be as high as 10%, depending on the patient's gender and underlying disease, sterility of the procedure, and ease of performing the catheterization. Therefore, every effort should be made to have the patients spontaneously void rather than undergo catheterization.

Tests for bacteriuria

Urinalysis that includes a Gram stain smear of the urine is useful as a preliminary test for diagnosing UTI. Pyuria in spun urine (five or more leukocytes per high-power field examination by light microscopy) has an accuracy of 65% to 70% in predicting the presence of bacteriuria. A Gram stain of either *unspun* urine that shows at least 1 bacterium per immersion oil field in several fields or of *centrifuged* urine that shows more than 20 bacteria per high-power field in several fields has approximately an 80% correlation with quantitative culture of at least 100,000 organisms/ml urine. Thus, in an ambulatory setting, a Gram stain smear of urine is useful as a preliminary screening test for bacteriuria until culture data become available.

Urine culture remains the sine qua non for the diagnosis of bacteriuria and UTI. For elderly patients who have genitourinary complaints that are consistent with UTI, a single urine culture yielding at least 100,000 colonies of a uropathogen/ml urine is highly reliable in confirming the presence of true UTI as opposed to urine contamination. In older women who are clinically asymptomatic, true bacteriuria is diagnosed when two urine specimens taken at least 24 hours apart show the same organism(s) in counts of at least 100,000 colonies/ml.[2] For asymptomatic older men, a single quantitative culture of at least 100,000 colonies of a uropathogen/ml urine is sufficient for the diagnosis of true bacteriuria.

Several simple culture techniques are available commercially that permit clinicians to perform urine cultures in the office and at a reasonable cost. These techniques permit screening for quantitative bacteriuria within 24 hours and also may be used to follow up with patients for the presence of bacteriuria (either as a test of cure after therapy or to follow the course of asymptomatic bacteriuria). Of the several available techniques, the dip-slide culture method appears to be the most reliable and simplest to use.[5] The dip-slide method utilizes a glass slide or plastic template that is coated with agar media on each side. Depending on the company (Uricult, Orion Laboratories, distributed by Medical Technology Corporation, Hackensack, New Jersey; Oxoid dip-slide, Flow Laboratories, Rockville, Maryland; Dipnoic, Stayne Diagnostics, East Rutherford, New Jersey; Clinicult, Smith Kline Laboratories, Philadelphia, Pennsylvania), the agar media vary, but they generally consist of a medium on one side for selective growth of gram-negative bacteria and a different medium on the other side for growth of gram-positive organisms. After collecting urine in a sterile container, the dip-slide is simply immersed in the urine. It then can be placed directly in an incubator (if one is available in the office) or be transported to a laboratory for processing. The results can be interpreted within 24 hours. By using a chart, physicians can match colony density on the slide to quantitative counts. The dip-slide method has a nearly 100% correlation with standard methods for quantitative urine culture; however, it does not permit identification of the species of the bacteria. Therefore, this test remains useful only as a screening test for the presence or absence of bacteriuria. Another feature of the dip-slide method is that isolated pathogens can be subcultured to standard plate culture methods and thus permit subsequent identification and antibiotic susceptibility studies.

INTERVENTION

Antibiotic treatment

Once a presumptive diagnosis of UTI is made, a decision must be made about either immediate empirical therapy or delayed specific treatment when culture data become available. Table 28-1 summarizes the recommended antibiotics for uropathogens that most commonly infect older adults. This information should be used only as guidelines.

When immediate empirical antibiotic therapy is considered, the antibiotic selection should be based on the patient's clinical history and most common uropathogens. For healthy, functionally independent, older persons who have no urinary catheters, histories of recurrent UTI, or underlying genitourinary abnormalities and who are clinically stable enough to justify outpatient therapy (uncomplicated UTI), initial treatment may begin with amoxicillin clavulanic acid, trimethoprim-sulfamethoxazole, or cefadroxil. (See Table 28-1 for the dosages.) The most likely uropathogens in this group will be *E. coli*, *Proteus mirabilis* (indole-negative), or *Klebsiella* sp. For aging patients with complicated UTI (i.e., hospital-acquired UTI, recurrent UTI, recent therapy with antibiotics, presence of genitourinary stones or other functional and anatomical genitourinary abnormalities, or indwelling bladder catheters), the causes of UTI will be more diverse and more resistant to standard antibiotics. For these patients in whom outpatient therapy is justified, treatment should be initiated with a quinolone such as norfloxacin or ciprofloxacin. (See Table 28-1 for dosages.)

Table 28-1 Treatment recommendations for pathogens causing urinary tract infection in older adults

Organism	Antibiotic*	Oral daily dose
Escherichia coli		
	Ampicillin	250-500 q 6 h
	Trimethoprim	100 mg q 12 h or 200 mg q 24 h
	Trimethoprim-sulfamethoxazole (TMP-SMZ)	160 mg TMP-800 mg SMZ q 12 h
	Cefadroxil	500 mg q 24 h
	Amoxicillin-clavulanic acid	250 mg (amoxicillin) q 8 h
	Cefixime	400 mg q 12-24 h
Proteus mirabilis (**indole-negative**)		
	Same as *E. coli*	
Klebsiella **sp.**		
	Cefadroxil	500 mg q 24 h
	Cefuroxime axetil	125 mg q 12 h
	Amoxicillin-clavulanic acid	Same as above
	TMP-SMZ	Same as above
	Cefixime	Same as above
Enterobacter **sp.**		
	Cefuroxime axetil	Same as above
	Amoxicillin-clavulanic acid	Same as above
	Norfloxacin	400 mg q 12 h
	Ciprofloxacin	250 mg q 12 h
Proteus **sp.** (**indole-positive**)		
	Same as *Enterobacter* sp.	
Morganella morganii		
	Same as *Enterobacter* sp.	
Serratia marcescens		
	Norfloxacin	Same as above
	Ciprofloxacin	Same as above
	Cefixime	Same as above
Providencia **sp.**		
	Same as *Serratia marcescens*	
Pseudomonas aeruginosa		
	Norfloxacin	Same as above
	Ciprofloxacin	Same as above

*Selection depends on antibiotic susceptibility data and clinician's preference. Some organisms may be resistant to the antibiotics listed and may require other drugs.

Table 28-1   Treatment recommendations for pathogens causing urinary tract infection in older adults—cont'd

Organism	Antibiotic*	Oral daily dose
Citrobacter sp.		
	Norfloxacin	Same as above
	Ciprofloxacin	Same as above
Enterococcus sp.		
	Ampicillin	Same as above
	Amoxicillin-clavulanic acid	Same as above
	Norfloxacin	Same as above
	Ciprofloxacin	Same as above
	TMP-SMZ	Same as above

When culture and antibiotic susceptibility data become available, therapy should be changed—if appropriate and feasible—to a less expensive, less toxic, or more narrow-spectrum antibiotic. Treatment should last a minimum of 10 days for older women with uncomplicated UTI. Infected older men as well as women who have complicated UTI should receive therapy for 14 to 21 days.

Table 28-2 describes precautions and recommendations for prescribing antibiotics for ambulatory elderly patients with UTI.

Follow-up

After antibiotic therapy has been prescribed, the patients should be contacted by telephone in 24 to 48 hours to determine their clinical statuses. If the patients report that they feel better and have no adverse drug reactions, treatment is continued. On days 3 through 6 of therapy, patients are instructed to bring urine specimens to the office or laboratory for either urinalysis or dip-stick culture to screen for bacteriuria (or patients may bring in dip-stick slide). If the patients continue to improve and their interim urine examinations show elimination of organisms, the patients are advised to return 7 to 10 days after completion of antibiotic therapy for a brief examination and repeat urine culture (proof of cure).

The alternative scenario is that the patients do not improve clinically 24 to 48 hours after initiation of antibiotics. These patients should be advised to return to their clinicians for reexamination and repeat urine culture (and urinalysis). If the patients appear clinically unstable, they should be immediately hospitalized and treated for urosepsis. However, if the clinical statuses of the patients appear stable, the patients may be managed on an outpatient basis. The antibiotic regimen should be changed empirically (after urine is collected for culture). The follow-up procedure would again be the same as previously outlined. All patients who have been suc-

Table 28-2 Precautions and recommendations for prescribing antibiotics in elderly patients with UTI

Drug	Pharmacological changes with age/adverse effects	Precautions and recommendations
Ampicillin and amoxicillin clavulanic acid	Reduced renal clearance; oral absorption unchanged	No dose reduction with creatinine clearance above 30 ml/min; avoid if there is allergy to penicillins
Carbenicillin	Same as ampicillin	Same as ampicillin; 23 mg sodium/387 mg tablet
Cefadroxil, cefuroxime, and cefixime	Reduced renal clearance; oral absorption unchanged	No dose reduction with creatinine clearance above 30 ml/min; cross-allergy may occur with penicillins
Trimethoprim-sulfamethoxaxole	Reduced renal clearance; oral absorption unchanged	No dose reduction with creatinine clearance above 30 ml/min; avoid if there is sulfa allergy or severe renal failure (creatinine clearance less than 10 ml/min)
Norfloxacin and ciprofloxacin	Renal clearance affected only with moderately severe renal impairment; nonrenal clearance mechanisms unaffected	Elevated serum theophylline levels with ciprofloxacin but not norfloxacin; antacids with calcium, magnesium, or aluminum reduce oral absorption

cessfully treated should have repeat urine cultures (dip-slide method would be suitable under these circumstances) 1 to 3 months after completion of therapy.

Asymptomatic bacteriuria

Since the natural history of asymptomatic bacteriuria in any one patient is quite unpredictable (many patients become abacteriuric spontaneously) and since the true risk of morbidity or mortality of this condition is unknown, antibiotic treatment of asymptomatic bacteriuria in older adults is generally not indicated. Nevertheless, under some select circumstances treatment may be considered. For example, patients with obstructive uropathy and chronic bacteriuria are at high risk for developing symptomatic UTI or urosepsis, as well as chronic pyelonephritis. Treatment of asymptomatic bacteriuria is warranted for these patients. Some patients may report intermittent but frequent bouts of symptomatic bacteriuria or UTI; such individuals may deserve antibiotic therapy in an effort to decrease the number of symptomatic episodes. Finally, some of these patients who have asymptomatic bacteriuria, especially men, should have further diagnostic evaluations of their genitourinary tracts (i.e., prostatic examination, residual volume of bladder urine, intravenous pyelography, or cystoscopy).

REFERENCES

1. Boscia JA, et al: Epidemiology of bacteriuria in an ambulatory elderly population, *Am J Med* 80:208, 1986.
2. Kunin CM, ed: *Detection, prevention, and management of urinary tract infections*, ed 4, Philadelphia, 1987, Lea & Febiger.
3. Lipsky BA, et al: Diagnosis of bacteriuria in men: specimen collection and culture interpretation, *J Infect Dis* 155:847, 1987.
4. Miriovsky MF: Office analysis of bacteriuria, *Am Fam Pract* (AFP) 19:121, 1979.

SUGGESTED READINGS

Abrutyn E, Boscia JA, Kaye D: The treatment of asymptomatic bacteriuria in the elderly, *J Am Geriatr Soc* 36:473, 1988.
Baldassarre JS, Kaye D: Special problems of urinary tract infection in the elderly, *Med Clin North Am* 75:375, March 1991.
Porush JG, Faubert PF, eds: Urinary infection. In *Renal disease in the aged*, Boston, 1991, Little, Brown.

CHAPTER 29

Common skin problems

ARNOLD W. GUREVITCH
KEITH GROSS

KEY POINTS

- The most common cause of itching for geriatric patients is dry skin.
- Intertriginous eruptions usually respond to a combination of a low-potency topical corticosteroid and an antifungal/anticandidal agent.
- Herpes zoster in elderly persons should be carefully assessed for possible dissemination.
- Suspect scabies in patients who itch and have contact with others who have itching.
- Ecchymoses limited to the dorsal arms and hands are a result of chronic sun exposure as are flat brown spots on the same areas.
- Basal cell carcinomas occur most commonly on the face, neck, and upper trunk.
- Actinic keratoses are persistent, rough-surfaced, reddish lesions on sun-exposed skin.
- Lentigo maligna melanoma occurs on chronically sun-exposed skin of elderly patients.
- Characteristics (A-B-C-D) of melanoma are *asymmetrical* lesion, *border* irregularity, *color* nonuniform, and *diameter* greater than 6 mm.

The human integument undergoes many changes with advancing age.[4] While many of these are related specifically to environmental factors such as chronic sun[19] and wind exposure, there are changes that are attributable solely to aging. Many of these structural and functional changes explain the different properties of aged skin. The degree to which all these changes affect any given individual is a function of the interrelated factors of environmental exposure and heredity. This chapter focuses on skin diseases that are most common among elderly persons or that present special and significant problems in this age group.

CZEMATOUS ERUPTIONS

Pruritus/Xerosis/Nummular Eczema

Clinical relevance. Itching, defined as a sensation that produces the desire to scratch, is the most common dermatological complaint of elderly persons. Chronic pruritus may be the presenting symptom of an internal disease; however, more commonly the cause is related to a primary cutaneous disorder or remains idiopathic.

Clinical manifestations. Pruritus may occur in a patient with or without visible skin lesions or in the absence of any skin problems. In the absence of either a primary skin disease such as atopic dermatitis or psoriasis or an associated internal disease, dry skin is the most likely explanation for pruritus. Many patients have scattered excoriations or scale crusts on a background of dry skin. However, extensive scratching or rubbing may induce a dermatitis, usually occurring as poorly defined, scaly, erythematous patches on the lower extremities. These areas also may exhibit superficial netlike cracking through the stratum corneum (asteatotic eczema [Figure 29-1]). Some patients develop more extensive eruptions consisting of round, red, scaly patches on the trunk and extremities (nummular eczema).

Diagnostic approach. Patients who have unexplained pruritus require a thorough history and physical examination that is directed toward a prior history of skin eruptions and possible underlying systemic diseases. The eczematous disorders previously

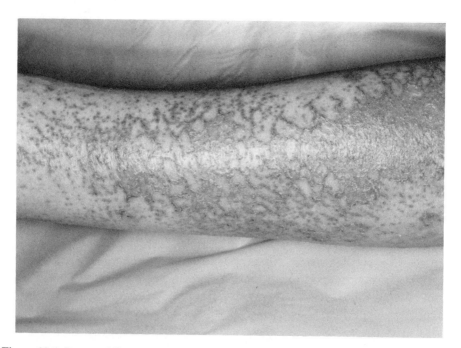

Figure 29-1 Dry crackling appearance of asteatotic eczema (eczema craqualé) on the anterior aspect of the lower extremities.

described are diagnosed on the basis of clinical appearance and trial of therapy if clinical evaluation provides no clue to the diagnosis. A lack of response to this therapeutic trial would necessitate additional diagnostic studies to exclude systemic diseases that cause generalized pruritus (i.e., uremia, hyperthyroidism, polycythemia vera, obstructive biliary disease, and internal malignancy, especially lymphoma). Diabetes mellitus as a systemic cause of pruritus is not well documented; it does cause pruritus vulvae or pruritus when associated with cutaneous candidiasis.[12]

Although eczematous eruptions are a more common cause of pruritus, other skin disorders must be considered, including folliculitis, scabies, pediculosis, fungal and yeast infections, as well as pruritis that is caused by drugs. Drugs, however, are an uncommon cause of chronic pruritus or pruritus without an eruption. In addition, depression and anxiety can be central factors in causing or exacerbating pruritus.

Intervention. For the patient with pruritus that is related to a systemic disease, treatment of the underlying disease often reduces the itching. However, in the majority of elderly patients who have xerosis and eczematous disorders, overdrying of the skin is the most important exacerbating factor. Therefore excessive bathing, especially with strong soaps and hot water, should be avoided. Patients should take short (5 to 10 minutes) lukewarm showers, using a mild soap such as Dove, no more than once daily and immediately apply emollients. Frequent use of mild nonsensitizing creams or lotions throughout the day is highly recommended. Topical antipruritic lotions such as Pramosone (pramoxine and hydrocortisone 1%) and Sarna (0.5% camphor and 0.5% menthol) are also very useful. When dermatitis is a prominent component, a topical medium-potency corticosteroid such as triamcinolone 0.1% ointment should be applied twice each day to the affected areas. It is best to avoid the systemic use of corticosteroids in all but the most extensive cases. Oral antipruritic agents such as the antihistamines hydroxyzine and diphenhydramine help control pruritus, probably through their central sedative effects rather than their blocking histamine receptors. Since pruritus in these conditions is not histamine mediated, the nonsedating antihistamines terfenadine and astemizole have not been very effective. If the skin appears secondarily infected, a 10-day course of an oral antibiotic such as dicloxacillin or erythromycin is indicated. The patient also should be made aware of external factors that may exacerbate the condition such as low humidity, cool air, contact with chemical irritants, and direct contact with wool.

Intertrigo and Perlèche

Clinical relevance. Intertrigo is a dermatitis of areas in which skin surfaces are opposed, such as genitocrural, inframammary, and axillary areas, resulting in increased moisture and friction. Predisposing factors, including obesity, diabetes mellitus, and incontinence, are common among elderly persons (especially the use of diapers). Perlèche or angular stomatitis is similar to intertrigo but occurs at the oral commissure. Among elderly persons, drooping of the cheeks may create an intertriginous area at the angles of the mouth.

Clinical manifestations. Initially there is erythema and slight tenderness or pruritus, followed by scaling, maceration, and fissure. These areas may become overgrown with yeast or bacteria. In candidal intertrigo, an erythematous, moist, or weeping eruption with surrounding vesicles or pustules is characteristic. The groin is the most common site for intertrigo, although obese patients often develop the problem in other body areas that have folds such as the abdomen and neck. Incontinent patients are more susceptible to intertrigo because urine and fecal matter increase the likelihood of maceration, fissure, and microbial invasion. This is not unlike the diaper dermatitis of infancy.

Perlèche is most common in edentulous patients or those with poorly fitting dentures. Saliva and food easily collect in the corners of the mouth, producing maceration and fissure followed by secondary infection with microorganisms, especially *Candida albicans*. This condition is often exacerbated by repeated licking of the area and by drooling, especially during sleep.

Diagnostic approach. The diagnosis of intertrigo and the related entities of diaper dermatitis and perlèche is based on clinical appearance, location, and history. Diagnostic evaluation for specific microorganisms, including fungal and bacterial cultures, potassium hydroxide preparation of skin scrapings for yeast and fungus, and Gram stain for bacteria, is important. Clinically, several other dermatological disorders may be confused with intertrigo. Inverse psoriasis and tinea cruris may affect similar sites but differ clinically because these conditions are more scaly and have sharply demarcated borders. Seborrheic dermatitis usually involves additional areas such as scalp, eyebrows, nasolabial creases, and chest. Irritant or allergic contact dermatitis also must be considered.

Intervention. Treatment of intertrigo must include elimination of the causative factors. The areas must be kept dry and well aerated. Preventing friction between skin surfaces and wearing loose clothing are essential. A low-potency topical corticosteroid cream such as hydrocortisone 1% should be used twice daily and rubbed in thoroughly. Highly potent topical corticosteroids should not be used on intertriginous areas since the natural occlusion in these sites may lead to atrophic changes. Topical antifungal/anticandidal medications in cream and/or powder form should be used in conjunction with the low-potency topical corticosteroid. If bacterial superinfection is suspected, the appropriate topical antibiotic should be added to the treatment regimen. In more severe or recurrent cases, it is often useful to include a topical paste such as zinc oxide, which decreases friction between skin surfaces and protects the skin from irritants.

Stasis dermatitis

Clinical relevance. Stasis dermatitis, an inflammatory skin condition of the lower extremities, is due to chronic edema from inadequate venous circulation. (See Chapter 54.) Early treatment of the dermatitis and associated edema is important in the prevention of cellulitis and leg ulcers.

Clinical manifestations. Poor venous circulation causes edema of the lower legs, which may result in inflammation of the involved skin, most often above the medial malleolus. A pruritic erythematous patch, which may be either weeping or dry and scaly, ultimately develops. The inflammatory process tends to recur and may be unilateral or bilateral. After repeated bouts, the skin of the lower legs becomes hyperpigmented and thickened.

Diagnostic approach. The patient often has a history of edema of the dependent leg and similar inflammatory episodes. Pedal edema is present when the patient is examined. Hyperpigmentation around the ankles, a history of thrombophlebitis and varicose veins help confirm the diagnosis. Bacterial cellulitis may be confused with acute stasis dermatitis; however, the former tends to be a unilateral process while the latter is often bilateral. Secondary infection of the dermatitic areas or of a resultant stasis ulcer may require bacterial culture. Acute contact dermatitis also may have a similar clinical appearance, necessitating a thorough history of all topical products used by the patient.

Intervention. Reduction of leg edema is critical to successful management of this condition. Reduction can be accomplished best by instructing patients to rest with their legs elevated. During acute dermatitis, the use of a midpotency topical corticosteroid cream is helpful. Oral antibiotics should be used for secondary bacterial infection as indicated by culture and sensitivities. Patients should wear support stockings on a regular basis to prevent recurrence.

INFECTIONS AND INFESTATIONS

Herpes zoster

Clinical relevance. Herpes zoster or shingles has a peak prevalence among the elderly population and represents a recurrent infection by the varicella zoster virus (VZV). Following the patient's initial infection with VZV causing chicken pox (varicella), the DNA virus resides within the satellite cells that encircle the neurons.[18] Subsequent reactivation of the virus spreads across the ganglia to multiple other satellite cells and neurons, causing a cutaneous eruption of dermatomal distribution (shingles).

Clinical manifestations. Typically, the patient experiences pain at the site of infection 4 to 5 days before the appearance of the eruption, which is characterized as grouped vesicles on an erythematous base over one or more contiguous dermatomes. As the vesicles age, they become pustular and then crust and heal within a few weeks, occasionally with scarring and pigmentary alteration. There is often regional adenopathy but no constitutional symptoms. In older patients, skin lesions occur primarily along the thoracolumbar dermatome distribution (50%) but are less prevalent in the sacral, cervical, and cranial nerve areas. When the cranial nerves are involved, there may be associated problems. For example, in the Ramsay Hunt syndrome the geniculate ganglion is involved and may produce facial palsy, hearing impairment, tinnitus, and vertigo with a rash involving the pinna, auditory canal, and anterior two thirds of the tongue. There is increased incidence of herpes zoster among patients who have immunological deficiencies either from disease (e.g., Hodgkin's disease) or drugs (e.g., cancer chemotherapy).

Important complications of herpes zoster in elderly patients include secondary bacterial infection, cutaneous and/or visceral disseminatioin, and postherpetic neuralgia. Cutaneous dissemination is manifested by the appearance of numerous varicella-like lesions at extradermatomal sites. Visceral complications of dissemination include pneumonitis and encephalitis. Postherpetic neuralgia is pain or dysesthesia that persists at the affected site for at least 6 weeks beyond healing of the skin lesions. More than one half of elderly persons who have herpes zoster are likely to experience this unfortunate sequela.

Diagnostic approach. Diagnosis of herpes zoster is clinically based on the appearance and distribution of the eruption. Careful assessment should be made to determine possible dissemination. Occasionally the diagnosis may require confirmation by laboratory tests. The Tzanck preparation is performed by scraping the roof and base of a vesicle with a scalpel blade, smearing this scraping on a glass slide, and staining the slide with the Wright, Giemsa, or Papanicolaou stains. The presence of multinucleated giant cells represents epithelial cells that are infected by viruses of the herpes family and is therefore not specific for VZV. A viral culture can distinguish between herpes simplex and VZV. Unfortunately, VZV is slow growing and may require 1 to 2 weeks before identification is possible. However, a recently developed fluorescein antibody test can identify VZV antigen within a 2-hour period. Additionally, a biopsy of a skin lesion can be studied by immunoperoxidase techniques to identify the presence of VZV antigen.

Intervention. The cutaneous lesions of herpes zoster should be treated with warm water compresses for their soothing and debriding effects. Associated pain usually can be controlled with mild analgesics. In addition, elderly patients with significant pain, serious zoster or involvement near the eyes, should receive oral acyclovir, 800 mg 5 times/day for 1 week, if it can be started within 72 to 96 hours of onset. Otherwise, antiviral therapy is not indicated. For many patients, treatment with acyclovir decreases the acute pain that is associated with the eruption, and it may shorten the clinical course by a few days. However, the incidence of postherpetic neuralgia is not reduced.[10] For immunocompromised older patients (e.g., with lymphoma), hospitalization and intravenous acyclovir is usually indicated. Some physicians advocate the use of systemic corticosteroids to decrease the incidence of postherpetic neuralgia for patients over the age of 55 who have herpes zoster. The evidence for this effect is inconclusive.

Scabies

Clinical relevance. Infestation with the scabies mite, *Sarcoptes scabiei*, produces an intensely pruritic rash that often is seen among nursing home residents. Scabies may occur in epidemics, so it is important to determine whether others in the family or same residence have similar rashes.

Clinical manifestations. Itching begins at least 2 weeks after infestation and is usually worse at night. The cutaneous findings are highly variable and pleomorphic, often consisting of several to hundreds of small red papules. Many of these lesions are covered with scale crusts. Other skin lesions include indurated inflammatory papules and nodules, vesicles on erythematous bases, eczematous changes, and excoriations. Uncommonly, the mite's burrow may be seen as a short wavy ridge. Among nursing home patients scabies lesions often are numerous on the back and buttocks, rather than the more typical sites such as volar wrists, interdigital webs, axillae, groin, gluteal cleft, nipples, and penis. This clinical distribution among nursing home patients indicates that contaminated bedding is a major factor in transmitting scabies. However, in most cases of scabies that occur in an ambulatory population, direct skin-to-skin transmission is the rule.

Diagnostic approach. The diagnosis of scabies can be confirmed by microscopic examination of skin scrapings. A scalpel blade is used to scrape or superficially shave the small papules or burrows. The specimen is then placed on a glass slide with mineral oil and a cover slip and examined at low power to identify mites, ova, or feces. Since the sensitivity of this procedure is less than 50%, a probable diagnosis depends on the patient's clinical history and physical examination.

Intervention. Effective treatment of scabies may be accomplished by one of several available scabicides. Commonly used agents include 1% gamma-benzene hexachloride lotion or lindane (Kwell) and 10% crotamiton (Eurax). However, recent studies indicate that 5% permethrin cream (Elimite) actually may be a more effective and less toxic scabicide and a superior agent for controlling scabies epidemics.[17,20] For the treatment of scabies, the topical agent of choice should be applied to all skin surfaces from the neck down, including the gluteal cleft, toe webs, and beneath fingernails. The faces of adult patients who have scabies are rarely affected, except for chronically ill and institutionalized patients. If lindane lotion or permethrin cream is used, it should be rinsed off 6 to 12 hours later and the treatment should be repeated in 1 week. Crotamiton is significantly less effective, even when applied for five consecutive nights. Following adequate treatment, the patient should not develop any new skin lesions. Since scabies generally is spread by skin-to-skin contact, all family members and others who have had physical contact with the patient also should be treated. Clothing and bedding should be washed thoroughly. Systemic antibiotic therapy may be necessary for patients with extensive excoriations and secondary bacterial infections. Topical corticosteroids may be used for symptomatic relief of severely eczematized skin. The patients should be advised that itching may persist for several weeks following successful treatment and may be controlled with oral antipruritic agents (hydroxyzine, diphenhydramine, etc.).

BENIGN SKIN LESIONS

Seborrheic keratosis

Clinical relevance. Seborrheic keratoses are benign skin tumors that usually begin to appear by the fifth decade and are quite common in older persons. These lesions vary in size from a few millimeters to several centimeters and may be worrisome for patients who believe that the lesions are skin cancers. The sudden onset of numerous seborrheic keratoses, the sign of Leser-Trelat, has a controversial association with internal malignancy that is not supported conclusively.[14] Malignant transformation of seborrheic keratoses is extremely rare but has been reported.

Clinical manifestations. Seborrheic keratoses vary in color from light tan to dark brown, and their morphology ranges from lesions that are barely raised above the skin's surface to thick papules or plaques. They are usually irregularly round or oval and are well demarcated, giving the appearance of their being "stuck on" the skin. Their surfaces may be dry and verrucous or smooth and shiny with follicular keratotic plugs (Figure 29-2). Seborrheic keratoses may be single or multiple and occur most commonly on the face and upper trunk, although they may be present on any area

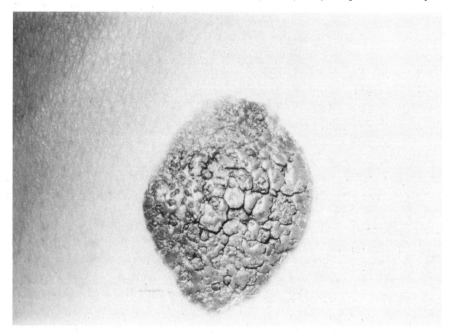

Figure 29-2 Hyperpigmented seborrheic keratosis with well-demarcated borders and stuck-on appearance.

with pilosebaceous follicles. The number of seborrheic keratoses tends to increase with age. These lesions may become inflamed (red) after trauma or irritation, thus altering their clinical appearance. Many patients complain of itching limited to sites of seborrheic keratoses. In darkly pigmented races, multiple small seborrheic keratoses of the face (dermatosis papulosa nigra) occur at a younger age than do ordinary seborrheic keratoses.

Diagnostic approach. The diagnosis of a seborrheic keratosis is based upon its characteristic clinical appearance. However, it may be difficult to distinguish a seborrheic keratosis from other pigmented lesions such as a benign nevus, malignant melanoma, or pigmented basal cell carcinoma. The patient's clinical history is often helpful in differentiating among the various possibilities. Age of onset is important

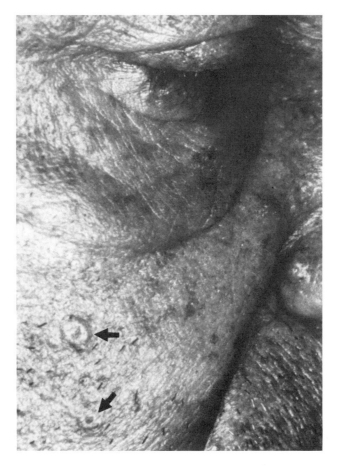

Figure 29-3 Umbilicated papules of sebaceous hyperplasia of the cheek. Lesion is generally yellow.

since seborrheic keratoses generally appear in the fifth decade, while acquired nevi usually appear before the age of 30. During examination of the patient, it also is useful to cross-light the lesion to accentuate its rough surface. Melanomas are usually more irregular in color, outline, and thickness. If the clinical diagnosis is uncertain, a biopsy of the lesion is indicated.

Intervention. Removal of seborrheic keratoses may be indicated because of the patient's discomfort that is due to the location or itching of the lesions or for cosmetic concerns. Various methods of treatment are effective, with their common feature being destruction of the keratotic lesion while minimizing damage to the surrounding and underlying normal skin. Preferred methods for treating seborrheic keratoses include liquid nitrogen cryotherapy or utilizing a sharp dermal curet to scrape the lesions, with or without prior electrodesiccation.

The accompanying box summarizes clinical information for other, common, benign, skin lesions that are found among the elderly population.

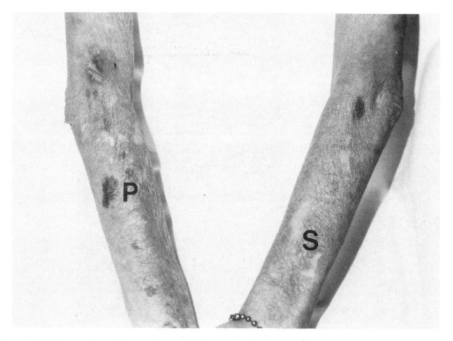

Figure 29-4 Large irregularly shaped violaceous solar purpura on dorsal forearms (*P*). Interspersed are white stellate pseudoscars (*S*).

COMMON BENIGN SKIN LESIONS OF ELDERLY PERSONS

Sebaceous hyperplasia (Figure 29-3)

Yellowish papules with central depressions; a few millimeters in diameter; found on face; single or multiple

Diagnosed clinically; may be confused with molluscum contagiosum, xanthomatous lesions, other benign sebaceous neoplasms, and basal cell carcinoma

Treatment by curettage, shave excision, or cryotherapy (liquid nitrogen) is for cosmetic reasons

Skin tags (acrochordons)

Overgrowth of normal skin with no malignant potential; possible correlation with internal polyps[6]

Flesh-colored or hyperpigmented papules on neck, axilla, eyelid, upper trunk, and groin; single or in clusters, 1 to 10 mm

May resemble nevi, neurofibromas, or soft tissue fibromas; biopsy if not certain of diagnosis

Treatment by excision, cryotherapy, or electrodesiccation is for comfort or cosmesis

Solar purpura (Figure 29-4)

Results from extravasation of red blood cells into the dermis because of mild trauma to chronically sun-exposed skin

Ecchymotic lesions of varying diameters, typically on dorsal forearm and hand; single or multiple and irregularly shaped

Coagulation studies are normal; no treatment required; avoid trauma and sun exposure

Cherry angioma

Red papules of 1 to 5 mm; found on trunk and proximal extremities; elevated or dome-shaped; do not blanch with pressure

Treatment with electrocoagulation or cryotherapy is for cosmetic reasons; be aware of complications of such treatment (postinflammatory pigmentary alteration or scarring)

Solar lentigo

Light tan to dark brown macules on face and dorsal forearm and hand; 0.5 cm to several centimeters in diameter; uniform pigmentation

Occasionally may be confused with melanoma and biopsy is required

Treatment with cryotherapy is for cosmetic reasons only

PREMALIGNANT AND MALIGNANT SKIN LESIONS

Actinic keratosis

Clinical relevance. Actinic or solar keratoses are premalignant lesions that are primarily seen in the middle-aged and elderly populations. Keratoses that are induced by ultraviolet light are more common in fair-skinned persons who do not tan easily. Since melanin provides significant protection from exposure to ultraviolet light, solar keratoses are rare in darkly pigmented persons. Untreated actinic keratoses may undergo malignant transformation, usually into squamous cell carcinoma. The probability of a given actinic keratosis transforming to squamous cell carcinoma is only a fraction of 1% per year. However, for the patient with many keratoses, the risk of their developing squamous cell carcinomas over a 10-year period may be as high as 10%.[3]

Clinical manifestations

Actinic keratoses are asymptomatic, erythematous or brownish, rough, scaly lesions on sun-exposed sites such as the face, ears, dorsal hands, and forearms, and lower lip (Figure 29-5). They are usually multiple and often occur in association with other signs of chronic actinic damage such as solar lentigines, telangiectases, solar

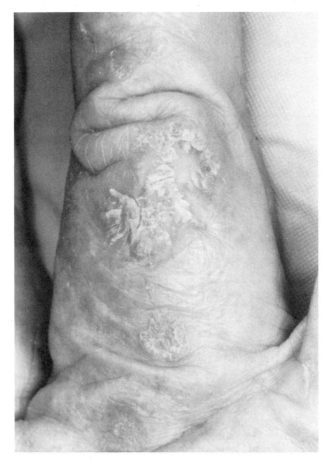

Figure 29-5 Multiple rough scaly actinic keratoses on sun-exposed dorsal aspect of hand.

cysts and comedones, and skin cancers. The patient is often aware of these persistent rough spots that are easily picked off or seem to resolve spontaneously, only to recur at the same site. Some actinic keratoses may become extremely hyperkeratotic and the presenting lesion is a cutaneous horn.

Diagnostic approach. Actinic keratosis is usually diagnosed clinically. If the lesion is large, atypical, or indurated, it actually may be a squamous cell carcinoma and a biopsy should be performed. The concurrent presence of seborrheic dermatitis may confound the diagnosis of actinic keratosis, since both conditions may occur on the face and bald scalp and both are erythematous and scaly. To identify the persistent actinic keratosis, it is first necessary to control the seborrheic dermatitis with topical medications. In some instances, benign keratotic lesions such as lichenoid or seborrheic keratoses may resemble actinic keratoses.

Intervention. Local destruction by one of several modalities is the preferred treatment for actinic keratoses. If there are only a few to several lesions, they may be treated easily with liquid nitrogen, electrodesiccation and curettage, or carbon dioxide laser and curettage. If actinic keratoses are numerous, treatment may be more complete and efficacious with dermabrasion, topical trichloroacetic acid, or topical 5-fluorouracil. Topical 5-fluorouracil is used twice daily on the face for 1 to 2 weeks or on the dorsal hands and arms for 2 to 6 weeks to treat multiple actinic keratoses that are apparent and those that are clinically inapparent. The endpoint of therapy is the appearance of inflammatory crusted lesions at the sites of the keratoses. This form of therapy is uncomfortable and unsightly. The severe inflammation may be decreased by the patient's concomitant use of topical corticosteroids. A recent study suggested that a more comfortable and equally effective regimen is the use of topical 5-fluorouracil once or twice weekly for an average of 6 to 7 weeks.[13] There is also evidence that treatment of actinic keratoses with topical tretinoin (Retin-A) is effective.[11] Important measures in preventing actinic keratoses are to avoid sun during peak hours (10 AM to 3 PM) and to use a sunscreen that provides adequate protection (a sun protection factor [SPF] of at least 15).[19]

Keratoacanthoma

Clinical relevance. Keratoacanthoma is a rapidly growing benign skin tumor of keratinizing squamous cells, usually of follicular origin. Both clinically and histologically it may resemble squamous cell carcinoma and rarely has been reported to develop into metastatic squamous cell carcinoma. There are several types of keratoacanthomas, with the solitary variety most commonly being seen among white patients in their sixth and seventh decades. This tumor is more common on sun-exposed areas and is rare in nonwhite patients. While this supports the hypothesis that keratoacanthoma is caused by exposure to ultraviolet light, this possibility has not been firmly established and other causal factors, including environmental exposure and viruses, have been proposed.

Clinical manifestations. The solitary form of keratoacanthoma is most common on the central face, dorsal hand and forearm, and lip. The initial presenting sign is a firm erythematous papule that enlarges rapidly. It may reach a diameter of 2 cm or more over the course of weeks to several months. The mature keratoacanthoma is a flesh-colored to pinkish dome-shaped nodule with a central crater that is filled with a crusted or keratinous plug. Untreated, most keratoacanthomas spontaneously involute in weeks to months, leaving residual hypopigmented scars. However, some lesions persist for a year or longer and can be extremely destructive to nearby structures.

Diagnostic approach. Because it may be extremely difficult to distinguish keratoacanthoma from squamous cell carcinoma, both clinically and histologically, it is important to obtain an adequate biopsy specimen for microscopic examination. The preferred biopsy techniques are either an incisional biopsy extending across the entire lesion or an excisional biopsy.

Intervention. Although keratoacanthomas often resolve without treatment, it is preferable to remove them since they are difficult to distinguish from squamous cell carcinomas and because their ultimate size and destructive potential is unpredictable. Surgical excision or curettage and electrodesiccation are effective definitive treatments. An alternative nonsurgical method is weekly intralesional injections of 5-fluorouracil for 3 weeks.

Bowen's disease

Clinical relevance. Bowen's disease is a slowly growing intraepidermal squamous cell carcinoma that is seen more commonly among elderly patients. If untreated for many years, this carcinoma may become an invasive and metastatic squamous cell carcinoma. In the past, an association has been made between the occurrence of Bowen's disease, especially on sun-protected areas, and internal cancer. However, this association is now highly doubtful.[15] Bowen's disease also has been associated with sunlight exposure, certain types of human papilloma virus, and arsenic ingestion.

Clinical manifestations. The characteristic lesion of Bowen's disease is a persistent, reddish, scaly plaque with a well-defined border. It may occur on any area of skin or adjacent mucous membrane. It is usually a solitary lesion that grows slowly and eventually becomes eroded and covered with scale crust.

Diagnostic approach. Clinically, Bowen's disease may be very difficult to distinguish from superficial basal cell carcinoma, and a biopsy is necessary to make the definitive diagnosis. Other entities that may resemble Bowen's disease are actinic keratosis, psoriasis, lichen simplex chronicus, nummular eczema, and dermatophytic fungal infection.

Intervention. Excision of the lesion and microscopic examination to confirm clearance is the treatment of choice. However, the size and location of the lesion in some cases make surgical excision difficult. In such situations, curettage and electrodesiccation, cryotherapy, and topical 5-fluorouracil may be used.

Basal cell carcinoma

Clinical relevance. Basal cell carcinoma is the most common human malignancy, with an annual incidence in the United States of 500,000 to 600,000 cases. The prevalence of basal cell carcinoma has increased in recent years, probably because of the population's increased exposure to the sun. Risk factors for developing basal cell carcinoma include fair skin, history of sunburn, family history of skin cancer, and outdoor occupation. Basal cell carcinomas are seen most commonly in elderly persons and are infrequent in darkly pigmented persons.

Clinical manifestations. Basal cell carcinoma occurs most frequently on the sun-exposed areas of the head and neck. Although related to chronic exposure to ultraviolet light, these tumors are rare on highly sun-exposed sites such as the dorsal hand and

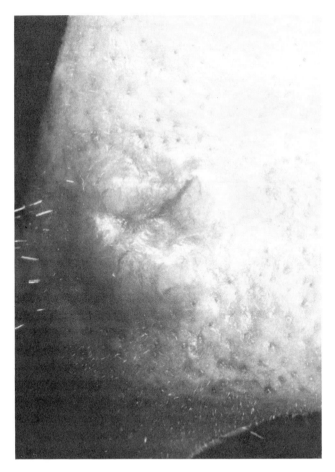

Figure 29-6 Noduloulcerative basal cell carcinoma of the nose with rolled pearly border, telangiectasia, and central depression.

forearm and are more frequently found on the upper trunk. On the face, basal cell carcinoma is especially common near the inner canthus, nasolabial fold, and post-auricular area. The typical noduloulcerative form of basal cell carcinoma is a pink papule or nodule with a translucent or pearly quality and overlying telangiectatic vessels. As the tumor enlarges, it becomes depressed in the center and the border appears rolled (Figure 29-6). Often there is central ulceration with an overlying scale-crust, which produces the typical "rodent ulcer." These tumors often bleed with minimal trauma. Basal cell carcinoma is a slow-growing tumor that is locally invasive and destructive over the course of many years. Its metastatic potential is extremely low, with several hundred cases of metastasis at most having been reported.

In addition to the noduloulcerative type, there are other clinicopathological patterns of basal cell carcinoma. The presenting symptoms of superficial basal cell carcinoma is a flat erythematous lesion that is usually scaly and well defined. It is often found on lesser sun-exposed areas such as the trunk. Another type of basal cell carcinoma is the pigmented variety, which is actually a pigmented noduloulcerative lesion that may resemble malignant melanoma (Figure 29-7). A fourth variant is the more locally infiltrative morphea-like or sclerosing basal cell carcinoma, which is a

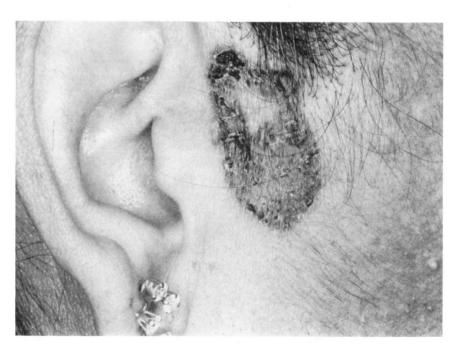

Figure 29-7 Pigmented basal cell carcinoma in preauricular location. Note difficulty in distinguishing from melanoma.

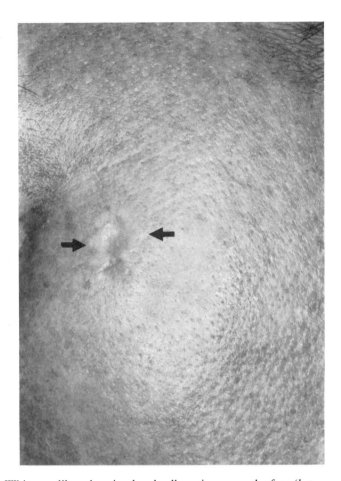

Figure 29-8 White scarlike sclerosing basal cell carcinoma on the face *(between arrows)*.

white, ill-defined scarlike plaque (Figure 29-8). In addition, basal cell carcinoma may appear at the sites of scars, burns, and radiation therapy.

Diagnostic approach. The diagnosis of basal cell carcinoma relies on clinical suspicion followed by biopsy of the lesion. The entity most commonly confused with typical nodular basal cell carcinoma is sebaceous hyperplasia. Superficial basal cell carcinoma is often difficult to distinguish from actinic keratosis, squamous cell carcinoma, Bowen's disease, and from benign conditions such as nummular dermatitis, tinea, or psoriasis. Morphea-like basal cell carcinoma must be distinguished from lesions of localized scleroderma and scars. It is often clinically difficult to differentiate between pigmented basal cell carcinoma and malignant melanoma.

Intervention. The most common forms of therapy for basal cell carcinoma are surgical excision, curettage and electrodesiccation, and Mohs surgery. It is important to individualize the treatment modality to the specific patient and lesion. Factors include the site and size of the lesion, histologic pattern, prior treatment if any, and general condition of the patient. The cure rate for basal cell carcinoma is greater than 90% after one procedure. Most recurrences are ultimately curable, with rare mortalities only from long-neglected cases. Other therapeutic modalities include radiation therapy, cryotherapy, and intralesional interferon.[1] Following treatment, it is important that these patients continue a scrupulous program to avoid the sun, use sunscreens, and undergo examination of the skin every 6 months.

Squamous cell carcinoma

Clinical relevance. Squamous cell carcinoma is the second most common skin cancer among white patients and the most common among black patients. These tumors occur more frequently in older adults and are definitely associated with cumulative exposure to sunlight.[5] The metastatic rate of squamous cell carcinoma varies between 0.5% and 16%, depending on the population group examined and site of the tumor.[2] Potential for metastatic spread is highest for tumors of the lip, temple, dorsal hand, and genitalia, as well as those squamous cell carcinomas arising from the sites of scars, chronic ulcerations, and radiation therapy.

Clinical manifestations. The clinical morphology of squamous cell carcinoma is rather variable. The lesions may appear as persistent keratotic plaques, erythematous indurated areas, or ulcerated nodules (Figure 29-9). Most commonly, squamous cell carcinoma occurs on chronically sun-exposed sites such as the face, ear, and dorsal hand and forearm. At times the lesions may be whitish or pearly with a raised border and central ulceration, resembling a basal cell carcinoma. These tumors also may arise in old burn scars, previously existing actinic keratoses, areas of chronic trauma (such as adjacent to a prosthetic limb), and sites of previous radiation therapy.

Diagnostic approach. The definitive diagnosis of squamous cell carcinoma depends on a biopsy and histologic confirmation. Clinically, it is often difficult to distinguish squamous cell carcinoma from basal cell carcinoma, chronic nonhealing ulcerations, actinic keratosis, and keratoacanthoma.

Intervention. The treatment modalities for squamous cell carcinoma are essentially the same as those for basal cell carcinoma. Cure rates for small previously untreated lesions are similarly high. Treatment with intralesional interferon is now being investigated. Depending on the site and size of the lesion and presence of palpable lymph nodes, it may be necessary for an oncological surgeon to perform a lymph node dissection and a medical oncologist to further evaluate the patient. Again, regular follow-up examination of these patients is important, as is emphasis on their need to avoid the sun and protect themselves by using an adequate sunscreen.

Melanoma

Clinical relevance. Malignant melanoma is a neoplasm that arises from melanocytes and may develop in the skin, mucosa, and eyes. Its prevalence is increasing in the

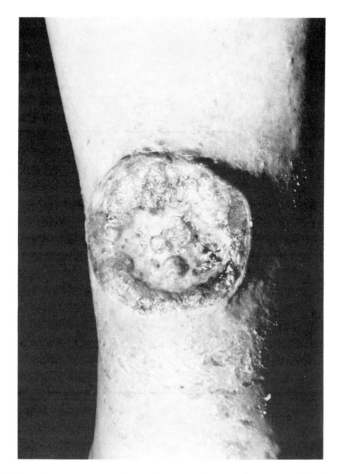

Figure 29-9 Ulcerating squamous cell carcinoma on the anterior aspect of the lower extremity.

United States, especially among the elderly population.[16] Recognition of melanoma is especially important since it is one of the few potentially fatal skin diseases.

Clinical manifestations. Patients at greater risk for developing malignant melanoma include those who have fair complexions and light-colored hair and eyes, those who were exposed to occasional intense sunlight, and those who had blistering sunburns during childhood or adolescence.[8] There are several clinical types of melanoma; the most common type found among the elderly population is lentigo maligna melanoma. This invasive tumor begins as an in situ (intraepidermal) lesion known as lentigo maligna, occurring most commonly on the chronically sun-exposed skin of the face and dorsal hands of elderly patients. Lentigo maligna initially appears as a flat tan macule resembling a solar lentigo. However, as it enlarges it develops variation in

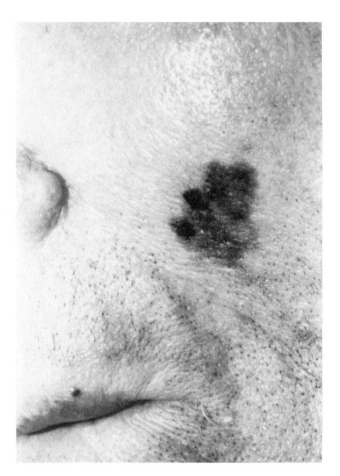

Figure 29-10 Flat irregularly pigmented lentigo maligna on cheek shows well-demarcated notched border.

color, from tan to dark brown, and often has a speckled appearance (Figure 29-10) Clinically, the variegate color helps to distinguish lentigo maligna from a benign solar lentigo. However, biopsy of the lesion is necessary for confirmation of the diagnosis. Development of dark brown or black areas of thickening within a lentigo maligna usually signifies progression to an invasive melanoma. Again, a biopsy is necessary to confirm the diagnosis and reveal the depth of invasion of atypical melanocytes.

Other forms of melanoma also occur in the elderly population. Nodular melanoma is usually a rapidly growing blue-black nodule that eventually ulcerates and bleeds. Acral lentiginous melanoma is a pigmented, irregularly shaped macule on the palms, soles, periungual areas, or nail beds. Like the lentigo maligna, it grows centrifugally and becomes thickened in areas when it penetrates the dermis. Of all patients who have primary invasive cutaneous melanoma, those who are 70 years of age or older are more likely to have nodular and acral lentiginous melanomas than are younger patients.[9] A fourth type of melanoma, superficial spreading melanoma, is a pigmented lesion often on the leg or back. It has variegate color, irregular borders (often with notching), and nonuniform surface elevation. Superficial spreading melanoma is more common among younger adults; however, older patients tend to have lesions of greater thickness and diameter.[16]

Diagnostic approach. Diagnosis of melanoma relies on the biopsy of clinically suggestive lesions. Existing pigmented lesions exhibiting an increase in size or change of color or newly discovered pigmented lesions, warrant close attention and may require a biopsy. A variety of pigmented lesions such as nevi, dysplastic nevi, blue nevi, lentigines, seborrheic keratoses, and pigmented basal cell carcinomas may be clinically similar to melanoma. Certain vascular lesions, including venous lakes, thrombosed hemangiomas, and pyogenic granulomas, also must be distinguished. It is advisable to do a complete excisional biopsy of a suspected melanoma, since a shave biopsy is usually not deep enough to permit histologic evaluation of the depth of the tumor. If an excisional biospy is not feasible because of the tumor's size or location, incisional biopsy or multiple punch biopsies may be satisfactory.

Intervention. Management of melanoma should be individualized for each patient, especially for the elderly population. The 5-year survival rate for all melanomas is approximately 83%, with survival being most closely related to depth of tumor invasion. The most recent information on surgical management indicates that a 1 to 2 cm resection margin, with the excision extending into the subcutaneous fat, is sufficient for melanomas less than 2 mm thick. Achieving a tumor-free margin of this size may be extremely difficult for large facial lesions or those lesions adjacent to a vital structure such as the eye. In such cases, Mohs surgery has been used successfully. Another alternative form of therapy is irradiation.[7] Elective dissection of lymph nodes remains controversial, and guidelines are based on tumor thickness and lymphatic drainage pattern from the melanoma site.[7] Treatment of metastatic melanomas requires a collaborative effort among several medical specialities that utilize modalities such as chemotherapy, immunotherapy, and various experimental regimens. Unfortunately, metastatic melanomas are almost uniformly fatal.

REFERENCES

1. Cornell RC et al: Intralesional interferon therapy for basal cell carcinoma, *J Am Acad Dermatol* 23:694, 1990.
2. Dinehart SM, Pollack SV: Metastases from squamous cell carcinoma of the skin and lip, *J Am Acad Dermatol* 21:241, 1989.
3. Dodson JM et al: Malignant potential of actinic keratoses and the controversy over treatment, *Arch Dermatol* 127:1029, 1991.
4. Fenske NA, Lober CW: Structural and functional changes of normal aging skin, *J Am Acad Dermatol* 15:571, 1986.

5. Gallagher MA et al: Trends in basal cell carcinoma, squamous cell carcinoma, and melanoma of the skin from 1973 through 1987, *J Am Acad Dermatol* 23:413, 1990.
6. Graffeo M et al: Skin tags: markers for colonic polyps, *J Am Acad Dermatol* 21:1029, 1989.
7. Ho VC, Sober AJ: Therapy for cutaneous melanoma: an update, *J Am Acad Dermatol* 22:159, 1990.
8. Koh HK: Cutaneous melanoma, *N Engl J Med* 325:171, 1991.
9. Loggie B et al: Invasive cutaneous melanoma in elderly patients, *Arch Dermatol* 127:1188, 1991.
10. McKendrick MW, McGill JI, Wood MJ: Lack of effect of acyclovir on postherpetic neuralgia, *Br Med J* 298:431, 1989.
11. Misiewicz J et al: Topical treatment of multiple actinic keratoses of the face with arotinoid methyl sulfone (Ro 14-9706) cream versus tretinoin cream: a double-blind, comparative study, *J Am Acad Dermatol* 24:448, 1991.
12. Neilly JB et al: Pruritus in diabetes mellitus: investigation of prevalence and correlation with diabetes control, *Diabetes Care* 9(3):273, 1986.
13. Pearlman DL: Weekly pulse dosing: Effective and comfortable topical 5-fluorouracil treatment of multiple facial actinic keratoses, *J Am Acad Dermatol* 25:665, 1991.
14. Rampen FHJ, Schwengle LEM: The sign of Leser-Trelat: does it exist? *J Am Acad Dermatol* 21:50, 1989.
15. Reymann F et al: Bowen's disease and internal malignant diseases: a study of 581 patients, *Arch Dermatol* 124:677, 1988.
16. Rivers JK et al: Age and malignant melanoma: comparisons of variables in different age groups, *J Am Acad Dermatol* 21:717, 1989.
17. Schultz MW et al: Comparative study of 5% permethrin cream and 1% lindane lotion for the treatment of scabies, *Arch Dermatol* 126:167, 1990.
18. Straus SE: Clinical and biological differences between recurrent Herpes simplex virus and Varicella Zoster virus infection, *JAMA* 262:3455, 1989.
19. Taylor CR et al: Photoaging/photodamage and photoprotection, *J Am Acad Dermatol* 22:1, 1990.
20. Yonkosky D et al: Scabies in nursing homes: an eradication program with permethrin 5% cream, *J Am Acad Dermatol* 23:1133, 1990.

SUGGESTED READINGS

Dodson JM et al: Malignant potential of actinic keratoses and the controversy over treatment, *Arch Dermatol* 127:1029, 1991.
Fenske NA, Lober CW: Structural and functional changes of normal aging skin, *J Am Acad Dermatol* 15:571, 1986.
Koh HK: Cutaneous melanoma, *N Engl J Med* 325:171, 1991.
Miller SJ: Biology of basal cell carcinoma (Part I). *J Am Acad Dermatol* 24:1, 1991.

CHAPTER 30

Pressure ulcers

DENNIS JAHNIGEN

KEY POINTS
- Successful management of pressure ulcers among outpatients requires attentive daily care and regular professional assessment
- In a high-risk patient, only 1 day of inadequate care is sufficient to lead to the development of a pressure ulcer.
- Relief of pressure is critical to both prevention and treatment of these ulcers.

CLINICAL RELEVANCE

Prevalence

Pressure ulcers are an important source of morbidity among debilitated elderly persons. Most of these individuals are sufficiently ill to require hospital or nursing home care. However, pressure ulcers may arise in homebound patients or patients in whom ulcer treatment is ongoing after a hospital or nursing home stay. Overall, the incidence among all elderly persons at home is less than 1%; however, among those who receive nursing care at their homes the rate is 5% to 10%.[3,5] In a large survey of funeral home directors in 1987, it was found that 24% of persons who expired had pressure ulcers at least at stage I, with stage II ulcers in over three fourths of these.[2]

Pressure ulcers are markers of underlying debility. Most patients with pressure ulcers will be in hospitals or nursing homes because of their need for intensive nursing care. Because it is labor intensive, management of pressure ulcers is expensive. In one study, the mean cost to heal a pressure ulcer (excluding base daily hospital and nursing charges) was $1,300, with a minimum duration of treatment of 16.5 days.[4] Precise cost of the care of pressure ulcers in ambulatory settings is unknown; however, 1987 Medicare hospital data show that for the 122,000 patients discharged with a primary or secondary diagnosis of pressure ulcer, total hospital charges were $1.5 billion.[4]

Morbidity and mortality

Pressure ulcers reflect serious underlying illness and directly contribute to morbidity and mortality. Ulcers rarely occur in otherwise healthy persons. The development of an ulcer is associated with a fourfold increase in 6-month mortality for both hospital and nursing home patients. Among nursing home residents in whom an ulcer fails to heal within 6 months, the mortality is six times as high. Although nearly all stage I ulcers can be successfully resolved, only half of all stage III or IV ulcers ever heal, regardless of treatment.

Pathophysiology

Four physical factors interact and lead to the development of pressure ulcers: (1) pressure, (2) friction, (3) shearing force, and (4) moisture.

Pressure. Unrelieved pressure is the essential ingredient for the patient's development of a pressure ulcer. Capillary filling pressure is only 32 mm Hg, which is easily exceeded over most bony prominences. A sustained pressure of only 70 mm Hg for 2 hours is sufficient to produce ischemia in underlying subcutaneous tissue or muscle. Pressure over the sacrum of a patient who is on a standard hospital mattress is often 150 mm Hg. Pressures often exceed 300 mm Hg over the ischial tuberosity while the patient is seated. This can lead to lymphatic and capillary obstruction, leakage of plasma into the interstitium, edema, autolysis, and finally tissue necrosis. Skin is somewhat less susceptible to pressure damage than muscle and subcutaneous tissue. Once surface tissue damage has been detected, a deep ulcer sometimes develops and worsens for several days, even if all pressure is relieved.

Shear. A shearing force is produced when the skin is against a fixed exterior surface while the subcutaneous tissues are subjected to lateral forces. These forces can stretch subcutaneous tissues, which have less elasticity than skin. In elderly persons, capillaries are particularly vulnerable to disruption from shearing. Sitting in the semi-Fowler position especially leads to greater shear stress over the sacrum and should be avoided in high-risk patients.

Friction. Friction of skin moving across a surface can abrade surface epithelium or even cause a friction burn. Normal aging of skin leads to its thinning and increased friability. For debilitated persons, transfers to and from bed easily lead to such injuries through inadvertent dragging of the back or pelvis across the bedsheet.

Moisture. Moisture can lead to tissue maceration with inflammation and increased friction. If urinary or fecal incontinence is present, this also can be a chemical irritant to open skin, which rapidly worsens an ulcer or makes healing difficult. Bacterial contamination of an open ulcer by feces can quickly progress to infection.

CLINICAL MANIFESTATIONS

Terminology

Many types of skin ulcers occur among older persons. The most common include neurotrophic (diabetic), vascular (arterial insufficiency), stasis (venous insufficiency), and pressure ulcers. Each of these is a distinct clinical entity, with different patho-physiology and treatment. This chapter focuses on pressure ulcers, which also are known as *decubitus ulcers, decubiti,* or *pressure sores.* The preferred term is *pressure ulcer,* which is more precise and emphasizes the primary cause.

Staging

Several methods of classification are used to describe pressure ulcers. The correct use of a staging system is important for prognosis and objectively describing a patient's response to therapy. One classification system that has been recommended by both the National Pressure Ulcer Advisory Panel and the National Association of Enter-ostomal Therapists is shown in the box below.

Risk factors

A number of risk assessment scales have been developed to identify those who are in need of special prevention measures. These scales have been used primarily in hospital or nursing home settings, but the predictors should have utility for outpatients as well. Areas of concern are the patient's general condition, mental status, activity level, mobility, and continence.[1] See the box below.

Physical findings

Over 95% of pressure ulcers occur on the lower half of the body. Although an ulcer can occur anywhere, the most common sites are the sacrum, ischial tuberosities, trochanters, heels, and lateral malleoli. It is important that the number, location, size, and stage of ulcers are recorded accurately in the office and home nursing records.

PRESSURE ULCER STAGES

Stage	Skin changes
I	Nonblanching erythema with intact skin
II	Partial thickness skin loss; penetration into subcutaneous tissue
III	Full-thickness lesion; penetration to fascia
IV	Deep full-thickness skin loss; penetration to muscle, tendon, or bone

---

RISK FACTORS FOR DEVELOPING A PRESSURE ULCER

Spinal cord injury	Hip fracture
Immobility	Fecal incontinence
Cognitive impairment	Malnutrition
Stroke	

Complications of pressure ulcers. Many complications may result from pressure ulcers. The most serious is sepsis. Infection of pressure ulcers is commonly poly-microbial with both aerobic and anaerobic bacteria (most often fecal flora). The mortality from sepsis associated with pressure ulcers is very high. Other complications include cellulitis, osteomyelitis, pyarthrosis, sinus tract formation, heterotopic cal-cifications, amyloidosis, and, rarely, tetanus. Ulcers with a large amount of exudate lead to loss of protein-rich fluid and contribute to malnutrition as a burn does.

DIAGNOSTIC APPROACH

The diagnosis of a pressure ulcer is normally clear cut, but fungal infections, cutaneous malignancies, and vasculitides have been confused with pressure ulcers. Occasionally, a biopsy is needed to clarify the condition. The most important initial determination is the assessment of comorbidities and the presence of contributory factors. If the patient's underlying condition is terminal, healing is not likely and prevention of new ulcers may be the best that can be achieved. Conversely, if the underlying disorder is reversible, complete resolution should be the objective. Another critical determination is whether the resources are present for adequate treatment in the home setting. Ulcers require inspection and treatment several times daily. An assessment by a visiting nurse once weekly is not adequate in the absence of a capable caregiver. If there is no caregiver, hospitalization of the patient must be considered. In all settings, efforts should be directed toward controlling the patient's pain and preventing the worsening of ulcers.

INTERVENTIONS

Although all pressure ulcers are "preventable" in theory, under some clinical circumstances they are virtually unavoidable even with aggressive nursing care. This does not diminish the importance of the clinician's attempt to reduce their occurrence. Several principles are common to both prevention and treatment of ulcers.

Step 1: Relieve pressure

The patient should be encouraged to improve mobility whenever possible. If the patient is bedbound, regular rotation is essential to relieve pressure. A 30-degree oblique position, left alternating with right, will keep the five most common sites (lateral malleolus, sacrum, trochanter, ischial tuberosity, and heel) pressure free. Pillows can be used to pad between the knees and the ankles and behind the back to prevent the patient from rolling to the supine position. If an ulcer already exists, it should not be placed in direct contact with the bed's surface. Heel and elbow protectors and chair cushions can be helpful in selected settings. Doughnut rings should not be used because they can concentrate pressure and diminish blood supply to tissue surrounding an ulcer. Special low-air-loss beds or air-fluidized beds have been used with some success in institutional settings but are rarely practical for patients who receive home care because of the high cost and complexity of operation. Foam mattress overlays, silicone gel pads, air mattresses, and waterbeds can reduce pressure and are economical.

Step 2: Control moisture

Perineal moisture can initiate the development of ulcers. For patients who have trochanteric or sacral ulcers, a bladder catheter may be used temporarily. Incontinent patients with intact skin do not need a catheter if they are kept dry. Absorbent adult diapers may be used but may require frequent changes. New protective skin "barriers" are available in sprays or lotions that are applied once or twice daily. Fecal incontinence can be a serious problem because the rapid transit of intestinal contents from diarrhea can be very irritating to skin. Occasionally, a constipating drug, rectal tube, or collecting pouch may be necessary.

Step 3: Clean and debride the wound surface

The ulcer should be kept clean with an appropriate cleansing agent such as Dakin's solution or very dilute povidone-iodine solution. These must be mild since either can be toxic to fibroblasts and epithelial cells. Strong solutions, heat lamps, or desiccating agents should be avoided since these remove moisture from all cells that are involved with wound repair. Necrotic tissue must be removed because it provides a culture medium for bacteria. An eschar on the surface of an ulcer may be suggestive of healing but should be removed since it will impair reepithelization. Several methods of debridement are available. The most widely used are wet-to-dry or wet-to-wet saline dressings. The drying gauze adheres to tissue and when removed, the gauze pulls off devitalized tissue. Since this method is often painful, wet-to-wet dressings are better tolerated. For fibrinous exudate, enzymatic debridement with streptokinase, desoxyribonuclease, or fibrinolysin can be used. A dental irrigator or saline-filled syringe removes some necrotic tissue or exudate. Surgical debridement while the patient is under general anesthesia is often necessary for deep ulcers to heal.

Step 4: Treat infection

Infected wounds do not heal or accept skin grafts. Bacteria are present both on the surfaces of wounds and intact skin. Cultures should be reserved for wounds that are obviously infected or worsening. Swab cultures of the wounds' surfaces are of little clinical utility. Cultures should be obtained from purulent material or tissue biopsy. Organisms most frequently recovered from early wounds are frequently gram-negative bacilli such as *Proteus mirabilis, and Escherichia coli,* as well as *Staphylococcus aureus.* Methicillin-resistant *S. aureus* is increasingly common in institutional settings. Anaerobes, along with gram-negative bacilli, are often present in chronic or deep wounds and their presence is suggested by their characteristic odor. Topical care with saline dressings is usually adequate to clean the surfaces of the wounds. If overt infection is present, dilute povidone-iodine (0.1%) or Dakin's solution (0.5% sodium hypochlorite) may be used. Systemic antibiotics usually are not required unless signs of sepsis, cellulitis, or osteomyelitis are present. A tetanus booster is advisable.

Step 5: Cover wound with a physiological dressing

Noninfected wounds heal fastest if they are kept covered in a warm moist environment. Such dressings also prevent external contamination. Every change of dressing causes some disruption of the architecture of a healing wound. Fewer changes of the dressing are preferred if the wound is clean. There are many synthetic dressings available that have different characteristics. (See Table 30-1.) All synthetic dressings have selective advantages for certain types of wounds; however, none of these advantages replace attention to the other steps.

Step 6: Treat general condition of the patient

Whether or not an ulcer heals depends on the underlying condition of the patient. If the primary disease is progressive, complete cure is often impossible. For any ulcer to heal, there must be careful attention to nutrition. Patients who have pressure ulcers are often malnourished at the time the ulcer develops. Nutritional intake must be adequate for the maintenance and new growth of tissue. Adequate total calories, protein, zinc, magnesium, calcium, copper, and vitamin C are all necessary. Supplemental water-soluble vitamins are advisable. Vitamin C in supplements of 500 mg twice daily have been reported to enhance healing. Zinc is essential for normal healing but supplements should not be added, unless the patient's serum zinc level shows a deficiency, since excessive amounts can impair healing. Other comorbid medical conditions should be optimized. Hypoxemia, congestive heart failure, anemia, hyperglycemia, and peripheral edema should be corrected.

Table 30-1 Topical treatments for pressure ulcers

Modality	Indication	Advantages	Disadvantages
Hydrocolloids	Low-exudate wounds	Provides cushioning	Impermeable to oxygen
Polyurethane films	Superficial lesions	Can see wound	Adherent to wound surface
Hydrogels	Superficial wounds	Infrequent changes	Hard to maintain in wound
Saline gauze	Any open wounds	Inexpensive	Frequent changes required

Step 7: Regularly monitor the condition of the ulcer

Skilled observation of the pressure ulcer in the home setting is critical to successful healing. The person performing the daily dressing changes must be able to determine if the wound is worsening. Weekly evaluations are essential by a skilled home-care nurse or by the physician, particularly in the early stages of treatment. For stage III or IV, a plastic surgeon should be part of the treatment team from the outset as such wounds often require surgical debridement or may be amenable to surgical closure. There are many reasons for failure of the ulcer to heal. Some include:

Unrelieved pressure

Worsening underlying condition

Local infection

SUMMARY

Pressure ulcers are more common among hospital or nursing home patients than those who are at home, but outpatient management is sometimes possible. An awareness of risk factors, precipitating events, and principles of treatment can provide a rational approach to the prevention and management of pressure ulcers.

REFERENCES

1. Allman RM et al: Pressure sores among hospitalized patients, *Ann Intern Med* 105:337, 1986.
2. Eckman KL: The prevalence of pressure sores among persons in the U.S. who have died, *Decubitus* 2:48, 1989.
3. Langemo DK et al: Incidence of pressure sores in acute care, rehabilitation, extended care, home health, and hospice in one locale, *Decubitus* 2:42, 1989.
4. Smith DM, Winsemius SK, Besdine RW: Pressure sores in the elderly: can they be improved? *J Gen Intern Med* 6:81, 1991.
5. National Pressure Ulcer Advisory Panel: Pressure ulcers: prevalence, cost, and risk assessment, *Decubitus* 2:24, 1989.

SUGGESTED READING

Allman RM: Pressure ulcers among the elderly, *N Engl J Med* 320:850, 1989.

CHAPTER 31

Falls

LAURENCE Z. RUBENSTEIN

<u>KEY POINTS</u>

- Falls are a major cause of mortality, morbidity, functional impairment, and nursing home admission among the elderly population.
- The most commonly cited precipitating causes for falls include environmental hazards, mobility disorders, dizziness, drop attacks, confusion, postural hypotension, and visual disturbances.
- The most important underlying risk factors for falls include muscle weakness, gait and balance problems, visual impairments, depression, and certain medications.
- A systematic postfall assessment is essential and can identify important underlying disorders that are amenable to treatment.
- Important components of all preventions include periodic identification and modification of risk factors and specific rehabilitation interventions.

CLINICAL RELEVANCE

The incidence of falls and severity of fall-related complications rise steadily after middle age. Accidents are the fifth leading cause of death for older adults, and falls constitute two thirds of these accidental deaths. In the United States, about three fourths of deaths from falls occur among 13% of the population aged 65 years and older. Approximately one third of this age group living at home will fall each year, and about 1 in 40 of them will be hospitalized. Of those who are admitted to a hospital after a fall, only about one half will be alive one year later. Repeated falls are a common reason for admissions of previously independent elderly persons to long-term care institutions.[1,4]

Incidence of falls varies among different settings and populations. The lowest rates (0.2 to 0.8/person annually, mean 0.49) are reported among generally healthy elderly persons who live in the community. Most of these falls produce no serious injuries, but about 5% of the victims sustain fractures or require hospitalization. As would be expected, persons living in long-term care institutions have the highest rates of incidence (0.6 to 3.6/bed annually, mean 1.7), and hospitals have intermediate rates (0.6 to 2.9/bed annually, mean 1.5).

However, the real problem of falls among elderly people is not just the high incidence, since young children and athletes have even greater rates, but the combination of high incidence and high susceptibility to injuries. The elderly person's propensity for injuries relates to the prevalence of clinical diseases and age-related declines such as osteoporosis and slower protective reflexes, which affect the elderly population and make even relatively mild falls particularly dangerous. In addition to specific injuries, falls can result in postfall disability syndromes and self-imposed functional limitations from the fear of falling.

CLINICAL MANIFESTATIONS: CAUSES AND RISK FACTORS

Table 31-1 lists the major causes of falls and their relative frequencies based on the major published studies. The relative frequencies of causes differ depending on the populations studied. Frail high-risk populations have higher rates of medical-related falls and higher incidences of falls of all types than do healthier populations. Accidents, gait and balance disorders, dizziness, and drop attacks are the four most frequent causes of falls.

Accidents, generally involving some environmental hazard, are the most common cause of falls, accounting for 30% to 50% in most series. However, many falls that are

Table 31-1   Causes of falls in elderly adults: summary of 12 studies that carefully evaluated elderly persons after a fall and specified a most likely cause

Cause	Mean (%)*	Range (%)†
Accident/environment-related	31	(1-53)
Gait/balance disorders or weakness	17	(4-39)
Dizziness/vertigo	13	(0-30)
Drop attack	10	(0-52)
Confusion and cognitive impairment	4	(0-14)
Postural hypotension	3	(0-24)
Visual disorder	2	(0-5)
Syncope	0.3	(0-3)
Other specified cause‡	15	(2-39)
Unknown	5	(0-21)

Modified from Rubenstein LZ et al: Falls and instability in the elderly, *J Am Geriatr Soc* 36:266, 1988.
*Mean calculated from the 3628 falls in the 12 studies.
†Ranges indicate the percentages reported in each of the 12 studies.
‡This category includes arthritis, acute illness, central nervous system disorders, drugs, alcohol, pain, epilepsy, and falling from bed.

attributed to accidents actually result from the combination of environmental hazards and the elderly person's increased susceptibility to these hazards because of the effects of aging or disease. Older people have stiffer and less coordinated gaits than do younger people. Posture control, body-orienting reflexes, muscle strength and tone, and height of stepping all decrease as individuals age and impair their abilities to avoid falling after trips or slips. Age-associated impairments of vision, hearing, and memory, tend to increase the number of trips and stumbles. In addition to the increased vulnerability of elderly people, environmental hazards commonly contribute to falls. Such hazards (e.g., throw rugs, poor lighting, unsafe stairs, objects on floor) must be carefully sought out. Published checklists exist that assist caregivers with accidentproofing the homes of older persons.

The broad category of gait problems and weakness is the second most common cause of falls. Gait problems and weakness can result from many factors. In addition to the purely age-related changes in gait and balance that were mentioned previously, ambulation problems can result from dysfunctions of the nervous, muscular, skeletal, circulatory, and respiratory systems, as well as from simple deconditioning following a period of inactivity. Muscle weakness is extremely common among elderly people; much of it results from disease and inactivity rather than aging per se. Common causes of weakness and gait problems include strokes, parkinsonism, fractures, skeletal abnormalities, arthritis, myopathies, and polyneuropathies.

The sensation of dizziness is an extremely common complaint of elderly patients who fall. (See Chapter 32.) This complaint necessitates a careful history from the patient because the description of dizziness is subjective and can reflect very different causes. True vertigo, a sensation of rotational movement, may indicate a disorder of the vestibular apparatus (e.g., benign positional vertigo, acute labyrinthitis, or Ménière's disease). Patients often describe symptoms of imbalances in their walking, which reflects gait disorders. Many patients describe a vague light-headedness that may reflect cardiovascular problems, hyperventilation, orthostasis, anxiety, depression, or side effects from drugs.

Drop attacks are sudden falls caused by unexpected leg weakness, without the patient's loss of consciousness or dizziness. Sudden change in head position is often a precipitating event. This syndrome has been attributed to transient vertebrobasilar insufficiency, although it is probably caused by diverse pathophysiological mechanisms. Leg weakness is usually transient but can persist for hours. Tone and strength sometimes can be restored more rapidly if patients push their feet against solid objects. Recent studies have found that substantially fewer falls result from drop attacks than earlier studies found, and the 10% average shown in Table 31-1 is considered to be too high an estimate by most current investigators.

Because in many cases a single specific cause for falling cannot be identified and because the origins of falls are usually multifactorial, many investigators have performed epidemiological case-control studies to identify factors that place individuals

Table 31-2 Important individual risk factors for falls: summary of eight controlled studies

Risk factor	Significant/ total*	Mean RR-OR†	Range
Weakness	8/8	5.1	1.9-10.3
Gait deficit	7/8	3.1	1.7- 4.7
Balance deficit	6/8	3.1	1.7- 4.7
Visual deficit	3/8	2.2	1.5- 3.5
Depression	3/3	2.0	1.7- 2.4
Postural hypotension	1/8	3.4	—
Cognitive impairment	1/7	2.3	—

Modified from Robbins AS et al: Predictors of falls among elderly people: results of two population-based studies, *Arch Intern Med* 149:1628, 1989.
*Number of studies with significant association/total number of studies that examined each factor.
†Relative risks (prospective studies) and odds ratios (retrospective studies).

at increased risk for falling.[2,3,6,7] These studies indicate that lower-extremity weakness, gait disorders, functional impairments, cognitive impairments, and polypharmacy (defined as taking five or more prescription medications) are the strongest risk factors for falls. Table 31-2 summarizes the data from eight studies that determined risk factors for falls. For example, persons with leg weaknesses have about a fivefold increase in fall risk, while persons with gait or balance impairments have about a threefold increase. Postural hypotension, impaired function, decreased vision, cognitive impairment, arthritis, and incontinence also have been identified as risk factors in several studies, although these associations are somewhat weaker. In addition, other case-control studies, which examined only single potential risk-factor associations, identified significant associations with polypharmacy, cardiac medications, psychotropic medications, and postprandial hypotension. Perhaps as important as identifying individual risk factors is appreciating the interaction and probable synergism between multiple risk factors. Several studies have shown that the risk of falling increases dramatically as the number of risk factors increases. For example, Tinetti, Speechley, and Ginter[7] showed that fall risk over a one-year follow-up period increased from 8% for elderly persons who had no identified risk factors to 32% for persons who had two risk factors to 78% for persons who had four or more risk factors. While few if any data exist to demonstrate whether strategies for reducing risk factors can effectively prevent falls, several studies are in progress and appear promising.

DIAGNOSTIC APPROACH

The physician's first objective when facing a patient who has fallen is to stabilize and treat any immediate medical problems that caused the fall (e.g., syncope due to cardiac arrhythmia) or complications of the fall (e.g., head injury, fractures). The physician then should identify the cause of the fall and any accompanying risk factors.

A careful and well-directed history is the most helpful part of the diagnostic process. Obtaining a full report of the patient's circumstances and symptoms surrounding the fall is crucial. Reports from witnesses are important because the patient may have poor recollection of these events. Historic factors that point to a specific cause or help the physician to narrow the diagnoses include reports of a sudden rise from a lying or sitting position (orthostatic hypotension), a trip or slip (gait, balance, or vision disturbance or an environmental hazard), an unexplained drop attack without loss of consciousness (vertebrobasilar insufficiency), looking upward or sideways (arterial or carotid sinus compression), and loss of consciousness (syncope or seizure).

Symptoms that are experienced when the fall occurs also may point to a potential cause—dizziness or giddiness (orthostatic hypotension, vestibular problem, hypoglycemia, arrhythmia, side effects from drugs), palpitation (arrhythmia), incontinence or tongue biting (seizure), asymmetrical weakness (cerebrovascular disease), chest pain (myocardial infarction or coronary insufficiency), or loss of consciousness (any cause of syncope). Medications and the existence of concomitant medical problems may be important factors. Other questions that might be raised during the history include the following:

1. How long was the patient on the ground?
2. What effect did the fall have on the patient's confidence, fear of further falls, and activity?
3. Are there any effects on the caregiver's expectations, fears, and plans for future activities?

The accompanying box outlines important findings to note during the patient's physical examination. Especially pertinent are orthostatic changes in pulse and blood pressure, presence of arrhythmias, carotid bruits, nystagmus, focal-neurological signs, musculoskeletal abnormalities, visual loss, and gait disturbances. Careful assessment of the patient's mental and functional statuses is crucial. Even if risk factors are discovered that did not cause the fall in question, their identification and treatment may reduce the likelihood of subsequent falls. It may be useful, under carefully monitored conditions, to reproduce circumstances that might have precipitated the fall (e.g., positional changes, head turning, urination, or carotid pressure). Gait and stability should be assessed by physicians as they closely observe the patients rising from their chairs, standing with eyes open and closed, walking, turning, and sitting down. Physicians should note particularly the gait velocity and rhythm, stride length, double support time (the time spent with both feet on the floor), height of stepping, use of assistive devices, and degree of sway.

The laboratory evaluation need not be extensive but should consist of a limited number of specific tests when the cause is not obvious, including complete blood count to search for anemia or infection; serum chemistries, especially sodium, po-

┌─────── **IMPORTANT FINDINGS TO NOTE ON PHYSICAL EXAMINATION** ───────┐

Vital signs

Postural pulse and blood pressure
   changes
Fever or hypothermia

Head

Nystagmus
Visual impairment
Hearing impairment

Neck

Motion limitation
Motion-induced imbalance

Chest

Rales

Heart

Arrhythmia
Murmur

Extremities

Arthritic changes
Motion limitations
Deformities
Fractures
Podiatric problems

Neurological

Altered mental status (dementia, de-
   lirium)
Focal deficits
Peripheral neuropathy
Muscle weakness
Rigidity
Tremor
Gait or balance abnormality

└──┘

tassium, calcium, glucose, and creatinine; electrocardiogram to document arrhythmia; and thyroid function tests, since occult thyroid disease may be difficult to diagnose clinically. Even then, the clinical evaluation and initial laboratory tests may not detect an intermittent problem that may have been the cause of the fall (e.g., orthostatic changes, arrhythmias, or electrolyte disturbances).

An ambulatory cardiac (Holter) monitor is advisable in cases in which transient arrhythmias are suggested by the patients' histories, for patients who have otherwise unexplained syncope, or for patients who experience unexplained falls, have histories of cardiac diseases, and take cardiac medications. The likelihood of physicians' finding suggestive abnormalities from the Holter monitors of elderly patients who fall is particularly high; however, since transient arrhythmias are prevalent among elderly persons, it is often unclear whether monitored abnormalities are related to the falls unless corresponding symptoms are noted. Therefore, it is essential that the patients are instructed to keep a careful diary of their symptoms during Holter monitoring.

For high-risk elderly patients, even those without histories of falls, thorough examinations may be helpful in identifying potentially correctable risk factors such as decreased vision, postural hypotension, diminished strength, and impaired gait. While the efficacy of screening a low-risk elderly population has not been evaluated, routine medical visits and the following periodic assessments might help prevent falls:

measurement of postural blood pressure, testing of visual acuity, evaluation of balance and gait, assessment of mental status, and review of medications and environmental risks.

INTERVENTION AND PREVENTION

The purpose of the previously outlined diagnostic approach is to uncover the direct or contributing causes of falls that are amenable to medical therapy or other corrective intervention. (For specific therapies, please refer to the appropriate chapters for each disorder.)

For patients with gait and balance disturbances, specific assistive devices are often helpful. These devices include walkers, crutches, canes, and even shoe modifications. Since the assistive devices must be modified to the patient's needs, physicians must be experienced in prescribing these devices or they should be prescribed in consultation with a physiatrist or physical therapist. (See Chapter 4.) Many patients— particularly those with strokes, hip fractures, arthritis, or parkinsonism—also benefit from a program of gait training under the supervision of a physical therapist. Focused exercise programs that increase strength and endurance among deconditioned persons are widely advocated and are being studied for their effectiveness. (See Chapter 21.)

Persons who are subject to drop attacks from vertebrobasilar insufficiency associated with head motion sometimes may be helped by cervical collars. The collars should be prescribed in consultation with a neurologist or rehabilitation specialist for proper fit because an ill-fitting collar can cause carotid compression.

A more difficult task is the management and prevention of recurrent falls by patients for whom specific causes cannot be identified or who have multiple or irreversible causes. A careful search for, and correction of, other risk factors that predispose the patients to falling (such as visual and hearing deficits) is essential. For disabilities that do not properly resolve with treatment of the underlying medical disorder (e.g., hemiparesis, ataxia, persistent weakness, or joint deformities), a trial of short-term rehabilitation along with consultation of a physiatrist or physical therapist may improve the patients' safety and diminish long-term disabilities. When irreversible problems exist, residual limitations should be explained and methods of coping developed.

Physicians should caution patients to eliminate home hazards such as loose or frayed rugs, trailing electrical cords, and furniture that is unstable or obstructs movement. Patients and their families should be advised about the importance of specific environmental improvements, including adequate lighting, bathroom grab rails, raised toilet seats, secure stairway banisters, beds at comfortable and safe heights for the individuals, and easily accessible alarm systems. Sometimes, furniture can be rearranged to provide support for unstable patients while they walk to the bathroom. A home evaluation can be performed by a visiting nurse or other experienced person who is qualified to suggest modifications. Numerous assessment forms and checklists for home safety are available to assist patients and their families in identifying and correcting home hazards. The accompanying box summarizes the most important items from these lists. (See Chapter 18.)

A comprehensive assessment of patients after they have fallen shows a high yield in terms of identifying important, correctable, medical problems and risk factors. In at least one randomized trial, these assessments proved to reduce subsequent hospitalizations. This result may reflect that the fall is a marker for other, underlying, serious conditions that can be improved through careful evaluation and timely intervention.[5]

Even older individuals who have not fallen can probably benefit from a systematic program that prevents falls. The assessment can be performed in the office setting as part of a periodic program for health maintenance. This program should include the following:

1. A discussion with patient (and caregiver, when appropriate) about the nature of the problem
2. A focused history and physical examination to assess risk factors

---

HOME SAFETY CHECKLIST

All living spaces

Remove throw rugs
Secure carpet edges
Remove low furniture and objects on floor
Reduce clutter
Remove cords and wires on floor
Check lighting for adequate illumination at night (especially bathroom pathway)
Secure carpet or treads on stairs
Eliminate chairs that are too low to sit in
Avoid waxing floors
Ensure telephone can be reached from floor

Bathrooms

Install grab bars in tub/shower and by toilet
Use rubber mats in tub/shower
Take up floor mats when tub/shower not in use
Install raised toilet seat if too low

Outdoors

Repair cracked sidewalks
Install handrails on stairs, steps
Trim shrubbery along pathway to house
Install adequate lighting by doorways and along walkways leading to doors

3. A discussion of home hazards and distribution of a checklist for hazards
4. A discussion and advice about exercise to improve gait and activities, with appropriate precautions concerning overexertion

Intervention programs to ameliorate single specific risk factors for falls (e.g., weakness, gait and balance impairments) as a means of preventing them are being established, and many studies are underway to examine their effectiveness. The content of these programs varies widely and includes exercise, rehabilitation, adjustment of medications, and assessment of environments. Although they have not yet proven effective in preventing falls, several of these programs have improved intermediate outcome variables. For example, several studies of interventions to improve patients' muscle strength, gait, and balance have shown positive effects on their strength and balance.

REFERENCES

1. Hogue C: Injury in late life. I. Epidemiology. II. Prevention, *J Am Geriatr Soc* 30:183, 276, 1982.
2. Nevitt MC et al: Risk factors for recurrent nonsyncopal falls: a prospective study, *JAMA* 261:2663, 1989.
3. Robbins AS et al: Predictors of falls among elderly people: results of two population-based studies, *Arch Intern Med* 149:1628, 1989.
4. Rubenstein LZ et al: Falls and instability in the elderly, *J Am Geriatr Soc* 36:266, 1988.
5. Rubenstein LZ et al: The value of assessing falls in an elderly population: a randomized clinical trial, *Ann Intern Med* 113:308, 1990.
6. Tinetti M, Williams TF, Mayewski R: Fall risk index for elderly patients based on number of chronic disabilities, *Am J Med* 80:429, 1986.
7. Tinetti ME, Speechley M, Ginter SF: Risk factors for falls among elderly persons living in the community, *N Engl J Med* 319:1701, 1988.

SUGGESTED READINGS

Kellogg International Workgroup on Prevention of Falls in the Elderly: The prevention of falls in later life, *Dan Med Bull* 34(suppl):1, 1987.
Weindruch R, Hadley EC, Ory MG, eds: *Reducing frailty and falls in older persons*, Springfield, Ill, 1991, Charles C Thomas.

CHAPTER 32

Dizziness and syncope

SCOTT L. MADER

KEY POINTS
- Hypotension is a common mechanism for both dizziness and syncope.
- A new episode of acute vertigo should be considered a cerebral vascular event until proven otherwise.
- Multiple sensory deficits are commonly associated with the symptom of dizziness.
- Syncope is often associated with multiple rather than single risk factors.
- The etiology of syncope differs between "young-old" and "old-old" patients.

DIZZINESS

Clinical relevance

The complaint of dizziness is frequent among elderly persons. It is the third most common reason why patients aged 65 years and older visit family physicians and the fifth most common reason why this age group visits general internists. It is the most common presenting complaint of patients aged 75 years and older.[10] Sloane and Baloh[10] reported on 116 patients who were over the age of 70 and referred to a neurootology clinic because of dizziness. After evaluation of the patients, these researchers made the following diagnoses: 46% peripheral vestibular disorders, 19% cerebrovascular disorders, 7% other central disorders (cerebellar atrophy, acoustic neuroma [previously diagnosed], drug toxicity), and 15% other disorders (anxiety, depression, multiple sensory deficits, vasovagal attack, cardiac arrhythmia, postcataract surgery). Causes were not determined for only 14%. Half of the patients with peripheral vestibular disorders were deemed to have benign positional vertigo, which is described in detail in the following discussion.

Clinical manifestations

Dizziness means different things to different people. When patients say they are dizzy, it generally can be categorized into one of the four following groups of symptoms: (1) vertigo, (2) presyncope, (3) imbalance, and (4) light-headedness (Table 32-1).

Table 32-1   Differential diagnosis of dizziness

1. Vertigo (sensation of being rotated or pushed)

Acute	*Recurrent*	*Positional*
Vertebrobasilar event	Ménière's disease	Benign positional vertigo
Toxic (illness or drug)	Migraine	Postinfectious
Infectious	Hypothyroid	Posttrauma
Trauma	Multiple sclerosis	Cervical
Tumor	Seizure	Central causes
Seizure	Syphilis	
	Vertebrobasilar insufficiency	

2. Presyncope (impending faint)

Orthostasis or near syncope
Hyperventilation

3. Imbalance (sensation localized to body and relieved by standing in a braced position or sitting or lying down)

Medication toxicity
Multiple sensory impairments
Cervical spine disease
Muscle weakness, unstable joints
Neurological disease (previous stroke, cerebellar degeneration, peripheral neuropathy myelopathy, parkinsonism)

4. Ill-defined light-headedness (cerebral sensation of wooziness, floating, or swimming)

Medications, visual disorders, previous stroke
Hyperventilation, psychiatric disorders
Carbon monoxide

After the patient describes the dizziness, especially the first episode, the following areas should be explored:

1. What do the patients mean when they say that they are dizzy?
2. How many kinds of dizziness do the patients have? (Forty percent of patients will have more than one type.)
3. What is the pattern of symptoms (acute, recurrent, positional, or continuous)? Are all of the episodes the same?
4. Are there any associated symptoms (hearing loss, tinnitus, nausea, sweating)?
5. What diseases do the patients have? Have there been recent acute illnesses or traumas?
6. What medications do the patients take (including alcohol, eye drops, and over-the-counter remedies) or what medications have they taken recently (especially aminoglycosides)?
7. What are the patients' general levels of activity and how have those levels been affected?

The initial task of the clinician is to clarify whether the patient has true vertigo as a cause of the symptoms. Sometimes patients who have vertigo feel like they are walking on uneven surfaces or being tossed in a boat. Sudden tilts of the environment or the feeling of being pushed or pulled can also represent vertigo. If patients have vertigo, it should be determined whether the vertigo is related to peripheral neurological dysfunction (e.g., labyrinth) or central neurological dysfunction (e.g., brain stem, cerebellum).

Vertigo of peripheral origin is generally the worst at onset, markedly aggravated by the patient's position, and often includes associated tinnitus or hearing changes. The severity of nystagmus often parallels the severity of the vertigo, whereas central neurological lesions may include impressive nystagmus with only minimal vertigo. The onset of vertigo in relationship to recent events helps physicians to associate symptoms with diagnoses (e.g., symptoms after a viral illness suggest vestibular neuronitis).

Vertigo of central origin usually has other neurological findings that are referable to the brain stem or cerebellum. The vertigo is more likely to be continuous, only variably affected by the patient's position, and probably not maximal at onset. The presenting symptom of vertebrobasilar insufficiency can be vertigo but it should not be considered unless clumsiness, weakness, ataxia, diplopia, or dysarthria are also present. The symptoms of patients who have cerebellar infarction and hemorrhage include vertigo, vomiting, headache, and inability to walk. Carotid artery disease, multiple sclerosis, and primary brain tumors or metastatic brain tumors are uncommon causes of vertigo. Even the presenting symptom of acoustic neuroma is not typically vertigo. Hearing loss, tinnitus, and neurological abnormalities frequently occur first.

A special category of vertigo is positional vertigo. Positional vertigo usually indicates a benign disorder and is almost always caused by a peripheral vestibular disturbance, although in rare cases it can be associated with a central lesion. The main historical features of benign positional vertigo (BPV) are that (1) symptoms occur only with changes in position, and (2) after a change in position, the symptoms last less than 1 minute. This allows BPV to be distinguished from the other conditions causing vertigo in which the sensation of rotation is generally continuous but exacerbated by movement. BPV is an episodic condition, lasting weeks to months but recurring frequently. It is often precipitated by lying down, rolling over in bed, or sudden head movements, which the patient often learns to avoid. BPV is usually idiopathic but can be secondary to previous infectious or traumatic insult. This type of vertigo can be distinguished from central positional vertigo by the Hallpike maneuver. (See the box on p. 308.)

If the problem is not vertigo, then the physician should determine whether the problem is one of presyncope, imbalance, or ill-defined light-headedness (Table 32-1). Patients who have orthostatic hypotension, hyperventilation, and cardiac disorders

---

HALLPIKE MANEUVER

1. Patient begins in a sitting position on the examination table
2. Examiner quickly but gently helps the patient to lie down with the head hanging over the back of the table at approximately a 30-degree angle and the face turned 45 degrees to the right; for a frail patient, hanging the head can be omitted
3. The patient is observed for nystagmus (eyes must be open and not fixed on a target) and asked about vertigo and reproduction of the symptoms; the head is held there for 1 minute
4. The patient is brought back to the sitting position and again observed for 1 minute
5. The test is then repeated with the head at 45 degrees to the other side; if vertigo is reproduced, the test should be repeated two or three times on the side that caused the greatest symptoms to determine if the nystagmus and symptoms fatigue

---

may have symptoms of presyncope. Patients can have cerebral hypoperfusion and dizziness without significant changes in orthostatic blood pressure.[8] This often can be clarified by asking patients whether their symptoms occur only after the patients stand or also while they lie down or roll over in bed. Hyperventilation is usually associated with light-headedness and circumoral and digital paresthesias. Patients who describe imbalance should be questioned about vision (glaucoma or refractive error), hearing, arthritis of the neck or extremities, alcohol use, and symptoms of peripheral neuropathy. The effect that support has on patients while they walk (e.g., canes or someone holds their elbows for support) is important because marked improvements in their stability with only minimal support are characteristic of multiple sensory deficits. The possibility of Parkinson's disease should be considered. Dilated cerebral ventricles or a midline cerebellar tumor also can produce these symptoms without other specific neurological findings. Ill-defined light-headedness is a symptom that usually does not suggest a serious underlying disorder. Light-headedness may be secondary to medication, hyperventilation, or a previous stroke. In the winter months, carbon monoxide poisoning should be considered as a cause of light-headedness for patients who also complain of headaches. Affective or anxiety disorders also can be associated with complaints about chronic light-headedness.

Time spent on a careful history can help the physician to focus the physical examination. The accompanying box summarizes important physical findings and maneuvers for patients who complain of dizziness.

Diagnostic approach

Special bedside testing may be necessary for some patients. The Hallpike maneuver can be useful for assessment of patients with true vertigo. Once patients are supine with their heads turned, those who have BPV experience a short *latency of 5 to 15 seconds* then complain of severe vertigo, and J-shaped rotatory nystagmus is observed.

PHYSICAL FINDINGS AND
MANEUVERS FOR PATIENTS WITH DIZZINESS

Blood pressure while patient is supine and after patient stands for 1 minute
Ear inspection for vesicles and wax; hearing test
Head turning (side to side/up and down)
Hyperventilation for 3 minutes
Valsalva maneuver

Neurological examination, including:

• Nystagmus (rotatory suggests peripheral; vertical suggests central lesion)
• Visual acuity; funduscopic (for papilledema)
• Evidence of previous stroke or parkinsonism
• Sensory testing, including joint position and sense of vibration
• Cerebellar testing (past pointing suggests vestibular lesion; intention tremor and abnormal alternating movements suggest cerebellar dysfunction)
• Romberg test
• Gait assessment
• Standing while braced; most easily performed when the patient stands with back against the wall and holds onto the back of a heavy chair; patients with multiple sensory deficits no longer feel dizzy

This condition *fades in less than 1 minute*. When the patients return to a sitting position, there again may be transient vertigo and nystagmus. When tested on their opposite sides, 20% of patients have recurrent symptoms and findings. *The vertigo fatigues with repeated testing.* During remissions or mild episodes of BPV the Hallpike maneuver may be negative, and the diagnoses must be made based on the patients' histories alone. A central lesion should be suspected if vertigo is dissociated from the nystagmus, and the nystagmus begins immediately when the patient is positioned, is primarily horizontal or vertical, lasts longer than 1 minute, or does not fatigue after repeated testing.

Laboratory testing depends on the presumptive diagnosis and the patient's symptoms. In the emergency room, routine glucose determination (for hypoglycemia) and monitoring of cardiac rhythm are useful for patients who are over 45 years old and have dizziness.[4] Because of the difficulties that physicians have in separating peripheral from central neurological findings, any new episodes of acute vertigo in elderly patients should be considered cerebrovascular events until proven otherwise.

In less acute settings, testing of patients who have vertigo should include blood or serum glucose for hyperglycemia, thyroid function, and serology for syphilis, which are potentially reversible causes. In cases where the diagnosis remains unclear, consultation with a subspecialist from either otolaryngology or neurology should be considered. Subspecialists may perform dynamic tests for the patient's vestibular function such as electronystagmography and caloric testing.

Patients who have presyncope should be evaluated similarly as those who have syncope. Patients with imbalance problems should receive tests that are dictated by their medical histories and physical findings. Persons with ill-defined light-headedness should have drug or carbon monoxide levels determined if appropriate.

Intervention

If an elderly patient without a previous history of vertigo develops an acute episode of moderate or severe vertigo, hospital admission for observation and control of the symptoms should be considered. It may be difficult to determine a brain stem or cerebellar infarction. Treatment of symptoms that are associated with acute vertigo usually includes medications with anticholinergic and antiemetic properties. A good initial choice is promethazine, which has both properties. It may be given orally, rectally, or intramuscularly in a dose of 12.5 to 50 mg. If the patient is excessively anxious, a benzodiazepine also may be useful adjunctive therapy. For patients with mild or moderate bouts of vertigo, promethazine can be used if nausea is present or meclizine if nausea is not present. One should start with a low dose of either medication (12.5 mg) at bedtime and gradually titrate up to tolerance. The scopolamine patch may cause severe anticholinergic toxicity for older patients and should not be used. In general, medication should be used for only short periods of time. Chronic therapy is rarely indicated. There are exercises that have been developed to shorten the duration and impact of BPV, and they have been used by elderly patients.[9]

For patients with presyncope, the specific causes should be addressed (e.g., orthostatic hypotension, hyperventilation). For patients with imbalance problems or multiple sensory deficits, referrals to physical therapists for gait evaluation and strengthening and assistive devices are important, as are audiological and ophthalmological screenings. Appropriate treatment for patients with ill-defined light-headedness begins with discontinuation of any offending medications and includes ophthalmological assessment. Psychiatric evaluation is appropriate if other symptoms suggest that patients may have psychiatric disorders. Physical therapy and exercise programs may be useful. Reassurance and regular follow-up are important.

SYNCOPE
Clinical relevance

The term syncope is used to denote a transient loss of consciousness and postural tone that resolves spontaneously, without resuscitative interventions and residual symptoms. This disorder must be differentiated from other states of altered consciousness such as cardiac arrest, coma, and seizure. Syncope is common for patients of all ages and increases with age. It accounts for approximately 3% of emergency room visits and 1% of medical admissions to a general hospital. A retrospective study of elderly nursing home residents showed a 10-year prevalence of 23%, an incidence of 6% for 1 year, and a recurrence rate of 30%.[6]

Two studies help us understand how the causes of syncope differ between young and old patients, and even more importantly between "young-old" and "old-old" patients. Kapoor evaluated 210 patients 60 years and older (mean age 71 years) from emergency rooms, clinics, and inpatient services and compared them to a younger group[5]. The most common etiologies of syncope for the young group were vasodepressor (15%), hypotension from orthostasis, situational stress, or drugs (19%), and ventricular tachycardia (7%). In the older group, hypotension was similar, but vasodepressor was rare, and ventricular tachycardia was twice as common. Overall, cardiovascular causes were much more common in the older group, and these notably included myocardial infarction, aortic stenosis, and carotid sinus syncope. When Lipsitz reported on 97 institutionalized elderly persons (mean age 87) with syncope[7], there were no vasodepressor events and no ventricular tachycardia. However, situational hypotension made up nearly 40% of their diagnoses. Again, they found that syncope was commonly caused by myocardial infarction or aortic stenosis (10%). These data suggest that the causes of syncope differ even among the broad category of "elderly", and when frail elderly patients present with syncope, one should look very closely at risks for hypotension and be alert to the possibility of a myocardial infarction or aortic stenosis.

There are some important additional observations from these studies. Elderly syncope patients are much more likely than controls to have multiple risk factors. Recurrence rates are approximately 30% for all etiologic classes of syncope, and did not greatly improve the likelihood of establishing a specific diagnosis in a patient who has previously undergone an evaluation. In the Kapoor study, one-third of patients from both groups sustained trauma, but it was more likely to be serious in the elderly subjects. The 2-year mortality was 25% in th elderly group which was 3 times higher than the younger group. An increased mortality was not seen when elderly nursing home residents with syncope were compared to residents without syncope[6].

Clinical manifestations

Initial evaluation for syncope begins with careful histories from the patients and any observers. Patients should be allowed to describe the events in their own words and encouraged to suggest possible causes. The accompanying box summarizes information that should be obtained from patients with syncope. The histories should also include careful review of patients' medications, alcohol use, and eye drops.[3] The past medical histories should focus on cardiovascular and neurological risk factors.

The physical examination should include blood pressure measurements in both arms (e.g., subclavian steal, aortic dissection) and a supine to standing orthostatic blood pressure measurement. After prolonged standing, walking, or climbing stairs, patients should have their standing blood pressures measured if suggested by their histories. Significant changes in orthostatic blood pressures (>20 mm Hg systolic pressure or 10 mm Hg diastolic pressure after 1 minute of standing) occur in ap-

_____ **IMPORTANT HISTORICAL INFORMATION ABOUT SYNCOPE** _____

1. How many times has this condition occurred? Has there been near-syncope as well as syncope?
2. How has the patient been feeling in the last few days? Has he or she been eating, drinking, and taking medications in the usual manner?
3. How did the episode begin? What activities was he or she doing? Were there any associated symptoms? Did it occur with standing (orthostasis), shaving (carotid sinus), defecation (reflex), recent meal or medication (hypotension), climbing stairs (hypoxia, aortic stenosis), chest pain (angina, myocardial infarction), palpitations (arrhythmia)? (Dizziness is frequently present in patients with syncope [70%], although it is more often associated with a psychiatric diagnosis.[11])
4. What occurred during the episode? Was there incontinence or tonic-clonic movements to suggest seizure?
5. How did the episode end? (Slow onset and slow recovery suggest hyperventilation or hypoglycemia. Sudden onset and slow recovery [>15 minutes] suggest a seizure disorder or transient ischemic attack.)
6. Was there any injury?

proximately 25% of patients with syncope, even when another cause of syncope is suspected. Therefore this finding should not be used exclusively to ascribe orthostasis as the cause.[1,5]

A careful cardiopulmonary examination should be done to determine volume status, aortic stenosis, hypertrophic cardiomyopathy, pulmonary embolism, or pulmonary hypertension. Stool guaiac and neurological examination should be performed.

Diagnostic approach

The differential diagnosis of syncope are shown in the box on p. 313. Laboratory testing should include complete blood count, blood chemistries, urinalysis for specific gravity, and electrocardiogram. Frequent ectopic beats, bradycardia, abnormal PR interval, long QT interval, conduction delay, or bundle branch block may suggest a rhythm disturbance as a cause, but it should be correlated with the patient's history.

With this data base, physicians will diagnose one third of the patients and the evaluation or treatment will proceed accordingly. If the diagnosis is unclear to a physician, carotid sinus massage can be performed to test the patient for carotid sinus hypersensitivity.[2] For patients with suspected defecation or micturition syncope or digitalis toxicity, the Valsalva maneuver can be performed and the patients monitored for bradycardia. If these evaluations are negative and a cardiac cause is still suspected, Holter monitoring and echocardiography can be useful.

Holter monitoring leads physicians to diagnoses in 17% of elderly subjects who

DIFFERENTIAL DIAGNOSIS OF SYNCOPE

Reflex

Vasovagal, carotid sinus, cough, defecation, micturition, swallowing

Hypotensive

Orthostatic, medications, postprandial, multiple diseases/impairments, volume depletion

Cardiac

Arrhythmias, valvular disease, myocardial infarction, cardiomyopathy (dilated or hypertrophic), pulmonary hypertension/embolism, aortic dissection, atrial myxoma

Central nervous system

Seizure, transient ischemic attack, tumor, subclavian steal, psychiatric disorder

Abnormal blood composition

Anemia, hyperventilation, hypoglycemia, hypoxia

---

are not identified after initial assessments.[5] The role of ambulatory blood pressure monitoring has yet to be determined, but may be useful. Computed tomography of the head and electroencephalography are low-yield studies for patients who have no clinical evidence of cerebrovascular disease or seizure.

Intervention

The goal of treatment is to prevent recurrence or death. If a specific cause of syncope is defined for the patient, such as aortic stenosis or heart block, then appropriate treatment options can be pursued. If orthostatic hypotension is present, it can be managed by the following four initial steps[8]:

1. Evaluate patient's medications
2. Increase patient's fluid, salt, and nutritional intake
3. Increase patient's activity level
4. Educate patient

Medications can be reduced, changed, or stopped completely. Patients with hypertension and orthostatic hypotension can be treated with vasodilator agents (calcium channel blockers, angiotensin-converting enzyme inhibitors, hydralazine) or beta blockers, which have a low risk of orthostatic side effects when given alone.

Diuretics and central sympatholytic (alpha-methyldopa) or peripheral alpha-adrenergic blockers (prazosin) should be avoided. In some instances, it may be difficult to stop the offending medications (e.g., antidepressant therapy, antiparkinsonian therapy). In these cases, treatment strategies, including elevating the head of the bed, salt tablets, and fludrocortisone may be instituted before or while patients take the offending medications. Since many older persons follow a low-salt diet, another useful measure is to increase salt intake (e.g., adding 1 g of salt at each meal) because adequate circulating volume is essential for the management of orthostasis. Time out of bed and exercise are extremely important. Even young healthy persons who are kept at bed rest have orthostatic hypotension, despite other treatment measures.

Education is important so that patients and families understand the cause and management of symptoms. Any unusual symptoms always should be treated initially with placement of the patient in the supine position. For the patient with persistent and troublesome symptoms, someone in the family should be taught to take blood pressures; these should be recorded and reviewed during office visits. They should be instructed to rise slowly from a supine to sitting position and to wait a few minutes before standing. They should stand only when there is support available to prevent their falling. Isometric tensing of the legs, arms, and abdominal muscles decreases venous pooling and helps maintain blood Isometric pressure while standing. A urinal or bedside commode should be provided so that patients do not have to walk to the bathroom at night. They should be instructed to take extra salt and fluid during times of volume stress such as airline flights, heat, febrile illness, or gastroenteritis.

For patients who do not respond to these simple measures, additional treatments are available. Tilting their heads upward at night while they sleep is effective and often easier for older patients who may sleep alone. This is done best with books or 2-inch x 6-inch blocks under the bed legs at the head of the bed. The bed can be raised in small increments to tolerance. Salt tablets (1 g) can be prescribed to patients with poor oral intake or questionable intake of salt. One gram of sodium chloride (NaCl) has 17 mEq of sodium, and treatment can start at 2 g twice daily and increased if necessary. Fludrocortisone acetate is an effective treatment, which acts by promoting salt retention and increasing the sensitivity of blood vessels to catecholamines. It can be started at 0.1 mg daily and increased every other day up to 0.5 mg twice daily. The most common side effects are hypokalemia (which can exacerbate orthostasis) and mild dependent edema (for which the patient should be warned). Precipitation of new congestive heart failure is a theoretical but uncommon occurrence. Adequate salt intake must be part of this regimen. Support hosiery is a widely recommended therapy for orthostatic hypotension, but the hose are difficult to put on and are effective only when waist-high fitted stockings are used. A common treatment regimen for "more difficult" patients would include fludrocortisone 0.2 mg twice daily, NaCl 2 g twice daily, KCl (potassium chloride) 8 mEq twice daily, and elevation of the head of the bed 4 inches on blocks. These patients should be monitored weekly for blood pressure and serum electrolytes until stable.

If no specific disorder is identified, then more general recommendations may be useful. Medications should be reviewed, especially for very elderly patients who take multiple medications. Common offenders include antihypertensives, vasodilators, ocular or systemic beta blockers, diuretics, antidepressants, and hypoglycemia agents. A regular exercise program should be initiated with supervision. Small frequent meals should be given with liberal water and salt. Extreme neck rotation and tight shirt collars should be avoided. Urination and showering should be performed while patients are seated. Prolonged, quiet standing should be avoided, as well as hypotensive stressors (hot tubs, saunas). After prolonged supine or sitting positions, patients should perform isometrical exercises of the upper and lower extremities and abdomen before they stand.

Patients should be monitored carefully and further episodes reported immediately. They should be instructed not to drive until their evaluations are completed. It is important to remember that the cause of syncope remains unknown for approximately one third of patients after their evaluations. Empirical therapy with pacemakers, digoxin, and antiarrhythmic or antiseizure medications is discouraged.

REFERENCES

1. Atkins D et al: Syncope and orthostatic hypotension, *Am J Med* 91:179, 1991.
2. Branch WT: Approach to syncope, *J Gen Intern Med* 1:49, 1986.
3. Davidson E et al: Drug-related syncope, *Clin Cardiol* 12:577, 1989.
4. Herr RD, Zun L, Mathews JJ: A directed approach to the dizzy patient, *Ann Emerg Med* 18:644, 1989.
5. Kapoor W et al: Syncope in the elderly, *Am J Med* 80:419, 1986.
6. Lipsitz LA, Wei JY, Rowe JW: Syncope in an elderly, institutionalized population: prevalence, incidence, and associated risk, *Quart J Med* 55:45, 1985.
7. Lipsitz LA et al: Syncope in institutionalized elderly: Impact of multiple pathological conditions and situational stress, *J Chron Dis* 39:619, 1986.
8. Mader SL: Orthostatic hypotension, *Med Clin North Am* 73:1337, 1989.
9. Norre ME, Beckers A: Benign paroxysmal positional vertigo in the elderly: treatment by habituation exercises, *J Am Geriatr Soc* 36:425, 1988.
10. Sloane PD, Baloh RW: Persistent dizziness in geriatric patients, *J Am Geriatr Soc* 37:1031, 1989.
11. Sloane PD et al: Clinical significance of a dizziness history in medical patients with syncope, *Arch Intern Med* 151:1625, 1991.

SUGGESTED READINGS

Baloh RW, Honrubia V, Jacobson K: Benign positional vertigo: clinical and oculographic features in 240 cases, *Neurology* 37:371, 1987.
Drachman DA, Hart CW: An approach to the dizzy patient, *Neurology* 22:322, 1972.
Kapoor WN: Evaluation and outcome of patients with syncope, *Medicine* (Baltimore) 69:160, 1990.

CHAPTER **33**

Weakness

RICHARD E. WALTMAN

KEY POINTS

- Weakness is a common complaint of older people.
- A key aspect of the evaluation is eliciting what the patient means by weakness.
- Major causes of weakness include lifestyle factors, depression, medications, and organic diseases or a combination of these.
- Weakness should not be dismissed as a trivial complaint of older people—a complete diagnostic evaluation should be initiated.
- Many treatable psychosocial and organic causes of weakness can be found.
- A thoughtful evaluation of this complaint will help physicians to formulate and solidify the physician-patient relationship.

CLINICAL RELEVANCE

Weakness is a common complaint of older people. The term *weakness* may mean different things to different people. To physicians, weakness usually connotes the decline in strength of a particular organ or anatomical structure. A literature search reflects this interpretation, since there are many listings for weaknesses of particular entities (e.g., weakness of a joint or weakness of a nerve) but only a few for weakness of the person. Despite its vague meaning, weakness is a very real complaint of many older people.

The patient's definition of weakness often varies. If five patients complain of weakness, their interpretations of the problem may be quite different. Weakness may mean lack of strength ("I'm so weak I can't carry my firewood anymore"), lack of energy ("I'm so weak I can't cut the grass anymore"), lack of interest ("I'm so weak I just don't feel like doing anything"), or fatigue ("I'm so weak I sleep all the time"). To others, weakness may actually indicate pain ("When I walk too long, I get a weakness in my heart").

Before the physician can address the complaint of weakness, the patient's interpretation of the word *weakness* must be explored. The evaluation of weakness is qualitatively different from, for example, the evaluation of a more defined clinical problem such as hematuria or pain in the left knee. Because this is a subjective and nonmedical term, some modification of the traditional diagnostic approach to an illness by the physician is required if this complaint is to be meaningfully recognized and managed. Rather than focusing on a specific organ system or a specific complaint, the physician must perform a more comprehensive evaluation, which includes some nontraditional parameters, and identify the cause or causes of this condition.

A unifying concept of weakness is the perception of change. The patient perceives a change, that is, something is different or something is wrong. Clinicians must understand what changes the patient perceives and ask family and friends to confirm or further characterize that perception.

Assessing weakness is important for at least three reasons. First, many causes of weakness can be identified and treated. Second, weakness may be a symptom that permits identification and treatment of a serious process at an earlier more treatable stage. Third, a thoughtful evaluation of weakness—whatever the outcome—can build and solidify a meaningful physician-patient relationship. Physicians must address weakness with the same care and respect that is given to other complaints, both to identify treatable causes and to satisfy the concerns of the patients.

CLINICAL MANIFESTATIONS

An older patient who complains of weakness may or may not look ill. How the patient looks is important, but looking well does not guarantee that problems are not present. Indeed many patients state that they resent being told how well they look "for their age" while they actually do not feel well.

The assessment of several factors and the responses to a series of questions help physicians to delineate what the complaint of weakness means to their patients.

Baseline level of function

A baseline level of function is a key measure for older people, particularly because there is wide variation of function for anyone of any chronological age in this segment of the population. To document any changes, physicians must know what the patients were like before they perceived that they were ill. Several standard measures of function exist, but generally a less formal approach can be used.[1] Ask the patients where they live and how much help they need, whether they drive, how much they walk, and how much they do on a daily basis. One open-ended question to establish a baseline is, If I had seen you before you began to feel weak, how would you have been?

Perception of change

Having established a baseline of function, a determination must be made of what has changed. Before ascribing anything to the aging process itself, the clinician should determine what has changed and if that change is compatible with normal aging. Key questions to raise therefore are (1) What can you no longer do?, and (2) Over how much time did that happen?

Presence of organic disease

Many older people have one or more chronic organic illnesses, and therefore it is important to assess whether these illnesses may be the causes of the weakness. A disease process may have progressed (e.g., renal dysfunction secondary to diabetes mellitus), complications of a disease may have occurred (e.g., dumping and malabsorption after gastrectomy), or side effects of treatment may have developed (e.g., anorexia secondary to digitalis toxicity). However, physicians must be careful not to ascribe weakness—or any other symptoms—to a known disease process without a thoughtful evaluation of the complaint.

Expectations and fears of the patient

While the physician may be inclined to identify organic disease, the older patient may have a different agenda. The patient may view weakness as a sign of a serious medical problem such as a malignancy or as evidence of progressive decline that is due to the aging process. Whereas the physician may be unsatisfied after identifying a chronic condition as a cause of weakness, the older patient when given that information may be quite pleased that a more malevolent process is not present. It is vital therefore that clinicians ask all older patients who have weakness as a complaint what *they* think is wrong. At times, their responses may lead to the correct diagnoses. In all cases, however, hearing the patients' concerns allows physicians to address those concerns and manage the patients' fears.[3]

CAUSES OF WEAKNESS

Causes of weakness can be divided into the following four categories: (1) lifestyle, (2) depression, (3) medication, and (4) organic. Although there is no meaningful statistical data on this subject and no numerical rendering of what causes predominate, the practitioner at least can know what disorders or processes can cause weakness and what evaluation is necessary to identify them. The assessment is an exclusionary evaluation, that is, the goal is to make certain that an identifiable and treatable entity is not being overlooked.

Based on my clinical experience, depression and other psychosocial problems are the primary causes of weakness. Side effects from medications are common causes as well. The organic causes most often seen are hypothyroidism, anemia, and cardiac arrhythmias.

Lifestyle factors

Various events and changes in an older patient's life may cause a sense of weakness and ill health. Included are behavioral and situational problems (see next section under "Life events,") which may cause these symptoms but are not due to clinical depression, dietary and nutritional problems, and exercise and conditioning. What is interesting about these three factors is that most physicians who are now in practice received little if any training about how to manage them.

Life events. It is reasonable to assume that being old in our society is difficult, and some of the normal aspects of aging may at times produce feelings of weakness and ill health. Even healthy older persons must encounter some life events that cause feelings of sadness, and their despair may be perceived as weakness. These include sickness and death of a spouse, loved one, or friend, family relationships and problems, changes in the community, financial problems, and anything that makes the older person feel stressed or overwhelmed. Counseling by the physician, a social worker, or other practitioner can be beneficial in helping older people through these episodes and stresses. If left unaddressed, these stressful life events may result in clinical depression or increased feelings of ill health for older people.

Diet and nutrition. Nutritional deficiencies are probably frequent causes of weakness among elderly persons. A nutritional assessment must be part of the evaluation, which should be done either by the physician or a dietician. (See Chapter 20.) For some patients the nutritional deficits are due to their inability to afford enough food. With the availability of meal sites and food supplement programs, this financial issue should be raised whenever unexpected nutritional problems and weight loss are seen.

Lack of exercise. When a younger person feels tired and slow, the intervention recommended most often is exercise. After getting involved in a regular exercise program, most younger people feel better once they are "in shape". Unfortunately, a tired younger person is told to exercise, whereas a tired older person is told to rest. The younger person gets better, the older person gets worse.

If there are no contraindications and the appropriate modifications are made, the older person who is poorly conditioned also benefits from an exercise program. (See Chapter 21.)

Depression

Older people are more likely to develop vegetative signs of depression (e.g., lack of energy, lack of interest) than to verbalize their feelings of depression. (See Chapter 36.) They also may be less able to identify depression than younger patients. Because meaningful interventions are available for depression, this diagnosis should be considered for any older person whose cause of weakness cannot be identified.

Medications

Many medications can cause weakness among older patients, when the medications are either at toxic or therapeutic levels. The use of many medications, including over-the-counter preparations, poor compliance, and both age-related physiological and disease-associated pathological changes in drug metabolism make side effects a rather common cause of weakness and other vague systemic symptoms for elderly persons. Bosker and Albrich[2] among others have clearly described the potential dangers of medications that older patients use. (See Chapter 3.)

Organic disorders

A wide variety of organic disorders can cause weakness. It is reasonable to say that almost *any* organic disorder can cause this symptom. The accompanying box lists the most common organic causes of weakness, based on isolated reports on this topic and my clinical experience.

DIAGNOSTIC APPROACH

Perhaps the most important aspect of the diagnostic approach for weakness is to believe that it is a real and serious clinical problem. The physician who believes that weakness is not a legitimate complaint does not evaluate it appropriately. Significant illnesses are not diagnosed, patients endure unnecessary discomfort and loss of function, and they lose confidence in their physicians. Weakness can and should be evaluated by the standard history, physical examination, and laboratory format, with some modifications because of the unusual nature of this complaint.

History and family involvement

The patients' histories are important, particularly to determine exactly what the patients mean when they complain of weakness. The most effective way to learn what

---

COMMON ORGANIC CAUSES OF WEAKNESS

Anemia
Cardiac disorders
Arrhythmia
Failure
Ischemia
Valve dysfunction

Diabetes mellitus
Infection
Malignancy

Metabolic disorders
Parathyroid disease
Parkinson's disease
Polymyalgia rheumatica
Renal failure
Thyroid disorders
Hyperthyroid
Hypothyroid

```
_____ EVALUATING WEAKNESS: QUESTIONS TO ASK _____

     1. What makes you weak?
     2. Are you weak all of the time or if not, when?
     3. How long have you felt weak?
     4. What do you do when you feel weak and want to feel better?
     5. What would you do differently if you did not feel weak?
     6. What do you think is wrong?
     7. Is the weakness worse or staying the same?
     8. Are you having pain or any other symptoms?
     9. Have other people in your family had the same problem?
    10. How can we help you?
```

weakness means to a patient is to ask the question, What do you mean when you say that you feel weak? Some very interesting responses may result. If the responses to this question do not point to a specific problem, additional queries listed in the box above may be posed.

With the consent of the patient, the closest family member or friend should be interviewed. In my opinion, that interview should almost always take place in the presence of the patient, unless the patient has advanced dementia.[4] The family member or friend may offer good insight about the patient. Family and friends know a patient's baseline status, can explain any real changes in the patient, notice physical or behavioral changes that the patient and physician may not realize, and are aware of stresses that the patient may not see or want to discuss.

Physical examination

Physicians should perform complete physical examinations and focus on clues that are suggested by the patients' histories and our knowledge of the most frequent organic causes of weakness. A rectal examination is almost always mandatory.

Laboratory testing

Laboratory testing should be moderately extensive for proper evaluation of weakness. Omitting potentially useful tests is often false economy. A wiser course for physicians is to perform a full laboratory evaluation and ascertain that piecemeal tests are not repeated elsewhere.

A panel of tests recommended for all patients with weakness in the absence of other diagnostic clues should include those listed in the box on p. 322. Selected tests should be considered based upon the patient's history and results of the physical examination (e.g., imaging scan, echocardiogram, Holter monitor). A complete diagnostic evaluation is not only necessary to ascertain the cause of weakness, but also to reassure and comfort the patient when all tests and evaluations are normal or negative.

RECOMMENDED LABORATORY
TESTS FOR EVALUATION OF WEAKNESS

Blood chemistry
Blood levels of medications
Chest x-ray
Complete blood count
Electrocardiogram
Erythrocyte sedimentation rate
Thyroid functions (include thyroid-stimulating hormone)
Urinalysis

INTERVENTION

Intervention depends upon what has been found. Diets may be improved and supplemented, exercise programs may be established, medication regimens may be modified, and organic diseases may be treated. Psychosocial problems may be addressed by the physicians if they are comfortable doing so, or these problems may be managed by other practitioners. Devoting attention to the complaint of weakness is probably the most important intervention of all.

At times, there are no identifiable explanations, organic or otherwise, for the subjective complaint of weakness. However, after completing a full evaluation, the physician still may have a positive impact. By initiating a complete evaluation for the weakness symptom rather than assuming that the complaint is "old age creeping in," the physician contributes to the patient's well-being by showing genuine concern and explaining negative findings. The older patient can be assured that no serious problem has been identified when the evaluation proves negative. Assurance itself can be a meaningful intervention if the patient is fearful of a terminal illness or an illness that produces loss of function and independence.

If at the end of the evaluation no cause for the weakness is identified, the patient should not be dismissed and told "nothing is wrong." Rather, an explanation should be offered to the patient that no cause was found, with emphasis that a serious illness fortunately was not present. A follow-up appointment should be scheduled, and the patient should be encouraged to call sooner if the weakness worsens or if other symptoms occur. If an organic problem is present, it may become more evident at a later date. If depression or another psychosocial problem is present, the patient may better identify and deal with the problem at a second appointment. Therefore, the physician conveys to the patients that their symptoms are legitimate and that he or she is concerned about the patients' well-being. That alone can be a meaningful therapeutic intervention.

REFERENCES

1. Applegate WB: Instruments for the functional assessment of older patients, *N Engl J Med* 322:26, 1990.
2. Bosker G, Albrich JM: Drug therapy: drug prescribing and systematic detection of adverse drug reactions. In Bosker G, ed: *Geriatric Emergency Medicine*, St Louis, 1990, CV Mosby.
3. Waltman RE: It never hurts to let patients second-guess you, *Med Economics*, p 78, July 1991.
4. Waltman RE: Seeing the patient first, *Geriatrics* 46(4):92-95, 1991.

SUGGESTED READINGS

Gordon M: Differential diagnosis of weakness: a common geriatric symptom, *Geriatrics* 41(4):75, 1986.
Waltman RE: Old age is not a diagnosis, *Senior Patient*, p 30, July 1989.
Wolf-Klein G: A new onset of fatigue in an active elderly man, *Geriatrics* 44(9):85, 1989.

CHAPTER 34

Confusion and delirium

MICHAEL E. MAHLER

KEY POINTS

- Acute confusional state (ACS) or delirium is a common syndrome of elderly persons.
- The clinical hallmark of ACS is a disturbance of attention.
- The specific historical and clinical pattern of ACS distinguishes it from other disorders of cognitive and behavioral function such as dementia.
- The syndrome can result from a variety of metabolic, toxic, infectious, and neurological diseases.
- Although it has a high mortality rate, ACS is usually reversible with a systematic approach to diagnosis and treatment.

CLINICAL RELEVANCE

To call a patient "confused" may itself be confusing since that word can mean different things to different observers. Many researchers have used more specific terms, including *acute organic brain syndrome, acute brain failure, organic* or *toxic psychosis, delirium,* and *acute confusional state,* to describe the acute mental disturbances accompanying many physical illnesses.

Following the example of Lipowski,[5] delirium and acute confusional state (ACS) will be used synonymously in this chapter. The definition of *ACS* is a rapidly developing yet fluctuating behavior change that is characterized by inattention and altered arousal; incoherent speech, thought, and action; global impairment of memory and intellectual processes; emotional lability; and perceptual disturbances, including illusions and hallucinations.[10]

The frequency of ACS increases with patients' advancing age,[5,6] and at least three factors account for this. First, older patients typically have multiple, chronic medical conditions superimposed upon age-related decline in the function of nearly all organs. This results in a fragile homeostasis that decompensates easily with additional stress. Second, many older persons use numerous medications, increasing their likelihood of adverse effects and toxicity. Third, the physiological, anatomical, and neurochemical changes of normal senescence increase the susceptibility of the aged brain to further insults.[2] These factors interact to increase the vulnerability of elderly persons to ACS.

There are no data about the actual incidence or prevalence of ACS in community populations. Among general medical and surgical wards, 20% of patients aged 65 years and older have ACS. This probably underestimates the true frequency since nongeriatricians may fail to recognize mild confusion in elderly persons. In geriatric centers, 35 to 80% of patients are hospitalized for confusion or develop it within the hospital.[5,6]

Because ACS so often occurs with serious illness, the mortality rate is high.[5] Between 25% and 37% of patients who have delirium die within one month. The oldest and those with the most impaired mental statuses have the worst prognoses. Among survivors, 80% recover within 1 month, and only 5% remain confused longer than 6 months. The time course for resolution is often more prolonged for the old than the young, and resolution of the precipitating illness may precede improvement in mental status. These numbers emphasize both the lethality and the potential reversibility of ACS.

CLINICAL MANIFESTATIONS

ACS develops rapidly over a few hours or days.[5,6] Fluctuations in a patient's attention, arousal, and activity are characteristic so that the illness appears to wax and wane. With appropriate treatment the condition usually subsides within 1 to 4 weeks, although older patients return to their baseline statuses more slowly. The accompanying box lists the major clinical features of ACS.

CLINICAL MANIFESTATIONS OF ACUTE CONFUSIONAL STATE

Impaired and fluctuating attention and arousal

Cognitive deficits

Disorientation
Poor memory
Incoherent thought
Incoherent speech, agraphia, anomia
Visuoconstructive deficits
Dyscalculia

Neuropsychiatric abnormalities

Hallucinations, illusions
Delusions
Mood changes

Motor system abnormalities

Psychomotor retardation or hyperactivity
Tremor, asterixis, myoclonus
Tone and reflex changes
Dysarthria

Neurovegetative symptoms

Autonomic dysfunction
Incontinence
Sleep disruption

Disorder of attention and arousal

The clinical hallmark of ACS is a disturbance of attention.[1,3,4,5,6,7,10] Attention refers to one's ability to maintain, focus, and selectively shift mental activity. It includes orientation to stimuli, exploration, concentration, vigilance, persistence, and freedom from distraction.[7] The clinician can best gauge a patient's attention with two simple tests.[3] First is the digit span, which assesses the patient's ability to focus attention briefly. The patient is asked to repeat in correct sequence a string of numerals of increasing length, immediately after hearing them. An average person can repeat seven digits but fewer than five is abnormal. The second test requires the patient to raise a hand whenever the examiner says the letter *a* in a random sequence of letters with about one fourth being *a*'s. Failure to respond appropriately indicates a deficit of sustained attention or vigilance.

For lethargic patients the disorder of attention is a decreased capacity to respond to stimuli or to mobilize mental processes. However, in agitated confusional states such as delirium tremens, the patients have increased levels of arousal and alertness with an inability to sustain or focus their attention selectively. Thus, the patients appear to be incoherent as they respond simultaneously or sequentially to the examiners and a variety of distracting stimuli.

An alteration of arousal is another common feature of ACS. Diminished arousal or clouding of consciousness is characterized by a patient's decreased responsiveness to the environment and varies from mild drowsiness to stupor or coma.[9] Increased arousal may occur as well, marked by a patient's hypervigilance, irritability, and excitability.

Agitated delirium may alternate with quiet lethargy, and there may be intermittent periods of incoherence and lucidity. Fluctuation between these extremes is characteristic of ACS regardless of its cause. With progression of the syndrome, stupor predominates and leads to coma.[9]

Other manifestations

In addition to the disturbance of the patient's attention, disorientation is common. Memory of both previously learned and newly presented information is poor, but accurate memory testing is difficult when the patient's attention is disturbed. The patient's speech may be slurred and incoherent, and decreased writing skills and verbal fluency are frequent language abnormalities.

Neuropsychiatric findings of hallucinations, illusions, and delusions are frequent in ACS.[5,6] Visual and auditory hallucinations are common but tactile and multimodality hallucinations may occur too. The hallucinations seem to be real with vivid colors and details. Illusions are misperceptions of real objects with distortions in the size, shape, number, or color of an object. Delusions that may have a paranoid quality occur. These are rarely as complex or systematized as in the functional psychoses.

Delirious patients often feel emotional distress and experience mood changes.[3,5,6,10]

Fear, anxiety, and rage are the most common emotions in ACS, but apathy, depression, and emotional lability occur too.

Motor system abnormalities

In addition to mental status changes, ACS often includes abnormalities of the motor system such as withdrawal and apathy or restless pacing and hyperactivity.[9,10] Other motor abnormalities depend on the site and extent of structural brain disease that is associated with ACS, as well as type and severity of metabolic encephalopathies.[2]

Vegetative functions are affected by ACS. Autonomic arousal often accompanies ACS with dilated pupils, rapid pulse, elevated blood pressure, and increased sweating.[5,6,10] Decreased food intake and incontinence occur frequently, sometimes because the patient is in restraints to control agitated behavior.

The normal sleep-wake cycle is interrupted so that a patient may be excessively drowsy during the day but awake, restless, and agitated at night.[5,6] Sleep itself is often fragmented with disruption of the usual progression of sleep stages.[10]

DIAGNOSTIC APPROACH

Differential diagnosis

Differential diagnosis of delirium or ACS involves two processes.[5] First, the physician recognizes the syndrome and distinguishes it from other types of confused behavior. Second, the physician determines the precise cause of ACS.

The onset, course, level of arousal, and other features usually allow the physician to separate an ACS from other syndromes such as dementia, aphasia, and primary mood disorders.[10]

Dementia has an insidious rather than rapid onset and does not fluctuate like ACS. Furthermore, in dementia the level of the patient's alertness is not impaired and, except for advanced cases of dementia, attention is generally preserved. The physician's difficulty in differentiating delirium and dementia occurs when a previously demented individual deteriorates further or when a patient with ACS fails to recover. Table 34-1 summarizes the distinctions between ACS and dementia.

In aphasia the pattern of neuropsychological deficits differs from that described for ACS, and there is no altered level of consciousness. However, an acute stroke or a mass lesion could cause both aphasia and a confusional syndrome.

Affective disease disturbs the patient's psychomotor activity but does not lead to fluctuations in the level of consciousness. Also, there may be a history of recurrent depression or mania. Similarly, schizophrenia does not first appear in elderly patients and does not compromise consciousness. However, an accurate history may not be available and a patient may not cooperate with the careful examination that is required for a full assessment. In that case, it is best to proceed on the assumption that an organic cause for ACS exists.

Table 34-1   Comparison of acute confusional state (ACS) and dementia

Feature	ACS	Dementia
Onset	Acute, hours to days	Slow, months to years
Course	Fluctuating during the day	Stable over the course of day
Mental status		
Attention	Impaired	Not affected
Arousal	Variable and fluctuating	Normal
Language	Dysarthric or incoherent, mildly anomic, dysgraphic	May be aphasic depending on cause
Memory	Impaired	Impaired
Hallucinations	Common	Less common
Motor system	Tremor, asterixis, myoclonus	Depends on cause; Alzheimer's disease normal until late
Sleep	Disrupted	May be disrupted
Electroencephalogram	Prominent slowing	May be normal until late

Common causes of ACS

The second step in differential diagnosis requires broad knowledge of the medical and neurological conditions that can cause ACS. Among elderly persons, diseases often have atypical presentations, and ACS may frequently be the initial manifestation. Perhaps the most frequent causes of ACS for elderly patients are those related to infections, drugs, hypoperfusion states (heart failure, shock, stroke), and metabolic disorders (hypoglycemia, dehydration, renal failure). A list of common causes of ACS is listed in the box on p. 329.

Evaluation

The clinician immediately should initiate a search for the causes of ACS whenever a patient comes to the office because of an acute change in mental status. Sometimes the initial symptoms may be subtle changes in personality or behavior; the astute clinician must have a high index of suspicion for ACS because of its high mortality. In addition to the patient's history and physical examination, a brief mental status examination that *emphasizes attention* is key to establishing the diagnosis as outlined previously. Inouye et al[4] have crystallized the essential diagnostic features of delirium into a quick and reliable algorithm for use by nonspecialists. This algorithm utilizes the history of an acute onset and fluctuating changes in a patient's mental status, an observation of the patient's difficulty in focusing attention, and the presence of either the patient's disorganized thinking or altered level of consciousness.

Clues to the specific cause of ACS are obtained from the history, physical, and laboratory evaluation. When the patient is incapable of giving the history, it should

_____ **COMMON CAUSES OF ACUTE CONFUSIONAL STATE** _____

Neurological

Mass lesion
Trauma
Vascular
• Hypoperfusion
• Acute stroke
CNS infections
• Abscess
• Meningitis
• Encephalitis
Seizures
Focal lesions
• Temporoparietal
• Brain stem

Systemic illness

Cardiac
Pulmonary
Anemia
Renal and electrolyte
Hepatic
Endocrine
Infection
Vitamin deficiency

Intoxication

Drugs
• Iatrogenic
• Drugs of abuse
Industrial exposures
• Volatiles
• Metals

Withdrawal

Drugs
Alcohol

Postsurgical
Psychiatric illness

Depression
Mania
Schizophrenia

be sought from relatives, hospital charts, and physicians and nurses who have known the patient because the past medical history contains the most likely causes. A relatively rapid development of symptoms is necessary to establish the syndrome, but a sudden onset would suggest cerebrovascular disease or seizure. Prior head trauma or recent surgery has obvious implications. The list of medications taken by the patient is vital, and it is equally important to consider the strength of the dose and frequency of prn and nonprescription drugs.

In addition to the usual information obtained from the patient's vital signs, respiratory changes often signal the underlying cause of a confused or stuporous state.[9] Damage to forebrain structures can result in posthyperventilation apnea or Cheyne-Stokes respiration, while midbrain damage results in central neurogenic hyperventilation and lower brain stem damage results in apneustic, cluster, or ataxic breathing. Metabolic encephalopathies also result in alterations of the respiratory pattern. Uremia, diabetic ketosis, lactic acidosis, certain poisons, and other causes of metabolic acidosis lead to compensatory hyperventilation. Hyperventilation with a primary respiratory alkalosis occurs with hepatic encephalopathy, sepsis, salicylism, and pneumonia. Hypoventilation should raise the physician's suspicion of sedative drugs, acute pulmonary insufficiency, or metabolic alkalosis from vomiting, diuretics, or Cushing's syndrome. The patient's breath may have characteristic odors because of hepatic encephalopathy and ketoacidosis.

Temperature elevations should not be overlooked. Conversely, it is important to remember that elderly persons are susceptible to hypothermia, especially with hypothyroidism or sepsis, and normal temperatures do not eliminate the possibility that serious infection is the underlying cause for ACS.

The general physical examination should focus on the presence of trauma, systemic organ disease, or evidence of prior surgery. The motor system's manifestations of ACS have been described. Autonomic arousal occurs in many types of delirium but it is especially prominent in alcohol or sedative withdrawal.

The initial diagnostic evaluation may take place in an office setting. If the ACS is mild and the cause is immediately recognized and easily treated (such as a drug intoxication), then outpatient management with close follow-up may be safe and effective. However, ACS is often associated with serious underlying medical illness and most patients require hospitalization.

Laboratory evaluation is important for physicians to determine the causes of ACS. The accompanying box lists necessary tests for the complete evaluation of ACS. This comprehensive assessment results in the identification of specific causes for 80% to 95% of patients who have ACS.[5]

LABORATORY EVALUATION FOR ACUTE CONFUSIONAL STATE

Initial testing in all cases

Complete blood count with white blood cell differential and erythrocyte sedimentation rate

Serum electrolytes, glucose, creatinine; blood urea nitrogen (BUN); serum calcium, phosphate, magnesium

Liver and thyroid functions, serum protein

Complete urinalysis with microscopical examination

Chest x-ray and electrocardiogram

Additional tests when indicated

Arterial blood gases

Blood, sputum, urine cultures

Serum vitamin B_{12} and folate

Toxicology screen and drug levels

Human immunodeficiency virus titers

Neuroimaging scans

Electroencephalography

Cerebrospinal fluid analysis

INTERVENTION

Treatment

Identification and treatment of the patient's underlying cause of ACS is the most effective therapy. While specific therapy is instituted, general measures help to keep the patient with ACS safe and comfortable. The environment should be adequately illuminated, and if the patient is ambulatory there should be a protected supervised area for walking. Caregivers should be calm and reassuring to alleviate the emotional distress of the confused individual. Appropriate nutrition and hydration are necessary for the patient.

A patient's habitual use of medications should be reevaluated and all nonessential medications should be stopped. Sedation may be necessary to reduce agitation and protect the patient and others, but it should not be done solely for the convenience of the caregivers. Low doses of short-acting sedatives such as oxazepam, lorazepam, or chloral hydrate should be used. Haloperidol, 0.5 to 2.0 mg given orally or intramuscularly, is often an effective tranquilizer that may not cause excessive sedation in elderly patients.[6] All sedatives should be used carefully to avoid exacerbating the patient's confusion.

Prognosis

Approximately one fourth to one third of the patients who have ACS die from the underlying illness. For those who survive, improvement in their mental statuses may occur gradually over several weeks, long after resolution of the precipitating events. Recovery from the syndrome is often more prolonged for older patients than it is for younger patients.

There are two reasons why some patients fail to recover fully from ACS. There may have been an incipient dementia from another cause, which was exacerbated by the superimposed delirium. Alternatively, the acute insult that caused the ACS may have resulted in permanent brain damage after the insult had resolved. However, even for chronic confusional states that fit the definition of dementia, the evaluation that was outlined previously may reveal a reversible component.[8]

REFERENCES

1. American Psychiatric Association: *Diagnostic and statistical manual of mental disorders*, ed 3, Washington, D.C., 1987.
2. Blass JP, Plum F: Metabolic encephalopathies in older adults. In Katzman R, Terry R, eds: *The neurology of aging*, Philadelphia, 1983, FA Davis.
3. Chedru F, Geschwind N: Disorders of higher cortical functions in acute confusional states, *Cortex* 8:395, 1972.
4. Inouye SK et al: Clarifying confusion: the confusion assessment method, *Ann Intern Med* 113:941, 1990.
5. Lipowski ZJ: Transient cognitive disorders (delirium, acute confusional states) in the elderly, *Am J Psychiatry* 140:1426, 1983.
6. Lipowski ZJ: Delirium (acute confusional states), *JAMA* 285:1789, 1987.
7. Mesulam M-M: *Principles of behavioral neurology*, Philadelphia, 1985, FA Davis.

8. Mahler ME, Cummings JL, Benson DF: Treatable dementias, *West J Med* 146:705, 1987.
9. Plum F, Posner JB: *The diagnosis of stupor and coma*, ed 3, Philadelphia, 1980, FA Davis.
10. Strub RL: Acute confusional states. In Benson DF, Blumer D, eds: *Psychiatric aspects of neurologic disease*, vol 2, New York, 1982, Grune & Stratton.

SUGGESTED READINGS

Cummings JL: *Clinical neuropsychiatry*, Orlando, Fla, 1985, Grune & Stratton.
Lipowski ZJ: *Delirium: acute confusional states*, New York, 1990, Oxford University Press.

CHAPTER 35

Dementia

DOUGLAS W. SCHARRE
JEFFREY L. CUMMINGS

KEY POINTS

- Dementia is a common disabling geriatric condition.
- Alzheimer's disease is the most common type of dementia accounting for 50% to 60% of cases; vascular dementias account for 10% to 30%.
- Reversible causes of dementia include hydrocephalus, meningiomas, subdural hematomas, medications, toxins, metabolic disorders, infections, and depression.
- A thorough history, physical examination, and detailed evaluation of mental status are essential for accurate diagnosis.
- Basic laboratory assessments and neuroimaging are indicated in every dementia evaluation to detect reversible causes and assist in management.
- Behavioral disturbances associated with dementia often respond to pharmacotherapy.
- Avoid polypharmacy and begin all medications at low doses.
- Prevent sensory and social deprivation and protect the patients from infection, dehydration, and environmental hazards.
- Caregivers of demented patients benefit from a review of goals of care, advance directives, and support services before crises occur.

CLINICAL RELEVANCE

Dementia is a common geriatric condition and an important source of disability among elderly persons. It is essential that physicians make an accurate and early diagnosis of dementia to facilitate appropriate treatment and care.

Approximately 5% to 10% of people aged 65 years and older are demented. Age-specific prevalence studies indicate that moderate to severe dementia is found in 3% of those aged 65 to 74 years old, 10% of those aged 75 to 84, and 30% of those aged 85 years and older.

Dementia is a nonspecific clinical syndrome produced by a variety of brain disorders. Alzheimer's disease is the most common type of dementia, accounting for 50% to 60% of the cases. Vascular dementias account for 10% to 30% of the cases, and 20% of dementia patients have both the vascular and Alzheimer type of pathology. Toxic and metabolic disorders account for about 18% of the cases and the dementia of depression accounts for about 5%. Hydrocephalic dementias occur with an incidence of 3% to 7% of the cases.

The impact on the health care costs for this ever-growing geriatric population with dementing diseases is considerable. Cognitive impairment necessitates adequate supervision and support systems that entail great expenses. It was estimated that in 1985 it cost $35.8 billion to care for the 2.4 million moderately to severely demented persons in the United States. By the year 2040, the estimated cost will reach $121 billion. Early accurate diagnosis leads to appropriate treatments that reduce cognitive impairments, facilitate the management of patients, and help contain costs.

CLINICAL MANIFESTATIONS OF DEMENTING DISORDERS

Dementia can be defined as a syndrome of acquired impairment of neuropsychological function with compromise in at least three of the following areas of mental activity: (1) language, (2) memory, (3) visuospatial skills, (4) personality or emotional state, and (5) cognition (abstraction, calculation, judgment). The dementia syndrome has many causes and a substantial number are treatable. The accompanying box presents a list of the principal causes of the dementia syndrome.

The key to accurate diagnosis is a thorough history and examination. The historical review must include information about the onset and clinical course of the problem. The onset is insidious in degenerative disorders and may be abrupt in vascular disorders. Progression is gradual in degenerative processes and stepwise in multiple stroke syndromes. Degenerative diseases are chronic, neoplasms and subdural hematomas may be subacute, and strokes are acute. Obtaining the patient's past medical history, including medical and psychiatric illnesses, is also critically important. Finally, a family history of dementia or psychiatric illness can provide useful information that helps guide the physician's diagnostic assessment.

After physical examination of the patient, a search for systemic illnesses or endocrine dysfunction is conducted. A complete neurological examination is critical. Are there any focal findings consistent with a localized lesion? Does the patient have an extrapyramidal syndrome indicative of a basal ganglia disorder? Is there ataxia and incontinence suggestive of normal pressure hydrocephalus?

The examination of the patient's mental status provides the most diagnostically useful information and should evaluate the domains of attention, language, memory, visuospatial skills (including constructional ability), abstraction, judgment, calculation, executive function, personality, and mood. Different profiles of cognitive deficits characterize the different dementia syndromes.

Dementing illnesses preferentially may affect cortical or subcortical structures. Alzheimer's disease and other *cortical dementia* syndromes are characterized by im-

---

CLASSIFICATION OF DEMENTIA SYNDROMES

Degenerative disorders

Cortical
- Alzheimer's disease
- Pick's disease

Subcortical
- Parkinson's disease
- Huntington's disease
- Wilson's disease
- Fahr's disease (idiopathic basal ganglia calcification)
- Progressive supranuclear palsy
- Spinocerebellar or striatonigral degeneration

Vascular dementias

Multiple large vessel occlusions
Lacunar state (multiple subcortical infarctions)
Binswanger's disease (white matter ischemic injury)
Mixed cortical and subcortical infarctions

Myelinoclastic disorders

Multiple sclerosis
Leukodystrophies

Traumatic conditions
Neoplastic dementias
Hydrocephalic dementias

Communicating obstructive (normal pressure hydrocephalus)
Noncommunicating obstructive

Inflammatory conditions

Arteritis (systemic lupus erythematosus, others)
Sarcoidosis

Toxic conditions

Prescription drugs
Alcohol or drug abuse
Metals (lead, mercury, manganese, arsenic, thallium)
Industrial agents and solvents

Metabolic disorders

Cardiopulmonary failure (hypoxia)
Uremia
Hepatic encephalopathy
Anemia and hematological conditions
Endocrine disorders (thyroid, adrenal, parathyroid)
Vitamin deficiencies (B_{12}, folate, niacin)

Infectious dementias

Syphilis
Chronic meningitis
Postencephalitic dementia syndrome
Acquired immunodeficiency syndrome (AIDS)
Jakob-Creutzfeldt disease
Progressive multifocal leukoencephalopathy

Depression

pairments in the patient's language (aphasia), learning (amnesia), visual perception (agnosia), and praxis (apraxia), with normal motor function. *Subcortical dementia* is a clinical syndrome characterized by the patient's forgetfulness, slowness of mental processing, impaired cognition, mood disturbances, and speech and motor system abnormalities.[2]

Specific neurological, neurobehavioral, and neuropsychiatric features characterize specific types of dementia or allow the development of diagnostic hypotheses that can be confirmed or excluded by laboratory tests and neuroimaging studies.

Alzheimer's disease

Alzheimer's disease almost always begins after one reaches the age of 50 years old, and it is increasingly common among elderly persons. It is found in about 5% to 10% of the population between 70 and 79 years of age and in 20% to 30% of those between 80 and 89 years of age. Typically there is an insidious onset and a gradually progressive clinical course. Remissions do not occur and plateau periods are rare. Death usually occurs 6 to 12 years after onset. In 25% to 40% of all cases, Alzheimer's disease is inherited as an autosomal dominant condition with age-dependent penetrance.

Alzheimer's disease is not a global disorder of the brain.[4] The primary visual, motor, and somatosensory cortical regions are relatively spared. Areas of the brain that are most affected include those cortical regions subserving language, memory, visual association, praxis, cognition, and executive function. Subcortical structures are not involved until late in the course.

Mental status changes occurring early in the disease include empty speech with a paucity of nouns, anomia manifesting as difficulty in naming objects, and poor generation of word lists (e.g., number of animals that can be named in one minute, with the normal number being 12 or more). New learning is difficult and recall of recent information is impaired. Copying two- or three-dimensional figures is difficult. Emotionally, the patient is usually unconcerned. Irritability, suspiciousness, or sadness may occur. Judgment becomes poor and carelessness is evident in work habits. Motor and sensory functions remain normal as do the electroencephalogram (EEG) and neuroimaging studies.

In the middle phase of the patient's illness, all intellectual functions continue to deteriorate. Fluent aphasia with paraphasic errors (substituting words with incorrect words or nonsense words), poor comprehension, and relatively preserved repetition is exhibited. Recent and remote memory are severely impaired. Figures cannot be copied. Calculations are poor and abstractions are concrete. The patient's inability to perform volitional acts on command or by imitation that can be performed spontaneously (apraxia) may occur. The patients are usually indifferent to their conditions. Delusions of infidelity, theft, or harm are common. Symptoms of depression occur in up to 40% of patients, but major depression occurs in only a few. Motor and sensory examinations remain intact. The patients may be restless and wander. EEGs show diffuse theta-range background slowing and computed tomography (CT) or magnetic resonance imaging (MRI) reveals cortical atrophy. Single-photon emission computed tomography (SPECT) demonstrates decreased parietal and temporal blood flow bilaterally, while positron emission tomography (PET) shows diminished metabolism in the same regions.

At the end stage of the disease, the patient's cognitive abilities are usually untestable. Mutism, palilalia (repetition of words or sentences), or echolalia (echoing what was spoken by another person) occurs. Urinary and fecal incontinence are present. The limbs become rigid and flexed and myoclonus may occur. EEGs show diffuse delta-range background slowing and neuroimaging (CT, MRI) studies show diffuse atrophy. PET and SPECT reveal decreased temporal, parietal, and frontal metabolism and perfusion.

Vascular dementia

Multiple cerebral infarcts are the second most common cause of dementia, after Alzheimer's disease. Typically the patient has a stroke with an abrupt onset and neurological impairments, including intellectual disturbances. Over time, stepwise progression of neurological insults results in a dementia syndrome. Usually there is a history of hypertension, heart disease, diabetes mellitus, or hyperlipidemia. Historical evidence of discrete vascular events or transient ischemic attacks is common but not invariably present, and a gradual course does not exclude the diagnosis of vascular dementia.

Vascular disease may result in either multiple large vessel occlusions involving primarily the cerebral cortex, multiple small vessel thromboses with subcortical infarctions (lacunar state), deep white matter ischemic injuries (Binswanger's disease), or mixed subcortical and cortical infarctions. The specific features of the vascular dementia syndrome depend on the location and amount of cerebral tissue that is infarcted.

The typical findings of left-hemisphere cortical infarctions include aphasia, poor verbal memory, impaired calculation abilities, and right hemiparesis, hemisensory loss, and hemianopsia. Findings in right-hemisphere cortical infarctions include poor nonverbal memory, visuospatial disturbances, and left hemiparesis, hemisensory loss, and hemianopsia. CT or MRI reveals multiple cortical infarcts. MRI is superior to CT for demonstrating ischemic cerebral injury.

Lacunar state results from multiple infarctions of subcortical structures including thalamus, basal ganglia, internal capsule, and brain stem. Spasticity, weakness, tremors, extrapyramidal signs, hyperreflexia, and gait difficulties are more common than sensory and visual impairments. Bladder and even bowel incontinence may occur. Pseudobulbar palsy is often present with dysarthria, dysphagia, bilateral facial paresis, brisk gag response, brisk jaw jerk, and exaggerated emotional displays. Memory is impaired, depression is frequent, paranoid delusions are common, and personality alterations may occur. Disorientation, poor judgment, and perseveration are characteristic features. MRI is more sensitive than CT for locating the small cavitary infarctions.

Binswanger's disease or subcortical arteriosclerotic encephalopathy involves the small penetrating vessels supplying the deep white matter. Hypertension is the usual cause. Unlike most other types of vascular dementia, a gradually progressive course rather than a stepwise progression is seen in the majority of cases of Binswanger's disease. Examination of the patient's mental status typically shows memory impairments, mood changes, poor judgment, lack of spontaneity, and perseveration. Weakness, ataxia, rigidity, dysarthria, and urinary incontinence are frequent neurological abnormalities. Bilateral periventricular white matter lucencies, dilated ventricles, and atrophy are common findings on the CT. MRI reveals hyperintensities in the periventricular areas and the deep white matter of the hemispheres. Binswanger's disease and lacunar state commonly coexist.

The dementia of Parkinson's and Huntington's diseases

Parkinson's disease and Huntington's disease exhibit the syndrome of subcortical dementia along with its characteristic motor abnormalities and depression.[2] Aphasia, agnosia, apraxia, and amnesia, typical in Alzheimer's disease and other cortical dementias, are not present.

Parkinson's disease is diagnosed by the patient's characteristic rest tremor, bradykinesia, rigidity, and gait instability. There is no genetic predilection for the disorder. About 30% of those with idiopathic Parkinson's disease have overt dementia and an additional 40% have subtle neuropsychological impairments. This dementia is largely distinct from Alzheimer's dementia.[5] Dementia is most common among patients who have postural instabilities and gait disturbances and least common among patients who have marked tremors. The intellectual decline is insidious and the clinical course is gradual. After examination of the patient's mental status, a typical subcortical dementia pattern is observed. Recognition of learned material is superior to spontaneous recall. Visuospatial deficits, including difficulties with constructions, are common. CT or MRI shows no characteristic findings.

Huntington's disease is an autosomal dominant condition. The average age of onset is 35 years, but it may occasionally begin in one's sixth decade. Chorea, subcortical dementia, and mood and personality changes characterize this disorder. The disease has a gradually progressive course until the patient's death. Patients who have Huntington's disease evidence difficulties in sustained concentration. Recent and remote recall is impaired and visuospatial skills are disrupted. Patients have disturbed planning and scheduling abilities. Apathy is prominent. Other behavioral changes include depression with suicidal ideation, mania, and intermittent explosive disorder. Mood and personality disorders may occur years before chorea or dementia. CT,

MRI, and PET studies of Huntington's disease reveal caudate nucleus atrophy and hypometabolism.

Hydrocephalic dementias

Hydrocephalus refers to an abnormal enlargement of the cerebral ventricles. This condition may occur either from the patient's loss of surrounding brain parenchyma or from obstruction of cerebrospinal fluid (CSF) outflow. Obstructive hydrocephalus may be either noncommunicating or communicating. Noncommunicating hydrocephalus occurs from a blockage of CSF flow within the ventricular system. Communicating hydrocephalus, also called normal pressure hydrocephalus (NPH), occurs when the CSF pathways within the ventricular system and from the ventricles to the subarachnoid space are open, but there is a barrier to CSF reabsorption into the venous sinuses. Causes include meningitis, encephalitis, subarachnoid bleeding, or trauma. Idiopathic cases also occur.

The triad of dementia, gait disturbance, and urinary incontinence characterize NPH.[1] Apathy, slowness of mental processing, memory abnormalities, impaired abstraction abilities, disturbed calculation skills, and disorientation are characteristic findings of the patient's mental status. The gait disturbance usually begins with clumsiness and spasticity. The patient's gait is typically slow, shuffling, and has a wide base. Difficulty with initiation of movement may be noticeable. Hyperactive reflexes and Babinski's signs are common. Urinary incontinence is a late finding.

CT and MRI show greatly enlarged ventricles with marked dilation of the temporal and frontal horns. The cortical sulci are not excessively widened. Periventricular hypodensity is seen on the CT and periventricular hyperintensity is seen on the MRI. Lumbar puncture temporarily may improve the patient's symptoms. Radionuclide cisternography reveals abnormal reflux of the tracer into the ventricles and failure of the tracer to evacuate the ventricles and be absorbed into the superior sagittal sinus by 72 hours. Use of CSF pressure monitors to demonstrate intermittent pressure elevations also has been helpful for diagnosis.

Toxic-metabolic dementias

Prescribed drugs are a common cause of dementia in the geriatric patient. Review of the patient's medication regimen and dosages may reveal a reversible cause of dementia. Nearly all medications can cause intellectual deficits but specific classes of agents, including anticholinergic drugs, antihypertensive agents, anticonvulsants, and psychotropic agents, are particularly likely to impair cognition.

Excessive and chronic alcohol intake can produce a dementia syndrome. Alcoholic dementia is characterized by the patient's loss of memory, slowness of mental processing, perseveration, disorientation, decreased attention, poor abstraction abilities, and constructional deficits. Language functions are spared. CT shows only generalized atrophy. Korsakoff's syndrome, related to thiamin deficiency, produces an amnestic disorder with abnormalities limited to memory and learning rather than a dementia syndrome. The syndrome occurs most commonly among alcoholics who have thiamin-deficient diets, but it may be seen in other patients who have malnutrition or gastrointestinal absorption disorders.

Intoxication from industrial solvents and heavy metals produces dementia only after one's prolonged exposure to the substances. A history of toxin exposure is present and progression of the patient's intellectual decline stops once the toxin is removed. A peripheral neuropathy is commonly associated with the dementia.

Systemic metabolic illnesses and nutritional deficiencies are common among elderly patients and may be associated with dementia. These dementias can be treated by physicians' recognizing and treating their patients' underlying conditions. Disorders causing metabolic encephalopathy include uremia, hepatic encephalopathy, anemia, hypothyroidism, hyperthyroidism, hypoparathyroidism, hyperparathyroidism, Addison's disease, Cushing's disease, and porphyria. Vitamin B_{12} or folate deficiency produces myelopathy, peripheral neuropathy, megaloblastic anemia, and dementia. The dementia occasionally may precede other systemic manifestations of the vitamin deficiency. Administration of the deficient vitamin may reverse the dementia. Anoxia or hypoxia from cardiac or pulmonary failure causes neuronal dysfunction and dementia.

On the examination of the patient's mental status, findings of metabolic encephalopathies include disorientation, decreased attention, fluctuating arousal, poor concentration, and impaired memory. Depression, agitation, delusions, and hallucinations may be observed. The neurological examination often reveals an action tremor, myoclonus, or asterixis. CT and MRI may be normal or show atrophy; EEG recordings reveal diffuse slowing.

Infectious dementias

A variety of infectious agents can produce dementia in geriatric patients. Dementia may result from chronic fungal or parasitic meningitis or may be the chronic residual of an acute viral infection such as herpes simplex encephalitis. Jakob-Creutzfeldt disease caused by prions is identified by intellectual decline, pyramidal and extrapyramidal signs, and myoclonus, with a progressive course to death in 6 to 12 months. A periodic polyspike discharge is present in the EEG in a majority of cases, but it may not appear until late in the clinical course. Acquired immunodeficiency syndrome (AIDS) can produce a subcortical type of dementia with a progressive course. CT and MRI may show periventricular white matter abnormalities. Lyme disease caused by the tick-borne spirochete *Borrelia burgdorferi* can result in a dementia that appears months to years after the patient's initial infection. Typical findings include memory loss, depression, anomia, and irritability. General paresis, which at one time accounted for up to 10% of all admissions to insane asylums, occurs sporadically. This syphilitic disorder is characterized by frontal lobe pathology with memory deficits, cognitive impairments, irritability, peculiar deportment, grandiose delusions, and Argyll Robertson pupils.

The dementia of depression

The typical features of depression are described in Chapter 36.

Substantial cognitive decline imitating a degenerative dementia occurs in some depressed patients. The onset is gradual; the clinical course is usually a few months in duration. The patient's intellectual impairment is reversible with successful treatment of the mood disorder. The patient's history of depression or a family history of depression are common.

The dementia of depression has the clinical features of subcortical dementia. Depressed mood, slowing of mental processes, poor memory, and cognitive dilapidation are seen. Immediate and delayed recall are poor, but the patient's recognition memory is usually unimpaired. Depressive psychosis, anxiety, and agitation commonly accompany the dementia.

The EEG is normal; CT and MRI are normal or show white matter abnormalities.

DIAGNOSTIC APPROACH

The dementia syndrome has many causes. These conditions often lack specific laboratory features. The first step in diagnosis is a careful history and examination, including a detailed evaluation of the patient's mental status. The clinical assessment is then supplemented by laboratory data and neuroimaging studies.

The *mini-mental state examination (MMSE)* was developed as a brief test to measure a patient's cognitive impairment.[3] The instrument assesses the patient's orientation, registration, attention, short-term memory recall, language, and constructional ability. The MMSE is well validated, useful as a brief screening tool, and appropriate for monitoring changes over the course of an illness. It is relatively insensitive to subtle changes and does not distinguish delirium, dementia, amnesia, or aphasia. Distinguished from the brief, standardized, mental status examinations, neuropsychological test batteries extensively evaluate the patients' cognitive functions. These tests provide more details but may be unduly fatiguing for elderly medically ill patients. These tests provide an excellent baseline with which future tests can be compared. Identification of the patients' early cognitive changes or focal deficits is also possible. These tests do not differentiate the various types of dementia.

Appropriate laboratory examinations are an essential part of the evaluation. Laboratory assessment is necessary to detect toxic, metabolic, and infectious dementias. Required examinations include a complete blood count, erythrocyte sedimentation rate and blood urea nitrogen; serum electrolytes, glucose, calcium, phosphorus, B_{12} and folate; thyroid and liver function tests; chest roentgenogram; and electrocardiogram. A serological test for syphilis is always indicated and should be the fluorescent treponemal antibody absorption (FTA-ABS) test because other screenings may be nonreactive in tertiary (late) syphilis.

CT and MRI provide images of the patient's brain structure. Algorithms developed to determine which patients require CT scanning have shown unacceptably low sensitivities in validation testing.[6] Therefore, at this time, a CT or MRI should be done on all dementia patients for whom a definite diagnosis has not been established by clinical or laboratory assessment. A CT scan of the patient's head detects neoplasms, abscesses, infarctions, white matter diseases, hydrocephalus, and subdural hematomas. MRI is superior to CT in most instances, particularly for characterizing infarctions and subcortical white matter disorders.

SPECT and PET are nuclear medicine imaging techniques that visualize the patient's cerebral blood flow or cerebral metabolism. They measure physiological rather than anatomical changes. They are the only tests that reveal characteristic patterns in degenerative diseases such as Alzheimer's disease and frontal lobe degenerations. PET is more sensitive than SPECT but more costly and has limited availability.

Additional optional tests should be considered in individual clinical circumstances. If the patient has a history of exposure to particular drugs, toxins, heavy metals, or industrial agents, then the appropriate assays are indicated. A lumbar puncture should be performed on all patients who have infectious, inflammatory, or demyelinating conditions. A human immunodeficiency virus (HIV) test or a *Borrelia* titer is indicated when the patient's symptoms are suggestive of one of these infections. EEG abnormalities are prominent in toxic and metabolic dementias and are normal in the early stages of Alzheimer's disease and the dementia of depression. Only as Alzheimer's disease progresses does generalized slowing of the EEG pattern occur. Jakob-Creutzfeldt disease has characteristic EEG findings. Computerized EEG (CEEG) may be useful as a means of graphically demonstrating the topographical distribution of electrocerebral changes, but its utility for the diagnosis of specific causes of dementia remains unproven. Cisternography or intracranial CSF pressure monitors are useful in diagnosing NPH.

INTERVENTION

Demented elderly patients are prone to many sources of disability. Patients with loss of memory underreport their symptoms and coincidental illnesses may be easily overlooked. Infection and dehydration are common. These must be carefully sought and treated. Adverse effects of medications and drug interactions are also common sources of disability. All medications must be reviewed to determine if they can be discontinued or the dosage reduced. Hazardous environmental situations may lead to falls and broken bones. Adequate supervision prevents accidents, medication errors, and improper nutrition. Social and sensory deprivation must be prevented by giving proper stimulation from caregivers and optimal hearing and vision care from physicians. Overstimulation may increase agitation and should be controlled. Support groups, family counseling, and social services help to educate and assist caregivers. Goals of care should be set with families; advance directives are especially important to address.

Disease-specific treatment

There is no consistently effective specific treatment for Alzheimer's disease. Ergoloid mesylates (Hydergine) have little effect. Cholinergic agents have been disappointing, but new preparations are being tested and some are promising.

Stroke prevention is aided by the daily use of 325 mg of aspirin and elimination of the sources of emboli. Cognition and cerebral perfusion both improve modestly among patients who have multiinfarct dementia when aspirin is taken, and the risk of recurrent stroke is reduced. Control of the risk factors of stroke such as hypertension, diabetes mellitus, hyperlipidemia, and smoking are critical.

The dementia of Parkinson's disease improves minimally with dopaminergic agents. In Huntington's disease genetic counseling is indicated. Dementia from subdural hematomas, meningiomas, and other tumors may reverse with surgical treatment. CSF shunting of patients who have NPH improves their ataxic gaits, urinary incontinence, and cognitive deficits. The gait abnormalities usually respond best. Surgical complications of shunt placement include subdural hematomas, shunt infections, and shunt blockage. Toxic dementias often resolve once the agent is removed. Intoxication from heavy metals can be reversed by chelation. Metabolic causes of dementia improve with specific treatment of the underlying condition. Syphilis, Lyme disease, and certain other infectious causes of dementia are treatable (but not necessarily reversible) with antibiotics. Progression of the AIDS dementia complex is slowed with azidothymidine. The dementia of depression responds to antidepressants or electroconvulsive therapy, resulting in resolution of both the depression and the dementia.

Behavioral management

Behavioral disturbances associated with dementing conditions are treatable. Table 35-1 lists precautions and recommendations for the drugs that are commonly used to treat behavioral disturbances associated with dementing conditions. Behavioral management regimens must be individualized and the patient's concurrent medical problems and medications must be taken into account.[7] Agents with anticholinergic properties may cause memory impairment, constipation, and urinary retention and should be avoided or used cautiously. All medications instituted should be started at a low dose and increased gradually to an optimal level. Periodically these medications should be reduced or stopped to determine if there is an ongoing need for the agent.

Agitation, suspiciousness, paranoia, sundowning, psychosis, or confusion are com-

Table 35-1 Precautions and recommendations for drugs commonly prescribed for elderly patients with dementia

Drugs	Pharmacological changes with age/adverse effects	Precautions and recommendations
Neuroleptics		
Haloperidol	Parkinsonism; sedation; falls; dyskinesia	Use low dose, 0.5-1 mg at bedtime; increase gradually
Thioridazine	Anticholinergic; orthostasis	Use low dose, 10-100 mg
Antidepressants		
Nortriptyline	Mild anticholinergic; sedation; orthostasis	Use low dose, 25-75 mg; check plasma levels
Trazodone	Sedation	Use low dose, 50-150 mg
Miscellaneous		
Lorazepam	Confusion; sedation; disinhibition; ataxia; rebound anxiety if stopped	Use low dose, 0.5-2 mg/day in divided doses; for mild dementia only
Propranolol	Bradycardia; hypotension	Doses 100-500 mg/day
Carbamazepine	Cognitive impairment; ataxia; leukopenia	Doses from 200 mg twice a day
Aspirin	Excessive bleeding; stomach irritation	use enteric coated aspirin, 325 mg/day

mon among patients who have dementia. Maintaining routines, avoiding unfamiliar environments, and correcting sensory impairments may ameliorate the patients' symptoms. If these actions are not successful, low-dose antipsychotics may be useful. Haloperidol and the high-potency phenothiazines have the least sedative and anticholinergic side effects. They may cause parkinsonism, akathisia manifested by increased restlessness and anxiety, and tardive dyskinesia. If parkinsonism or akathisia are excessive, a trial of thioridazine is indicated.

Anxiety usually can be treated by correcting patients' underlying physical problems such as pain, sensory impairment, urinary urgency, or dyspnea. If anxiety is chronic, then a low dose of a short-acting benzodiazepine such as lorazepam is indicated. Propranolol may provide relief of symptoms for some patients.

When aggression or violence occurs, a search for patients' underlying physical ailments should be undertaken. Treatment options include a low dose of an antipsychotic agent, trazodone, propranolol, or carbamazepine.

Insomnia accompanied by agitation is best treated with a sedating antipsychotic or short-acting benzodiazepine and when accompanied with depression is best treated with an antidepressant such as trazodone. Treatments for isolated insomnia include lorazepam, thioridazine, or trazodone.

Wandering is best managed by providing a safe contained environment for the patients. Planned regular exercise may reduce wandering. Hyperoral behavior necessitates removing items that could be ingested by the patients.

REFERENCES

1. Benson DF: Hydrocephalic dementia. In Vinken PJ, Bruyn GW, Klawans HL, eds: *Handbook of clinical neurology*, vol 2, Amsterdam, 1985, Elsevier.
2. Cummings JL, Benson DF: Subcortical dementia: review of an emerging concept, *Arch Neurol* 41:874, 1984.
3. Folstein MF, Folstein SE, McHugh PR: Mini-mental state: a practical method for grading the cognitive state of patients for the clinician, *J Psychiatr Res* 12:189, 1975.
4. Katzman R: Alzheimer's disease, *N Engl J Med* 314:964, 1986.
5. Mahler ME, Cummings JL: Alzheimer disease and the dementia of Parkinson disease: comparative investigations, *Alzheimer Dis Assoc Disord* 4:133, 1990.
6. Martin DC et al: Clinical prediction rules for computed tomographic scanning in senile dementia, *Arch Intern Med* 147:77, 1987.
7. McDonald WM, Krishnan KRR: Pharmacologic management of the symptoms of dementia, *Am Fam Physician* 42:123, 1990.

SUGGESTED READINGS

Cummings JL, Benson DF: *Dementia: a clinical approach*, ed 2, Stoneham, Mass, 1992, Butterworth.
Cummings JL, ed: *Subcortical dementia*, New York, 1990, Oxford University Press.

CHAPTER 36

Common psychiatric disorders

MICHAEL PLOPPER

KEY POINTS

- Depression may be masked by patients' physical symptoms.
- Suicide is common among elderly patients and depressed elderly patients should be questioned regarding suicidal thinking.
- Antidepressants are underused and anxiolytics overused in the treatment of mood disorders among elderly patients.
- History from family or friends should be obtained while physicians evaluate older patients.
- Elderly females with depression and physical illnesses are the most likely patients to be receiving long-term benzodiazepine treatment.
- Psychotropic medications should be discontinued if they are no longer truly necessary.
- Tardive dyskinesia secondary to neuroleptic medications is more common among older patients.

Elderly patients who have psychiatric disorders are commonly encountered in physicians' offices. Their psychiatric symptoms complicate the clinical presentations of medical illnesses and make the treatment process far more difficult. Alternatively, medical illnesses may produce or mimic psychiatric symptoms and true physical illnesses may be misdiagnosed. Careful evaluation of these symptoms and appropriate treatment or referral greatly benefit elderly patients who have medical illnesses, psychiatric symptoms, and social causes or consequences of these symptoms.

MOOD DISORDERS

Clinical relevance

One of the most common symptoms encountered by phy
medical outpatients is alterations in their patients' moods. Up
based elderly persons report depressive symptoms[1], while 4% to 10% o
adults clearly meet defined criteria for depressive disorders. These patients are ov
represented in clinical settings because more depressed elderly patients suffer significant physical illnesses than do their nondepressed counterparts. While overrepre-
sented, this population of depressed elderly patients tends to be undertreated for a
variety of reasons. Lack of recognition of the mood disorder or devaluation of patients'
psychological symptoms contributes to this undertreatment, as does the fact that
elderly depressed patients are less likely than their younger counterparts to seek
treatment for their mood disorders.

The accompanying box summarizes important facts about depression that compel
physicians to evaluate their patients' mood disorders adequately.

Clinical manifestations

The mood disorders consist of *major depression, dysthymic disorder* and *bipolar
disorder.* Somatization is a related disorder that will be addressed as well. The *Diagnostic and Statistical Manual of Mental Disorders*[4] provides specific diagnostic criteria
for these disorders. The following descriptions are consistent with these criteria but
include information that is more specific to elderly persons.

Major depression is the most clinically significant of these disorders and can be
quite disabling; yet, it is the most amenable to treatment by somatic therapies. The

IMPORTANT FACTS ABOUT DEPRESSION
IN OLDER ADULTS

Older persons are far more likely to commit suicide than are younger persons.
Several studies have demonstrated a higher mortality rate over time among depressed
elderly patients or those suffering severe grief responses.
Depressed older adults are less likely to have the emotional or physical capacity to fol-
low through with recommended medical treatment.
Many physical illnesses produce depressive symptoms.
Depression may be masked by patients' physical symptoms.
Depression may worsen the course of physical illness.
Depression leads to loss of physical function and social withdrawal.
Depression is eminently treatable through somatic therapy, psychotherapy, and social
intervention.

st prominent psychological symptom is either a depressed mood or anhedonia, a ss of interest or pleasure in nearly all activities. Elderly patients often do not complain of depression but express their distress through depressive equivalents or physical symptoms that mask the depressed mood. Direct questioning regarding a patient's mood may lead to absolute denial of any emotional discomfort; yet, the patient may complain of abdominal symptoms, back pain, headache, dizziness, or a variety of other physical symptoms that seem inconsistent with demonstrable physical illness. When depressed mood is evident, a diurnal variation may be present such that the patient's mood varies predictably over the course of the day, with mornings usually being the most vulnerable period.

Besides depressed mood or anhedonia, vegetative symptoms of impaired sleep, altered appetite with significant weight change (most often weight loss), and fatigue are evident among patients who have major depression. Psychomotor agitation or retardation, anxiety, poor concentration, feelings of worthlessness, and recurrent thoughts of death or suicide may be present. Psychotic symptoms, particularly delusions with nihilistic content, may be prominent in the patient's thinking.

Major depression may occur as a single episode or may be recurrent. The onset is usually rather acute, developing over a matter of weeks to months, and may last from 6 months to as long as 2 years without treatment. Chronic physical illness predisposes the elderly patient to major depression and is the most significant factor leading to persistence of depressive symptoms.[6]

The elderly patient suffering major depression may have a cognitive disturbance, usually memory impairment, as a prominent symptom. While mild memory problems may accompany normal aging, especially among those elderly persons who are more than 75 years old, depressed older persons may perceive themselves as having significant memory disturbances, which they demonstrate on their cognitive tests. Depression may occur as a concomitant to dementia, including Alzheimer's disease and multiinfarct dementia, at any stage in the course of the dementing illness. The differentiation of *depressive pseudodementia* from depression that is associated with dementia is essential. Otherwise, elderly patients with depression falsely may be presumed to suffer from dementia.

Depression occurring in the context of medical illness provides a troublesome problem for the clinician. A number of medical illnesses produce symptoms similar to the vegetative symptoms of major depression. These and other medical illnesses directly may produce depressed moods through neurochemical pathways. Disorders notably associated with depression include the endocrinopathies, renal disease, coronary artery disease, chronic obstructive pulmonary disease, viral infections, cancer, Parkinson's disease, chronic pain, and stroke. For example, 60% of patients with strokes who were evaluated 6 months after their strokes were found to have depression, with more severe depression following left hemispheric lesions.[6] Medications known to contribute to depressed moods include prednisone, cimetidine, levodopa, the antihypertensives clonidine and propranolol, many of the psychotropic medications, and others.

For elderly patients who seem to be suffering reactive depression and whose symptoms are less severe than those of major depression, the proper diagnosis is *dysthymic disorder, secondary type*. Dysthymic disorder is characterized by a chronically depressed mood that is evident for at least 2 years and may be accompanied by altered sleep and appetite, fatigue, low self-esteem, poor concentration, and hopelessness. These symptoms are of lesser intensity yet greater duration than are those of major depression. In *dysthymic disorder, primary type*, there is no preexisting condition (i.e., physical illness) that seems to be producing the depressive symptoms. Individuals suffering dysthymic disorder, primary type, usually were depressed throughout their lives and responded to any stressor with withdrawal and pessimism. It is to be noted that major depression also may be reactive to an individual's life events. In contrast to dysthymic disorder, major depression tends to be episodic and the patient has periods of normal functioning between episodes.

In *bipolar disorder*, there are manic episodes consisting of euphoric mood, grandiosity, pressured speech, racing thoughts, decreased sleep, and excessive spending or other acts of poor judgment. These episodes are usually interspersed with major depressive episodes. The onset is usually sudden, developing over days or weeks, and often follows a significant stressor. Elderly patients rapidly fatigue during these episodes, and those with significant physical illnesses are at great risk for further morbidity or mortality.

Somatization disorder is evident when elderly patients complain of recurrent and multiple physical symptoms for which there are no apparent physical causes. These patients seek medical attention, often from multiple physicians, over a number of years for their symptoms. The patients tend to be females who have had chronic but fluctuating courses of illness over much of their adult lives. When pain is the predominant symptom and there is an absence of demonstrable physical findings, the condition is referred to as *somatoform pain disorder*. These two disorders are to be distinguished from *hypochondriasis*, a condition in which patients are preoccupied with fears of their having a specific disease or multiple diseases. These are common problems in the health care setting and provide continuing sources of frustration for physicians.

Diagnostic approach

The determination of the presence and severity of a mood disorder is based on focused history taking, rational use of laboratory tests to exclude medical causes, and adequate examination of the patient's mental status.

Most medical causes for a patient's apparent depression can be excluded by a complete physical examination and an inexpensive battery of tests for common medical problems. These include complete blood count (CBC), thyroid function tests, serum electrolytes, standard chemistry panel, urinalysis, electrocardiogram, and chest x-ray. Serum folate and B_{12} levels may be indicated if the CBC is abnormal. A toxicology screening should be performed if a patient is suspected of taking unknown psychotropic medications. There have been great efforts in the past decade to define biological markers for the presence of major depression, with the test for dexamethasone suppression receiving the most attention. Unfortunately these tests have so far proved unreliable for clinical practice.

A complete history must be obtained and, whenever possible, information from family members or other observers should be sought. Important data to be obtained include the patient's history of depressive episodes or other psychiatric disturbances, the family's history of depression and/or substance abuse, and the patient's prior responsiveness to treatment for depression. A recent history of stressors such as family conflict, displacement from home, financial loss, or loss of a loved one may indicate reactive depression. The patient should be questioned about vegetative symptoms and suicidal thinking. If the patient has suicidal thoughts, it is imperative to ask if the patient has thought of plans for suicide. A patient's history of suicide attempts, the family's history of suicide, and statements reflecting the patient's hopelessness are important indicators of increased risk. Elderly persons are far more likely than younger adults to commit suicide, and the suicide rate among the elderly population is increasing markedly. The elderly patient who has suicidal thoughts should be referred for urgent psychiatric consultation and possibly hospitalization. Other indicators for psychiatric referral are listed in Table 36-1.

Further history should include the use or abuse of alcohol and/or prescription medications. Alcohol dependence is strongly associated with depression, and psychotropic medicines, particularly the benzodiazepines, are important contributors to depressed mood.

Table 36-1 Indications for psychiatric consultation

Indication	Reason
Statements of suicide or harm to others	Strong potential for suicide; need for hospitalization
Recent onset of impulsive behavior	May need hospitalization to prevent self-harm or harm to others
Major depression	Need for close monitoring and/or change in medication; may need hospitalization
Persistent paranoia	Resistance to treatment; may need hospitalization
Substance dependence	Withdrawal in hospital; need for recovery program
Persistent anxiety	May become dependent on sedatives
Prolonged grief	High physical and psychiatric morbidity without treatment
Recent onset of cognitive changes	May represent depressive pseudodementia
Onset of anxiety, agitation, psychosis, or depression in dementia patient	Differential diagnosis; range of medications

---

_____ INDICATORS OF DEPRESSIVE PSEUDODEMENTIA _____

Depressive symptoms often predate the onset of cognitive disturbances

Acute onset of symptoms over weeks to months, instead of the more gradual onset of dementia, particularly Alzheimer's disease, or the more sudden onset of delirium

Greater apathy and inattention during testing, although this behavior may be seen among patients with delirium as well

Variable performance in cognitive testing upon patient's reevaluation, although this variation may be seen among patients with delirium as well

Patient's history of depression

Family's history of depression

Patient's responsiveness to a trial of antidepressant medication

---

If the patient's presenting symptoms are cognitive dysfunction and apparent depression, the clinician's task is to differentiate depressive pseudodementia from dementia or delirium. (See also Chapters 34 and 35.) Again, independent history from family or other observers is most helpful. Factors that indicate depressive pseudodementia are shown in the box above.

Often a final determination of whether the patient suffers from depression, early dementia, or delirium is made over time as the patient's complex of symptoms evolves and efforts at treatment are undertaken.

An examination of the patient's mental status should be performed and is described in Chapter 13.

Intervention

The principal modes of interventions for elderly patients who have mood disorders are psychotherapy with the patient and family, pharmacotherapy, and electroconvulsive therapy (ECT).

Elderly patients are good candidates for psychotherapy, even those who are initially reluctant to enter into psychotherapeutic situations. Most psychotherapy with elderly patients is conducted by the physician, in the office. The physician may be the most influential person in the older patient's life, particularly if the patient is isolated. More importantly, the physician may be the only person with whom the patient comes into physical contact. A friendly pat on the back or hug may have great therapeutic impact, even more so than some of the medications that are prescribed.

Pharmacotherapy for elderly patients with mood disorders can provide great relief and help patients to lead productive and worthwhile lives. Antidepressant medications are the cornerstone of effective treatment. However, at the same time, their approach can be a source of morbidity and even mortality among these patients because of potential adverse drug side effects.

INDICATIONS FOR ANTIDEPRESSANT MEDICATIONS
Apparent major depression, particularly if vegetative symptoms are present
Strong suspicion of masked depression is evident, and probable medical causes for the presenting symptoms have been excluded
Apparent depressive pseudodementia, particularly if delirium seems unlikely
Dementia with significant depressive symptoms
Dysthymic disorder, particularly if insomnia is present

Indications or conditions for which a trial of antidepressant medications is justified are listed in the box above. The use of psychotropic medicines by older patients is restricted by age-related pharmacokinetic and pharmacodynamic changes that alter the distribution and metabolism of these drugs. Older patients have decreased lean body mass, increased body fat, reduced total body water, and decreased plasma protein, which all affect the binding and activity of a drug. Many antidepressant medications are primarily lipophilic and distribute into fat tissue, prolonging the half-life of these medications and increasing the risk of toxicity for aging adults. Many antidepressants are protein bound and because older patients have less plasma protein available, more of the drug is available to act freely at receptor sites. Depending on metabolic pathways, hepatic clearance may be reduced, leading to a greater concentration of antidepressants and antipsychotics that is metabolized by the liver. Renal clearance is diminished; therefore, active metabolites of the antidepressant medications are less efficiently excreted and drugs such as lithium, which is primarily eliminated by renal excretion, are present in higher concentrations. (See Chapter 3.) Therefore it is imperative that (1) the doses of antidepressants for elderly patients should be significantly lower than those for younger adults, (2) close monitoring of the patients should be undertaken, and (3) drugs should be discontinued if they no longer truly are needed.

Plasma levels of antidepressant medications appear to be of great value to physicians as they monitor pharmacotherapy for their elderly patients. However, therapeutic levels correlating with clinical responsiveness have been well established only for nortriptyline (Pamelor) and somewhat less so for imipramine (Tofranil) and its active metabolite desipramine (Norpramin). Plasma levels should be obtained when these medications are prescribed and when physicians are concerned about the toxicity of any antidepressant medications. When lithium carbonate is prescribed, serum levels always should be obtained.

The choice of an antidepressant medication for an elderly patient is determined by the patient's complex of symptoms and side effects of the medication, which are correlated with the probable tolerance of the patient for these side effects. Historically, the most commonly used antidepressants have been the tricyclic antidepressants. Amitriptyline (Elavil) has been used with great frequency among older patients;

however, its strong anticholinergic properties and potential to produce orthostatic hypotension limit its usefulness. The anticholinergic effects of dry mouth, constipation, blurred vision, potential urinary retention, and central anticholinergic syndrome are particularly troubling side effects for older persons. Orthostatic hypotension is a great contributor to falls and is more likely to occur in dehydrated patients or those who are taking antihypertensives. Nortriptyline is a useful antidepressant for elderly patients because it is less sedating and has fewer anticholinergic side effects than other antidepressants, and there are established therapeutic plasma levels for this drug. Desipramine is also of value for the same reasons. However, both of these medications still produce troubling side effects, particularly for elderly patients who are prone to side effects for other reasons. Doxepin (Sinequan) is used frequently by aging patients; however, it has strong anticholinergic and sedative properties. Zoloft (Sertraline) is a selective serotonin reuptake inhibitor that causes little sedation or anticholinergic side effects. Recommended doses for preferred antidepressant medications are listed in Table 36-2.

If any one of the following side effects occurs while the patient takes a tricyclic antidepressant, the medicine should be discontinued:

1. Central anticholinergic syndrome, comprising the acute onset of confusion, hallucinations, and agitation
2. Significant orthostatic hypotension
3. Cardiac arrhythmia
4. Urinary retention

Lithium carbonate is most useful in the treatment of bipolar disorder and helps to prevent recurrence of major depression. It can be of benefit in the treatment of a major depressive episode, particularly as a potentiator of tricyclic antidepressants. Its major side effect is lithium toxicity, which occurs among older patients who have far lower serum levels than younger patients. Lithium requires close monitoring of the patients' serum levels. The therapeutic and toxic levels that have been established for clinical use among adults should not be deemed as appropriate guidelines for monitoring elderly patients.

The patient's presenting signs and symptoms, in addition to the profile of the medication's side effects, determine which antidepressant the physician should prescribe for the elderly patient. For the agitated patient, a more sedating agent such as trazodone, amoxapine, or doxepin may be used. If the patient has a significant sleep disturbance, the largest dose of the medication should be taken at bedtime unless the patient has orthostatic hypotension. The patient with psychomotor retardation responds better to nortriptyline, desipramine, fluoxetine, or bupropion. The patient who has psychotic symptoms in association with major depression may respond better to amoxapine or a combination of antidepressant and neuroleptic medications. For the patient with post stroke depression, nortriptyline has shown to be of benefit. If dementia and depression are evident, the less-anticholinergic agents, trazodone, fluoxetine, or bupropion, are preferred. For dysthymic disorder with insomnia, trazodone

Table 36-2 Advantages and precautions for preferred psychotropic medications for elderly patients

Medications	Advantages	Precautions	Doses
Antidepressants			
Bupropion (Wellbutrin)	No sedation; no anticholinergic effects	Can cause seizures if predisposed	75-300 mg
Fluoxetine (Prozac)	No sedation; no anticholinergic effects	May cause anxiety, insomnia, nausea	20-60 mg
Nortriptyline (Pamelor)	Therapeutic plasma levels	Some anticholinergic effects; orthostasis	10-100 mg
Desipramine (Norpramin)	Therapeutic plasma levels	Some anticholinergic effects; orthostasis	10-100 mg
Doxepin (Sinequan)	Sedating; useful at bedtime	Sedating; significant anticholinergic effects	10-150 mg
Trazodone (Desyrel)	Sedating; useful at bedtime	Sedating	50-200 mg
Amoxapine (Asendin)	Sedating; mild antipsychotic effects	Strong anticholinergic effects; potential for orthostasis	25-200 mg
Neuroleptics			
Perphenazine (Trilafon)	Less sedating; less orthostasis	Causes extrapyramidal side effects	2-8 mg
Haloperidol (Haldol)	Less sedating; less orthostasis	Causes extrapyramidal side effects	1-6 mg
Trifluoperazine (Stelazine)	Less sedating; less orthostasis	Causes extrapyramidal side effects	2-8 mg
Thiothixene (Navane)	Less sedating; less orthostasis	Causes extrapyramidal side effects	2-5 mg
Lithium carbonate	Plasma levels to prevent toxicity	Toxicity can occur at lower doses for older rather than younger patients; keep levels less than 1.2 mEq/L	300-1,200 mg
Anxiolytics			
Alprazolam (Xanax)	Short half-life	Causes dependence, sedation, ataxia	0.25-1.5 mg
Lorazepam (Ativan)	Short half-life	Causes dependence, sedation, ataxia	0.5-2 mg
Buspirone (BuSpar)	No addiction potential; no sedation	May cause dizziness; nausea	10-60 mg

at bedtime has shown to be of benefit.

With all of the antidepressants, a major cause of failed treatment is premature discontinuation of the medications. Unless the patient is troubled by side effects, the medication should not be stopped until at least a 4-week trial at adequate doses has been completed. If the patient has not responded to the medication by that point, an antidepressant of another class is warranted.

ECT is indicated for patients with major depression who do not respond to adequate trials of antidepressants or are at great risk without immediate treatment. ECT remains the most effective treatment for patients with severe major depression.[7] Often, patients who have major depression that is associated with psychotic features require ECT. ECT generally is a safe and effective treatment with relatively low morbidity. Transient confusional states or memory disturbances frequently occur after ECT; however, these side effects are of insufficient significance to forgo treatment of seriously ill patients.

ANXIETY DISORDERS

Clinical relevance

Anxiety as a symptom is frequently seen by all physicians in outpatient practice. In fact 44% of elderly patients manifesting anxiety disorder are treated by primary care physicians.[8] Twenty-two percent of elderly men and 17% of elderly women in the community report anxiety symptoms.[5] The prevalence of phobic disorders decreases only slightly in late life (occurs in more than 10% of community-based elderly persons). While generalized anxiety disorder in late life has not been well studied, clinical experience indicates that this disorder is common in late life as well. Anxiety in late life is associated with significant comorbidity, as well as medical and psychiatric disorders. Multiple medical disorders include anxiety as a part of the patient's complex of symptoms, either through direct autonomic arousal as a pathophysiological component of the disorder or through a fear response to the symptoms that the patient experiences. The persistence of anxiety carries great import for the course of medical illnesses (e.g., anxiety-associated labile hypertension and its ultimate vascular consequences).

Older adults encounter myriad anxiety-provoking life experiences at a time when their mastery and control of self and environment may be diminished. *State anxiety*, associated with one's transitory anxiety responses to stressors, appears to increase in late life, while *trait anxiety*, associated with one's predisposition to anxiety as a function of a personality disorder, remains relatively constant throughout life. Contributing to this increase in state anxiety are multiple losses and changes that, although experienced by people when they were younger, carry greater ramifications for loss of function and independence now that those people are older. The stressors most often perceived as anxiety-provoking in late life are threats to physical health.[5]

Clinical manifestations

Anxiety includes physical and psychological symptoms, which, like the mood disorders, can present a difficult diagnostic challenge to the clinician. The physical symptoms represent either autonomic arousal or somatic manifestations of anxiety. The autonomic symptoms may consist of palpitations, tachycardia, sweating, rapid shallow breathing, restlessness, tremulousness, or insomnia. The somatic manifestations tend to cluster around specific organ systems. The anxious elderly patient may complain of symptoms that are specific to the gastrointestinal tract such as nausea, abdominal discomfort, diarrhea, or a "lump in the throat." Another patient may be more focused on possible neurological symptoms such as light-headedness, dizziness, faintness, tingling sensations, numbness, and so forth. Any of the organ systems can be foci of discomfort for the elderly patient, and of course the patient may complain of symptoms pertaining to more than one system. But most often these anxiety symptoms are specific to one system.

The psychological symptoms vary and may relate to anxiety, such as a sense of fear and vigilance or feeling "on edge," or an exaggerated startle response. Other symptoms are more vague and easily misdiagnosed such as a feeling of unreality, distractability and poor concentration, or inability to sit still.

The anxiety disorders seen most often in late life are *phobic disorder* and *generalized anxiety disorder*. *Obsessive compulsive disorder* persists into late life but is less pertinent to the office-based physician and will not be discussed here. *Panic disorder* per se is not seen frequently in late life; yet, its associated symptom of agoraphobia frequently is seen. The interpretation of this symptom is mitigated because older persons have more bona fide reasons to be fearful of situations outside their homes or where help may be unavailable.

Phobic disorder is the fear of exposure to specific stimuli or situations that are seen as harmful or embarrassing. As distinguished from younger patients, older adults with phobic disorder include people who have become isolated and shut in as a result of physical problems, estrangement from family and friends, or other social factors. These people gradually develop a fear of social interaction, and simply forays outside their homes such as visits to their doctors' offices provoke great anxiety.

Generalized anxiety disorder is characterized by excessive worry or anxiety about life's circumstances and is associated with autonomic arousal and psychomotor tension. Elderly patients with this disorder are chronically anxious and bothered by anxiety symptoms more often than they are not bothered by these symptoms. There is a high comorbidity with physical illnesses for these patients, and it is often difficult to differentiate somatic manifestations of anxiety from their symptoms of physical illnesses. These are the patients who become frequent users or abusers of benzodiazepines.

Diagnostic approach

Because there is a strong association between physical illness and anxiety among elderly persons, the major focus of differential diagnosis is the exclusion of specific medical causes for the anxiety symptoms. Several medications can produce anxiety. Theophylline, amantadine, bromocriptine, metoclopramine (Reglan), methylphenidate (Ritalin), and anticholinergics are among the medications that produce anxiety. The patient's use of caffeine and alcohol should be explored. Minor withdrawal states from alcohol and/or sedatives frequently occur in the intermittent abuser of these drugs. Akathisia, a common extrapyramidal side effect of the neuroleptic medications, includes intense restlessness or the inability to sit still, and is frequently misinterpreted as anxiety. This misinterpretation often leads to an increase in the offending medication.

Illnesses that cause hypoxia may produce anxiety. Thyroid disorders frequently are associated with anxiety. Hypoglycemia rarely causes anxiety but is often cited as the problem for patients who have vague psychiatric complaints. Mild delirium from any cause may include anxiety-like symptoms. Mitral valve prolapse is strongly associated with intense anxiety symptoms.

Anxiety is a prominent presenting symptom of many psychiatric disorders. These psychiatric disorders include the mood disorders, dementia, psychotic states, and substance dependence, among others. Usually with an adequate history and examination of the patient's mental status, a physician differentiates these disorders from a primary anxiety state. Elderly patients with somatization disorder may complain of nervousness but tend not to have the autonomic arousal that is seen in primarily anxious patients with somatic manifestations of anxiety.

Intervention

The treatment of the anxiety disorders often produces greater morbidity than the disorders themselves. The benzodiazepines are the most frequently prescribed medications for anxiety, and the most likely patients to receive long-term benzodiazepine treatment are elderly females who have physical illnesses and depressive symptoms.[2] The benzodiazepines are associated with physical dependence, sedation, respiratory depression, memory disturbance, and ataxia. Older persons are particularly at risk when these complications occur; therefore, like the antidepressant medications, doses for older patients should be far lower than those for younger patients. The benzodiazepines with long half-lives such as diazepam (Valium) and chlordiazepoxide (Librium) undergo multistep hepatic biotransformations that produce active metabolites. Because of elderly patients' reduced hepatic metabolic capacities, the elimination half-lives of these drugs may be two or three times longer for elderly patients. For this reason, the benzodiazepines with shorter half-lives such as alprazolam (Xanax) or lorazepam (Activan) are preferred. Recommended doses are listed in Table 36-2.

Benzodiazepines should be prescribed on an as needed, *not continuous*, basis and for a *limited period* of time. Elderly patients should be educated about the drug's potential for producing dependence and should be cautioned not to drink alcohol while taking benzodiazepines. If it is determined that the patients may require long-term treatment, an antidepressant such as trazodone or desipramine in relatively low divided doses may produce adequate anxiolytic action. Meprobamate, once a popularly prescribed sedative, is strongly associated with dependence and should no longer be prescribed.

Buspirone (BuSpar) is a newer anxiolytic, chemically unrelated to the benzodiazepines. It does not produce physical dependence or sedation. This drug's onset of action is gradual, requiring 2 to 4 weeks before the patient responds. The half-life of buspirone is short, and the drug should be given three times a day. Its principal side effects are dizziness or light-headedness and sometimes nausea, which occurs early in the treatment. However, these side effects are usually not significant enough to discontinue the medication.

Most elderly patients who are anxious respond best to a combination of time-limited psychotherapy, anxiolytic medication, and any intervention that provides greater mastery and control over their physical or environmental stressors. Greater involvement in treatment considerations, educational approaches to specific physical illnesses, advice regarding exercise and diet, social services' assistance, physical and occupational therapies, and promotion of leisure activities are examples of interventions that significantly help patients to relieve anxiety.

THE PSYCHOTIC DISORDERS

Clinical relevance

Symptoms of psychosis, particularly paranoid delusions, occur with moderate frequency among the geriatric population. Surveys indicate that approximately 4% of community-based elderly persons suffer delusional symptoms.[3] Of those elderly patients who have symptoms of delusional thinking and do not suffer from dementia, most are women who have significant hearing loss. Clearly, perceptual disturbance that is due to significant deafness contributes to the onset of paranoid thinking. The majority of these patients were not schizophrenic when they were younger. The florid symptoms of schizophrenia may give way to social withdrawal and emotional detachment in late life. *Schizophrenia* is a heterogenous disorder with different pathways and outcomes, which are influenced by many factors, and is quite distinct from late-onset *paranoid disorder*. About one half of community-based elderly persons with delusional thinking have cognitive disturbances, and the other one half, about 2% of the elderly population, have functional psychoses.

Clinical manifestations

Paranoid disorder consists of the onset of delusions that are usually persecutory in nature. The elderly patients feel spied upon, followed, and harassed, often by individuals whom they know or with whom they have come into contact. They may believe that they are being poisoned or physically manipulated by sophisticated machinery such as lasers or electronic devices. These patients often believe that they have been watched or violated in a sexual manner. Sometimes hallucinatory experiences accompany the delusional thinking. Generally these people are of good intellect and function reasonably well, other than in their social contacts. They often resent that family or friends do not understand or are unsympathetic to their suffering. The course usually waxes and wanes. When paranoid disorder is severe, there is ongoing vigilance, impaired sleep, and inadequate food intake, especially if food is deemed to be poisoned. These patients often have had good premorbid functioning in work or outside interests; however, the patients frequently are described by their families as having been emotionally cold or overbearing in adult life.

Other disorders may have psychotic features as well. Major depression may be associated with delusions but rarely hallucinations. Often these delusions are nihilistic or involve a great sense of guilt or having done wrong. Elderly patients with bipolar disorder can have delusions, often with grandiose content. In dementia, particularly early on, there may be persecutory delusions. Later in the course of dementia, psychotic symptoms may change rapidly and become memory disturbances or misinterpretations of environmental stimuli. In delirium, disturbances of patients' visual or tactile perceptions may be prominent.

Diagnostic approach

The proper diagnosis of the elderly patient who has psychotic symptoms usually can be made with an adequate history (including that from outside sources), mental status examination, and laboratory tests when delirium is suspected. Patients with paranoid disorder may seem quite lucid until questions about their delusions arise. Even then the patients may be reluctant to discuss their beliefs because they may be deemed crazy. Often a family member or friend can elaborate on the patient's preoccupation with delusions. The aging schizophrenic has a history of psychiatric hospitalizations or serious social dysfunction during adult life. The elderly patient with major depression and psychotic features has a history of severe mood disturbances and these symptoms preceded the onset of delusions.

If the patient is suspected to have delirium, a toxicology screening and routine battery of tests will exclude many causes of delirium. (See Chapter 34.) The central anticholinergic syndrome, secondary to antidepressants and/or neuroleptics, is a common cause for delirium among elderly patients who have hallucinations, agitation, and confusion.

Intervention

The pharmacotherapeutic approach to psychotic disorders rests primarily with the neuroleptic medications. Patients with paranoid disorder respond well to neuroleptics and experience at least a significant attenuation of their symptoms, if they can be convinced to take the medications. Psychotic symptoms that are associated with mood disorders and delirium respond to the neuroleptics, if the symptoms are not due to central anticholinergic syndrome. The preferred medications for elderly patients are the high-potency neuroleptics such as perphenazine (Trilafon), haloperidol (Haldol), trifluoperazine (Stelazine), and thiothixene (Navane). These neuroleptics are safer overall because they have fewer anticholinergic effects and are less likely than the lower-potency neuroleptics such as thioridazine (Mellaril) and chlorpromazine (Thorazine) to cause orthostatic hypotension or sedation. However, the high-potency neuroleptics are more strongly associated with extrapyramidal side effects such as akathisia and dystonia. Tardive dyskinesia, a condition marked by involuntary repetitive mouth movements, is a permanent neurological consequence of neuroleptic medication and is more common among elderly persons, particularly elderly women. This condition is associated with increased doses of the medication and duration of treatment. The best preventive technique for this condition is the "drug holiday," a lengthy period of time (at least weeks) when the patient completely stops taking the medication. The patient's continued use of neuroleptics, like all psychotropic medications, frequently should be reevaluated. Recommended doses are listed in Table 36-2.

SUBSTANCE ABUSE

Clinical relevance

Patients' dependencies on alcohol and prescription drugs are common problems facing the office-based physician. Many alcoholics die by late life; however, others begin heavy drinking only in late life. Those who are alcoholics early in life are socially isolated by late life and estranged from family and friends. Those who are alcoholics late in life are widowed, depressed, and suffering from physical illnesses. Older alcoholics are less likely than younger alcoholics to suffer occupational or legal consequences because of their drinking behavior, and therefore their drinking is more often hidden. Most alcoholism becomes apparent when the elderly patients are treated for physical illnesses.

Elderly patients who are dependent on prescription drugs have developed their problems by undergoing treatment from well-meaning physicians. The most commonly abused drugs are the sedative hypnotics and the less abused are the narcotic analgesics. When initially treated, these patients tend to be anxious, depressed, and suffer sleep disturbances. Many suffer true mood disorders and are not given trials of antidepressant medications. A number of factors contribute to the patient's development of a drug dependency, including passivity when the patient relates to the physician, inadequate understanding by the patient about the potential for a drug addiction, multiple physicians who prescribe different drugs for the patient, and noncompliance with the physicians' recommendations.

Clinical manifestations

The patient's obvious signs of intoxication, hepatic and hematological changes, and clinical signs that are determined by the physical examination all indicate a patient's alcohol dependency. Elderly patients who are dependent on sedatives may be less conspicuous. In the office, they may be calm, alert, and responsive, yet tolerant of and dependent on benzodiazepines. When the medications are not available, they become anxious, irritable, sleepless, and may suffer frank withdrawal syndromes. Other patients demonstrate lethargy, depression, and confusion secondary to benzodiazepine dependence. The withdrawal syndromes associated with alcohol and the sedative hypnotics are similar in many ways and both can result in seizures. The withdrawal syndrome of elderly patients who depend on both alcohol and sedative hypnotics can be quite dangerous and difficult to manage.

Diagnostic approach

Efforts to diagnose patients who are dependent on both alcohol and prescription drugs are usually hampered by patients' denials of their problems. A patient's history as it relates to number of drinks per day, binging versus regular abuse, and types of medication and frequency of use should be obtained if possible. Memory disturbance secondary to alcohol or benzodiazepines, in addition to a patient's denial, may interfere with an accurate history. A complete physical examination and routine laboratory tests reveal much about the seriousness and consequences of alcoholism for the elderly patient. Because alcoholism and drug dependencies coexist with other psychiatric disorders in many elderly patients, examination of the patients' mental statuses, with attention toward other psychiatric symptoms, is essential.

Intervention

Withdrawal of alcohol or sedative hypnotics, especially from patients who are highly dependent on these substances, may be extremely difficult and may cause serious medical complications. Therefore withdrawal therapy should be undertaken in a hospital setting. Once withdrawal has been accomplished by the patient, efforts toward continuing recovery and abstinence must begin. For the elderly patient with another psychiatric disorder, adequate treatment of that disorder should commence immediately. The alcoholic patient, without memory disturbance and with motivation and reliability, may benefit from disulfiram (Antabuse) early in recovery as an adjunctive measure to ensure sobriety. When possible, the family should be involved in treatment planning and educated about the patient's problem. Alcoholics Anonymous and Pills Anonymous provide essential support, education, and social interaction for people to share their experiences. Many elderly persons resist these groups and require great encouragement to participate. If they refuse, the likelihood of ongoing sobriety diminishes. However, if these patients become reinvolved with their families and sober friends and have stimulating social environments, recovery can be achieved.

REFERENCES

1. Blazer D, Hughes D, George L: The epidemiology of depression in an elderly community population, *Gerontologist* 27:281, 1987.
2. Catalan J et al: General practice patients on long-term psychotropic drugs: a controlled investigation, *Br J Psychiatry* 152:399, 1988.
3. Christenson R, Blazer D: Epidemiology of persecutory ideation in an elderly population in the community, *Am J Psychiatry* 141:1088, 1984.
4. *Diagnostic and statistical manual of mental disorders*, ed 3, Washington, DC, 1987, American Psychiatric Association.
5. Himmelfarb SW, Murrell S: The prevalance and correlates of anxiety symptoms in older adults, *J Psychol* 116:159, 1984.
6. Robinson R, Starr C, Price T: A two-year longitudinal study of mood disorder following strokes: prevalence and duration at six months follow-up, *Br J Psychiatry* 144:256, 1984.
7. Scovern A, Kilmann, P: Status of electroconvulsive therapy: review of the outcome literature, *Psychol Bull* 87:260, 1980.
8. Yates W: The National Institute of Mental Health Epidemiologic Study: implications for family practice, *J Fam Pract* 22:251, 1986.

SUGGESTED READINGS

Busse EW, Blazer DG, eds: *Geriatric psychiatry*, Washington, DC, 1987, American Psychiatric Press.
Diagnostic and Statistical Manual of Mental Disorders, ed 3, Washington, DC, 1987, American Psychiatric Association.

CHAPTER 37

Movement disorders

MICHAEL E. MAHLER

KEY POINTS

- Parkinson's disease is characterized by resting tremor, rigidity, bradykinesia, and gait disturbance.
- Although not curable, Parkinson's disease is treatable. Dopaminergic therapy with Sinemet or direct dopamine agonists is the mainstay of symptomatic treatment; selegiline appears to protect patients against the disease's progression.
- Causes of tremor in older persons include parkinsonism and exaggerated physiological, essential, and cerebellar tremors; nonparkinsonian tremors tend to be action tremors.
- Hyperkinetic movement disorders of dyskinesia and dystonia in elderly persons are primarily due to drugs and structural brain lesions.

PARKINSON'S DISEASE AND PARKINSONISM

Parkinsonism refers to a clinical syndrome that comprises tremor at rest, rigidity, bradykinesia, and gait disturbance. When this syndrome results from a specific degenerative disorder, it is called *Parkinson's disease (PD);* when it is caused by other definable diseases, it is called *secondary* or *symptomatic parkinsonism.*

Clinical relevance

PD is important to clinicians who care for older patients for two reasons. First, it is a common cause of morbidity in elderly persons. Second, PD may be complicated by dementia or depression; the association between the movement disorder and the behavioral syndrome must be understood for correct diagnosis and treatment.

Epidemiology. The age-adjusted annual incidence of PD is approximately 20/100,000 population, with a prevalence between 100 and 170/100,000.[10] The age-specific incidence peaks at 120/100,000 population around age 70 years old and then declines, while the age-specific prevalence increases almost exponentially beyond age

65 years old. Thus, PD most often strikes the "young old" but is most prevalent among the "old old", affecting 1% to 2% of the population who are more than 80 years old. Men and women are equally likely to develop PD.

Incidence and prevalence rates for *secondary* parkinsonism vary widely, depending on patients' underlying disorders. Drug-induced parkinsonism is quite common, as is that due to cerebrovascular disease. Many of the neurodegenerative diseases associated with parkinsonism are quite rare.

Pathology and pathogenesis. There are many theories on the cause of PD, including genetics and toxins such as methylphenyltetrahydropyridine (MPTP).[3,6,11] A detailed discussion is beyond the scope of this chapter. The pathology of PD involves the loss of pigmented neurons and the presence of Lewy bodies in the substantia nigra and ventral tegmental area (VTA). This causes denervation of the nigrostriatal and VTA-mesocortical dopaminergic pathways. Dopamine deficiency in the striatum is the major factor in the pathogenesis of both PD and secondary parkinsonism. Clinical symptoms occur when there is approximately 80% depletion of the striatal dopamine.

Clinical manifestations

Physical features. Although more than one half of all PD patients have tremors, other features of the disease are usually present at the time of diagnosis. PD is often mildly asymmetrical at first, but eventually it affects both sides of the body relatively equally. The tremor is typically between 4 and 7 Hz (hertz) and consists of coarse, alternating agonist-antagonist muscle movements. The tremor is present when the patient is at rest and alert but not moving volitionally. With purposeful movements, the tremor decreases. Some PD patients have an additional high-frequency-low-amplitude action tremor.

The rigidity of PD consists of an increase in resistance of the muscles to passive stretching throughout the range of motion. The superimposed tremor, especially in the arms, gives rise to the cogwheel phenomenon. Rigidity is also evident in the stooped posture of PD patients, with flexion of their necks, trunks, hips, and knees. Despite the rigidity, there is no loss of muscle strength.

Bradykinesia is probably the most disabling feature of PD. The slowness of movement affects almost all voluntary and many involuntary actions. PD patients also have difficulties in initiating their movements. The bradykinesia and paucity of movements cause the masklike expressionless face (emotional grimace and decreased eye blinks), drooling (decreased swallowing), hypophonia (soft speech), and micrographia (small, illegible handwriting).

Abnormal gait and postural instability occur frequently enough to warrant separate consideration. The PD patient walks with a forward stooped posture, shortened shuffling steps *(marche à petit pas)*, decreased arm swings, and tendency to propel forward with increasing speed (festination). When turning, the patient does not pivot but takes several small steps and turns *en bloc*. The balance is unsteady, especially when the patient turns. This imbalance can be severe enough to impair standing and even unsupported sitting. Falls are frequent and often bring the patient to medical attention.

PD patients often experience symptoms of autonomic dysfunction, including hyperhidrosis, orthostatic hypotension, impotence, constipation, and incontinence. Many PD patients also complain of insomnia, and many have subjective sensory complaints such as burning pain or tingling in the extremities.

Neurobehavioral features. Although James Parkinson wrote that the senses and intellect of PD patients are uninjured, most contemporary investigations demonstrate cognitive decline. More than 40% of these patients have an obvious dementia syndrome, while more than 90% have subtle but measurable neuropsychological deficits.[1] The cognitive impairment is characterized by poor memory with retrieval deficits, slowing of information processing, and difficulty with executive tasks of the frontal lobe, but impairment spares the language function. The dementia syndrome of PD is heterogeneous, and some PD patients probably have coincidental Alzheimer's disease.[7] However, the pathology of PD by itself is sufficient to cause intellectual and motor system abnormalities.

Depression affects 40% to 60% of PD patients and is not directly related to severity of or disability from the disease. The depression in PD is indistinguishable from primary affective disorders, and treatment with antidepressants may be necessary.

Diagnostic approach

Differential diagnosis. The key to the diagnosis of parkinsonism is recognition of the cardinal features of resting tremor, rigidity, bradykinesia, and gait disturbance.

Mild PD must be distinguished from the effects of normal aging on locomotion. With normal aging, the gait becomes more hesitant and there is a forward-stooped posture, decreased stride, and diminished arm swings. Also, many elderly individuals exhibit a degree of psychomotor slowing. Although qualitatively similar to some of the symptoms of parkinsonism, these normal changes of aging generally do not cause functional disability, and rigidity and tremor are not present in normal elderly persons.

It may be difficult to differentiate PD and secondary parkinsonism. The box on p. 366 lists some of the causes of secondary parkinsonism. The resting tremor is less prominent in arteriosclerotic and drug-induced parkinsonism. Marked asymmetry of symptoms, limb weaknesses, and abnormal reflexes are likely to be present in arteriosclerotic parkinsonism. The patient's history of exposure to drugs or toxins that are capable of producing the syndrome is necessary to establish those causes; however, it is not possible to be certain about a diagnosis of PD within 6 months of the patient's exposure to an offending medication. Progressive supranuclear palsy (PSP) closely mimics PD, but in the former there is the characteristic and defining supranuclear ophthalmoplegia, pseudobulbar palsy, and axial rigidity. PSP patients also usually have few tremors. The other degenerative conditions are multisystem disorders that display combinations of extrapyramidal, corticospinal, and spinocerebellar signs.

SECONDARY PARKINSONISM

Postencephalitis	Hydrocephalus
Arteriosclerosis	Basal ganglia tumor
Drug induced	Basal ganglia arteriovenous malformation
• Neuroleptics	Basal ganglia calcification
• Lithium	Progressive supranuclear palsy
• Metoclopramide	Striatonigral degeneration
• Reserpine	Olivopontocerebellar atrophy
• Methyldopa	Parkinson-dementia complex (of Guam)
Intoxications	Cortical Lewy body disease
• Carbon monoxide	Wilson's disease
• Manganese	Alzheimer's disease
• Methylphenyltetrahydropyridine	Jakob-Creutzfeldt disease
Hypoparathyroidism	Shy-Drager syndrome
Hypothyroidism	Acquired immunodeficiency syndrome
Post-head trauma	

Other tremor syndromes of elderly patients should not be mistaken for parkinsonism. In all other tremor syndromes, including essential tremor, the tremors are more prominent when the patients are active rather than at rest, and the frequency of the tremors is usually faster.

Laboratory evaluation. Laboratory testing of patients with newly discovered parkinsonism helps physicians to distinguish those cases resulting from metabolic abnormalities or structural lesions of the basal ganglia. (See the box above.) Serum chemistries and screenings for metals are indicated, as are thyroid function tests. Brain imaging also is indicated, except when there is a clear history of drug-induced parkinsonism. Magnetic resonance imaging (MRI) is more sensitive than computed tomography (CT) for the detection of cerebral ischemic lesions that are associated with parkinsonism. Imaging also detects calcifications and structural lesions of the basal ganglia. Selective atrophy of the midbrain may be noted for patients with PSP and selective atrophy of the cerebellum and brain stem may be noted for those with olivopontocerebellar atrophy. Despite the utility of laboratory evaluations, PD is primarily a clinical diagnosis.

Intervention

Pharmacotherapy. Symptomatic pharmacological treatment is necessary when tremor and bradykinesia begin to interfere with the patient's occupational and social

Table 37-1 Recommendations for pharmacotherapy of elderly patients with Parkinson's disease

Drugs	Pharmacological changes with age/adverse effects	Precautions and recommendations
Sinemet (Carbidopa/levodopa)	Nausea; dizziness; confusion; psychosis; dyskinesia when high doses used long term; tachyphylaxis with chronic use (possible receptor changes)	Initial symptomatic relief ½ tablet (25 mg carbidopa, 100 mg levodopa) daily to start; increase gradually to total 800-1000 mg levodopa/day
Dopamine agonists	Same as Sinemet	Adjunct to levodopa; bromocriptine 2.5 mg or pergolide 0.05 mg; start 1 tablet/day and increase gradually
Selegiline (Eldepryl)	Insomnia; confusion	Protective therapy to start with diagnosis; 5 mg twice daily

functioning, independence, and self-care activities. Table 37-1 provides recommendations for drug therapy of PD in elderly patients.

For young patients with mild symptoms, anticholinergic medications provide partial relief. Anticholinergics are more effective for the tremor of PD than for rigidity or bradykinesia. However, because of the increased prevalence of serious side effects from these agents (urinary retention, delirium, blurred vision), anticholinergics should be used with caution, if at all, by elderly patients.

Similarly, amantadine (100 mg twice or thrice daily) is useful for mild symptoms or as an adjunct to levodopa; however, the efficacy appears short lived and elderly patients frequently experience ankle edema and, more seriously, confusion.

Since the late 1960s, dopamine replacement has been the mainstay of treatment. The combination of levodopa and carbidopa in Sinemet is the most efficient way to get dopamine into the brain. Dopamine does not cross the blood-brain barrier but levodopa does, and it is converted to dopamine through decarboxylation. The carbidopa inhibits only the peripheral decarboxylation of levodopa; this reduces the peripheral side effects and enhances the central action of dopamine. Several strengths of Sinemet are available, so doses can be accommodated to individual needs. Levodopa is dramatically effective; bradykinesia and rigidity improve markedly, and tremors respond well but variably.

The initial dose of Sinemet for elderly patients should be lower than the three-times-a-day dose of the 25/100 (25 mg carbidopa, 100 mg levodopa) tablet, which is recommended for younger adults. Elderly patients may start with only ½ tablet twice a day, since they almost always can tolerate that dose. The dose should be increased every *week* by daily increments of ½ to 1 tablet. The serum half-life of levodopa is 3 hours, so a four-times-a-day or more frequent schedule is necessary as the daily dose increases. Most patients experience satisfactory initial improvement with a total daily dose of levodopa between 300 and 600 mg. The 10/100 or 25/250 Sinemet tablets should be substituted when the dose is more than six tablets a day of the 25/100 tablets, since 75 to 100 mg/day of carbidopa maximally inhibits peripheral decarboxylase.

The short-term side effects of levodopa are nausea, dizziness, confusion, and psychosis; these problems are limited by careful titration of the dose. After several years of therapy and because of progression of the illness, altered pharmacokinetics or receptor changes, the response to levodopa decreases and new problems emerge. These complications include dose-related dyskinesias (chorea, dystonia, myoclonus), end-of-dose or wearing-off effects, and unpredictable motor fluctuations (the on-off phenomenon). The use of the lowest dose that controls symptoms early in the disease may forestall the development of these disabling and difficult-to-manage fluctuations of response. The controlled release preparation, Sinemet-CR 50/200, may reduce the wearing-off phenomenon.

When symptoms are unresponsive at a level of 800 to 1000 mg/day of levodopa, dopamine agonists are added to the regimen.[9] Bromocriptine, pergolide, and other dopamine agonists act directly on the presynaptic and postsynaptic dopamine receptors. These agents are not as effective as levodopa when used alone: however, when these agents are used in conjunction with levodopa, they may improve efficacy and smooth out the motor fluctuations. The dopamine agonists have the same side effects as levodopa. The initial dose of bromocriptine should be 1.25 mg twice a day, and increases in the dose should be made every *week*, or longer, in 1.25 to 2.5 mg/day increments. Some patients may require doses of 20 to 30 mg/day, but few can tolerate this level.

The discovery that MPTP is toxic only after oxidation to the free radical, MPP+, led to a new use for an old drug. Deprenyl, now called selegiline, selectively inhibits monoamine oxidase-B and protects pretreated animals from developing parkinsonism after their exposure to MPTP. A large, multicenter study recently concluded that selegiline delays the progression of PD symptoms and postpones the time when symptomatic therapy becomes necessary.[8] It is not clear yet whether this benefit continues throughout the course of the illness. The effective dose of selegiline is 5 mg twice a day, with the second dose being taken by patients in the early afternoon to avoid insomnia. Some patients become confused when they take selegiline; one half of the dose may be tolerated. No dietary restrictions are necessary. All newly diagnosed PD patients should begin taking selegiline for its neuroprotective effect; levodopa should be added later if symptoms worsen. In advanced cases of PD, selegiline may not be of benefit.

The management of secondary parkinsonism depends upon the precise cause in each case. In arteriosclerotic parkinsonism and many of the degenerative disorders, treatment is symptomatic as it is in PD. However, the patients who have these other conditions respond less to therapy than those patients who have PD.

While appropriate therapy may provide symptomatic relief to patients for many years, the underlying pathology of PD progresses. At a certain point, medications prove ineffective against the advancing illness and all the manifestations of PD worsen inexorably. This pessimistic scenario may prove incorrect if the neuroprotective effect of selegiline persists long term.

The progressive immobility of PD patients makes them susceptible to infection, inanition, and death. Untreated PD advances to death within 8 to 10 years, but treatment has improved the survival of patients with PD to a life expectancy of about 15 years following diagnosis.

TREMORS

Clinical relevance

The incidence of essential tremor is more than double that of PD, with estimates ranging from 380 to 5500/100,000 in various populations.[10] Furthermore, many drugs and systemic disorders cause tremors. Not all who shake have parkinsonism, and other causes of tremor are often misidentified and mistreated as PD.

Clinical manifestations

A tremor is an involuntary, rhythmic, oscillatory movement. Careful observation of the frequency, amplitude, distribution, and action characteristics of the tremor leads to accurate classification of a tremor.[4] Table 37-2 describes the features for the four major types of tremors.

Table 37-2   Clinical classification of tremors

Feature	Parkinsonian	Exaggerated physiological	Essential	Cerebellar
Frequency (Hz)	4-7	6-12	6-12	3-5
Amplitude	Coarse	Fine	Variable	Variable
Tremor at rest	+ + + +*	+	+	+
Tremor with action				
Postural	+ +	+ + + +	+ + +	+ + +
Contraction	+	+ +	+ + + +	+ +
Intention	+ +	+ +	+ +	+ +
Distribution	Limbs, jaw, tongue	Limbs	Hands, head, voice	Limbs, head

*Range of prominence or severity; +, least; + + + +, most.

Exaggerated physiological tremor. An *exaggerated physiological tremor* occurs when a toxin or metabolic disturbance magnifies the minute tremor that is normally present in all people. In older individuals, the frequency of this tremor is lower and overlaps with the slower parkinsonian tremor. Anxiety, fatigue, and caffeine also cause this type of tremor. Hypoglycemia, thyrotoxicosis, and pheochromocytoma are pathological causes of a physiological tremor. The tremors caused by lithium, tricyclic antidepressants, amphetamines and other stimulants, bronchodilators, and alcohol withdrawal are also of this type. Catecholamine excess may be a common pathophysiological mechanism in these conditions. Usually, treatment is directed at the underlying cause, but if a medication such as lithium cannot be stopped, a beta blocker may ameliorate the tremor.

Essential tremor. The term *essential tremor* is sometimes used synonymously with *action tremor*, but essential tremor is only one of several entities with action-induced tremors. (See Table 37-2.) Essential tremor may be hereditary or sporadic, with onset at any age. The incidence of essential tremor rises with age and since it is not fatal, the prevalence also rises with age. Although a similar tremor occasionally may be seen with degenerative neuropathology, it is called *essential* because the condition is usually not associated with other symptoms or pathology. The dominant frequency of the tremor diminishes with age. Because the tremor particularly affects voluntary movements, it interferes with one's writing and eating, as well as performing in a highly skilled occupation. The tremor can be heard during speech. Small amounts of alcohol may suppress essential tremor, but this is not usually effective therapy.

Cerebellar tremor. Cerebellar tremors are not so common among elderly persons because the usual causes (multiple sclerosis, spinocerebellar degenerations, etc.) occur infrequently in the geriatric population. However, tumors or strokes affecting the cerebellum and its connections may cause this infrequent tremor. Associated symptoms such as ataxia, nystagmus, and dysmetria also indicate the cerebellum's involvement.

Diagnostic approach

The most important initial approach to the differential diagnosis of a tremor is to classify it as either parkinsonian, exaggerated physiological, essential, or cerebellar because the spectrum of disorders varies according to tremor type. A careful evaluation of a patient's medications is important since so many drugs are responsible for tremors. Serum chemistries and metabolic studies, particularly thyroid function tests, are necessary in the evaluation. Masked hyperthyroidism in elderly patients can be difficult to diagnose because the patients may appear to have PD along with psychomotor slowing and tremors. Brain imaging is indicated when the tremor is cerebellar or when it is associated with other neurological signs or symptoms.

Intervention

The centrally active beta blockers such as propranolol and nadolol lead to significant improvement in more than one half of the cases of essential tremor. The necessary dose of propranolol is 40 to 320 mg/day, but few older persons can tolerate the higher doses without mental dullness, severe bradycardia, or hypotension. Primidone in doses from 50 to 750 mg/day (average 125 to 250 mg/day) is also effective. The side effects of drowsiness, dizziness, and nausea limit tolerance, but they may be prevented by careful titration of the dose.[5] Clonazepam or another benzodiazepine is a third-choice drug for essential tremor. Appropriate caution should be exercised when physicians prescribe benzodiazepines for older patients.

DYSKINESIA AND DYSTONIA

A *dyskinesia* is a relatively rapid involuntary movement and a *dystonia* is one with a more sustained posture; both are forms of hyperkinetic movement disorders. The two occur together, in varying proportions, in a variety of disorders. (See the box below.) When multiple involuntary movements affect the trunk and proximal muscles it is called *chorea; athetosis* affects the distal extremities. Some older adults, especially edentulous ones, have involuntary, chewing, jaw movements sometimes called *senile chorea*.

Drug-related dyskinesias are common in elderly persons. Some medications, including levodopa, bromocriptine, tricyclic antidepressants, isoniazid, phenytoin, and stimulants can cause acute choreiform movements that disappear when the drug is stopped. *Tardive dyskinesia (TD)* is a persistent dyskinesia or dystonia of the face,

---

HYPERKINETIC MOVEMENT DISORDERS

Chorea

Tardive dyskinesia
Drug induced
Posthemiplegic
Postanoxic
Hypoparathyroidism
Wilson's disease
Huntington's disease
Acquired immunodeficiency syndrome

Ballismus

Dystonia

- Meige's syndrome
- Torticollis
- Tardive dystonia
- Hypocalcemia

Myoclonus

- Dementias
- Encephalopathies

Tic disorders

mouth, and hands (other parts of the body also may be affected) following patients' more prolonged exposures to neuroleptics and related drugs such as metoclopramide. Older adults and those with brain disorders are more susceptible to the development of TD. Once it begins, TD may be irreversible. Treatments for TD are partially effective at best, but perhaps one half of all cases improve gradually if the offending agent is discontinued.

Other dyskinesias result from structural lesions within the basal ganglia. Strokes or tumors may cause posthemiplegic chorea in the distribution of the affected limb. When the movement is a large-amplitude movement of one arm (e.g., a throwing motion) it is termed *hemiballismus*. This usually results from a lesion of the subthalamic nucleus.

Meige's syndrome is a regional dystonia with onset in the middle to late years. It is characterized by contractions of the face, jaw, and neck muscles; blepharospasm is prominent. No specific pathology is associated with Meige's syndrome. In torticollis, the dystonia affects the neck only. Oral anticholinergic medications may be partially effective, when they are tolerated. More recently, botulinum toxin injections into the affected muscles have become the treatment of choice for many cases of blepharospasm and torticollis.[2]

REFERENCES

1. Cummings JL: Intellectual impairment in Parkinson's disease: clinical, pathologic and biochemical correlates, *J Geriatr Psychiatry Neurol* 1:24, 1988.
2. Hall WH: Clinical use of botulinum toxin: NIH consensus development conference statement (11/12/90), *Arch Neurol* 48:1294, 1991.
3. Golbe LI: The genetics of Parkinson's disease: a reconsideration, *Neurology* 40 (suppl 3):7, 1990.
4. Jankovic J, Fahn S: Physiologic and pathologic tremors: diagnosis, mechanism, and management, *Ann Intern Med* 93:460, 1980.
5. Koller WC: Essential tremor. In Johnson RT, ed: *Current therapy in neurologic disease-3*, Philadelphia, 1990, BC Decker.
6. Langston JW, Ballard P, Tetrud JW: Chronic parkinsonism in humans due to a product of meperidine-analog synthesis, *Science* 219:979, 1983.
7. Mahler ME, Cummings JL: Alzheimer disease and the dementia of Parkinson disease: comparative investigations, *Alzheimer Dis Assoc Disord* 4:133, 1990.
8. Parkinson Study Group: Effect of deprenyl of the progression of disability in early Parkinson's disease, *N Engl J Med* 321:1364, 1989.
9. Rinne UK: Combined bromocriptine-levodopa therapy early in Parkinson's disease, *Neurology* 35:1196, 1985.
10. Schoenberg BS: Epidemiology of movement disorders. In Marsden CD, Fahn S, eds: *Movement disorders 2*, London, 1987, Butterworth.
11. Tanner CM, Langston JW: Do environmental toxins cause Parkinson's disease?, *Neurology* 40 (suppl 3):17, 1990.

SUGGESTED READINGS

Klawans HL: Emerging strategies in parkinson's disease *Neurology* 40 (suppl 3):1, 1990.
Koller WC: *Handbook of parkinson's disease*, New York, 1987, Marcel Dekker.

CHAPTER 38

Headache

PATRICIA LANOIE BLANCHETTE

<u>**KEY POINTS**</u>

- Headache is a common problem among elderly persons and the coexistence of several causes for headache is to be expected.
- Headache that is of acute onset and rapidly progressive should be treated as a medical emergency. Common causes are accelerated or malignant hypertension and subarachnoid hemorrhage.
- While primary brain tumors are not common in elderly persons, patients frequently fear that occult tumors are the cause of their headaches.
- A collateral history, daily diary, and an examination of mental status are important to the evaluation of headache in elderly persons.
- A number of medications may cause headache as a side effect for elderly patients.

CLINICAL RELEVANCE

Acute, recurrent, and chronic headaches are among the most frequent complaints in primary care medicine. Although there is a reported decline in the prevalence of headache from early adulthood to advanced old age, headache remains one of the most frequently experienced health problems of older people. Estimates for the incidence of headache among outpatients aged 65 years or older is about 8%, with 13.9% of headaches affecting women and 6.5% affecting men.[3,6] Epidemiologically, headaches are strongly associated with patients' joint pain, depression, bereavement, wakefulness during the night, use of eyeglasses, symptoms of temporomandibular dysfunction, and poor self-assessment of health.[2]

373

CLASSIFICATION OF HEADACHE BY ACUITY OF ONSET IN ELDERLY PATIENTS

Acute/subacute

Accelerated hypertension
Giant cell arteritis
Ischemic/thrombotic stroke
Subarachnoid hemorrhage
Intracranial tumors
Intracranial infection
Herpes zoster

Recurrent

Trigeminal neuralgia
Cluster headache
Hypnic headache syndrome

Chronic

Migraine
Muscle contraction headache
Cervical radiculopathy
Temporomandibular joint syndrome
Chronic open-angle glaucoma
Medication-related headache
Parkinson's disease
Thyroid disorders
Chronic sinus headache
Headache associated with psychiatric
  conditions (e.g., conversion cephalgia,
  depression, hypochondriasis)

CLINICAL MANIFESTATIONS

Since headache is a symptom, it may be classified in several different ways[1] such as primary or secondary type or by acuity of onset. (See the box above.) In the primary type, head pain is the principal manifestation. Examples include migraine, muscle contraction headache, and trigeminal neuralgia. In the secondary type, headache is a consequence of systemic conditions, including hypertension, cervical arthritis, or those related to medications. When the diagnosis is not known, it is useful to classify the headache by acuity of onset and associated symptoms. It is also helpful to distinguish the patient who ages and has a long history of recurrent or chronic headaches from the patient who has an acute onset.

Table 38-1 provides a concise summary of clinical features of some of the more important types and causes of headaches in older persons.

DIAGNOSTIC APPROACH

The best approaches to the accurate diagnosis and management of headaches for elderly persons are meticulous histories and physical examinations, along with carefully selected laboratory and imaging studies.

History

For older people, the key to diagnosis is frequently in the histories that are obtained both from the patients and family members who have observed the episodes of headaches. The clinician must inquire about type of onset, location, quality of pain, duration, frequency, precipitating, aggravating, or ameliorating factors, and associ-

Table 38-1 Clinical features of various types and causes of headaches in older persons

Type/cause of headache	Characteristics of headache	Other features
Acute/subacute		
Accelerated hypertension	Generalized; throbbing	Rapid rise in blood pressure; chronic type is occipital headache
Giant cell arteritis	Variable location; variable quality	Tenderness over arteries; jaw pain with chewing; systemic symptoms may be present; more common in women
Ischemic/thrombotic stroke	Variable quality	More common if there is history of headache; neurological deficits
Subarachnoid hemorrhage	Sudden onset; moderate to severe intensity	Associated with hypertension, trauma, aneurysm; high mortality; meningeal irritation; blood in cerebrospinal fluid; necessitates neuroimaging scan (CT, MRI)
Intracranial tumors	Recent onset; increasing frequency and intensity; present when patient awakens; worse with head movement	Headache often absent with primary or metastatic brain tumors
Intracranial infection	Variable quality; variable location	Other signs more important: fever, meningeal signs, confusion, etc.
Herpes zoster	Cranial nerve involvement; unilateral	Dysesthesia along cranial nerve distribution; vesicular lesions; malaise; low-grade fever
Recurrent		
Trigeminal neuralgia (tic douloureux)	Unilateral; lightning-like stabbing along trigeminal nerve distribution; during waking hours	May see motor or sensory changes in face due to brain stem or gasserian ganglion lesion; also may be idiopathic
Cluster	Episodic; unilateral; excruciating; around the eye	80% are men; severity may make patient consider suicide; patient should avoid alcohol and smoking
Chronic		
Migraine	Unilateral; pulsating; moderate to severe; lasts hours to days	Nausea, photophobia, intolerance to noise; aura or prodrome; family history in 50-70%; more common in women
Muscle contraction (tension)	Begins in muscle units of head or neck and spreads over entire head; trigger point or tenderness over muscle involved	Caused by physical and psychological stress that makes muscle units contract

Continued.

Table 38-1 Clinical features of various types and causes of headaches in older persons—cont'd

Type/cause of headache	Characteristics of headache	Other features
Cervical radiculopathy	Begins as cervical spine pain; spreads to occipital area and becomes generalized; worse with neck movement	Caused by osteoarthritis; neck radiographs show characteristic changes
Medication related	Generalized; variable intensity and quality, depending on medication	Establish temporal relationship when patient takes medication; any medication may be a potential cause
Chronic sinus	Begins early in day; improves during day with sinus drainage; pressurelike or aching may be over sinus areas or generalized	History of chronic sinusitis; possible allergies must be excluded; may have tenderness over sinus area

ated symptoms. A history of similar episodes may be particularly helpful. Family histories are not often contributory to the diagnosis for elderly persons but may be helpful regarding vascular events or clues about the patients' fears. Social histories are important, especially concerning patients' financial losses or bereavement. Inquiry about the patients' personality traits, daily habits, and routines also may give the physician some insight into patients' problems.

Diary

Patients may be unable to relate from memory the elements of their histories that are critical to accurate diagnosis. For patients who have chronic headaches, keeping a daily diary may be quite helpful both for diagnosis and as a guide to effective treatment. In addition to symptoms, the patients or their family members should be asked to record medications, meals, and sleep-wake times. If migraine is suspected, food and beverages ingested by the patients should be recorded in an attempt to find triggers. Severity of the pain should be recorded on a Likert-type scale (e.g., from 0 to 10) to help assess progress of the patients.

Physical/neurological examination

A meticulous physical and neurological examination is necessary, with particular attention directed toward the following: orthostatic blood pressure and pulse; scalp or facial tenderness; eye examination, including visual acuity; oral cavity, especially ill-fitting dentures and occult abscess; temporomandibular joint; cervical range of motion; wasting of upper extremity muscles; cranial nerves; and sensorimotor examination.

Mental status examination

A particularly helpful part of the examination of older patients is a screening test for their mental statuses. Several short well-validated tests are available, which can be administered in 10 to 15 minutes.[3] (See Chapter 13.) In the evaluation of headache, it is particularly helpful to examine older patients for abnormalities of attention, which may suggest systemic illness or depression; memory, which may suggest unreliable history; or language skills, which may indicate the possibility of past stroke. The test for mental status is probably most useful for longitudinal assessment of patients, as a screening for decline in their cognitive function, or as a measure of their improvement as a result of treatment.

Laboratory tests

Because of the possibility of systemic illness and the likelihood of contributing comorbid conditions, certain routine laboratory tests are indicated in the evaluation of a patient with headaches. These tests include complete blood count, chemistry profile, urinalysis, erythrocyte sedimentation rate (ESR), and thyroid function. Analysis of cerebrospinal fluid is required in cases of suspected infection or subarachnoid hemorrhage.

Carefully selected imaging studies may be particularly helpful, even lifesaving, in the diagnosis of headache. Depending on the patient's presenting symptoms, tests may include computed tomography (CT), magnetic resonance imaging (MRI), and cerebral angiography. CT is particularly useful for patients with acute conditions, especially when the physician suspects intracranial or subarachnoid hemorrhage. The sensitivity of CT is superior to that of MRI for hyperacute hemorrhage. CT is usually readily available in large hospitals, and patients who are ill enough to require monitoring equipment can be accommodated. The continued availability of CT is important for older people because they are more likely to be affected by the contraindications to MRI for patients who have embedded metallic objects (i.e., cardiac pacemakers, surgical ferromagnetic clips, ocular metallic foreign bodies, and cochlear implants). Alternatively, MRI is particularly useful in cases of chronic headache for the identification and localization of structural lesions below the resolution of the CT scanner. There is better visualization of deep structures and the posterior fossa. Cerebral angiography is the best mechanism for identifying abnormalities of the vasculature such as aneurysms, vascular tumors, occlusive strokes, and vascular malformations. Because of the risks associated with intravascular injections of radiopaque dyes, including stroke, this test has been reserved for patients for whom there is a strong likelihood of surgically correctable lesions. Noninvasive angiography using MRI technology is of special interest for older patients who, being at greater risks for complications, are the most likely to benefit from noninvasive studies.

INTERVENTION

Communication with the patient

In the management of all patients, especially those with chronic headaches, it is important to communicate to patients that they have been heard. It is also important to elicit any fears or beliefs that they may have about their headaches and to allay those fears once a proper evaluation has been conducted. When treatment is undertaken, it is important to help patients understand the goal of various therapies, including basic anatomical, physiological, and psychological factors.

Physical treatments

Given the potential problems with comorbidity, side effects from drugs, and polypharmacy among older people, adjunctive physical measures to treat their headaches should be attempted for appropriate conditions. Some examples of these adjunctive measures include moist heat treatments and massage for muscle contraction headaches; brief periods of wearing a cervical collar and intermittent traction for cervical radiculopathy; localization and interruption of physical trigger points with local anesthetics; capsaicin cream; acupuncture; or transcutaneous electrical nerve stimulation (TENS) unit.

Biofeedback and self-regulatory treatment

For tension, mixed, and migraine headaches, various combinations of relaxation, measures for cognitively coping with stress, and biofeedback may offer excellent relief for selected patients.[4]

Drug therapy

Minor analgesics. The management of many forms of headaches among elderly patients is greatly facilitated with the use of minor analgesics such as acetaminophen or aspirin. Pain is better managed with standing doses of medication that are administered at fixed intervals rather than an intermittent as-needed basis. (See Chapter 39.) It is surprising how many patients complain of headaches and have not taken minor analgesics to help control them. The appropriate use of these drugs should be encouraged. The long-term daily use of acetaminophen should be avoided by patients because it has been associated with transient elevations of hepatic transaminases. However, for short-term treatment of pain acetaminophen is safe, effective, and usually the best choice for elderly patients.

Management of chronic headache pain. One of the most troubling problems in primary care practice is the management of patients with chronic headaches who have become addicted to narcotic analgesics. Narcotic analgesics are contraindicated for patients other than those who are terminally ill and in chronic pain, since these drugs lose their effectiveness relatively soon and do nothing to treat the underlying pathology. Older patients are particularly prone to prescription drug abuse because they may receive care from several physicians. These patients do not arouse suspicion because they do not fit the image of the typical drug-addicted individual. If addiction is present, it is important to establish one provider who manages the addiction and is the sole source of prescriptions for narcotic analgesics as they are withdrawn. (See Chapter 36).

Antidepressants. Antidepressants should be used for headaches that are related to depression. A detailed description about appropriately prescribing antidepressants for older patients appears in Chapter 36.

Lithium. Available in oral form as lithium carbonate, lithium is an element best known for its use as an antimanic agent in bipolar manic-depressive disorder. It also has been used in the treatment or prophylaxis of refractory cluster headache and migraine. Because it is a particularly difficult drug for elderly patients to use, caution must be exercised by the physician who prescribes lithium. (See Chapter 36).

Beta blockers. Beta blockers are used commonly for cluster and migraine prophylaxis. Beta blockers are usually categorized according to their relative lipid or water solubility and cardioselectivity. The drug most thoroughly tested and most commonly used for prophylaxis is propranolol, a noncardioselective beta blocker. Older people may be at greater risk for the mentally depressive and bronchospastic adverse reactions to propranolol. It is likely that newer, water-soluble, cardioselective beta blockers in low doses may be equally effective for headache and better tolerated by elderly patients. (See Chapters 52 and 53).

Methysergide. Methysergide also has been used in migraine prophylaxis and is used in difficult cases of cluster headaches. However, patients must be monitored closely for retroperitoneal and cardiopulmonary fibrosis, and methysergide is contraindicated for patients with coronary artery disease. Newer treatments for both cluster headache and migraine are likely to result in rare use of methysergide for refractory cases.

Management of certain headache pain syndromes

Mixed headache syndrome. It is not unusual for headache to have more than one cause in the same patient. It is important for both the patient and physician to understand this fact so that a proper interpretation of response to treatment may be obtained. The initial approach should be to identify and treat the dominant component first, which usually is muscle contraction headache in most patients.[5]

Acute and chronic anxiety disorders. Headache may occur as a result of acute or chronic anxiety. Chronic anxiety disorder usually is managed with appropriate psychotherapy buspirone, or benzodiazepines. Chapter 36 discusses management of anxiety disorders.

Migraine headache. Treatments for migraine headache include prevention and pain medications, sedatives, and antiemetics to ameliorate the discomfort. To *prevent* migraine headache, it may be possible to identify and deter certain triggers such as oversleeping, caffeine, alcohol, bright light, foods high in tyramine (chocolate, nuts, aged cheeses), citrus fruits, onions, legumes (navy and lima beans), nitrites (prepared or smoked meats), monosodium glutamate, eggs, yogurt, fried foods, and foods that are identified by individualized food-challenge testing. Medications used for *prophylaxis* of attacks include beta blockers, calcium channel blockers, monoamine oxidase (MAO) inhibitors, nonsteroidal antiinflammatory drugs (NSAIDs), and methysergide. The standard for *abortive treatment* of acute attacks is ergotamine, which is available in many forms, including inhalants, oral tablets, suppositories, sublingual capsules, and injectable preparations. Ergotamine commonly causes or increases nausea, so the patient may need an antiemetic. The absorption of oral ergotamine is facilitated by caffeine, and many believe that the two drugs are synergistic. For elderly patients, the vasoconstrictive properties and the effects of overdosage of ergotamine are particularly dangerous. Ergotamine is contraindicated for patients with peripheral vascular disease, coronary artery disease, hypertension, impaired renal or hepatic function, and sepsis. It is not recommended for patients who have had recent serious infections. These contraindications exclude many older people. One alternative drug is Midrin, a combination drug including isometheptene mucate, dichloralphenazone, and acetaminophen. NSAIDs also have been used effectively. Future therapies are expected to include serotonin agonists and antagonists. For older patients, treatment with analgesics beyond the abortive phase is similar to that for younger adults but includes lower doses of medication and particular caution regarding oversedation, constipation, fecal impaction, and accidental overdosage from repeated self-administration.

Cluster headache. Drugs commonly used for migraine prophylaxis such as beta blockers may be helpful for cluster headache. Prophylaxis should be initiated when cluster attack occurs. The drug can be discontinued when there have been no headaches for 3 to 6 months. Aerosolized ergotamine at the first sign of headache may be helpful. Oxygen inhalation (6 to 8 L of 100% oxygen) for 5 to 15 minutes has been reported to be helpful early in an attack. Newer treatments such as intranasal lidocaine or capsaicin cream 0.025% (Zostrix, formerly Axsain) applied to the nostril that is on the same side of the head as the headache have proven to be useful. Ergotamine tartrate (Cafergot) 1 mg 3 times/day or 2 mg at bedtime is commonly used. Other potential treatments include prednisone in tapering doses over 3 weeks, starting with 40 to 60 mg/day; indomethacin, 50 to 100 mg in divided doses; and cyproheptadine (Periactin) 4 to 20 mg/day. Methysergide 4 to 12 mg/day also has been used in difficult cases, but patients must be monitored closely for adverse effects. Methysergide is contraindicated for patients with coronary artery disease. Lithium carbonate may be effective, but toxicity and adverse effects limit its usefulness for the treatment of elderly patients. Another treatment of potential benefit in recalcitrant cases is pressurized oxygen in special hyperbaric compression chambers. These chambers are costly and are not widely available, but they may be found in military facilities, medical schools, research institutes, or wherever treatment for deep diving injuries is available.

Trigeminal neuralgia. For trigeminal neuralgia, carbamazepine (Tegretol) in low doses may be helpful, but sometimes high therapeutic serum levels are required to realize an effect. Because of the rare phenomenon of aplastic anemia that occurs with the use of carbamazepine, complete blood counts should be obtained for the patients before and after onset of treatment and periodically thereafter. Topical capsaicin cream 0.025% applied 3 or 4 times daily also may be helpful. Phenytoin (Dilantin) may be helpful. Other possible treatments include combined carbamazepine and phenytoin, chlorphenesin (Maolate), or baclofen (Lioresal). Neurosurgical sectioning of the nerve root proximal to the ganglion may be required in refractory cases.

Postherpetic neuralgia. As with other dermatomes, persistent head or facial pain may remain following an occurrence of herpes zoster. Postherpetic neuralgia is particularly difficult to treat effectively. Analgesics, antidepressants, and a TENS unit may offer some relief. Anesthetic nerve blocks may be very effective but inconsistently so. Newer treatments for postherpetic neuralgia that also may be effective include capsaicin cream 0.025% applied topically 3 or 4 times daily. Care should be taken by patients not to get the cream into their eyes or onto broken skin. Carbamazepine (Tegretol) may provide excellent relief for some patients. Doses of carbamazepine that are required for treatment may vary. The hematological adverse effects of carbamazepine were discussed previously, and the dosage should be carefully monitored.

REFERENCES

1. Ad Hoc Committee on the classification of headache, *JAMA* 179(9):717, 1962.
2. Cook NR et al: Correlates of headache in a population-based cohort of elderly, *Arch Neurol* 46(12):1338, 1989.
3. Hale WE et al: Symptom prevalence in the elderly: An evaluation of age, sex, disease, and medication use, *J Am Geriatr Soc* 34(5):333, 1986.
4. Kabela E et al: Self-regulatory treatment of headache in the elderly, *Biofeedback Self Regul* 14(3):219, 1989.
5. Sims TJ: Headaches in women: management strategies, *The Female Patient* 16(5):25, 1991.
6. Solomon GD et al: Demographics of headache in elderly patients, *Headache* 30(5):273, 1990.

SUGGESTED READINGS

Baumel B, Eisner LS: Diagnosis and treatment of headache in the elderly, *Med Clin North Am* 75(3):661, 1991.
Black P: Brain tumors. I., *N Engl J Med* 324(21):1471, 1991.
Black P: Brain tumors. II., *N Engl J Med* 324(22):1555, 1991.

CHAPTER 39

Pain

BRUCE A. FERRELL

KEY POINTS
- Pain is not normal as patients age.
- Always ask patients about pain. Many elderly patients do not like to complain, even though pain may affect their functional status, mood, and quality of life.
- As analgesics, nonsteroidal antiinflammatory drugs (including acetaminophen) are limited by a ceiling effect. Serious complications, including gastric bleeding and renal insufficiency, are more common among elderly patients.
- Elderly people (especially those who have not been recently exposed to opiate drugs) are more sensitive to analgesic effects and the side effects of opiate drugs.
- Fears of tolerance, addiction, and other side effects do not justify withholding narcotics and prolonging needless suffering.
- Family and informal caregivers' support is extremely important in the overall management of chronic pain.

CLINICAL RELEVANCE

Pain is the most common symptom of disease and the most common complaint in physicians' offices. Population-based studies have estimated that 25% to 50% of community-dwelling elderly people suffer important pain problems. In a survey by Crook, Rideout, and Browne[2] of 500 randomly selected households in Burlington, Ontario, 16% of the total population aged 18 to 105 years old reported a "significant" painful problem in the preceding 2 weeks. In this study, the age-associated morbidity for pain was twofold greater (250/1000 versus 125/1000) among those over the age of 60 years old compared with younger subjects.

It has been recognized that a number of painful diseases are more common among elderly patients. Arthritis may affect 60% of people aged 65 years and older, and most suffer significant pain. Among cancer patients, one third of patients with active disease and two thirds with advanced disease have significant pain. Other specific pain syndromes that are known to affect the geriatric population disproportionately include herpes zoster, temporal arteritis, polymyalgia rheumatica, and atherosclerotic peripheral vascular disease.

Possible outcomes of pain are widespread among the elderly population. Depression, decreased socialization, sleep disturbance, impaired ambulation, and increased health care utilization and costs each have been associated with the presence of pain among older adults. Though less thoroughly explored, deconditioning, gait disturbances, falls, slow rehabilitation, polypharmacy, cognitive dysfunction, and malnutrition are among the many geriatric conditions that are potentially worsened by the presence of pain. Finally, pain and its management have major implications for quality of life and quality of care, especially for frail elderly persons and those with terminal illnesses. Although comfort and control of chronic disease symptoms are salient goals in geriatric care, it is ironic that little research has focused on pain in elderly persons.

CLINICAL MANIFESTATIONS

Pain is a complex experience derived from sensory stimuli but modified by individual memory, expectations, emotions, and behavior. Neuroanatomical and neurochemical findings now indicate an overwhelmingly complex central nervous system for nociception and psychological responses to painful stimuli. Although elderly persons often may have presenting symptoms that are altered, including painless myocardial infarctions and painless intraabdominal catastrophes, whether these clinical observations represent distinct age-related changes in pain perception remains controversial. Using a variety of methods to stimulate pain in "normal" volunteers, studies have resulted in mixed conclusions. In the final analysis, age-related changes in pain sensitivity and tolerance remain difficult to document and are of questionable validity since induced pain may not be analogous to clinically experienced pain.[5]

DIAGNOSTIC APPROACH

With no biological markers, pain can be a perplexing problem for physicians to assess. Because pain is such an individual experience, physical, functional, and psychological evaluations are often necessary to ensure accurate assessment. Ultimately, pain assessment should be viewed from the patient's perspective. In fact, clinicians can rely simply on the patient's report for accurate pain assessment in the majority of cases.

Assessment of any complaint of pain should begin with a thorough history and physical examination. Special attention should be directed toward the musculoskeletal and nervous systems. For frail elderly patients, any history of trauma should be thoroughly evaluated. Older patients may present special problems for physicians who must obtain accurate histories of pain. Depression, failures in memory, and sensory impairments may hinder history taking. More importantly, underreporting of symptoms may result because patients often expect pain to be associated with aging. In addition, they may not report pain because they fear the meaning of pain or they think that pain cannot be relieved. Many elderly patients do not want to complain about pain, despite their having severe pain that affects their mood and functional status.

Many elderly patients suffer concurrent diseases; however, physicians must avoid attributing new pain to patients' preexisting chronic illnesses. Furthermore, chronic pain is usually not constant. Both the characteristics and intensity of chronic pain may fluctuate with time. Injuries that are due to trauma or acute disease such as gout are easily overlooked in some situations. Only astute questioning and comprehensive evaluation can prevent these pitfalls.

As part of the physical examination it is important to palpate for trigger points and inflammation. Trigger points may result from tendonitis, muscle strain, or nerve irritation. Specific maneuvers that reproduce the pain such as straight leg raising and joint motion may be useful for diagnosis and functional assessment. A thorough neurological examination should be focused on signs of autonomic, sensory, and motor deficits that are suggestive of neuropathic conditions and nerve injuries.

Evaluation of function is important as an outcome measure for pain management so that mobility and independence are maximized for elderly patients in pain. Functional assessment may include information from the history and physical examination and several scales that are available for functional assessment or measurement. (See Chapter 13.) For patients in the ambulatory setting, instrumental activities of daily living and "elective" activities such as ambulation, psychosocial function, and quality of life may correlate clinically with the presence and severity of pain.

Psychological evaluation should be conducted because psychological problems are often associated with chronic pain. Most patients with chronic pain have significant depressive symptoms or anxiety at some time and may benefit dramatically from psychological or psychiatric intervention. Cognitive impairment also may be exacerbated by pain and its treatment. Psychological assessment therefore should include at least a thorough mental status examination. Formal psychological tests, which have been validated for use among older populations, may help physicians to identify patients who might benefit from specific psychological or psychiatric therapy.

Both qualitative and quantitative pain scales (e.g., the McGill pain questionnaire) have been developed to help clinicians and researchers more accurately measure, document, and communicate patients' pain experiences.[1] For ambulatory elderly patients, a pain diary may be particularly helpful. Recent work has attempted to validate behavioral responses to pain, including body language and agitation, as valuable indicators of pain. This is an important area for further study because cognitively impaired patients may be unable to verbally communicate their pain.

INTERVENTION

Despite that pain management may entail special risks for elderly patients, there have been few pain management strategies designed specifically for older people. For the most part, principles of pain management have been extrapolated from younger populations and those with pain because of cancer.

The control of most acute and postoperative pain relies initially on treatment of the underlying condition and short-term administration of analgesic drugs. Chronic pain, however, often may require a combination of nonpharmacological interventions, as well as analgesic and adjuvant drug therapies. Patients with cancer pain usually respond well to constant administration of opiate analgesics. However, long-term use of narcotic analgesics for chronic pain that is not due to cancer remains more controversial. Neuropathic pains such as herpes zoster and poststroke thalamic pain may not respond to traditional analgesic drugs but may respond to adjuvant drugs such as tricyclic antidepressants or anticonvulsants. Multiple trials with various combinations of pharmacological and nonpharmacological strategies may be required for optimum pain relief.

Prescribing analgesic drugs for older patients

The most common treatment for pain is oral analgesic medications. A review of individual drugs is beyond the scope of this chapter, but several good articles by other authors already exist.[7,8] However, several important principles should be considered when physicians prescribe analgesic drugs for their elderly patients.

Nonsteroidal antiinflammatory drugs (NSAIDs) act peripherally in the nervous system, affecting pain receptors, nerve conduction, and inflammatory conditions that may stimulate pain. Table 39-1 lists recommendations and precautions for prescribing NSAIDs for older patients. Individual drugs in this class vary widely in their analgesic properties, metabolism, excretion, and profiles of side effects. The analgesic activity of these drugs is limited by a low ceiling effect. A ceiling effect is a level at which increasing the dose results in no further increase in analgesia. These drugs often work well when given alone or in combination with narcotic analgesics for metastatic bone pain and inflammatory conditions. More importantly, NSAIDs have no habit-forming properties of their own. However, the NSAIDs have been associated with a variety of adverse effects among the older patients, including peptic ulcer disease, renal insufficiency, and bleeding diathesis. Among frail elderly persons, constipation, cognitive impairment, and headaches have been associated with NSAIDs. Although

Table 39-1 Precautions and recommendations for prescribing nonsteroidal antiinflammatory drugs for elderly patients

Drugs	Pharmacologic changes with age/ adverse effects	Precautions and recommendations
Acetaminophen	Hepatotoxic at high dose	Keep dose to less than 4 g/24 hr
Aspirin	Gastric bleeding; abnormal platelet function	Avoid high dose for prolonged periods of time★
Diflunisal (Dolobid)	Weak antiinflammatory activity; side effect profile similar to other NSAIDs	Usually requires a loading dose followed by continuous dosing for maximum effectiveness
Ibuprofen (Motrin, etc.)	Gastric, renal, and platelet abnormalities may be dose and time dependent; constipation, confusion, and headaches may be more common in elderly patients	Avoid high dose for prolonged periods of time★
Naproxen (Naprosyn)	Similar toxicity to ibuprofen	Avoid high dose for prolonged periods of time★; may require a loading dose
Sulindac (Clinoril)	Similar toxicity to ibuprofen	Avoid high dose for prolonged periods of time★
Salsalate (Disalcid)	Prolonged half-life of 8-12 hr; similar toxicity to ibuprofen; classic salicylate toxicity may develop at high dose	Salicylate levels may be occasionally necessary to avoid toxicity★
Trisalicylate (Trilisate)	Prolonged half-life of 12-24 hr; may have less gastric, renal, and platelet abnormalities; also may have less analgesic and antiinflammatory activity	Avoid drug accumulation with every 24-hr dose
Indomethacin (Indocin)	Highest prevalence of gastric and other toxicities	Avoid entirely for elderly patients or keep to minimum doses for very short periods of time★

★Gastric toxicity partially may be prevented by the concomitant use of misoprostol (Cytotec).

NSAIDs have been considered the safest form of analgesia for mild to moderate pain, recent studies question their overall safety when used by frail elderly patients.[8]

When administered systemically, opiate analgesic medications act on the central nervous system (brain and spinal cord) to decrease the perception of pain. Some of these drugs (including morphine) also may act as local anesthetics and are used in widespread epidural administration. Opiate drugs have no ceiling to their effects and relieve all types of pain. Short-term studies have shown that elderly patients are more sensitive to the pain-relieving properties of these drugs than are younger patients. This is true for postoperative and chronic cancer pain. Advanced age is associated with a prolonged half-life and altered pharmacokinetics for opiate drugs. Thus, elderly patients may achieve pain relief from smaller doses of opiate drugs when compared with younger patients.

It is well known that opiate drugs have the potential to cause cognitive disturbances, respiratory depression, constipation, and habituation among older persons. Clinical experience suggests that opiate drugs (as with most psychoactive drugs) occasionally may produce paradoxical excitement and agitation. Morphine remains the standard by which all other analgesic drugs are compared. Morphine's effects remain the best understood and most predictable. Thus, morphine may be the leading opiate of choice for severe pain. Physicians' reluctance to prescribe opiate drugs probably has been overly influenced by recent political and social pressures against illicit drug use. In fact, among patients taking morphine (for both malignant and nonmalignant diseases), recent studies have observed that (1) drug tolerance is usually related to worsening disease; (2) drug addiction is exceedingly rare; and (3) when drug dependency does occur, it is surprisingly easy to manage.[6] This does not imply that morphine and other opiates can be used indiscriminately, but dependency and other side effects do not justify the failure to treat pain in elderly patients.

Tolerance also occurs to some side effects of opiate drugs. This tolerance may have a beneficial effect on patients by reducing their risks for respiratory depression and drowsiness. Analgesic drugs should be administered on a continuous basis (as opposed to prn or as needed) whenever possible. It is now recognized that continuous administration results in reduced overall drug consumption, continuous analgesia, and tolerance to drowsiness and respiratory depression. However, some side effects of opiates such as constipation and perhaps nausea do not diminish with time. These side effects make overall pain management more difficult. It is therefore important that patients begin bowel regimens early, when opiates are first started. Increased fluids, bulk agents, lubricating agents, and bowel stimulants may be required while opiates are administered. Nausea results from direct stimulation of a chemoreceptor trigger zone in the brain. Although antiemetic drugs (e.g., antihistamines and phenothiazines) have been the mainstay for preventing nausea in younger patients, it is important to remember that elderly patients are especially sensitive to anticholinergic side effects from these drugs, including bowel or bladder dysfunctions, delirium, and movement disorders.

A variety of opiate drugs are available, and they differ widely in their analgesic potencies and side effects among the elderly. Table 39-2 lists precautions and recommendations for prescribing opiate drugs for elderly patients.

Adjuvant analgesic drugs are medications without inherent analgesic properties themselves, but they are helpful in treating certain types of chronic pain. These drugs include antidepressants, anticonvulsants, and some sedatives. Tricyclic antidepressants and anticonvulsants are sometimes helpful in controlling neuropathic pain. Tic douloureux, herpes zoster, diabetic neuropathies, and thalamic (poststroke) pain syndromes sometimes respond uniquely to these drugs. Finally, mild sedatives or tranquilizers are also sometimes helpful in reducing anxiety, stress, and tension, as well as allowing the patient to sleep well. Chronic pain is an exhausting experience, and patients often cope better with adequate sleep.

Table 39-2 Precautions and recommendations for prescribing opiate analgesic drugs for elderly patients

Drugs	Pharmacologic changes with age/adverse effects	Precautions and recommendations
Morphine sulfate	Short half-life; elderly people are more sensitive to side effects than are younger people	Start low and titrate to comfort; give continuously (q3-4h); avoid prn use; anticipate and prevent side effects
Sustained release morphine (MS Contin)	Potency and toxicity similar to plain morphine sulfate	Use q12h (q8h rarely required); escalate dose slowly to avoid accumulation (daily or every other day); avoid frequent doses
Codeine (Tylenol with Codeine No. 3 and other combinations)	NSAID combinations limit maximum dose; constipation a major issue	Avoid high doses; anticipate and prevent NSAID side effects; begin bowel program early
Oxycodone (Percodan)	NSAID combinations limit maximum dose; toxicity similar to codeine	Avoid high doses; anticipate and prevent NSAID side effects; begin bowel program early
Hydromorphone (Dilaudid)	Half-life may be shorter than morphine (3 hr); toxicity similar to morphine	Similar to morphine; start low and titrate to comfort; give continuously (q3-4h); avoid prn use; anticipate and prevent side effects
Opiate drugs to avoid for elderly patients		
Meperidine (Demerol)	Extremely low oral potency; metabolite and normeperidine may accumulate, causing confusion, agitation, and seizure activity, especially among patients with renal impairments	Choose a drug with higher oral potency; there are no advantages for choosing either oral or parenteral meperidine over other opiate drugs
Pentazocine (Talwin)	Mixed opiate agonist-antagonist activity often leads to CNS excitement, confusion, and agitation	Avoid entirely for frail elderly patient
Propoxyphene (Darvon)	Potency no better than aspirin; significant potential for abuse and renal injury	Choose a NSAID or weak opiate
Methadone (Dolophine)	Plasma half-life may be extremely prolonged in elderly people; analgesic half-life relatively short	Sustained release morphine appears to be a better choice

Nonpharmacological strategies for pain management

Clinical experience suggests that many nonpharmacological techniques are quite effective in individual cases. The value of physical methods, including heat, ice, and massage, should not be underestimated. Such measures relax tense muscles and are soothing for a variety of complaints. These methods can be applied by the patients, giving the patients and their families a sense of control over the symptoms and treatments. Precautions should be taken to avoid skin and soft tissue damage during prolonged use of either heat or ice. Physical therapy directed toward stretching and strengthening specific muscles and joints also may be useful in improving muscle spasms and allowing enhanced functional activity. Referrals to trained physical therapists may be appropriate for patients' safe and effective rehabilitation from most painful conditions.

Transcutaneous electrical nerve stimulation (TENS) has been used successfully for a variety of chronic pain conditions in older patients. Painful diabetic neuropathies, shoulder pain or bursitis, and fractured ribs respond to TENS therapy. Although some patients have experienced relief for years, the effectiveness of TENS usually diminishes with time and strong placebo effects are associated with its use.[3] An important issue in the success of TENS therapy is the appropriate placement of the electrodes and adjustment of the current. This involves a meticulous search for the best settings that optimize an individual's comfort. Also, care must be taken by the patients to avoid skin irritations and possible burns from the electrodes, especially among cognitively impaired patients.

Some psychological maneuvers may be quite effective in controlling pain. Biofeedback, relaxation, and hypnosis may be helpful for some patients when a trained psychologist or therapist administers these techniques. These methods usually necessitate patients with high levels of cognitive function.

Pain management and rehabilitation clinics are effective for the treatment of patients with chronic pain, apparently because these clinics provide an interdisciplinary program for individual pain problems.

Finally, a variety of distractions may be effective in decreasing patients' perceptions of pain. Many patients find comfort in prayer, meditation, or music. Involvement in activities, exercise, and recreation should be encouraged, as much as can be tolerated by the patients. Inactivity and immobility may contribute extensively to depression and worse pain.

Family and informal caregivers in pain management

Family caregivers are critical providers of support for patients with chronic pain. Family caregivers provide physical, emotional, social, and economic support so that elderly and chronically ill patients can remain ambulatory in the comfort of their homes and avoid institutionalization. Caregivers often decide what medications should be taken and when they should be taken and are gatekeepers against drug abuse and overdosage. The control of patients' chronic pain is a problem that may have important implications for caregiver stress. (See Chapter 6.) Increased anxiety, depression, marital and family conflicts, embarrassment, guilt, resentment, low morale, and severe emotional and physical exhaustion are commonly reported by distressed caregivers. Indeed pain management may present unique kinds of stress for caregivers. For example, pain management often requires the administration of hazardous drugs, which must be monitored carefully to achieve maximum control of patients' pain, safely and with minimum side effects. Caregivers often struggle with questions about the causes of pain, side effects of medications, drug addiction, and pain as a metaphor for advanced illness and death of the patients. These unanswered questions often lead to increased anxiety, stress, and overall caregiver burden. More importantly, caregiver stress may translate to inadequate pain management for the patients. Education and support for caregivers cannot be overemphasized in the management of pain for ambulatory elderly people.[4] Thus, physicians should be aware of caregiver burden associated with pain management and help to establish a reasonable, simplified, and feasible plan of care, based on the resources and skills that are available to caregivers.

Finally, it should be remembered that inpatient hospitalization or respite care is sometimes necessary to alleviate the patients' pain and support the caregivers. Respite for the caregivers can be accomplished while the patients are hospitalized and major modifications are made to the treatment plans.

REFERENCES

1. Chapman RC, Syrjala KL: Measurement of pain. In Bonica JJ, ed: *The management of pain*, Philadelphia, 1990, Lea & Febiger.
2. Crook J, Rideout E, Browne G: The prevalence of pain complaints among a general population, *Pain* 18:299, 1984.
3. Deyo RA et al: A controlled trial of transcutaneous electrical nerve stimulation (TENS) and exercise for chronic low back pain, *N Engl J Med* 322(23):1627, 1990.
4. Ferrell BR et al: Family factors influencing cancer pain, *Postgrad Med J* 67(suppl 2):S64, 1991.
5. Harkins SW, Kwentus J, Price DD: Pain in the elderly. In Benedetti C, ed: *Advances in pain research and therapy, vol 7*, New York, 1984, Raven Press.
6. Melzack R: The tragedy of needless pain, *Sci Am* 262(2):27, 1990.
7. Portenoy RK: Drug treatment of pain syndromes, *Semin Neurol* 7(2):139, 1987.
8. Roth SH: Merits and liabilities of NSAID therapy, *Rheum Dis Clin North Am* 15(3):479, 1989.

SUGGESTED READINGS

The American Pain Society: *Principles of analgesic use in the treatment of acute pain and chronic cancer pain: a concise guide to medical practice*, 3 ed, Washington, DC, 1990.
Ferrell BA: Pain management in elderly people, *J Am Geriatr Soc* 39:64, 1991.
Ferrell BA, Ferrell BR: Pain management at home, *Clin Geriatr Med* 7(4):765, 1991.
Portnoy RK, Fakash A: Practical management of nonmalignant pain in the elderly, *Geriatrics* 43(5):29, 1988.

CHAPTER 40

Joint problems

EDWARD MONGAN

KEY POINTS
- The cardinal symptom of osteoarthritis is pain after joint use which is relieved by rest.
- Osteoarthritis cannot be diagnosed for a given joint unless characteristic radiographic findings are present.
- Nonsteroidal antiinflammatory drugs must be used cautiously by elderly patients because of the drugs' gastrointestinal and renal side effects.
- Patients with polymyalgia rheumatica respond dramatically to oral corticosteroid drugs.
- Gout is the most frequently overdiagnosed type of arthritis.

Musculoskeletal diseases are a major cause of disabilities, especially for elderly persons. Most of these conditions are diagnosed and treated in an outpatient setting. This chapter focuses on common musculoskeletal disabilities in elderly persons.

OSTEOARTHRITIS

Clinical relevance

Osteoarthritis is a noninflammatory disorder of movable joints that is characterized by deterioration and abrasion of articular cartilage and by formation of new bone on the surfaces of the joints. Osteoarthritis is the most common type of arthritis among the general population and elderly persons. In a sample of 6672 adults 18 to 79 years of age in the United States, 37% of the individuals who were examined had radiographic evidence of osteoarthritis.[6] All levels of severity of radiographic osteoarthritis increased steadily with age, from 4% among persons 18 to 24 years of age to 85% among individuals 75 to 79 years of age. Males were affected more commonly than females before they reached age 45, but the sex ratio reversed thereafter. However, moderate or severe involvement was nearly twice as common for females (11%) than males (6%).

PATTERN OF JOINT DISTRIBUTION
CLASSICALLY SEEN IN PRIMARY OSTEOARTHRITIS

Distal interphalangeal joints of the hands	Large weight-bearing joints (hips and knees)
Joints around the base of the thumb	Great toe joints
Lower cervical spine	Temporomandibular joints
Lumbosacral spine	

Osteoarthritis is traditionally divided into the following two categories:
1. *Primary osteoarthritis,* which arises de novo
2. *Secondary osteoarthritis,* which results from the effects of an injury or mechanical derangement of the joint

The primary form is the most common type of osteoarthritis in older adults and usually becomes symptomatic after adults are 50 years old. While secondary osteoarthritis can occur in any joint, primary osteoarthritis favors certain target sites.[1] (See the box above.) Because the cause of primary osteoarthritis is unknown, there currently is no effective form of prevention.

Secondary osteoarthritis may arise as a direct consequence of trauma to a joint such as a fracture with subsequent malalignment. Other causes of secondary osteoarthritis are congenital anomalies such as dislocation of the hip, local damage to a joint caused by a bacterial infection, metabolic diseases such as acromegaly, and neurological abnormalities leading to neuropathic joints as in tabes dorsalis or syringomyelia. Even low-grade trauma over a number of years can lead to secondary osteoarthritis.[3]

Clinical manifestations

The cardinal symptom of osteoarthritis in younger or older adults is pain, which is relieved by rest, after they use their joints. Later the pain occurs with minimum motion or even while the individual is at rest. Stiffness of short duration, aches at times of inclement weather, and crepitation with motion are other symptoms that are frequently found but are nonspecific because they also are found in many other types of arthritis. While the affected joints may be tender and enlarged, signs of inflammation are uncommon except for effusion. Range of motion, which may be limited, is particularly helpful to physicians for diagnosing osteoarthritis of the hips. Osteophytes can be palpated on the dorsal lateral aspect of the proximal and distal interphalangeal joints, and malalignment of an extremity because of asymmetrical involvement of the joints is common.

The pattern of joint involvement is similar in men and women, until they are 55 years old. Among older individuals, distal interphalangeal, proximal interphalangeal.

and first carpal metacarpal joints are more frequently affected in women and the hips are more frequently affected in men. There is a well-known familial predominance of distal interphalangeal joint involvement (Heberden's nodes) and proximal interphalangeal joint involvement (Bouchard's nodes) in women.

Diagnostic approach

For elderly patients with clinical and radiographic evidence of osteoarthritis, it is unnecessary and not cost effective to order routine rheumatological blood tests (e.g., rheumatoid factor) for diagnostic purposes. Synovial fluid from osteoarthritic joints is a type I or noninflammatory fluid (i.e., only a slight increase in the number of white blood cells and most cells are mononuclear). The one consistent abnormality in osteoarthritic joints is the radiographic findings. Osteoarthritis probably cannot be diagnosed in a given joint unless characteristic radiographic findings are present. These findings include irregular joint space narrowing, subchondral bony sclerosis, marginal osteophyte formation, and, occasionally, bone cysts. However, only 30% of joints that show radiographic evidence of osteoarthritis are symptomatic.

Intervention

Treatment of osteoarthritis must be individualized. Many older patients only require reassurance that they have no generalized crippling form of arthritis. Rest of the involved joints and protection of the joints from overuse is important, especially for the weight-bearing joints. Forces on the lower extremities increase threefold when individuals shift their weight to each leg as they walk. For this reason weight reduction should be carried out by obese elderly patients because if they are successful, a significant reduction in their pain can be achieved.[2] Canes or walkers are beneficial for protection of the joints, when necessary. Physical therapy to relieve pain and associated muscle spasm and maintain range of motion for the joint is important.

For patients with mild pain from osteoarthritis, analgesic drugs such as acetaminophen or propoxyphene hydrochloride may be effective when used on an as-needed basis. Narcotic preparations should be avoided, especially by older patients. In moderate to severe cases of osteoarthritis, nonsteroidal antiinflammatory drugs (NSAIDs) are often beneficial. Aspirin is effective for elderly patients, but it is more hazardous to older persons than to younger persons. Even small doses of aspirin may cause bleeding from the gastrointestinal tract; therefore, the total daily dose for older adults should not exceed 2.5 g/day and enteric-coated preparations are recommended. Other NSAIDs are effective in osteoarthritis, even when they are used in small doses. Unfortunately the following two types of significant side effects must be monitored:

1. The gastrointestinal side effects of NSAIDs include gastritis and gastric ulcer, which are sometimes associated with acute bleeding. (See the box on p. 394.) Moreover, these conditions are difficult to diagnose because they can occur

RISK FACTORS FOR GASTROPATHY FROM NONSTEROIDAL ANTIINFLAMMATORY DRUGS

Old age
Use of corticosteroids
History of gastrointestinal side effects
    from NSAIDs

Prior hospitalization for gastrointestinal
    disorders
Use of high doses of NSAIDs

without any abdominal symptoms to warn patients or their physicians. For patients who have a significant risk of gastric ulcers, misoprostol (Cytotec), a synthetic prostaglandin analog, can be added to the NSAID to reduce this complication. Misoprostol is given in doses of 100 to 200 mg 4 times a day with food. Routine reduction of the dose is not necessary for older adults or patients with renal impairments.

2. Although it is far less frequent than gastrointestinal complications, renal failure may occur with long-term administration of NSAIDs. Such manifestations are more likely to occur among older persons and patients with preexisting renal diseases; therefore, these drugs should be used with caution by all such patients.

Judicious intraarticular injections of corticosteroids may be beneficial in the management of acute joint flare-ups for patients with osteoarthritis. The improvement is only temporary, rarely lasting more than 4 to 6 weeks. Injections should be infrequent, especially into weight-bearing joints. As a general rule, a given joint should not be injected with corticosteroids more than 3 times in 1 year.

The prognosis for patients with osteoarthritis is good. Even for elderly patients with chronic pain from arthritis, careful medical management generally provides significant relief and helps them to maintain function. In 1% to 2% of patients with advanced osteoarthritis of a weight-bearing joint, an orthopedic procedure may be beneficial. In the past 20 years the judicious use of total joint arthroplasties in the hips and knees have resulted in marked symptomatic improvements for most patients, including older adults, by providing striking pain relief and improved range of motion. If ambulatory elderly patients who have osteoarthritis complain of hip or knee pain at night when they are not bearing weight, referral to an orthopedic surgeon for evaluation and, possibly, elective joint surgery is indicated.

POLYMYALGIA RHEUMATICA

Polymyalgia rheumatica is a syndrome of older patients that is characterized by pain and stiffness in the neck, shoulders, and pelvic girdle, persisting for at least a month, without weakness or atrophy. This syndrome usually is accompanied by a rapid (high) erythrocyte sedimentation rate.[5] The disease is rare in patients who are less than 50 years old, and it is reported twice as often in women than it is in men. Almost all of the patients who are reported to have the disease are white. The patients complain of severe pain in the neck, back, shoulders, upper arms, and thighs; the onset of symptoms is often abrupt. Weakness is not prominent, but morning stiffness is marked. Nonspecific symptoms include fever, anorexia, weight loss, apathy, and depression. Despite the severity of the complaints, there are few physical findings. The patients have no arthritis, muscle weakness, or muscle atrophy. Radiographs of the joints are usually normal. The erythrocyte sedimentation rate is almost always above 50 mm/hr. A certain percentage of patients with polymyalgia rheumatica also suffer from temporal arteritis, frequently with involvement of the ophthalmic arteries. The most satisfactory way to confirm the diagnosis of polymyalgia rheumatica is a trial of prednisone (10 to 15 mg/day). The response of polymyalgia rheumatica to corticosteroids is truly dramatic; some patients are almost entirely well the next day. The improvement is so invariable that if a response is not seen within a week, the diagnosis should be doubted. After several weeks, the dose is reduced to a daily maintenance dose of 5 to 7.5 mg of prednisone while the clinical response is monitored. Patients with polymyalgia rheumatica often need to stay on low-dose prednisone therapy for 2 or more years. If the patients develop any eye symptoms or tenderness over the temporal arteries, a temporal artery biopsy to exclude the diagnosis of temporal arteritis is indicated. If temporal arteritis is present, the patient should immediately be placed on high doses of prednisone (60 to 80 mg/day) for at least a month to prevent vision loss.

GOUT

The diagnosis and treatment of gout in older adults is no different than it is in younger patients. However, the following two circumstances alter the way that older patients with gout are treated:

1. While there is conclusive evidence that a medication to reduce serum uric acid levels and a prophylactic medication to prevent acute attacks are worthwhile, patients who are more than 70 years old and develop their first attacks of acute gout may be treated differently. Since the chances of recurrent attacks of gout leading to chronic tophaceous gout are so small for elderly men, physicians may elect just to treat acute attacks because their patients probably will not live long enough to develop chronic tophaceous gout. The average time from the first attack of acute gout to the onset of chronic tophaceous gout is more than a decade.[4]

2. Now that there are a large number of individuals living into their 80s and 90s, more elderly women have acute gout. Males develop gout approximately 20 to 30 years after the normal increase in their serum uric acid levels occurs at

puberty. The finding explains the prevalence of gout among 40- to 60-year-old men. In women, serum uric acid levels do not rise until menopause. Not only is gout usually not considered as a disease of elderly women, but also the symptoms of the disease do not present as classically as they do for middle-aged men. However, if gout is suspected, it can be as readily diagnosed in women by the appropriate blood and synovial fluid studies as it can for men. Moreover, treatment for women is as successful as it is for men.

One final clinical point is that gout is the most frequently overdiagnosed type of arthritis that rheumatologists see. The reason for this overdiagnosis is that some physicians equate hyperuricemia and joint symptoms of any kind as being suggestive of gout. Only if there are compatible clinical features and hyperuricemia should gout be suspected. The diagnosis of gout is absolutely confirmed by demonstrating that the involved joint has uric acid crystals.

REFERENCES

1. Bluestone R: *Rheumatology*, Boston, 1980, Houghton Mifflin.
2. Felson DT et al: Obesity and knee osteoarthritis, *Ann Intern Med* 109:18, 1988.
3. Handler NM et al: Hand structure and function in an industrial setting: influence of three patterns of stereotyped repetitive usage, *Arthritis Rheum* 21:210, 1978.
4. Hench PS: Diagnosis of gout and gouty arthritis, *J Lab Clin Med* 22:48, 1936.
5. McCarty DJ: *Arthritis and allied conditions*, ed 11, Philadelphia, 1989, Lea & Febiger.
6. Roberts J, Burch TA: Prevalence of osteoarthritis in adults by age, sex, race, and geographic area, United States—1960-1962. [National Center for Health Statistics: vital and health statistics: data from the national health survey.] United States Public Health Service Publication No. 1000, Series II, No. 15, 1966. Washington DC: United States Government Printing Office.

SUGGESTED READINGS

Allen NB, Studenski SA: Polymyalgia rheumatica and temporal arteritis, *Med Clin North Am* 70(2):369, 1986.
Corman LC: Clinical spectrum and treatment of rheumatic syndromes in the elderly, *Med Clin North Am* 73:1371, 1989.
Fam AG: Osteoarthritis in the geriatric patient, *Geriatr Med Today* 6(4):18, 1987.
Hamerman D, ed: Rheumatic disorders, *Clin Geriatr Med* 4(2):241, 1988.

CHAPTER 41

Foot care

ARTHUR E. HELFAND

KEY POINTS
- Foot problems are common among elderly persons.
- Foot problems may be the first symptom or sign of a systemic disorder.
- Problems related to the foot impact older patients' functional ability, mobility, and independence.
- Disorders of the foot arise primarily from local skin and nail problems, biomechanical abnormalities, and selected systemic diseases.

GENERAL CONSIDERATIONS

Foot health and the patient's ability to remain ambulatory are prime considerations in the ambulatory management of the older patient.[2,3] Although the foot itself is seldom the direct cause of mortality. However, morbidity, disability, and limitation of activity can arise because of foot problems.

The effects of chronic systemic disease are often first demonstrated in the foot.[4] For instance, an ulcer on the toe may be the first sign that the patient has diabetes mellitus. The status of foot health can provide significant insight into the medical and social needs of the patient. The patient's ability to retain ambulation and mobility may determine the need for institutionalization, help prevent depression, and reduce the need for social assistance.[6]

Foot health care for the older patient should be directed toward the following three primary goals[5]:

1. Limit the patient's disability
2. Preserve the patient's maximum level of functional ability
3. Restore the patient's highest possible level of independent activity

RISK FACTORS FOR
_____ FOOT PROBLEMS IN ELDERLY PERSONS _____

Changes in gait
Prior foot care and management
Environmental factors
Emotional factors
Current medications and therapeutic
  programs
Associated systemic and local disease
  processes

Past foot conditions
Changes in mental status that enhance
  neglect
Atrophy of muscles and associated musculoskeletal and neurovascular diseases

Older persons are at great risk for the development of foot problems. The box above summarizes the risk factors for foot problems in elderly persons. Certain diseases are associated most notably with foot problems. (See the box below.) Special attention to the assessment of foot health should be provided to patients with these disorders.

COMMON FOOT PROBLEMS

Nail disorders

Onychauxis. Onychauxis is hypertrophy, thickening, and hardening of toenails, resulting in discomfort and pain. Onychauxis is associated with aging, recurrent trauma, inflammation, local infection, nutritional disturbances, and degenerative diseases that decrease the vascular supply to the nail matrix and bed. Hypertrophy is accompanied by discoloration and loss of translucency of the nail plate. This problem is magnified for the patient who is obese and unable to bend over or who has a loss

_____ DISORDERS ASSOCIATED WITH FOOT PROBLEMS _____

Ischemia
Lymphedema
Buerger's disease
Arteriosclerosis obliterans
Venous stasis
Chronic thrombophlebitis
Peripheral neuropathies
Posttrauma
Chronic cellulitis

Diabetes mellitus
Congestive heart failure
Edema
Neurosyphilis
Gout
Scleroderma
Degenerative joint disease
Rheumatoid arthritis

of vision and manual dexterity. Neglecting the toenails creates excessive pressure in the shoe, which results in potential ulceration of the nails, as well as limitation of the patient's ambulation. Debridement should be completed every 30 to 60 days. Mild keratolytics such as 20% urea preparations help to soften and reduce associated keratosis.[7]

Onychogryphosis. Onychogryphosis or ram's horn nail is a severely deformed and hypertrophic nail that follows the curvature of the toe because of pressure. Management is similar to that of onychauxis. When the nail deformity is extensive, the total and permanent removal of the nail and matrix may be advised. The choice of surgical excision or avulsion and chemical destruction of the matrix rests with the clinician; however, avulsion without concern for the matrix results in a new nail that may be more hypertrophic than the previous one. In addition, with avulsion only, tissue retraction occurs and produces anterior pressure as the new nail regenerates 4 to 8 months later.

Subungual hemorrhage. Sudden trauma to the toenail can result in subungual hemorrhage. Idiopathic subungual hemorrhage can be identified in patients with diabetes mellitus, recent stroke, chronic renal failure, as well as those patients who take anticoagulants. Pain may be significant and bleeding can be identified under the nail plate. If the trauma was recent, drainage may be required. Using an 18-gauge needle or a surgical burr, the physician can drill the nail. With residual hemorrhagic areas, which appear dark blue-black, pain is not a significant factor and drainage is usually not required. Radiographic examination should be considered to exclude a fracture. The nail plate may autoavulse or the color change may persist until the entire nail is replaced (usually 6 to 10 months). Should the nail become loose, it should be debrided.

Onychophosis. Onychophosis is diagnosed when the patient has incurvated, involuted, or pincer toenails. It is the result of repeated microtrauma to the nail plate. Xerosis or the presence of mycosis adds to the development of hyperkeratotic tissue. Management includes debriding hyperkeratotic tissue, thinning the nail plate, removing external pressure, and using keratolytics or emollients such as 15% salicylic acid or (Carmol 20, Keralyt Gel, or Lac-Hydrins). Nail removal may be necessary when pain is severe.

Ingrown toenail. Onychocryptosis or ingrown toenail occurs when a segment of nail penetrates the nailfold. Onychocryptosis can result from nails that have been cut too short or from external trauma. Inflammation, swelling, infection, and, if the nails are protracted, periungual ulcerative granulation tissue result. Marked curvature of the nail plate predisposes individuals to onychocryptosis. For patients who have associated diseases such as diabetes mellitus or arterial insufficiency, complications from these diseases can lead to amputations. Antibiotics alone, without the removal of the nail from the soft tissue, do not resolve the condition. Initial management includes drainage of the superficial abscess and partial avulsion or excision of the penetrating nail segment. Saline or povidone-iodine compresses can be used. When a patient has significant infection, radiographic and laboratory studies are necessary and appropriate antibiotic therapy should follow. If the problem becomes chronic, surgical excision and/or chemical cautery of a segment of nail matrix should be considered. Periungual granulation tissue can be managed with chemical cauterization such as 75% silver nitrate or with excision of the deformed nail segment and matrix. These procedures usually are completed while the patient is under regional field block anesthesia.

Subungual corn. Subungual heloma (corn) results from localized pressure on the nail bed and may be associated with subungual bone spurs. The lesion usually appears subungually as a dark spot and is painful when it is palpated. Pressure from a nail deformity can precipitate a subungual ulceration, which may have similar characteristics. Management includes debridement of the lesion and removal of pressure both externally from the shoes and internally from the bone deformity. Footwear with a high toe box and soft leather upper is indicated. Tube foam or lamb's wool also can be used to help reduce pressure to the area.

Fungal infection. Onychomycosis (fungal infection of the nails) is extremely common in old age. Predisposing factors include moisture, poor footwear, recurrent trauma, and diabetes mellitus. Onychomycosis is often associated with tinea pedis. The toenails become thickened, deformed, and discolored. While different parts of the nails can be affected, the entire nail plates and subungual tissues of elderly patients are usually involved. The nails become granular and dry, crumble, and have characteristic musty odors. Discomfort and pain are related to the deformity and resultant shoe pressure. Autoavulsion and traumatic avulsion are not uncommon. Paronychia can develop with trauma and systemic diseases such as diabetes mellitus or peripheral vascular insufficiency.

Clinical management includes debridement (mechanical, surgical, and chemical) and topical antifungal agents. Systemic antifungal drugs must be taken for many months and are associated with significant side effects; hence, they are rarely used by elderly patients. Complete cure is unlikely. Debridement usually is required about every 2 months.

Dermatological disorders

Age-related changes of the foot include dryness, scaliness, and atrophy. There is diminished sebaceous activity and hydration, as well as dysfunction in keratin formation. There is associated loss of hair on the foot and elasticity of the skin, and the toenails may become striated and brittle. These changes are magnified by arteriosclerotic changes.

Pruritis. Pruritis is related to dryness, scaliness, environmental changes, disturbed keratin formation, decreased sebaceous activity, and defatted skin as a result of multiple hot baths. (See Chapter 29.) Chronic tinea pedis and neurogenic and emotional dermatoses should be excluded. Treatment should be directed toward moderation of the patients' bathing procedures and use of emollients to lubricate and hydrate the skin. If tinea is present, topical antifungals should be used. Antihistamines in titrated doses may be effective in breaking the patients' scratch reflex but may cause side effects in older patients. Oil and water baths may be of value but must be used sparingly.

Fissured heels. Fissured heels can become a serious complication when they are associated with vascular insufficiency. Tinea should be considered when there is diffuse keratosis. Atrophy of the skin and repeated microtrauma cause stress marks in the heel area and are the early signs of calcaneal fissuring. Emollients and heel cups to reduce pressure should be employed. Poly-foam or plastic cups are often useful. Topical antifungals are indicated for mycotic infection. Antibiotic therapy and reducing weight bearing on the foot should be considered when there is infection. With vascular insufficiency, physical modalities such as tepid whirlpool and exercise can be employed. Limited topical enzymes are valuable in the chemical debridement of the fissured areas. Local tissue stimulants such as compound tincture of benzoin or gentian violet may improve epithelialization.

Hyperhidrosis. Hyperhidrosis may be associated with tinea, faulty footwear, stockings that lack absorptive qualities, orthotic coverings, and emotional factors. Local management includes proper foot hygiene, cotton socks, and absorbent foot powder. Peroxide, alcohol, and 10% formalin solutions or Drysol are indicated when appropriate.

Bromhidrosis. Bromhidrosis is characterized by a foul odor, which is due to the biochemical decomposition of sweat. The treatment is similar to hyperhidrosis. Deodorants and topical neomycin powder may prove beneficial during the initial period of management. Shoes should be changed daily and permitted to air dry in sunlight, whenever possible.

Tinea pedis. Tinea pedis is common among elderly persons. In the acute stages, astringent compresses and topical antifungals should be employed. When secondary bacterial infection is present and cellulitis is noted, appropriate systemic antibiotics should be given. Antifungal foot powders are an appropriate preventive approach, particularly in the presence of hyperhidrosis.

Foot ulcers. Foot ulcers are associated with pressure, biomechanical dysfunction, and concomitant systemic disease such as diabetes mellitus or peripheral arterial insufficiency. The older patient is particularly at risk because of residual foot deformities and gait changes. Associated angiopathy, dermopathy, and neuropathy are major risk factors. Radiographic studies and imaging scans may be necessary to exclude associated osteomyelitis. Initial management should include bed rest, management of the related disease process, and early hospitalization to prevent the need for amputation. Judicious debridement and drainage may be required. Topical enzymes are sometimes of value. Antibiotics are necessary when there is clinical evidence of local or systemic infection. Whirlpool and muscle stimulation may assist the healing phase. All measures of removing weight bearing from the ulcerative site should be instituted, including Plastazote, Thermold, and appropriate orthotic inserts. Special shoes such as Extra Depth Inlay or Darco shoes are helpful. These measures all facilitate the changing of dressings. Contact casts aid in the healing process and reduce the risk of amputation.

Biomechanical considerations

The older patient often has significant changes in gait patterns due to deformity, paralysis, weakness, or spasticity. Consequently, hyperkeratotic lesions often develop. Excessive pressure on a localized area of the foot leads to keratosis and pain. The pressure may result from a bony abnormality, foot-to-shoe incompatibility, deformity such as hammer toe or bunion, last hallux valgus or change in the method of weight bearing.

Hyperkeratosis. Calluses are broad-based (tylomas) or circumscribed (helomas) hyperkeratotic lesions. The formation of hyperkeratotic lesions represents the normal reaction of the body to external or internal pressure on the skin. The degenerative loss of the plantar fat pad, as well as digital contractures, spur and hyperostosis formations, arthritic changes, and functional adaptations are significant factors in the development of hyperkeratotic lesions.

Management includes debridement, emollients or mild keratolytics, and silicone molds or other orthotic devices to reduce local pressure and help modify the alignment and weight-bearing forces. Weight-bearing radiographs are of value to assess the patient's functional factors. Surgical revision may be considered when there is intractable pain, failure of conservative measures, and recurrent infection and ulceration.

Patients should be advised not to apply any commercial "corn cure" products that contain strong concentrations of acid because inappropriate use can produce a second-degree chemical burn or a loss of tissue and can increase the potential for infection.

Footwear also should be considered in the management of keratotic lesions, regardless of their causes. When there clearly is a shoe-related incompatibility, changes should be recommended. The Extra Depth Inlay, Thermold, Ambulator, and Bunion lasts, the classic or orthopedic last, and a standard shoe that has been relasted are available but expensive alternatives. Commercial athletic or walking shoes offer an alternative for many elderly patients.

Hammer toe. Digitus flexus or hammer toe deformity results from a complex interaction of multiple factors. Pain is usually the result of inflammatory changes that are associated with bursitis, capsulitis, or tendonitis. Heloma formation is common both dorsally and distally and is related to foot-shoe last incompatibility. Ulceration and sinus formation are potential results of continuous pressure.

Bunion. Hallux valgus or bunion deformity is one of the most common reasons that older people seek podiatric care. There is an inward deviation of the first meta-tarsal (varus), outward deviation of the great toe (valgus), lateral displacement of the plantar sesamoids under the first metatarsal head, tendon contracture, adventitious bursa formation, rotation of the great toe, and bony enlargement. These deformities often alter gait and balance and cause pain.

Hallux limitus and Tailor's bunion. Hallux limitus often is associated with bunion deformity. It appears clinically and radiographically as a monoarticular degenerative arthritis of the first metatarsal-phalangeal joint. Clinically, there is marked limitation of extension of the great toe because of dorsal and/or lateral lipping and spur formation in the periarticular segments of the joint. Movement creates inflammation and locking, resulting in pain and limited mobility.

Digitus quintus varus or Tailor's bunion involves an inward deviation or varus of the small or fifth toe and an outward deviation or valgus of the fifth metatarsal.

Management of these deformities is directed toward relief of pain, care of the secondary keratotic and ulcerative lesions, change in footwear, and consideration of surgical revision of the deformity when conservative measures fail. Radiographic evaluation is necessary as a baseline. Orthoses and shields can modify pressure, antiinflammatory drugs may help with pain, and local corticosteroid injections can be helpful. Physical modalities such as protective orthoses, crest molds, and silicone molds are also of benefit.

Metatarsalgia. Diffuse pain in the ball of the foot is referred to as *metatarsalgia*. It may be caused by abnormal, long, bony architecture, loss of the anterior metatarsal fat pad, inflammation of the bursa, tendon, or capsule, and trauma. Patients with chronic arthritis of any kind frequently have this problem.

Management includes study of comparative radiographs of the weight-bearing and non–weight-bearing foot; physical modalities, including mild heat, hydrotherapy, and electrical stimulation, as indicated; analgesics, nonsteroidal antiinflammatory drugs, and local corticosteroid injections; and orthoses and/or shoe modifications. Existing deformities such as hammer toe and increased plantar pressure through subluxed joints also should be corrected.

Morton's neuroma. Interdigital neuritis and neuroma (Morton's neuroma) produce pain that is exaggerated by compression, usually from unsuitable footwear. The patient usually complains of a burning or radiating pain, extending from the metatarsal head area to the distal portion of the toe, that feels like an electric shock. Neuritis generally responds to conservative management, which includes local anesthetics, local corti-costeroid injections, and physical modalities. Orthoses also can be employed to change the relationship between the metatarsal heads. A change in shoe last and size to remove the compression factor also should be considered. Neuromas that do not respond to conservative management usually require surgical intervention.

Heel pain. The causes of heel pain are numerous. Plantar calcaneal spurs often are demonstrated on the patient's x-ray but may not always be the cause of the pain. Pain can be related to subcalcaneal bursitis and chronic plantar myofasciitis. Gradual loss of subcutaneous fat also can increase heel sensitivity.

The management of plantar heel pain includes physical modalities such as ultrasound, whirlpool, radiant heat, and electrical stimulation to reduce inflammation and pain. Local corticosteroid injections, as well as a medical approach, are indicated during the acute phase when point tenderness is found. Analgesics can be used to control pain. Heel pads, heel cups, shoe modifications, and orthoses to reduce the pull on the plantar fascia and to reduce the percentage of weight bearing on the medial tuberosity of the calcaneus are indicated. The primary biomechanical consideration is to provide some elevation of the heel. Shock-absorbing materials such as PPT, Spenco, Sorbathane, Plastazote, and other similar products are indicated to reduce shock to the plantar structures.

SYSTEMIC DISEASES ASSOCIATED WITH FOOT PROBLEMS

Many patients who have other diseases initially complain of symptoms of the feet. Elderly patients are prone to multiple conditions that sometimes manifest confusing symptoms and signs. Complaints are often motivated by the patients' inability to walk or the presence of painful feet. Many times, care is not provided until complications arise or pain becomes significant.[8,9]

Osteoarthritis

Osteoarthritis is a common cause of foot problems. (See Chapter 40.) The relationship between chronic trauma and obesity is well reflected in the weight-bearing joints of the foot.

The primary findings in the foot include pain, stiffness, swelling, limitation of movement, and deformity. The older person's ambulation and transfers are often affected. Clinically, findings include plantar fasciitis, calcaneal erosion and/or spur formation, stress fractures, tendonitis, and tenosynovitis.

Gout

Although it may commonly affect the great toe (podagra), gouty arthritis may produce symptoms in any joint of the foot and should always be suspected where intense pain is present without trauma. The primary manifestations include chronic painful and stiff joints, soft tissue tophi, loss of bone substance, deformity, and functional impairment. (See Chapter 40.)

Rheumatoid arthritis

The presenting symptoms of rheumatoid arthritis are exacerbations of pain, joint swelling, stiffness, muscle wasting, and deformity. Long-standing disease creates residual deformities of the forefoot including hallux rigidus (severe form of hallux limitus), arthritis of the first metatarsal-phalangeal joint, hallux valgus, cystic erosion, sesamoid erosion, metatarsal-phalangeal dislocation, hyperkeratosis, digitus flexus (hammer toe), extensor tenosynovitis, displacement, and ganglion. Rheumatoid complications of the rearfoot include talonavicular arthritis, rigid pronated foot, ankle arthritis, subtalar arthritis, tarsal arthritis, subachilles bursitis, subcutaneous nodule, plantar fasciitis, spur, and Achilles tendon shortening.

Diabetes mellitus

Diabetes mellitus is complicated by multiple pedal manifestations. Foot problems even may be the first presenting symptoms. Paresthesia, sensory impairment, muscle and soft tissue atrophy, and diminished or absent pedal pulse are frequently seen. Secondary problems may include tinea pedis, chronic infection, ulceration, and terminal necrosis or gangrene. Nail problems such as diabetic onychopathy also are very common. Idiopathic subungual hemorrhages commonly occur before other hemorrhages develop in the eye.[1] (See Chapter 43 for general management of diabetes mellitus.)

Patients who are at risk for ulceration include those with histories of ulcerations, neuropathies, peripheral vascular diseases, structural changes (such as hammer toe, bunion, or Charcot's joint), callous formations, abnormal gaits, and improper shoes.

Peripheral vascular insufficiency

Peripheral vascular insufficiency is present to some degree in many elderly patients. (See Chapter 54.) Overt manifestations of decreased arterial supply include muscle fatigue, cramps, claudication, pain, coldness, pallor, paresthesia, burning, nail disorders, absent pedal pulses, atrophy of soft tissue, and dryness from xerosis and loss of hair. Calcification may be demonstrated during the course of an incidental diagnostic radiographic study. Arch pain can be mistaken for pathomechanical changes when the real cause is ischemia. The result of severe arterial occlusion is gangrene that is usually self-demarcating.

Edema

Edema caused by cardiac hypothyroid or renal disease also may cause foot problems. Edema that is due to a combination of inactivity, dependency, immobilization, pain, and/or venous insufficiency may give rise to difficulties. Chronic stasis, ulceration, and associated dermatological manifestation are seen. (See Chapter 54.)

REFERENCES

1. American Diabetes Association: *Therapy for diabetes and related disorders*, Alexandria, Va, 1991.
2. Calkins E, Davis PJ, Ford AB, eds: *The practice of geriatrics*, Philadelphia, 1986, WB Saunders.
3. Eisdorfer C, ed: *Annual review of gerontology and geriatrics*, vol 4, New York, 1984, Springer.
4. Helfand AE, ed: *Clinical podogeriatrics*, Baltimore, 1981, Williams & Wilkins.

5. Helfand AE, Bruno J, eds: *Rehabilitation of the foot: clinics in podiatry*, vol 1 (2) Philadelphia, 1984, WB Saunders.
6. Helfand AE, ed: *Public health and podiatric medicine*, Baltimore, 1987, Williams & Wilkins.
7. Jessett DF, Helfand AE: Foot problems in the elderly. In Pathy MSJ, ed: *Principles and practice of geriatric medicine*, ed 2, Edinburgh, 1991, John Wiley & Sons.
8. Steinberg FU, ed: *Care of the geriatric patient*, ed 6, St. Louis, 1983, CV Mosby.
9. Williams TF, ed: *Rehabilitation in the aging*, New York, 1984, Raven Press.

SUGGESTED READINGS

American Diabetes Association: *Therapy for diabetes and related disorders*, Alexandria, Va, 1991.
Helfand AE: Nail and hyperkeratotic problems in the elderly foot, *Am Fam Physician* 38:101, 1989.
Helfand AE, ed: *Public health and podiatric medicine*, Baltimore, 1987, Williams & Wilkins.

CHAPTER 42

Osteopenia: osteoporosis and osteomalacia

KENNETH W. LYLES

KEY POINTS

- In most cases, osteoporosis is a diagnosis of exclusion; other diseases must be excluded.
- Generally, osteoporosis is a silent disease and patients become aware of the diagnosis when they have fractures, routine radiographs, or bone mass measurements.
- Prevention of osteoporosis is the only cost-effective approach to this disease.
- Patients with hip and vertebral compression fractures have significant impairments in function, which can be improved with target physical therapy.
- Osteomalacia is a disease that must be considered if this diagnosis is to be made.
- Most common causes of osteomalacia in older patients can be treated with vitamin D replacement and phosphate supplementation or by stopping offending drugs.

OSTEOPENIA

The term *osteopenia* means a reduced amount of bone and traditionally refers to the finding of diminished amounts of bone on the patients' radiographs. Osteopenia can result from an actual reduction in the bone mass or from a failure of the bone matrix to mineralize normally. Osteopenia can be misdiagnosed as the result of an overpenetrated radiograph. This chapter focuses on *osteoporosis*, a reduction in the amount of bone mass such that a subject is at risk for skeletal fractures with minimal trauma, and *osteomalacia*, a failure of the osteoid matrix to mineralize normally.

OSTEOPOROSIS

Clinical relevance

Osteoporosis has reached epidemic proportions in the United States, with 25 million people affected by the disease. There are over 1.3 million osteoporotic fractures annually, and the cost of care for these fractures is $10 billion.[4] This figure does not account for the excess morbidity patients suffer and the services that impaired patients must purchase after they have developed skeletal fractures.

A number of factors potentially reduce an individual's bone mass, including ethnicity (whites, Asians), poor nutrition (especially calcium and vitamin D intake), alcohol, cigarette smoking, and prolonged immobility. A number of diseases and drugs also affect the skeleton. Common conditions associated with osteoporosis are castration, gastrectomy, hyperthyroidism, hyperparathyroidism, rheumatoid arthritis, Cushing's syndrome from both disease and iatrogenic causes, and, possibly, diabetes mellitus. Glucocorticoids frequently are associated with osteoporosis, and other drugs such as anticonvulsants and heparin also cause bone loss. Obesity appears to protect individuals from bone loss, possibly because of an increase in skeletal loading or estrogen levels. Several studies have shown that thiazide diuretics may have a protective role in osteoporosis, presumably because diuretics conserve renal calcium.

Osteoporosis is a heterogeneous disease. In most cases osteoporosis is primary, and no other disease causing bone loss can be diagnosed. Primary osteoporosis can be divided into several types that are listed in Table 42-1.

The majority of patients with primary osteoporosis have what is classified as involutional osteoporosis with two subcategories: (1) type I or postmenopausal osteoporosis, and (2) type II or senile osteoporosis.[4] Type I osteoporosis is found in women, usually 15 years after menopause. The prevalence of type I osteoporosis in women is six to eight times higher than that in men. The patients' presenting symptoms include fractures of trabecular bone such as the vertebrae or distal forearms.

Type II or senile osteoporosis occurs in men or women who are more than 70 years old. There is a female-to-male ratio of 2:1 or 3:1. Patients usually have fractures of the hips and vertebrae, although fractures of their pelvises, proximal humeri, ribs, and tibias also occur. These skeletal sites contain both cortical and trabecular bone. Measurements of bone mass in these patients are in the lower part of the normal range when those measurements are adjusted for age, race, and sex. The mechanisms for bone loss may affect all older people. Increased bioactive parathyroid hormone and decreased osteoclast function are two of the factors that effect this type of bone loss. Many fractures result from falls or traumas that occur frequently among these older people. There are few differences between the measurements of hip bone mass for patients, more than 80 years old, who have or have not had hip fractures. Thus, falls or other traumas, as well as reduced bone loss, play roles in the causes of these fractures.

Table 42-1 Classification of osteoporosis

Primary	Secondary
Juvenile	**Acquired**
Idiopathic	
Involutional	Hypogonadism
Type I, postmenopausal	Hyperparathyroidism
Type II, senile	Hyperthyroidism
	Cushing's syndrome
	Prior gastrectomy
	Chronic liver disease
	Alcoholism
	Intestinal malabsorption
	Immobilization
	Hypercalciuria
	Adult hypophosphatasia
	Scurvy
	Systemic mastocytosis
	Diabetes mellitus
	Drugs
	Glucocorticoids
	Anticonvulsants
	Heparin
	Thyroid hormone
	Inherited
	Glycogen storage disease
	Osteogenesis imperfecta
	Homocystinuria due to cystathionine synthetase deficiency
	Wilson's disease

There are other diseases and medications that are associated with reduced bone formation or accelerated bone loss. These diseases and medications are listed as secondary causes of osteoporosis in Table 42-1.

Clinical manifestations

Generally, osteoporosis is an asymptomatic disease, and patients become aware of the problem when they have skeletal fractures, when their physicians note reduced bone densities on the routine radiographs, or when their physicians measure bone mass. Vertebral compression fractures occur with minimal traumas such as bending at the waist to pick up an object, coughing, falling, or sitting down hard. Most vertebral compression fractures affect the lower thoracic and upper lumbar spine. The pain of the vertebral compression fracture is severe, and the patient generally can localize the pain over the compressed vertebrae. Pain may radiate bandlike around the thorax or abdomen. Movement may make the pain worse. Occasionally the pain is severe enough to cause an ileus.

With fractures of the lower thoracic and upper lumbar spine, a deformity known as a dowager's hump may develop in the curve of the thoracic spine. There is flattening of the natural lumbar lordosis. With vertebral compression fractures, loss of height occurs. This vertebral compression occurs in the thorax, so the patients may notice that their blouses or shirts become much larger. With more fractures, the abdomen may protrude and patients may complain of early satiety. With recurrent fractures, the rib cage may come to rest on the iliac crest. Patients with multiple vertebral fractures may complain of unsteadiness in gait and may be at risk for more falls. Vertebral compression fractures can cause significant impairments in physical functioning and in carrying out activities of daily living and instrumental activities of daily living.

The most devastating osteoporotic fracture is the hip fracture. The prevalence of hip fractures doubles every 6 years for those who are more than 40 years old. Most hip fractures result from traumas. Recent studies show that it is rare for the hip to fracture and cause a fall. Thus, not only is reduced bone density important to the cause of fracture, but also the fall, the nature of the fall, the amount of soft tissue that can decrease the impact, and the patient's response to the fall are very important. Fractures of the proximal femur can be divided into two classes: (1) subcapital fractures, which occur in one third of the cases, and (2) trochanteric fractures, which comprise the remainder.

Diagnostic approach

Osteoporosis is such a common disorder that most older patients who are seen in an ambulatory geriatric practice have some degree of involutional osteoporosis. Involutional osteoporosis is a diagnosis of exclusion, and a woman in her 70s may have components of both type I and type II osteoporosis. When osteoporosis is diagnosed either because of a compression fracture or because of the finding of osteopenia on a radiograph, a complete history and physical examination and functional assessment are warranted.

Since osteoporosis is generally irreversible, all patients should be evaluated at least once to determine treatable causes. This can be accomplished by a fasting multichannel chemistry panel, complete blood count, thyroid panel, and urinalysis to check for sulfosalicylic acid precipitable protein. Further evaluations for diseases such as asymptomatic hyperparathyroidism should follow if an elevated serum calcium level is found. Neoplasia of several types can cause osteoporosis. Multiple myeloma, lymphoma, leukemia, or carcinoma may result in bone loss, particularly from the vertebral column, and this bone loss may occur without the presence of hypercalcemia. Since multiple myeloma is a disease that is prevalent among the aged, this diagnosis should be considered for elderly patients with compression fractures and anemia.

In the absence of clinically apparent fractures, conventional radiographs are not useful measurements of bone mass since 30% to 60% of the bone mineral must be lost before osteopenia can be detected. Nevertheless, conventional radiographs can provide other valuable information about the skeleton (e.g., compression fracture).

Over the past 2 decades, new methods have been developed to quantitate the amount of bone mass. These include single- and dual-energy photoabsorptiometry, dual-energy x-ray absorptiometry, quantitative computed tomography, and neutron activation analysis. Each of these methods is an improvement over previously available methods such as standard radiographs. Each method provides different information, and quality control during the measurement is essential. Measurements of bone mass are useful for both clinical practice and research studies.[3] For screening asymptomatic patients, these measurements are not warranted. However, the Scientific Advisory Board of the National Osteoporosis Foundation recently suggested the following four indications for bone mass measurements:

1. To diagnose significantly low bone mass in estrogen-deficient women and to make decisions about hormone replacement therapy
2. To diagnose spinal osteoporosis in patients with vertebral abnormalities or osteopenia that shows on their roentgenograms and to make decisions about further diagnostic evaluation and therapy
3. To determine low bone mass in patients who are receiving long-term glucocorticoid therapy and to adjust their therapy
4. To diagnose low bone mass in patients with asymptomatic primary hyperparathyroidism and to identify those who are at risk for severe skeletal disease and may be candidates for surgical intervention; bone biopsy and histomorphometrical studies are not routinely used

Intervention

Prevention. Prevention is the only cost-effective approach to osteoporosis. Unless there is a history of hypercalciuria or calcium-containing kidney stones, the calcium content of the diet should be increased to 1000 mg/day for young adults and 1200 mg/day for adolescents. Postmenopausal women should have a daily calcium intake of 1200 to 1500 mg.[1] Physical exercise should be encouraged, and cigarette smoking and heavy alcohol consumption should cease.

The decision for estrogen replacement should be made by the woman and her physician. Use of estrogen appears to be the most effective therapy to prevent postmenopausal bone loss in the vertebrae, wrists, and hips. Epidemiological evidence suggests that estrogen decreases the frequency of fractures for women.[7] A low dose of estrogen is effective; higher doses provide no additional benefits and increase complications and noncompliance. Estrogen should be initiated as soon as possible after menopause. Women who are postmenopausal by 10 to 15 years may benefit from estrogen therapy but not as much as if it was initiated in the perimenopausal period. It is unknown how long estrogens should be continued but at least 10 years is advised; some authorities suggest the therapy should be lifelong.

Although there are many benefits of estrogen therapy, there also are risks. Estrogens are associated with an increase in endometrial hyperplasia and uterine cancer, as well as more abnormal vaginal bleeding and breast enlargement and tenderness. (See Chapter 26.) Several recent metaanalyses investigated the risk of breast cancer associated with estrogen replacement therapy. One study concluded that postmenopausal estrogen in a conjugated dose of 0.625 mg/day is not associated with an increased risk of breast cancer.[2] Another study concluded that there is an increased risk of breast cancer with more than 5 years of estrogen replacement.[5] Patients with hypertension should be monitored. Estrogens also may increase the prevalence of gallstones and venous thrombosis.

An estrogen-treated woman who still has a uterus should receive a progestational agent. This agent can be given for 10 days each month and results in a menstrual period. Smaller doses can be given throughout the month, with the estrogen and spotting usually cease after several months. Any patient who receives hormone replacement therapy should have a uterine dilatation and curettage to investigate abnormal bleeding episodes. Use of progesterone decreases the incidence of hyperplasia and endometrial cancer. However, progestins may blunt some of the positive effects that estrogen has against cardiovascular disease. At present, no data suggest that progestational agents should be given to the estrogen-treated woman who has had a hysterectomy. Some authorities believe that once compression fractures have occurred, estrogen treatment is not useful in protecting bone mass, although this area necessitates further study.

Therapy. Currently, three drugs are approved by the Food and Drug Administration for the treatment of osteoporosis: (1) calcium, (2) estrogen, and (3) calcitonin. These drugs act by decreasing bone resorption. With these agents, bone mass can be maintained or the rate of bone loss decreased. These forms of therapy are most effective for patients with increased bone resorption, which occurs in approximately two thirds of patients with type I osteoporosis.

For patients who have osteoporosis, calcium therapy should be given daily in 3 to 4 divided doses of 1000 to 1500 mg of elemental calcium. Choices of the various forms that are available (e.g., carbonate, gluconate) should be guided by considerations of the cost (e.g., generic calcium carbonate is considerably less expensive than other alternatives) and of the patient's tolerance. The major contraindications to this therapy are hypercalcemia and nephrolithiasis. The absorption of calcium can be improved by adding 400 U of vitamin D to the regimen. No increased efficacy has been demonstrated for 1,25-dihydroxyvitamin D. For achlorhydric patients, calcium is better absorbed after meals. Once calcium and vitamin D treatment is initiated, serum and urine calcium levels should be monitored on an annual basis.

Calcitonin can prevent bone resorption, and some research has shown that calcitonin can relieve some of the associated pain of the disease. Recent studies suggest that calcitonin can prevent postmenopausal bone loss, so this therapy should be considered for women who must be made menopausal as part of the therapy for breast cancer. At the present time, the major drawback of calcitonin is that it must be given by injection. The use of a nasal spray to administer the drug may make this a more attractive form of therapy for perimenopausal patients for whom estrogens are contraindicated.

Recently, two clinical trials showed that the bisphosphonate etidronate, when given to postmenopausal women for 2 weeks and followed by 2½ months of calcium supplementation at 1000 mg daily, increased bone mass and reduced vertebral fracture rates.[6,7] The drug appears to act as an antiresorptive agent. The two clinical trials are ongoing. Etidronate is still under review by the Food and Drug Administration as a therapy for osteoporosis. No significant side effects are noted.

Exercise is another form of therapy for all types of osteoporosis. (See Chapter 21.) Although studies have shown that exercise can improve bone mass and patients' sense of well-being, no studies have shown that exercise reduces fracture rates. For patients with type II osteoporosis, preventing falls and other traumas may be as beneficial as therapy that is aimed at preventing further bone loss. Psychotropic medications are associated with increased risks for hip fractures.

Fluoride directly stimulates osteoblasts. In doses of 40 to 80 mg/day it can increase trabecular bone volume, but there is no effect on cortical bone. Fluoride has significant side effects such as nausea and gastric irritation, which occur in most patients. Approximately 10% of patients have lower-extremity pain, which can be from stress fractures or tendonitis. Some studies suggest that hip fractures are prevalent among patients receiving fluoride, while other studies do not show any prevalence. At present, sodium fluoride should be restricted for use in clinical trials.

OSTEOMALACIA

Clinical relevance and clinical manifestations

A second cause of osteopenia is osteomalacia, a syndrome of bone pain, myopathy, and fracture. Osteomalacia is characterized by impairment in the mineralization of remodeling bone. Patients with osteopenia caused by osteomalacia have increased bone pain in their backs and weight-bearing bones. There can be proximal muscle weaknesses, as well as bone fractures. Unless a clinician thinks of the diagnosis of osteomalacia and searches for its cause, the syndrome can go undiagnosed for years. When the diagnosis of osteomalacia is made, therapy can be instituted. Frequently the patient's condition can be improved with therapy, and sometimes the patient can be totally cured. Most of the causes of osteomalacia are deficiencies or abnormalities in vitamin D and/or phosphate metabolism.

The box on p. 414 lists causes of osteomalacia. Excluding patients with chronic renal failure, most older patients have an acquired form of osteomalacia, either from vitamin D deficiency or renal phosphate wasting. Vitamin D deficiency is uncommon

_____ **CAUSES OF OSTEOMALACIA** _____

Acquired forms of osteomalacia

Vitamin D deficiency
• Nutritional deficiency
• Malabsorption
• Hepatobiliary disease
Renal phosphate wasting
• Oncogenic osteomalacia
• Adult onset hypophosphatemic osteo-
  malacia
• Multiple myeloma
• Light chain nephropathy
• Renal phosphate wasting after renal
  transplantation
• Toxins
• Cadmium toxicity
• Outdated tetracycline

Drug-induced osteomalacia
• Phosphate-binding antacids
• Etidronate
• Sodium fluoride
• Phenytoin (with vitamin D deficiency)
• Aluminum (with chronic renal failure)
• Total parenteral nutrition
Chronic renal failure
• Osteomalacia
• Aluminum-induced osteomalacia

Inherited forms of osteomalacia

Renal phosphate wasting
• X-linked hypophosphatemic rickets
  (with osteomalacia)
• Fanconi's syndrome
• Renal tubular acidosis
Vitamin D disorders
• Vitamin D-dependent rickets
Miscellaneous forms of osteomalacia
• Axial osteomalacia

in the United States because of fortification of the diet with vitamin D; however, some recent studies suggest that housebound elderly people who have no dairy products in their diets and do not take multivitamins may have osteomalacia. Drugs can cause osteomalacia. Continual use of phosphate-binding antacids have caused osteomalacia in approximately a dozen reported cases. Patients do not absorb adequate amounts of phosphate from their diets because of the phosphate-binding antacids. The drug etidronate was first developed to treat Paget's disease of the bone. Now the drug is being used in several clinical trials for osteoporosis. Etidronate can cause osteomalacia when the drug is taken in doses of 10 mg/kg for longer than 6 months at a time. This drug inhibits mineralization when it is taken for prolonged periods and leads to osteomalacia. Sodium fluoride, another experimental agent for the treatment of osteoporosis, has been shown to cause osteomalacia. The anticonvulsant phenytoin can cause a low-turnover type of osteoporosis, and when patients who take this drug have vitamin D deficiencies, they also develop osteomalacia.

Diagnostic approach. The diagnosis of osteomalacia is made when it is considered in the differential diagnosis of osteopenia. Vitamin D deficiencies, phosphate losses, potential diseases, or drugs should be considered when a patient has bone pain, osteopenia, or skeletal fracture. If vitamin D deficiency is sought, measurement of serum levels of 25-dihydroxyvitamin D or calcifediol give an accurate measurement of vitamin D stores. Levels below 15 ng/ml in the United States show vitamin D deficiency, as long as there is not a loss of vitamin D-binding protein in the urine (e.g., nephrotic syndrome). In addition to low vitamin D levels, serum calcium, phosphorus, and alkaline phosphatase should be measured. Calcium levels are usually normal, phosphorus levels are usually low, and alkaline phosphatase levels are usually high. Parathyroid hormone levels should be measured to determine whether there is secondary hyperparathyroidism as a result of the vitamin D deficiency. If hypophosphatemia is found, a fasting serum phosphorus level should be repeated and the threshold for renal phosphate reabsorption should be determined. This is done by measuring the clearance of phosphate, divided by the clearance of creatinine, and can be completed by measuring a 2-hour fasting urine specimen, with serum creatinine and phosphorus levels drawn at the midpoint of the urine collection. Values below 2.5 mg/dl suggest renal phosphate wasting and should lead to searches for disorders that cause phosphate wasting.

A careful drug history and toxin screening can exclude drug-induced causes of osteomalacia. For patients with chronic renal failure who have or have not been receiving dialysis, osteomalacia should be considered as a cause of bone pain. Radiographs are useful for diagnosing osteomalacia, and they can show osteopenia. Areas associated with pain should be examined for pseudofractures or loosers zones, thin cortical radiolucent lines, or stress fractures at right angles to the bone shaft. They are often symmetrical and bilateral. If the diagnosis of oncogenic osteomalacia is considered, a thorough examination for tumor masses should be performed, including palpation of the skeleton, x-ray of the lung to exclude carcinoma, examination of the prostate to exclude prostate cancer, and x-ray of the sinus to exclude neoplasm.

To make the diagnosis of osteomalacia, a bone biopsy may be necessary. This is done by removing a piece of anterior iliac crest. The patient is generally under local anesthesia. To measure the mineral apposition rate prior to the biopsy, the patient receives 2 doses of 250 mg tetracycline at intervals that are separated by 10 to 14 days. The biopsy is obtained 3 days after the second dose of tetracycline. If vitamin D deficiency is the diagnosis that is being considered, this can be confirmed by low vitamin D levels and elevated serum parathyroid hormone levels; therefore, a biopsy is usually not necessary. However, when the disorders of renal phosphate wasting are being considered, as well as some of the more unusual types of osteomalacia such as those that are seen in inherited forms or in chronic renal failure, then a biopsy can provide valuable information about the extent of the disease and can serve as a baseline for therapy once it is initiated. For drug-induced osteomalacia, a biopsy is probably not necessary when phosphate-binding antacids, etidronate, phenytoin along with vitamin D deficiency, or sodium fluoride are the causes. However, aluminum-induced osteomalacia along with chronic renal failure, as well as osteomalacia from total parenteral nutrition, probably warrant a bone biopsy to document extent of disease.

Intervention

Treatment of osteomalacia depends on the underlying cause. When simple vitamin D deficiency is found, administration of vitamin D in the form of ergocalciferol, either orally or parenterally, effectively can replenish vitamin D stores in a short period of time. This can be 50,000 U of vitamin D given twice a week for 6 to 8 weeks. A 25-hydroxyvitamin D level should be repeated to confirm the efficacy of the replacement. Supplements of 400 U/day then can be used.

Patients with osteomalacia from uncorrectable renal phosphate wasting should take neutral or acid phosphate supplements, generally 1 to 2 g/day in 4 divided doses. Since phosphate supplementation can induce secondary hyperparathyroidism, it is necessary to use a form of vitamin D. Currently, calcitriol is the drug of choice. For the treatment of oncogenic osteomalacia, 1.5 μg of calcitriol is given in divided doses daily. Hypercalcemia and hypercalciuria must be closely monitored for patients with oncogenic osteomalacia. For drug-induced forms of osteomalacia, stopping the drug is generally an effective way to treat the osteomalacia. For patients receiving long-term phenytoin therapy, supplements of vitamin D (400 to 1000 U daily) are recommended. When oncogenic osteomalacia is diagnosed, cure is achieved only with resection of the underlying neoplasm. For unresectable neoplasms, treatment with oral phosphates and calcitriol (Rocaltrol) can significantly improve the patients' bone pains and normalize the bone biopsies so that these patients can become functional and perform normal daily activities.

REFERENCES

1. Dawson-Hughes B: Calcium supplementation and bone loss: a review of controlled clinical trials, *Am J Clin Nutr* 54:274S, 1991.
2. Dupont WD, Page DL: Therapy and breast cancer, *Arch Intern Med* 151:67, 1991.
3. Johnston CC Jr et al: Clinical indications for bone mass measurements, *J Bone Miner Res* 4(2):1, 1989.
4. Riggs BL, Melton LJ III: Involutional osteoporosis, *N Engl J Med* 314:1676, 1986.
5. Steinberg KK et al: A metaanalysis of the effect of estrogen replacement therapy on the risk of breast cancer, *JAMA* 17:265, 1991.
6. Storm T et al: Effect of intermittent cyclical etidronate therapy on bone mass and fracture rate in women with postmenopausal osteoporosis, *N Engl J Med* 322(18):1265, 1990.
7. Watts NB et al: Intermittent cyclical etidronate treatment of postmenopausal osteoporosis, *N Engl J Med* 323:73, 1990.

SUGGESTED READINGS

Dawson-Hughes B: Calcium supplementation and bone loss: a review of controlled clinical trials, *Am J Clin Nutr* 54:274, 1991.
Johnston CC Jr et al: Clinical indications for bone mass measurements, *J Bone Miner Res* 4(2):1, 1989.
Riggs BL, Melton LJ III: Involutional osteoporosis, *N Engl J Med* 314:1676, 1986.

_____

CHAPTER 43

Diabetes mellitus

LINDA A. MORROW
JEFFREY E. HALTER

KEY POINTS

- Diabetes mellitus affects 15% to 20% of individuals aged 65 years and older; fully one half of these cases are undiagnosed.
- Most diabetes in older people is the non–insulin-dependent type; however, insulin-dependent diabetes can occur at any age.
- Elderly people with diabetes mellitus are at risk for all of the long-term diabetes complications.
- Diabetes mellitus in elderly persons frequently persists with asymptomatic hyperglycemia or with a complication of diabetes.
- Initial assessment should focus on the presence of complications and the risk factors for complications.
- Goals for glycemic control should be either prevention of long-term complications (fasting serum glucose <140 mg/dl and mean serum glucose 110 to 140 mg/dl) or prevention of symptomatic hyperglycemia (mean serum glucose approximately 200 mg/dl).
- Patients should be encouraged to do blood glucose monitoring at home.

CLINICAL RELEVANCE

Carbohydrate metabolism is altered with age among different races and cultures. For older individuals without diabetes mellitus, fasting plasma glucose changes little with age (perhaps 1 to 2 mg/dl/decade after the age of 30), but postprandial glucose elevates 6 to 15 mg/dl/decade. These changes are considered to be within the normal range for older adults.

417

Large epidemiological studies in the United States have revealed a prevalence of diagnosed diabetes mellitus of at least 8% among individuals aged 65 to 74 years old. When the medical history was accompanied by oral glucose tolerance testing for individuals who had no history of diabetes, the prevalence of diabetes mellitus, based on currently accepted criteria as developed by the National Diabetes Data Group (NDDG), more than doubled to almost 20%.[4,9] Impaired glucose tolerance (defined by NDDG criteria) also increased with age, so nearly one half of individuals aged 65 years and older had abnormalities in carbohydrate metabolism that met the diagnostic criteria for either diabetes mellitus or impaired glucose tolerance.

Impaired glucose tolerance predisposes a person to the development of overt diabetes mellitus. For individuals aged 70 years and older with normal glucose tolerance, their risk of developing diabetes mellitus is .04% per year. The risk is at least 2% per year for older individuals who have glucose intolerance.[1]

CLINICAL MANIFESTATIONS

Diabetes mellitus may present as a health problem in a variety of ways. (See the box on p. 419.) After routine screenings are performed, many older individuals are found to have asymptomatic hyperglycemia. Other presenting symptoms of hyperglycemia are urinary frequency, nocturia, incontinence, as well as changes in the patient's vision. Other patients may have symptoms from long-term complications of diabetes mellitus such as cataracts, neuropathies, or myocardial infarctions when diabetes has not been previously recognized.

Impaired glucose tolerance

While patients with impaired glucose tolerance have no recognizable symptoms or signs, the condition is significant clinically for several reasons. Individuals with impaired glucose tolerance may have fasting blood sugars elevated above the normal range (but <140 mg/dl [7.8 mM]). These patients also may have evidence of associated coronary artery disease. Individuals with glucose intolerance may become markedly hyperglycemic during physiological stress from, for example, a systemic infection or myocardial infarction.

Acute hyperglycemia

The clinical presentation of diabetes mellitus in older adults includes two life-threatening disorders that are associated with extreme elevations in plasma glucose: (1) diabetic ketoacidosis (DKA), and (2) hyperglycemic hyperosmolar nonketotic coma (HHNC). Although only a small percentage of older adults with diabetes mellitus have insulin-dependent diabetes mellitus, DKA can be the initial presenting symptom. For those individuals who develop HHNC, up to two thirds have not had a previous diagnosis of diabetes mellitus.

CLINICAL PRESENTATION OF
DIABETES MELLITUS IN ELDERLY PERSONS

General symptoms

Weight loss
Malaise
Weakness
Confusion
Fatigue
Falls

Symptoms secondary to hyperglycemia

Altered mental status
Visual blurring
Thirst
Urinary symptoms: frequency, nocturia,
    incontinence

**Symptoms and signs secondary to
complications**

Central nervous system
• Stroke
• Dementia
• Transient ischemic attack
Ophthalmological
• Visual blurring
• Visual field deficits
• Flashing lights
• Blindness

Cardiovascular
• Angina pectoris
• Congestive heart failure
• Dysrhythmia
• Dyspnea with exertion
• Peripheral edema
• Claudication
• Ischemic ulcers
Renal
• Renal failure
• Proteinuria
• Peripheral edema
Peripheral and autonomic nervous system
• Orthostatic hypotension
• Gastrointestinal symptoms: vomiting,
  diarrhea, constipation, fecal incontinence
• Genitourinary symptoms: urinary incontinence, urinary retention, impotence
• Peripheral neuropathy with pain,
  numbness, or dysesthesias in the extremities
• Mononeuropathy
• Charcot joint
• Lower extremity ulceration

Both DKA and HHNC have mortality rates that approach 50% among elderly persons. DKA, a rare illness among elderly persons, has presenting symptoms that are typical of those seen among younger adults. However, HHNC occurs almost solely in individuals who are more than 50 years old. The typical patient is nearly 70 years of age and has an underlying illness that either interferes with the patient's access to oral fluids or enhances dehydration. HHNC usually develops slowly over several days, and all of the patients are markedly dehydrated. The primary management of HHNC is hospitalization and volume replacement.

Chronic complications

Older adults with diabetes mellitus are subject to all of the complications, both macrovascular and microvascular, that are observed in younger patients with diabetes. The complications of diabetes are responsible for substantial morbidity and mortality.

Macrovascular disease is manifested as cerebrovascular, cardiovascular, or peripheral vascular disease. Stroke occurs almost twice as frequently in those individuals aged 65 to 74 years old with diabetes, compared to those in the same age range without diabetes, and stroke is associated with higher morbidity and mortality.

The risk for cardiovascular disease for older diabetics is double that of older nondiabetics. Following myocardial infarctions, the mortality rates for diabetic patients exceed those of nondiabetic patients. Particularly for women with diabetes, the risk of their dying is more than twice that of nondiabetic women. While silent myocardial infarction is considered to be common among diabetic individuals, recent studies show that chest pain is still the most common presenting symptom of myocardial infarction in diabetic elderly patients who are admitted to the hospital.[3] In addition to silent myocardial infarction, silent ischemia occurs frequently in diabetic patients. While diabetic patients without severe neuropathy can have silent ischemia, patients with autonomic neuropathy may be at greater risk.[8]

The risk of lower-extremity amputation for diabetic patients aged 65 years and older is greater than 10 times that of nondiabetics of the same age. In addition, age increases the risk for amputation among diabetic patients. Diabetic individuals aged 65 years or older have seven times the risk of amputation than that of diabetic individuals who are less than 45 years old.[6] Major risk factors for amputation include peripheral vascular disease and peripheral neuropathy. Other risk factors are those typically associated with the development of peripheral vascular disease, including hypertension, hypercholesterolemia, cigarette smoking, and infection.

Ophthalmic disease as a complication of diabetes is responsible for a significant proportion of blindness in elderly people. Approximately 3% of patients aged 65 years and older with non-insulin-dependent diabetes mellitus (NIDDM) are legally blind.[5] While retinopathy (both proliferative and nonproliferative) occurs in up to 40% of diabetics over the age of 60 who do not use insulin (prevalence is higher among insulin users), cataracts are the most common causes of visual impairments among the older population with diabetes. Glaucoma, which appears to occur more frequently among older adults with diabetes than among those without diabetes, and macular degeneration, an age-associated disease, also contribute substantially to loss of vision.

While the risks of diabetic nephropathy and subsequent renal failure have long been recognized for individuals with insulin-dependent diabetes, only recent studies have revealed that the risks for those with non–insulin-dependent diabetes are similar. The prevalence of end-stage renal disease in NIDDM increases with age, and most individuals with diabetes who develop end-stage renal disease are, in fact, elderly patients with NIDDM.[7]

Diabetic neuropathy manifests in both younger and older diabetic patients as distal symmetrical polyneuropathy, mononeuropathy, or autonomic neuropathy. The prevalence of neuropathy appears to increase with age, but the additional risk for older diabetics has not been clearly defined. Diabetic neuropathy can interact with age-related sensory impairments, thereby magnifying the clinical importance. For example, sensory neuropathy can have particular impact on an older patient with significant hearing or visual impairment. One neuropathic syndrome, diabetic neuropathic cachexia, occurs most frequently in older men. These individuals have severely painful extremities and marked weight loss but may have mild diabetes and only minimal evidence of distal symmetrical polyneuropathy. The disorder is usually self-limited, with the pain and weight loss resolving within months.

DIAGNOSTIC APPROACH

Diagnostic criteria

Despite changes in carbohydrate tolerance that occur as part of normal aging, the diagnostic criteria for diabetes in elderly persons are the same as those for younger adults. The diagnosis of diabetes is made based on the following three criteria:

1. Random hyperglycemia >200 mg/dl (11.1 mM) with the classic symptoms of diabetes mellitus (polyuria, polydipsia, polyphagia, and weight loss)
2. Fasting hyperglycemia >140 mg/dl (7.8 mM) on at least two occasions
3. Two oral glucose tolerance tests that meet diagnostic criteria for diabetes mellitus

The best screening for diabetes mellitus is a fasting serum glucose. This test is inexpensive and easy to perform. However, when a fasting serum glucose level is inconvenient to obtain in the office, a random serum glucose can be a useful if not diagnostic alternative. Any random serum glucose >120 mg/dl (6.7 mM) should be followed up by a fasting serum glucose. The oral glucose tolerance test (OGTT) is not a good screening test for diabetes because the results can be affected by a variety of factors, including diet, intercurrent illness, and medications. Because of the variability of the OGTT, abnormal results on two OGTTs are required to establish the diagnosis. The OGTT should be reserved for those patients with fasting plasma glucose between 115 mg/dl (6.4 mM) and 140 mg/dl (7.8 mM) and those patients for whom the approach to management will change because their results meet the diagnostic criteria for diabetes. Although not recommended by everyone, screening for diabetes mellitus with a fasting or random serum glucose should be performed on an annual basis for all patients aged 65 years and older. (See Chapter 22.)

The terminology to describe the types of diabetes can be confusing. The terms *insulin-dependent* (or type I) and *non–insulin-dependent* diabetes (or type II) should be used to describe clinical syndromes for which insulin is either required or not required to prevent ketoacidosis. Many individuals are treated with insulin to control their blood sugar but do not develop ketoacidosis if insulin is withdrawn. These individuals are properly described as having non–insulin-dependent diabetes. The terms *juvenile-onset* and *adult-onset* diabetes have been discarded because it is clear that older adults can develop insulin-dependent diabetes. About 5% of older adults with newly diag-

INITIAL EVALUATION OF ELDERLY DIABETIC PATIENTS

Complete history with special emphasis on the following:

Symptoms and complications of diabetes
(See the box on p. 419.)
Date of onset of symptoms
Current diet
Exercise habits
Weight changes
Medications
Risk factors for atherosclerosis
Tuberculin and immunization status

Complete physical examination with special attention to:

Complications of diabetes, especially changes in vision (refer to ophthalmologist for baseline reference and future management)
Feet

Skin
Arterial circulation
Neurological deficits

Multidimensional assessment

Activities of daily living
Instrumental activities of daily living
Cognitive function
Psychosocial and environmental factors

Laboratory

Fasting serum glucose
Glycosylated hemoglobin or fructosamine
Fasting lipid profile
Urinalysis
Electrocardiogram

nosed diabetes have insulin-dependent diabetes. There are also some older adults who initially appear to have non–insulin-dependent diabetes mellitus and subsequently become insulin-dependent. In general, elderly individuals who have ketosis will require insulin for treatment, although a small number will be managed with oral hypoglycemic agents following initial therapy with insulin.

Initial evaluation of elderly diabetics

The American Diabetes Association recently published guidelines for the care of diabetic patients.[2] With only slight modifications, the guidelines can be used by physicians for the treatment of most elderly patients. The above box summarizes the evaluation that is recommended for elderly diabetic patients.

INTERVENTION

Treatment goals

In general, treatment goals for older adults with diabetes should be directed toward the signs and symptoms that directly relate to hyperglycemia and toward the prevention of chronic complications from diabetes. Uncontrolled diabetes may exacerbate other medical illnesses that are common in older adults and may precipitate common geriatric syndromes such as incontinence and falls. A strong argument can be made for the treatment of symptomatic hyperglycemia in any geriatric patient. The degree

TREATMENT FOR OLDER ADULTS WITH DIABETES

Basic care

Goals

- Prevent symptomatic hyperglycemia (average serum glucose <200 mg/dl [11.1 mM] and no glycosuria)
- Maintain patient's comfort and minimize intercurrent illness
- Detect and treat complications of diabetes early
- Prevent hypoglycemia

Assessment

- Screening for diabetes complications
- Screening Geriatric assessment
- Risk factors (hypertension, smoking, hypercholesterolemia)
- Immunization and tuberculin statuses

Management

- Basic diabetes education
- Ad-lib diet or no concentrated sweets
- Exercise as tolerated
- Oral hypoglycemic agents or insulin, as required to meet goals for glycemic control
- Monitor by intermittent random blood glucose to assess level of glycemia and need for modification of therapy (3 times/wk and less frequently when patient is stable)
- Annual visit and complete physical examination, including feet, eyes, and teeth; assess urinary protein and update immunizations

Aggressive care (additions to basic care)

Goals

- Maintain near-normal glycemia (fasting blood or serum glucose between 115-140 mg/dl [6.4-7.8 mM]; postprandial <180 mg/dl [10 mM])
- Prevent complications of diabetes mellitus

Management

- Early and in-depth education about all aspects of diabetes
- Low-fat high-carbohydrate diet (± caloric restrictions as indicated)
- Regular aerobic exercise at least 3 times/week if tolerated
- Oral hypoglycemic agents or insulin, as required to maintain near-normal glucose levels
- Monitor blood glucose at home frequently with intensive monitoring [4 times/day]) for newly diagnosed patients and for those on new treatment regimens; monitoring may be less frequent as glycemia stabilizes

of hyperglycemia that is associated with symptoms may vary among individuals because of their different renal thresholds for glycosuria. In general, consistently elevated random blood sugar >200 mg/dl (11.1 mM) should be considered as an indication for active intervention for any older adult with diabetes, even one who has a short life expectancy. While some arguments remain regarding the efficacy of tight diabetes control to prevent long-term complications, it seems prudent to recommend more stringent control for the youngest and healthiest of the elderly diabetic patients who have life expectancies of more than 10 years. Ongoing clinical trials may provide more definitive answers regarding this issue.

Treatment goals for geriatric patients are divided into basic care and aggressive care. The above box outlines treatment goals and recommended management for both categories.

Therapeutic interventions

There are four standard modalities of treatment: (1) diet, (2) exercise, (3) oral hypoglycemic agents, and (4) insulin. Most patients are treated with some combination of these, either diet, exercise, and oral hypoglycemic agents or diet, exercise, and insulin. The choice of therapy is dependent upon glycemic goals. In essence, therapy is modified (usually with the addition of oral hypoglycemic insulin) until the glycemic goal is attained.

Diet. Most patients with NIDDM should be considered for a trial of dietary management before pharmacological agents are used. The American Diabetes Association recommends a diet for diabetic patients that contains 50% to 60% carbohydrates, 20% proteins, and less than 30% fats. In addition, the fat content should be less than 10% saturated fat. Caloric restriction is important to individuals for whom weight loss is a treatment goal, but weight loss may be difficult for older adults. (See Chapter 45.) While one study shows that dietary therapy leads to weight loss and improved glycemic control for elderly diabetic patients,[10] dietary therapy alone is frequently unsuccessful for restoring normoglycemia in both older and younger patients. The best diet for an older diabetic is not only one that limits fat or excess calories and provides adequate nutrition, but also is one that can be successfully followed.

Exercise. While exercise has been well documented to improve glucose tolerance in both diabetic and nondiabetic individuals, the effectiveness that exercise has in lowering plasma glucose is unclear. In addition, the benefits of exercise disappear rapidly (within days to weeks) after patients discontinue their exercise programs. Elderly patients are frequently unable to exercise because of other medical illnesses such as arthritis, peripheral vascular disease, and pulmonary or cardiovascular disease. A recent study found that more than 80% of newly diagnosed older men with diabetes were unable to participate in regular training programs because of other medical illnesses or treatments.[12] Certainly the cardiovascular benefits that accompany exercise make it an important addition to the overall regimen for any older individual with diabetes who is physically able to exercise. (See Chapter 21.)

Oral hypoglycemic agents. Oral hypoglycemic agents, specifically the sulfonylureas, have been important additions to the therapeutic armamentarium for older individuals with diabetes. More than 70% of the prescriptions written by office-based physicians for sulfonylureas are written for patients who are over the age of 60. The ease of administration and once- or twice-daily doses have made these drugs the usual first line of therapy for individuals with NIDDM who have failed diet therapy alone or diet and exercise therapy. Table 43-1 describes the six oral agents on the market in the United States, as well as their dosage schedules and durations of action.

The major risk of sulfonylurea therapy is hypoglycemia, and older patients appear to be at greater risk than younger patients. There is evidence that long-acting sulfonylureas may be responsible for more episodes of hypoglycemia than the short-acting ones, but long-acting sulfonylureas have been more widely prescribed. Risk

Table 43-1 Oral hypoglycemic agents

Drug	Duration of action (hours)	Recommended starting dose (mg)	Daily dose range (mg)
Tolbutamide (Orinase)	6-12	500	500-3000
Acetohexamide (Dymelor)	12-18	250	250-1500
Tolazamide (Tolinase)	12-16	100	100-1000
Chlorpropamide (Diabinese)	40-72	100-125	100-500
Glipizide (Glucotrol)	8-12	2.5	2.5-40
Glyburide (DiaBeta, Micronase)	24	1.25	1.25-20

factors for hypoglycemia that potentiate the effects of oral hypoglycemic agents include abnormalities in hepatic and renal functions, which interfere with drug metabolism and clearance, and drug interactions, which lead to decreased protein binding (salicylates, warfarins, sulfonamides) or competition for metabolic enzymes (monoamine oxidase inhibitors). Another risk associated with the use of oral hypoglycemic agents is hyponatremia (primarily with chlorpropamide, although all the agents have been implicated), particularly when hypoglycemic agents are combined with thiazide diuretics.

Insulin. When treatment goals for glycemic control have not been achieved with other modalities, insulin therapy should be instituted. While many practitioners have reservations about insulin therapy for older adults, there are no studies indicating that older patients cannot safely and effectively use insulin. Insulin is relatively inexpensive, even when the cost of frequent blood glucose monitoring is added. A single daily dose of long-acting insulin may be appropriate for elderly patients for whom the goal of treatment is the prevention of symptomatic hyperglycemia. However, a split-mixed regimen (multiple doses of short- and long-acting insulin) may be required to achieve more normal levels of glycemia. As necessary, insulin should be administered to achieve treatment goals.

There are special considerations for prescribing insulin to elderly diabetic patients. The patients or caregivers must be able to provide both medications and meals on a regular schedule. Insulin must be drawn up and administered properly. Home monitoring of blood glucose is essential for patients who take insulin. Thus, either the patients or caregivers must be able to monitor blood glucose competently.

Follow-up care

Older patients with diabetes are seen frequently for follow-up visits in the outpatient setting. The routine visit should include a brief history, review of therapy (diet, exercise, and medication) and glucose diary, search for symptoms of hypoglycemia, and search for any other symptoms of diabetic complications. The routine examination should include measurements of weight and blood pressure, an examination of the feet, and an examination directed toward any specific complaints. Routine laboratory assessments are not indicated necessarily, particularly if the patients are performing home monitoring of blood glucose. However, the reliability of these measurements should be checked in the physicians' offices, with the patients performing the tests on their own machines. When glucose diaries are not available, fasting blood glucose or glycosylated hemoglobin or fructosamine may provide information to assess the efficacy of treatment. Older patients with diabetes should have in-depth evaluations as previously described (See the box on p. 422.) and preventive health care on an *annual basis*. (See Chapter 22.)

Monitoring is an important part of ongoing care of diabetic patients. Most older patients with diabetes should be taught home monitoring of blood glucose and should be encouraged to monitor their blood glucose as frequently as necessary to meet treatment goals. They also should be taught to monitor during times of illness or decreased oral intake. They also should be encouraged to maintain blood glucose diaries. Monitoring urine glucose has a less important role in the ongoing care of diabetics since such monitoring is unreliable and may provide misleading information. Simple and relatively inexpensive glucometers are now widely available.

Hypoglycemia is a risk for any patients who are treated with oral hypoglycemic agents or insulin, and elderly patients may be less tolerant of hypoglycemia than are younger patients. Older adults, subject to impaired drug metabolism and excretion, are at substantial risk for the development of hypoglycemia.[11] Symptoms of hypoglycemia in elderly patients are shakiness, diaphoresis, hunger, and weakness, but hypoglycemia also may present as disorientation, confusion, or coma. While glucose is clearly the treatment for any acute episode of hypoglycemia, prevention is the key to limiting morbidity and mortality. The risk of hypoglycemia can be reduced in several ways. The first is through blood glucose monitoring to ensure that treatment is adequate and that fasting glucose levels are >100 mg/dl (5.6 mM). An occasional 2 AM or 3 AM blood glucose may provide valuable information and help to prevent nocturnal hypoglycemia. Education of patients is another means for reducing their risks of hypoglycemia. The patients and their caregivers must understand the importance of regular meals and medication, as well as the danger of missed meals. Patients and caregivers also should be educated regarding the symptoms of hypoglycemia and its treatment. A third approach to reducing the risk of hypoglycemia is using the patients' social networks to maintain frequent (at least daily) contact with elderly diabetic patients who live alone.

REFERENCES

1. Agner E, Thorsteinsson B, Eriksen M: Impaired glucose tolerance and diabetes mellitus in elderly subjects, *Diabetes Care* 5(6):600, 1982.
2. American Diabetes Association: Standards of medical care for patients with diabetes mellitus, *Diabetes Care* 12(5)365, 1989.

3. Day J et al: Myocardial infarction in old people: the influence of diabetes mellitus, *J Am Geriatr Soc* 36(9):791, 1988.
4. Harris MI et al: Prevalence of diabetes and impaired glucose tolerance and plasma glucose levels in the U.S. population aged 20-74 years, *Diabetes* 36:523, 1987.
5. Herman WH: Eye disease and nephropathy in NIDDM, *Diabetes Care* 13(suppl 2):24, 1990.
6. Herman WH, Teutsch SM, Geiss LS: Closing the gap: the problem of diabetes mellitus in the United States, *Diabetes Care* 8(4):391, 1985.
7. Humphrey LL, Ballard DJ: Renal complications in non–insulin-independent diabetes mellitus, *Clin Geriatr Med* 6(4):807, 1990.
8. Murray DP et al: Autonomic dysfunction and silent myocardial ischemia on exercise testing in diabetes mellitus, *Diabetic Med* 7(7):580, 1990.
9. National Diabetes Data Group: Classification and diagnosis of diabetes mellitus and other categories of glucose intolerance, *Diabetes* 28:1039, 1979.
10. Reaven GM: Beneficial effect of moderate weight loss in older patients with non–insulin-dependent diabetes mellitus poorly controlled with insulin, *J Am Geriatr Soc* 33(2):93, 1985.
11. Seltzer HS: Severe drug-induced hypoglycemia: a review, *Compr Ther* 5:21, 1979.
12. Skarfors ET et al: Physical training as treatment for type II (non–insulin-dependent) diabetes in elderly men: a feasibility study over 2 years, *Diabetologia* 30(12):930, 1987.

SUGGESTED READINGS

Froom J: *Diabetes mellitus in the elderly, Clin Geriatr Med* 6(4):693, 1990.
Halter JB, Christensen NJ: Diabetes mellitus in elderly people, *Diabetes Care* 13(suppl 2):1, 1990.
Morrow LA, Halter JB: Carbohydrate metabolism in the elderly. In Sowers JR, Felicetta JV, eds: *The endocrinology of aging*, New York, 1988, Raven Press.

CHAPTER 44

Thyroid disorders

DAVID B. REUBEN

KEY POINTS

- Screening for hypothyroidism or hyperthyroidism is not cost effective in general populations of older persons; the value of case findings in this age group is controversial.
- The most common clinical manifestations of thyrotoxicosis in older persons are weight loss and nonspecific failure to thrive.
- In older persons with thyrotoxicosis, tachycardia is less common and atrial fibrillation is more common compared with younger persons who have thyrotoxicosis.
- Hypothyroidism may be *overt* or *subclinical*, depending on the presence of typical clinical findings and abnormalities of thyroid function tests.
- Treatment of hypothyroidism for older persons requires lower doses of thyroxine compared with those doses required for younger persons.
- The sensitive thyroid-stimulating hormone (STSH) is the best test for monitoring thyroid replacement and thyroid suppression therapy.
- The evaluation of a solitary thyroid nodule in euthyroid patients should begin with a fine-needle aspiration biopsy.

CLINICAL RELEVANCE

Thyroid diseases deserve special consideration when physicians care for older persons because of the increased frequency of disease (hypothyroidism and thyroid nodules) and the altered presentation of disease (hyperthyroidism and hypothyroidism). The diagnosis and management of thyroid disorders occur primarily in ambulatory settings for several reasons. First, only rarely do thyroid disorders cause clinical symptoms that are acute or severe enough to warrant hospitalization. Second, the treatment of nearly all of these disorders can occur in the ambulatory setting. Finally, testing in ambulatory settings may be preferable because non-thyroidal acute illnesses that precipitate or occur during hospitalization may confound the interpretation of thyroid function tests.

Hyperthyroidism

Hyperthyroidism in older persons probably occurs at approximately the same rate as in younger persons. Data from population surveys indicate that the incidence of unsuspected cases of overt thyrotoxicosis ranges from 2 to 20 cases/1000 persons.[6] Although Graves' disease remains the most common cause of hyperthyroidism among older persons, toxic multinodular and uninodular goiter assume increased importance. Among the less frequent causes of hyperthyroidism in older adults include TSH-producing pituitary tumors, metastatic thyroid follicular carcinoma, iodine-induced hypothyroidism, subacute lymphocytic and radiation thyroiditis, prior treatment for Hodgkin's disease, medications (e.g., amiodarone), and exogenous hyperthyroidism (due to thyroid overreplacement)—the latter is particularly important.

Hypothyroidism

Hypothyroidism occurs more commonly in older persons and affects women two to five times more often than men. The terms *overt* and *subclinical* have been used to describe hypothyroid patients. The latter refers to those who have elevated thyrotropin (thyroid-stimulating hormone [TSH]) and normal thyroxine levels. Patients with overt hypothyroidism may be subclassified as those who have elevated TSH and low thyroxine levels but do not have identifiable symptoms, and those who have these biochemical abnormalities and clinical manifestations that are attributed to diminished thyroid hormone. The reported incidence of unsuspected overt hypothyroidism among older persons ranges from 0 to 7/1000 men and from 3 to 18/1000 women.[6] The definition of subclinical hypothyroidism has varied among studies and the reported prevalence of this disorder ranges from 1% to over 10% depending on the threshold of TSH used to establish the diagnosis. Hypothyroidism is usually due to primary diseases of the thyroid, especially autoimmune thyroiditis, but also commonly results from treatment of Graves' disease, especially when it is treated with iodine-131. Treatment of Hodgkin's disease with radiation recently has been associated with high rates (44% by 25 years) of overt or subclinical hypothyroidism, most commonly identified during the second and third years after treatment.[5] Occasionally, medications, especially lithium, amiodarone, and iodine, may cause hypothyroidism. Less common causes of hypothyroidism include iodine deficiency and secondary to hypopituitarism and hypothalmic failure.

Thyroid nodules

The prevalence of thyroid nodules increases linearly with age, with thyroid nodules occurring in approximately 5% of persons who are 60 years of age or older. As with other thyroid diseases, the prevalence of thyroid nodules in women far exceeds the prevalence of thyroid nodules in men. Prior exposure to ionizing radiation is associated with the increased prevalence of both benign and malignant nodules. The majority of nodules (80-90%) are benign. Nevertheless, the incidence of thyroid cancer has been increasing steadily over the last half century, with age-adjusted incidence rates exceeding 5/100,000/yr. Thyroid carcinomas are usually epithelial in origin and these are classified as follicular, papillary, medullary, and undifferentiated (anaplastic). Of these carcinomas, papillary cancer is most common and represents 40% to 70% of all thyroid malignancies in those patients aged 65 years and older. Papillary cancer is associated with a poorer prognosis for persons aged 65 years or older compared with the prognosis for younger persons. Similarly, follicular carcinoma that occurs in older persons, which accounts for approximately 15% to 20% of thyroid cancers, tends to be more aggressive and invasive compared with follicular carcinoma that occurs in younger persons. Anaplastic cancers, which are rapidly invasive and carry a poor prognosis, are also more common among older persons. The so-called small cell cancer of the thyroid is not of epithelial origin; however, it is more accurately classified as malignant lymphoma. Rarely, thyroid cancer may be metastatic from other organs.

Table 44-1   Symptoms attributable to thyrotoxicosis in young and old patients

	Old-old	Young-old	Young
Number	25	85	247
Mean age (yrs)	81.5	68.6	40.0
Range (yrs)	79-95	60-82	5-73
Symptoms (%)			
No symptoms	8	—	—
Weight loss	44	35	85
Palpitations	36	42	89
Weakness	32	28	70
Dizziness, syncope	20	—	—
Nervousness	20	38	99
Memory loss	8	—	—
Tremor	8	—	—
Local symptoms	8	11	—
Pruritus	4	4	—
Heat intolerance	4	63	89

Modified from Tibaldi JM et al: Thyrotoxicosis in the very old, *Am J Med* 81:620, 1986. (Reprinted with permission.)

Table 44-2 Clinical findings attributable to thyrotoxicosis in young and old patients

	Old-old	Young-old	Young
Number	25	85	247
Mean age (yrs)	81.5	68.6	40.0
Range (yrs)	79-95	60-82	5-73
Physical signs (%)			
None	8	—	—
Pulse >100	28	58	100
Atrial fibrillation	32	39	10
New onset atrial fibrillation	20	—	—
Lid lag	12	35	71
Exophthalmos	8	8	—
Fine skin	40	81	97
Tremor	36	89	97
Myopathy	8	39	—
Hyperactive reflexes	24	26	—
Gynecomastia	1	1	10
Thyroid (%)			
Impalpable or normal	68	37	—
Diffusely enlarged	12	22	100
Multinodular goiter	12	20	—
Isolated nodule	8	21	—

Modified from Tibaldi JM et al: Thyrotoxicosis in the very old, *Am J Med* 81:620, 1986. (Reprinted with permission.)

CLINICAL MANIFESTATIONS

Hyperthyroidism

Presenting symptoms of hyperthyroidism in older persons tend to be cardiovascular, gastrointestinal, psychiatric, or neuromuscular. Table 44-1 compares symptoms among thyrotoxic patients of three different age groups.[10] Of importance are the weight loss and nonspecific symptoms, often termed *failure to thrive*. Clinical findings also differ between age groups, especially the presence of atrial fibrillation (Table 44-2) and lower frequency of sinus tachycardia in hyperthyroid persons who are 75 to 95 years of age. In two studies of elderly patients with Graves' disease, the prevalence of goiter has been highly variable, ranging from 14% to 73%.[7,10]

Hypothyroidism

Hypothyroidism in elderly persons frequently presents with clinical manifestations that are different from those occurring in younger persons. In one large study, less than half of the patients had any clinically recognized signs of hypothyroidism. More often, the nonspecific presenting symptoms are fatigue, lethargy, depression, and constipation. Not only are these symptoms common among the older population, these symptoms are no more common in older women who have TSH levels >10 mU/L compared with those women who have TSH levels <10 mU/L. Concern has been raised that subclinical hypothyroidism may be a risk factor for coronary artery disease. One study demonstrated unfavorable low-density and high-density lipoprotein-cholesterol levels among persons who had subclinical hypothyroidism and were compared with controls who were matched for age, sex, and body mass index.[1]

Thyroid nodules

Most thyroid nodules are asymptomatic and are discovered through routine physical examinations. Less commonly, hemorrhage into a benign or malignant nodule may cause sudden swelling, painfulness, or tenderness of the gland. Compressive symptoms such as an abnormal sensation when the patient swallows more often accompany diffuse or multinodular goiters than solitary nodules. Tracheal obstruction, dysphagia, and hoarseness may occur with either multinodular goiter or thyroid carcinoma, and these symptoms are not valuable in distinguishing benign and malignant diseases. Anaplastic carcinomas and lymphomas tend to be rapidly enlarging thyroid masses, which are often rock hard. However, physical examination generally is not reliable in distinguishing benign and malignant thyroid masses.

DIAGNOSTIC APPROACH

The sensitive thyroid-stimulating hormone (STSH) is an accurate test for identifying older persons with both hyperthyroidism and hypothyroidism. However, questions about the cost-effectiveness of STSH screening and case finding, as well as the use of STSH as the initial diagnostic test have been raised, particularly questions regarding the benefits of early diagnosis on patients' outcomes.

The choice of which initial test to use to investigate possible hyperthyroidism or hypothyroidism remains controversial. Many physicians currently begin with a sensitive thyrotropin test, although a strategy that begins with measurement of total thyroxine (T_4) appears to be more cost effective.[3,6] However, the sensitivity and specificity of the STSH (95% and 92%, respectively) are better than those of total T_4 (76% and 90%, respectively) or free thyroxine index (FT$_4$I [78% and 93%, respectively]). Costs of thyroid function tests may differ between institutions and may influence the preferred order of diagnostic tests.

The interpretation of thyroid function tests may be clouded by the effects of diseases and medications (e.g., the euthyroid sick syndrome (ESS), which includes the low-T_3 syndrome, low-T_4-and-T_3 syndrome, and high-T_4 syndrome). Although these syndromes do not signify abnormal thyroid status, they may mislead physicians and prompt unnecessary treatment. The *low-T_3 syndrome* is associated with congestive heart failure, diabetes mellitus, cirrhosis, renal failure, malnutrition, and febrile illness.

Drugs such as dexamethasone, propranolol, amiodarone, and propylthiouracil, may also cause this disorder. The basic disturbance is diminished extrathyroidal conversion of T_4 to T_3. Serum T_4 and TSH are usually normal as is the thyrotropin response to thyrotropin-releasing hormone (TRH). The *low-T_4-and-T_3 syndrome* is characteristically found in severely ill, often moribund, patients with a variety of systemic illnesses. As with the low-T_3 syndrome, serum TSH and TSH response to TRH are normal. The *high-T_4 syndrome* is seen in some patients who have acute psychiatric or medical (e.g., hepatic disease) illnesses or in patients who take estrogen or tamoxifen free. T_4 and FT_4I values are normal; serum T_3 and free T_3 may be low or normal.

Hyperthyroidism

The diagnosis of hyperthyroidism is usually established by an elevated T_4, FT_4I, *and* a low or undetectable STSH. Rarely, a serum T_3 level is necessary to establish the presence of T_3 toxicosis. However, the presence of a suppressed STSH alone is not suggestive of thyrotoxicosis.[4] Several studies have demonstrated that a minority (and perhaps a majority) of persons who have low STSH do not have thyrotoxicosis and will not develop the disorder during a 4-year-follow-up period. In the Framingham cohort, the most common cause of a low serum STSH was therapy with thyroid hormone.[9] Other causes of low STSH include central hypothyroidism, acute psychiatric illness, and medications, particularly glucocorticoids and dopamine. If T_4, FT_4I, *and* STSH are elevated, thyrotoxicosis that is induced by thyrotropin-producing tumors must be suspected.

Hypothyroidism

The diagnosis of hypothyroidism is made by the demonstration of low T_4 and FT_4I *and* high STSH level. Serum T_3 level is unnecessary. If the T_4 and FT_4I are low without an elevated STSH, the diagnosis of pituitary hypothyroidism is suggested. Conversely, STSH may be elevated in states other than hypothyroidism. For example, during the recovery phase of non-thyroidal illness, transient hypothyroxinemia may occur along with increased STSH response, both of which return to normal upon subsequent testing. Sensitive thyrotropin also may be elevated in states of generalized resistance to thyroid hormone.

Thyroid nodules

The presence of a difficult or multinodular goiter should be evaluated with thyroid function tests to exclude hyper- or hypothyroidism. Thyroid nodules should be evaluated to detect and treat possible thyroid malignancy. Radionuclide imaging has been used based on the presumption that "warm" or "hot" nodules are unlikely to be malignant. In one series, however, 9% of warm and 4% of hot nodules were malignant. Similarly, ultrasound cannot reliably distinguish malignant from benign nodules. As many as 12% of mixed solid and cystic lesions and 7% of cystic lesions are malignant.

Therefore, this evaluation is probably best approached by fine-needle aspiration or large-needle biopsy, by experienced physicians who can perform and interpret the biopsy accurately.

INTERVENTION

Hyperthyroidism

The treatment of hyperthyroidism for elderly persons is similar to that for younger persons. Graves' disease is usually treated with radioactive iodine, although hypothyroidism may occur in up to three fourths of these patients over the ensuing decade. Toxic multinodular goiter is especially resistant to radiotherapy and may be managed best with a surgical approach. Prior to definitive therapy, antithyroid drugs, either propylthiouracil or methimazole, are given to the patient to restore a euthyroid state and deplete the gland of hormone stores, thereby preventing the possibility of hyperthyroidism resulting from acute radiation-induced thyroiditis.

Hypothyroidism

For older patients, the treatment of hypothyroidism is different from the treatment of hypothyroidism for younger patients in that the replacement doses are likely to be lower because of age-related changes in the older patients' thyroid hormone disposal. Levothyroxine preparations should be used because of their long (1 week) half-lives, which provide stable blood levels, and because thyroxine permits peripheral tissues to generate triiodothyronine in a manner that stimulates normal physiology. Replacement therapy is begun at low doses (usually 0.025 mg/day). The dosage can be increased by 0.025 mg every 2 to 4 weeks, as needed, to reach full replacement dosages, which are usually in the 0.050 to 0.100 mg/day range. Full clinical recovery may take as long as 6 months, despite the return of serum thyroxine to normal and occasionally elevated levels. The STSH may remain elevated for up to a year and the optimal time to begin monitoring is uncertain; some experts have suggested 6-12 months.

Although the optimal frequency of monitoring patients who are receiving replacement therapy is unknown, some experts recommend yearly monitoring with STSH. If patients are asymptomatic (clinically euthyroid), a normal STSH requires no adjustments to the dosages. An undetectable TSH suggests that the patients[7] are overreplaced with thyroxine and the dosages should be reduced regardless of the T_4 or FT_4I levels. Conversely, elevations of STSH >10 mU/L imply undertreatment, presuming that the patients are compliant, and the dosages should be increased. The significance of mildly elevated STSH (6 to 10 mU/L) in patients who are being treated with thyroid replacement is uncertain.

Subclinical hypothyroidism

The management of subclinical hypothyroidism is controversial. If STSH levels >6 mU/L are used to define subclinical hypothyroidism, its progression to overt hypothyroidism is extremely rare when STSH levels are within the range of 6 to 10 mU/L. Studies of persons with subclinical hypothyroidism who have STSH levels >10 mU/L have demonstrated variable rates, ranging from 1% to 20%/yr, of progression to overt hypothyroidism. Higher values of STSH and high titers of antimicrosomal antibodies (>1:1600) appear to be predictive of this decline. Whether treatment of subclinical hypothyroidism is associated with clinical benefit is also uncertain. Trials of thyroxine treatment for subclinical hypothyroidism have not demonstrated benefits on serum cholesterol levels. Nevertheless, in one study, summary scores of nonspecific symptoms (e.g., dry skin, poor energy, easy fatigability) improved.[2] In another study, a minority of subjects stated that they "felt better" while they took the hormone, and a small percentage improved after neuropsychological testing was performed.[8]

Thyroid nodules

The treatment of thyroid nodules depends upon the pathology that is discovered in the diagnostic evaluation. Needle aspiration suffices for approximately half of the patients with thyroid cysts. Those patients who have nodules with blood or thick brown fluid or nodules that are larger than 4 cm, as well as patients who have postaspiration masses for which biopsies cannot be performed, should be considered for surgery. Treatment of thyroid cancer varies by cell type. Papillary and minimally invasive follicular carcinomas are usually managed surgically and followed by thyrotropin suppression with exogenous thyroxine. A single undetectable STSH predicts a suppressed response to TRH and undetectable TSH levels over a 24-hour period. Aggressive follicular carcinomas are treated with total or near-total thyroidectomy, followed by iodine-131 ablation. Medullary carcinoma is treated surgically and anaplastic carcinoma is approached with combination-modality therapy (surgery, radiotherapy, and chemotherapy.) At some centers, benign adenomas are excised because of the difficulty physicians have in distinguishing benign from malignant disease after fine-needle aspirations are performed. Hyperfunctioning (hot) nodules are often treated with iodine-131 if they are small (less than 3 cm) but usually are removed surgically if they are large.

REFERENCES

1. Althaus BU et al: LDL/HDL-changes in subclinical hypothyroidism: possible risk factors for coronary heart disease, *Clin Endocrinol* 28:157, 1988.
2. Cooper DS et al: L-Thyroxine therapy in subclinical hypothyroidism, *Ann Intern Med* 101:18, 1984.
3. de los Santos ET, Starich GH, Mazzaferri EL: Sensitivity, specificity, and cost-effectiveness of the sensitive thyrotropin assay in the diagnosis of thyroid disease in ambulatory patients, *Arch Intern Med* 149:526, 1989.

4. Ehrmann DA, Sarne DH: Serum thyrotropin and the assessment of thyroid status, *Ann Intern Med* 110:179, 1989.

5. Hancock SL, Cox RS, McDougal IR: Thyroid diseases after treatment of Hodgkin's disease, *N Engl J Med* 325:599, 1991.

6. Helfand M, Crapo LM: Screening for thyroid disease, *Ann Intern Med* 112:840, 1990.

7. Nordyke RA, Gilbert FI, Harada ASM: Graves' disease: influence of age on clinical findings, *Arch Intern Med* 148:626, 1988.

8. Nystrom E et al: A double-blind cross-over 12 month study of L-thyroxine treatment of women with "subclinical hypothyroidism". *Clinical Endocrinology* 29: 63-76, 1988.

9. Sawin CT et al: Low serum thyrotropin (thyroid-stimulating hormone) in older persons without hyperthyroidism, *Arch Intern Med* 151:165, 1991.

10. Tibaldi JM et al: Thyrotoxicosis in the very old, *Am J Med* 81:619, 1986.

SUGGESTED READINGS

Helfand M, Crapo LM: Monitoring therapy in patients taking levothyroxine, *Ann Intern Med* 113:450, 1990.

Mazzaferri EL, de los Santos ET, Rofagha-Keyhani SR: Solitary thyroid nodule: diagnosis and management, *Med Clin North Am* 72:1177, 1988.

Rojeski MT, Gharib H: Nodular thyroid disease, *N Engl J Med* 313:428, 1985.

Surks MI et al: American Thyroid Association guidelines for use of laboratory tests in thyroid disorders, *JAMA* 263:1529, 1990.

CHAPTER 45

Weight problems

JOHN E. MORLEY

KEY POINTS

- Weight loss is a more important problem than weight gain for older persons.
- Depression and medications are the most common treatable causes of weight loss in older persons.
- Unusual attitudes toward eating and body image are not rare among older persons and these attitudes can interfere with the management of weight problems.
- Metabolic causes of weight loss in older persons include hyperthyroidism, hyperparathyroidism, and pheochromocytoma.
- Early treatment of weight loss includes nutritional supplements and referrals to Meals On Wheels programs.
- Major indications for treatment of obesity for older persons are the presence of diabetes mellitus, hypertension, or osteoarthritis.
- Exercise and moderation in diet are the cornerstones of treatment for obesity.
- Aggressive treatments for obesity (e.g., drugs and surgery) should be avoided for older persons.

WEIGHT LOSS

Clinical relevance

Weight problems are extremely common among older persons and yet these problems are rarely adequately treated in the outpatient setting. In general, being underweight or losing weight is a greater problem with graver medical consequences for older persons than is being overweight. It is imperative that physicians pay careful attention to weight changes that occur in older patients between their outpatient visits. Early recognition and intervention in cases of weight loss are the best management strategies.

437

Protein energy malnutrition is an extremely common problem among older individuals. Approximately 16% of individuals between 65 and 75 years of age ingest less than 1000 Calories/day. This calorie intake is insufficient to maintain body weight or to ingest sufficient quantities of essential nutrients to meet the recommended daily allowances. The situation is even worse among minorities. Eighteen percent of older black Americans ingest less than 1000 Calories per day.

Despite the importance of protein energy malnutrition in older persons, few studies have emphasized its occurrence in the outpatient setting. Thompson and Morris[8] reported that only 45 out of 10,000 patients aged 63 years and older had billing diagnoses of "weight loss" and losses of at least 7.5% in their baseline body weights in a 6-month time period. This almost certainly represents an underdiagnosis of the problem. However, Miller et al[3] reported that 22% of outpatients more than 70 years of age in a Veterans Affairs hospital had some evidence of malnutrition. In this study they found that 100% of the physicians had failed to recognize the presence of a nutritional problem prior to their assessments of the patients. Other studies assessing the prevalence of malnutrition in the outpatient setting have failed to separate middle-aged from old persons. There are no data on health outcomes associated with malnutrition in the outpatient setting.

Malnutrition has been associated with a variety of other conditions, which are listed in the box below. For example, malnutrition clearly can lead to immune dysfunction with the development of T-cell defects and anergy. This in turn can predispose the patient to infections, including acute infections (e.g., urinary tract infection and pneumonia) and chronic infections (e.g., tuberculosis).

No studies have specifically examined the impact of malnutrition on activities of daily living (ADLs), but it would seem that the associated weakness would lead to a

---

EFFECTS OF PROTEIN ENERGY MALNUTRITION

Immune dysfunction	**Decreased cognition**
Anergy	
Infection	**Depression**
	Low serum albumin
Increased falls	Peripheral edema
Hip fracture	Increased drug toxicity
	Elevated ionized serum calcium
Poor wound healing	Increased drug-drug interactions
Postural hypotension	
Anemia	**Euthyroid sick syndrome**
Muscle weakness	**Male hypogonadism**
Fatigue	

Table 45-1   Early detection of persons at high risk for protein energy malnutrition

Parameter	Score*	
	1 point	**2 points**
Sadness	YGDS† 10-15	YGDS >15
Serum cholesterol	<180 mg/dl	<160 mg/dl
Serum albumin	<4 g/dl	<3.5 g/dl
Loss of weight	2 lb in 1 mo	6 lb in 6 mo
Eating problems	Either cognitive problems or physical limitations	Both cognitive problems and physical limitations
Shopping problems	Inability to shop for or prepare a meal	—

*Score of 3 or greater indicates major risks.
†Yesavage Geriatric Depression Scale.

decrease in all of the basic ADLs. One study has suggested a correlation of low body mass with instrumental activities of daily living (IADLs).[1]

Clinical manifestations

Numerous patients are at high risk for developing protein energy malnutrition. To allow early detection of persons who are at nutritional risk for protein energy malnutrition, a useful screening tool has been developed (Table 45-1). This screening tool also should allow the early implementation of preventive interventions.[4] Any score of 3 or greater puts the patient at major risk for developing protein energy malnutrition. While other nutritional screenings have been developed, they are generally nonspecific because they attempt to identify all persons with illnesses or impaired ADLs rather than specify those persons who are at nutritional risk. Both depressed and demented patients are likely to score high on this screening tool because of their generally low scores on food IADLs (i.e., ability to feed themselves, ability to shop for food, and ability to prepare food).[1]

The causes of protein energy malnutrition are multifaceted and generally can be remembered best in the outpatient setting by the mnemonic "Meals On Wheels." (See the box on p. 440.) In a more rigorous approach, Table 45-2 compares the causes of weight loss that are identified in three studies.[6-8] Only one of these studies was strictly a geriatric series but all three included predominantly older persons. The major point to be derived from these studies is that cancer is not the cause of weight loss in the majority of these patients.

From a pathophysiological perspective, anorexia and weight loss can be considered to be due to *social, psychological, medical,* and/or *age-related* causes.

Social causes. Human beings are social beings who, on the whole, tend to eat

MEALS ON WHEELS MNEMONIC FOR THE
CAUSES OF PROTEIN ENERGY MALNUTRITION

M—Medications
E—Emotional problems (depression)
A—Anorexia tardive
L—Late-life paranoia
S—Swallowing disorders

O—Oral problems
N—No money (poverty)

W—Wandering and other dementia-related behaviors
H—Hyperthyroidism, hyperparathyroidism
E—Entry problems (malabsorption)
E—Eating problems
L—Low-salt, low-cholesterol diet
S—Shopping and meal preparatory problems

more in social situations. Isolation therefore can play an important role in leading to decreased food intake. Social isolation also may cause depression, further aggravating the situation.

Certainly many older persons cannot shop for food or adequately prepare food. For anyone who experiences weight loss, these issues need to be carefully explored. Some older persons, particularly those living in the inner city, may have inadequate facilities to prepare food (e.g., a malfunctioning freezer). Poverty is also a major factor in producing decreased food intake. This is particularly important when an older person on a fixed income is prescribed an expensive medication and needs to choose between buying food and adhering to the physician's instructions. The patient's level of education also has been related to an increased consumption of calories, iron, thiamine, and niacin. Women are less likely to consume adequate nutrients than are men.

Psychological causes. Depression is a major cause of weight loss for older persons. (See Chapter 36.) Depression in older persons often presents atypically and weight loss in not a rare presenting symptom.

Bereavement often leads to anorexia, especially among older males. Grieving-associated dysphoria leads to reduced food intake, which in turn results in ketosis. The ketone bodies produce further appetite suppression, thus triggering a vicious cycle.

Alcoholism can have its first onset in old age and may result in the late-life squalor syndrome. For a disheveled older person who is losing weight, alcoholism should be suspected. Depression may be associated with alcoholism for older alcoholics.

Table 45-2 Causes of unintentional weight loss

	Number of persons affected in each study*		
	Thompson and Morris, 1991	Rabinovitz et al, 1986	Morton, Sox, and Krapp, 1981
Sample size	45	154	91
Age (mean or range) in yrs	63-83	64.2	59
Idiopathic	24	23	26
Cancer	16	36	19
Psychiatric	18	10	9
Gastrointestinal	11	17	14
Medication	9	—	2
Infection	2	6	3
Hyperthyroidism	9	3	1
Diabetes mellitus	—	3	1
Neurological	7	—	2
Cholesterol phobia	2	—	—
Nutritional/alcohol	2	—	8

*See References 6, 7, and 8.

Recently it has been recognized that anorexia nervosa or anorexia tardive is not a rare phenomenon in older persons. I have encountered a number of older women who have had episodes that were compatible with their having histories of anorexia nervosa as teenagers, and who, at age 60 years or older have had recurrent episodes. In some cases these women have been weight restrictors all their lives. Also, there are some women whose husbands have told them that they were overweight for much of their adult lives, and these women become excessively happy when at last they lose weight in their old age.

Another group of older people appear to develop abnormal attitudes toward feeding at the end of their lives.[2] These malnourished individuals, who are often men, claim to enjoy having their stomachs empty, express fear of their being overweight, and continue their dieting behaviors in the presence of severe weight loss. They often are convinced that they are overweight. This condition is perhaps best termed *anorexia tardive*. Some of these persons appear to be searching for life extension through dietary restriction.

Late-life paranoia can lead to weight loss. In some instances paranoic individuals believe that their food is being poisoned. In other instances they become so preoccupied with their paranoic delusions that they have little time to prepare and eat food. For example, a patient may spend all her time rushing to the door to prevent the neighborhood children from ruining her plants. Late-life mania can result in weight loss that is due to sleeplessness and continuous pacing.

Some older men who have spent most of their lives subtly abusing their spouses may find that the "tables are turned" when they become frail because of illnesses, and their wives begin to assert control over them. To regain their loci of control, these men may refuse to eat, while recognizing that failure to eat their wives' cooking will be hurtful to them. Refusal to eat also may be a ploy to obtain increased sympathy and attention.

Weight loss is a common concomitant of dementia. To feed demented persons, a large amount of time is required. They often fail to recognize the need to eat or the fact that they have missed a meal. Some demented patients develop apraxia of swallowing and need to be reminded to swallow after each mouthful. Pica, resulting in the ingestion of a variety of nonnutritious objects, is not rare among demented patients. Some demented patients wander incessantly, causing marked increases in their caloric requirements. Despite claims to the contrary, there is little documentation that demented patients have increased metabolic rates.

Finally, it should be recognized that some older persons decrease their food intake in the last few months before death. It would seem that, for these individuals who are at the extreme of old age, life has come to be excessively burdensome and they choose not to eat as a way to exit this life. These individuals appear to be making a rational decision and have no evidence of depression.

Medical causes. Medical causes of weight loss that is due to increased metabolism include hyperthyroidism, pheochromocytoma, and Parkinson's disease. Pheochromocytoma occurs as commonly in older persons as it does in younger persons and should be suspected for any person whose hypertension does not ameliorate with severe weight loss. Hyperthyroidism may develop apathetically in older persons, with the major presenting symptoms being weight loss, muscle weakness, heart failure, and atrial fibrillation. The eyes may be hooded rather than their having the classical proptosis.

Anorexia can result from a variety of conditions, including esophageal candidiasis (characterized by pain when the patient swallows), abdominal ischemia (early satiety), hyperparathyroidism, esophageal dysmotility syndrome, and cancer. Numerous medications can result in anorexia; the more common offenders are digoxin, psychotropics, cimetidine, and theophylline. Vitamin A or D, which both commonly are taken as over-the-counter drugs, may produce hypercalcemia resulting in anorexia. Laxative abuse can lead to dehydration and malabsorption. High-fiber diets, particularly when taken with inadequate fluids, can lead to early satiety.

While breathing, patients with chronic obstructive pulmonary disease increase their utilization of energy because they use their accessory muscles excessively. Many of these patients develop dyspnea while they eat, and eating has been demonstrated to cause a fall in Po_2 (arterial oxygen tension) in these individuals. Cardiac cachexia occurs in persons with severe heart failure. They often have a protein-losing enteropathy, as well as severe anorexia.

Zinc deficiency can lead to anorexia. It is more likely to occur in homebound rather than ambulatory elderly persons. Persons with cirrhosis of the liver or type II diabetes mellitus or those who take diuretics are at greater risk for developing zinc deficiency.

Dysphagia can lead to weight loss. It may occur in association with cerebrovascular accidents. Malabsorption syndromes need to be considered for older persons. In particular, some consideration should be given to late-onset gluten enteropathy and lactose deficiency. Persons with severe weight loss and muscle fasciculations may have a diagnosis of motor neuron disease (amyotrophic lateral sclerosis).

Numerous older persons with medical problems are placed on diets such as low-salt, low-cholesterol, or diabetic diets. In some cases these diets can trigger excessive weight loss. It needs to be recognized that dietary changes in older persons may have major consequences and when these dietary changes are indicated, older persons need to be carefully monitored for the development of malnutrition.

Finally, repeated low-grade infections (e.g., chronic sinusitus) can result in anorexia and weight loss.

Age-related causes. Older persons have decreases in taste and smell, both of which decrease the pleasurable qualities of food. Loss of teeth can lead to a decrease of approximately 100 Calories/day in food intake. Deterioration in vision can lead to problems in food preparation.

In addition, basic science studies have suggested that as people age, they experience mild anorexia. This appears to result from a lack of the opioid feeding drive and an excessive anorectic effect of the peripheral satiety hormone cholecystokinin.

Diagnostic approach

The diagnosis of protein energy malnutrition is made by the demonstration of (1) a decrease in body weight that is below 90% of the average body weight, when age-adjusted tables are used, or (2) a serum albumin that is below 3.5 g/dl. The presence of anergy, leukopenia, low serum cholesterol, low serum levels of transferrin, and prealbumin or retinol-binding protein may help to confirm the diagnosis. For patients with abnormal water metabolism, measurements of midarm circumferences may be used to replace measurements of body weight.

Diagnosing the cause of protein energy malnutrition relies on a careful history and examination to determine treatable causes. All persons losing weight should be screened for depression with the Yesavage geriatric depression scale and for dementia with the Folstein mini-mental State test. A full medication history, including over-the-counter medications should be obtained; the relationship of the introduction of new medications to the onset of weight loss should be explored. A history of faddish food diets also should be taken.

A minimum laboratory assessment for a person who has malnutrition includes a full chemistry panel, especially to determine hypercalcemia, renal failure, liver dysfunction, or uncontrolled diabetes mellitus. All persons with weight loss should have their serum thyroxine, thyroid stimulating-hormone (TSH) and triiodothyronine (T_3) measured. (See Chapter 44.) A T_3 in the upper normal range is suggestive of T_3 toxicosis because T_3 should be suppressed below the normal range in the presence of malnutrition. A fecal sample should be examined qualitatively for the presence of undigested meat fibers and fecal fat, which may suggest malabsorption. If the person has gastrointestinal complaints, it is necessary to examine the bowel fully, including the upper and lower gastrointestinal tract. If patients have dysphagia or other unusual symptoms as they eat, esophageal manometry should be performed to determine esophageal dysmotility problems. A formal swallowing evaluation by a speech therapist is indicated for the patient if there is a history of aspiration. If the person has hypertension that does not improve with weight loss, 24-hour urine samples for vanillylmandelic acid and metanephrine should be obtained to determine pheochromocytoma. If no positive diagnosis can be made, a workup to exclude cancer should be undertaken.

Intervention

Prevention of protein energy malnutrition requires that physicians and dieticians reinforce to older persons their need for adequate caloric intake. For older persons, there is a need to deemphasize the American mania for dieting. It is necessary to stress that dietary principles, which may be useful for middle-aged persons, have much less significance for older persons. Prohibiting dramatic dietary changes for older persons is a cornerstone of prevention. Early detection of weight loss should immediately trigger aggressive treatment.

Treatable causes should be identified and appropriate management instituted. In particular, abnormal attitudes toward food intake should be identified because they will interfere with appropriate dietary counseling. The patient should be referred to appropriate community resources such as Meals On Wheels and community meal centers. Referrals for help with the patients' shopping should be considered. The specific food likes and dislikes of the patients should be identified. Persons who have weight loss should be encouraged to eat as much of their favorite snack foods as possible.

Caloric supplements should be used early if the patients cannot be encouraged to increase their caloric intake. It must be remembered that supplements can be expensive and may be beyond the budgets of some older persons. The older patients must be counseled to ingest supplements between meals and not to use supplements as substitutes for meals.

Patients with weight loss that is due to psychiatric or psychological causes should have the underlying condition treated. (See Chapter 36.)

A number of drugs have been used experimentally in the attempt to stimulate patients' weight gain. These drugs include medroxyprogesterone acetate and cyproheptadine, an antiserotoninergic agent. Recombinant growth hormone has been used to treat severely malnourished persons and its safety for administration to healthy older persons has been demonstrated. While extremely expensive, recombinant growth hormone may prove to be cost effective for some severely malnourished older persons.

OBESITY

Clinical relevance

Approximately 26% of white American males aged 65 to 76 years old are overweight. Thirty-seven percent of white American females are overweight.[5] Obesity is even more prevalent among black Americans. Older persons tend to have more abdominal fat and less peripheral weight, with an increase in waist-to-hip ratio.

With one's advancing age, the mortality trend tends to decrease as one's weight increases, even if the individual is severely overweight. However, obesity in old age is associated with hypertension, diabetes mellitus, sleep apnea, pulmonary embolism, gallbladder disease, diagnostic problems, and increased surgical risks. Obesity is a problem particularly for older persons with osteoarthritis. Obesity also can lead to bedsores if the patient is immobile. Functional status can be greatly impaired for older persons with massive obesity.

Clinical manifestations

Most overweight older persons reach obesity by lifelong habits of eating more calories than they burn off by exercising. Older persons tend to have less physical activity than younger persons, further aggravating the situation.

Most acquired forms of obesity are not commonly seen in older persons. Hypothyroidism is an exception and should be considered as a possible cause of overweightness for older persons. Cushing's syndrome is rarely seen in older persons. Male hypogonadism is not rare among older persons and may aggravate obesity. Hypopituitarism also is associated with obesity in younger persons, but underweightness is more commonly seen in older persons.

Diagnostic approach

Overweight persons should be carefully questioned regarding their food intake and should have 24-hour dietary recall performed by a dietician. The physician should probe for the social use of alcohol. A history of exercise should be taken. For some persons who believe that they are exercising, a pedometer may be useful to demonstrate the reality. A history of preferred forms of exercise should be taken. Factors that may prevent the institution of an exercise program should be explored. (See Chapter 21.)

Obese persons should have a fasting blood or serum glucose level or a serum fructosamine level measured every 6 months to screen for diabetes mellitus. All obese persons should have a fasting blood screen for hypertriglyceridemia. Blood pressure should be measured with a large cuff. If abdominal pain occurs, an ultrasound should be ordered to exclude cholecystitis. A serum TSH should be obtained to exclude hypothyroidism.

Intervention

The prevention of obesity is a lifelong struggle in which a person is counseled to limit calorie intake and increase exercise to maintain body weight within reasonable limits. The physician should be particularly aware that one's weight often increases sharply between the ages of 40 to 50 years old (middle age spread) and should provide advice about increasing one's exercise at this time. Weight often increases at the time of menopause. Retirement with its associated decreased activity is another time when the risk of weight gain is increased.

I recommend that weight reduction should be attempted by all older persons who are more than 30% above average body weight and by persons with diabetes mellitus, hypertension, and osteoarthritis of weight-bearing joints who are more than 10% above average body weight. In most cases an exercise program is the first approach recommended for overweight seniors. (See Chapter 21.)

For older persons who require weight reduction diets, never prescribe less than 1000 Cal/day; supplement these diets with multivitamins. Older persons who diet often develop dehydration; therefore, they should be advised to drink eight glasses of fluids every day. Increasing fiber content in the diet also may help with weight loss.

Behavioral modification techniques should be used by older persons who attempt to alter lifelong dietary habits. These techniques include putting the fork down between bites, not snacking between meals, and eating only in one designated place. Attitude techniques include learning how to recognize high-risk situations and cravings and learning how not to become depressed following a relapse. Rewards such as praise from the physician are an important part of a successful behavioral modification program. Finally the patient should be educated about recognizing the caloric value of different foods.

Any weight reduction program for older persons requires the support of their spouses. It is essential that spouses agree not to pressure the dieters to eat. Obvious attempts by the spouses to thwart weight loss programs need to be openly confronted. The spouses should be encouraged to exercise along with their partners.

A number of weight-loss drugs have been prescribed for younger persons. Of these the most effective are the serotonin uptake reblockers fenfluramine and fluoxetine. These agents are potentially dangerous for older persons and should be avoided. Thermogenic drugs such as thyroid hormone and beta-adrenergic agents can result in myocardial ischemia and cardiac arrhythmias for older patients.

Surgical treatments for obesity such as gastric restriction and jejunoileal bypass are not recommended for persons who are more than 60 years of age.

REFERENCES

1. Berlinger WG, Potter JF: Low body mass index in demented outpatients, *J Am Geriatr Soc* 39:973, 1991.
2. Miller DK et al: Abnormal eating attitudes and body image in older undernourished individuals, *J Am Geriatr Soc* 39:462, 1991.
3. Miller DK et al: Formal geriatric assessment instruments and the care of older general medical outpatients, *J Am Geriatr Soc* 38:645, 1990.
4. Morley JE: Why do physicians fail to recognize and treat malnutrition in elderly persons?, *J Am Geriatr Soc* 39:1139, 1991.
5. Morley JE, Glick Z: Obesity. In Morley JE, Glick Z, Rubenstein LZ, eds: *Geriatric nutrition: a comprehensive review*, New York, 1990, Raven Press.
6. Morton KI, Sox HC, Krapp JR: Involuntary weight-loss: diagnostic and prognostic significance, *Ann Intern Med* 95:568, 1981.
7. Rabinovitz M et al: Unintentional weight loss, *Arch Intern Med* 146:186, 1986.
8. Thompson MP, Morris LK: Unexplained weight loss in the ambulatory elderly, *J Am Geriatr Soc* 39:497, 1991.

SUGGESTED READINGS

Chernoff R; ed: *Geriatric nutrition*, Gaithersburg, Md, 1991, Aspen.

Mobarhan S, Trumbone LS: Nutritional problems of the elderly, *Clin Geriatr Med* 7:191, 1991.

Morley JE, Glick Z, Rubenstein LZ; eds: *Geriatric nutrition: a comprehensive review*, New York, 1990, Raven Press.

_____

CHAPTER 46

Anemia

DAVID A. LIPSCHITZ

KEY POINTS

- Anemia is common in elderly persons. The most common causes are iron deficiency and the anemia of chronic disease.
- For a patient who has mild anemia (hemoglobin 10.5 to 12 g/dl), a normal complete blood count (except anemia), normal physical examination, and negative occult blood in the stool, an intensive evaluation to identify the cause of anemia may be unnecessary.
- It is important to accurately diagnose an iron deficiency prior to initiating an extensive gastrointestinal workup to identify the cause of blood loss.
- Iron deficiency is diagnosed by the presence of iron deficient erythropoiesis (microcytosis, low serum iron, and low transferrin saturation) and absent iron stores (low serum ferritin and high total iron-binding capacity).
- The anemia of chronic disease is diagnosed by the presence of iron deficient erythropoiesis and *increased iron stores* (normal or high serum ferritin and low total iron-binding capacity).

CLINICAL RELEVANCE

Studies of hospitalized patients have shown that anemia is very common among elderly persons. For example, an analysis of admissions to the geriatric evaluation unit at the John L. McClellan Veterans Hospital revealed that 65% of elderly males had hemoglobin values <14 g/dl (14 g/dl is the usual reported lower limit of hemoglobin for men) and 25% had hemoglobin concentrations <12 g/dl. For men, a definite increase in the prevalence of anemia is found among the older age groups. In contrast, the prevalence of anemia among women older than 59 years of age has been approximately equal to that found among women of childbearing age in some studies. Studies from Great Britain are important because they have determined the prevalence of anemia in large numbers of older subjects.[3] Among men and women, the prevalence of anemia increased significantly with each successive decade. A recent analysis of the second National Health and Nutrition Education Survey (NHANES 2) demonstrated a significant reduction in hemoglobin levels for apparently healthy elderly males and a minimal although significant reduction in hemoglobin levels for elderly females.[8] Based upon a lower normal limit of 14 g/dl, a very large percentage of elderly males were found to be anemic. This study proposed that the reduction in hemoglobin levels for males was a consequence of aging and suggested that age-specific reference standards for hemoglobin concentrations for elderly persons should be adopted.

Etiology of anemia

A rational approach to the differential diagnosis of anemia for elderly persons is to classify the disorder on the basis of the abnormality in erythropoiesis.[4]

Hypoproliferative anemia is caused by a decreased production of red cell precursors by the bone marrow. *Hemolytic anemia* results from an increased peripheral destruction of mature red cells. Maturation abnormalities of red cell precursors result in cells that are unable to egress from the marrow, and this result is referred to as *ineffective erythropoiesis.* Using this diagnostic approach, physicians have found that mild anemia of apparently healthy elderly subjects is due primarily to the *hypoproliferative* type. A careful assessment of hematopoiesis in these individuals revealed mild marrow failure.[5,6] The cause of this mild marrow abnormality remains to be determined. A major unanswered question is whether or not this decline in hemoglobin is a consequence of the normal aging process or reflects some yet-to-be-defined abnormality. Based upon data from longitudinal studies that demonstrated no reduction in red cell mass with age for healthy elderly subjects and experiments in animals, it seems highly likely that the decrease in hemoglobin seen commonly among the elderly is not a consequence of the normal aging process.[1,2,7]

DIAGNOSTIC APPROACH

From a clinically relevant perspective, hemoglobin concentration of 12 g/dl is considered the lower limit of normal for elderly men and women. For elderly men with hemoglobin concentration of 12 to 14 g/dl, a cause is rarely found. Even at the borderline level of 12 g/dl, clinical judgment should determine how aggressively a physician should evaluate the patient. The complex nature of the problems that older individuals have and the high risk of multiple pathologies occurring simultaneously make this evaluation much more critical. However, the principles involved in assessment and evaluation of older patients with low hemoglobin are very similar to those that are used to assess and evaluate patients of any age group. The causes of the various anemias seen in elderly patients are described in subsequent discussions.

The initial diagnostic approach for an older patient with anemia must include a complete history and physical examination, as well as a complete blood count (CBC). The CBC permits evaluation of the size and production rate of red blood cells. Microcytosis, defined as a mean corpuscular volume (MCV) <84 fl (femtoliters [Coulter counter]), indicates an impairment of hemoglobin synthesis. Macrocytosis, defined as an MCV >100 fl, frequently is caused by an abnormality in nuclear maturation but less commonly is caused by reticulocytes. The reticulocyte production index estimates the level of red cell production.[4] Hemolytic anemia usually has a reticulocyte index >3, whereas a failure of production is indicated by a reticulocyte index <2. An elevated serum lactic dehydrogenase (LDH) and indirect hyperbilirubinemia result from the increased destruction of red cell precursors in the marrow, and these results may be used to distinguish ineffective erythropoiesis from hypoproliferative anemia.

Observation may be a reasonable approach for the older individual who has a mild decrease in hemoglobin (10.5 to 12 g/dl), a normal reticulocyte index, a normochromic normocytic index, no leukocyte or platelet abnormality, and no occult blood in the stool. Further investigation is indicated if the anemia worsens or a change in the peripheral blood pattern occurs. For the individual with mild anemia and a hypochromic microcytic index or more severe anemia and a normochromic normocytic index, a more extensive evaluation is required. Similarly the presence of macrocytosis warrants additional investigation.

For older patients with hypoproliferative anemia (iron deficiency and chronic disease), serum iron, total iron-binding capacity (TIBC), and ferritin should be obtained. With macrocytosis, serum B_{12} and folate levels should be reviewed. Other tests (e.g., hemoglobin electrophoresis) should be ordered, depending on clinical findings and initial screening laboratory data.

SPECIFIC ANEMIAS

Hypoproliferative anemias

Iron deficient erythropoiesis. The majority of anemias in elderly persons are of the hypoproliferative type, which most commonly is associated with inadequate iron supply for erythropoiesis. (See the box on p. 451.) This type of anemia is diagnosed by the presence of a decreased serum iron and a reduced transferrin saturation (serum iron divided by the TIBC expressed as a percent; <20% is abnormal). Absolute iron deficiency (blood loss) is the most common cause of iron deficient erythropoiesis for younger patients. For elderly patients, the cause of iron deficient erythropoiesis is more likely to be the anemia of chronic disease or anemia associated with inflammation. Iron deficient erythropoiesis in elderly patients results from a defective ability of the reticuloendothelial system to reuse iron that is derived from senescent red cells. Thus tissue iron stores are normal or high, resulting in a serum ferritin concentration >50

ANEMIAS CAUSED BY IRON DEFICIENT
ERYTHROPOIESIS IN ELDERLY PERSONS

Blood loss
(low serum iron, high serum TIBC, low transferrin saturation [<20%], low serum ferritin [<20 ng/ml])

Neoplasm
Angiodysplasia of large bowel
Diverticular disease
Drugs
Epistaxis
Hematuria
Uterine bleeding
Platelet and coagulation abnormalities

Chronic disease and inflammation
(low serum iron, low serum TIBC, low transferrin saturation [<20%], normal serum ferritin [>50 ng/ml])

Acute infection
Chronic infection (e.g., tuberculosis)
Neoplasm
Tissue necrosis (e.g., pressure ulcer)
Collagen vascular disease
Arthritis (e.g., osteoarthritis)

ng/ml and a low TIBC. This contrasts with a low serum ferritin and a high TIBC, which reflect absent iron stores in blood loss anemia. (See the box above.)

Anemia from blood loss, anemia of inflammation, anemia of chronic disease, and anemia associated with protein energy malnutrition are the most prevalent anemias among the elderly population. For men and women, a progressive increase in iron stores occurs with advancing age. In older men, tissue iron stores average 1200 mg and in women, iron stores increase from a mean of 300 mg to approximately 800 mg over the decade following menopause. Thus *nutritional* iron deficiency is very rare among elderly persons, despite the prominence of other nutritional problems. When unexplained iron deficiency does occur, it is *almost exclusively due to blood loss from the intestinal tract,* even if bleeding is not detected by repeated stool examinations for blood. Other routes of bleeding may occur but are easily recognizable (epistaxis, hematuria, abnormal uterine bleeding). The causes of blood loss in elderly persons include drugs (aspirin) and neoplasms. Angiodysplasia of the large bowel and diverticular disease are frequent causes of blood loss, but these causes only should be considered once neoplasms have been excluded from the diagnosis. Rarely, iron deficiency results from malabsorption of iron or urinary losses of iron, which occur along with intravascular hemolysis. Clinical manifestations of blood loss may be subtle or not apparent if hemorrhage is chronic. Fatigue, falls, cognitive impairment, loss of appetite, and others may be the presenting symptoms. Treatment should be directed toward the underlying cause of bleeding and toward iron replacement.

For elderly persons, inflammation is a second, and perhaps a more frequent, important cause of anemia or iron deficient erythropoiesis. Etiological factors of inflammation include bacterial infection, immune reaction, tissue necrosis, or neoplasm. In contrast to the iron block that results from iron deficiency, the iron block that results from inflammation is less severe and there is usually minimal microcytosis. The hemoglobin concentration is generally moderately decreased. In some instances, these hematological findings may be present with little or no evidence of inflammation. Inadequate food intake and increased tissue breakdown may contribute to the severity of the anemia through decreased erythropoietin stimulation. Clinical manifestations usually reflect the underlying inflammatory process. Treatment should be directed toward the underlying disease. Only rarely is anemia severe enough to necessitate transfusion. Iron therapy is usually ineffective because of the limited absorption of iron in the presence of inflammation and because of the trapping of parenteral iron in the macrophage.

The term *anemia of chronic disease* is often used to explain an anemia that is associated with some other major disease process. Examples include cancer, collagen vascular disorder, rheumatoid arthritis, and inflammatory bowel disease. Generally, clinical manifestations of the chronic disease mask the signs of anemia if the hemoglobin concentration is only moderately low. However, occasionally the anemia may be the initial manifestation of an occult disease. It is critical for the clinician to be aware of this possibility and to ensure that a rational appropriate search for a treatable cause of the anemia is made. Management of the anemias of both inflammation and chronic disease also should include adequate nutrition.

Lack of erythropoietin. Nutritional deprivation in the aged generally results in a normocytic normochromic anemia and an essentially normal peripheral smear. For the hospitalized patient, evidence of iron deficient erythropoiesis (low transferrin saturation) is common and the serum ferritin is evaluated. There is usually a history of weight loss, and laboratory studies indicate a reduced serum albumin and a decreased TIBC (<240 g/dl). This disorder is particularly important because there is evidence that correction of the nutritional deficiency and its underlying cause can result in significant improvement of the hemoglobin level and other hematopoietic parameters (stimulation of erythropoietin).

For frail older patients who have multiple medical problems, a multifactorial etiology of anemia is more likely. A typical example is an older patient with active rheumatoid disease who takes aspirin and has an anemia of chronic inflammation and an anemia from blood loss (aspirin). Another example is an older patient who has protein energy malnutrition or blood loss that aggravates the anemia associated with cancer. The possibility of a multifactorial etiology should be considered when the anemia of chronic disease or inflammation is associated with a hemoglobin <10 g/dl. In this circumstance the laboratory investigations frequently give equivocal results, hence, a bone marrow examination may be required.

Stem cell dysfunction. Bone marrow failure, due to interference with proliferation of hematopoietic cells, occurs in elderly persons. The disorder is generally associated with suppression of all marrow elements and is suggested by the presence of peripheral pancytopenia. Common etiological factors include drugs, immune damages to the stem cell population, intrinsic marrow lesions and marrow replacements by malignant cells or fibrous tissues. The latter is usually associated with a myelophthisic blood picture (nucleated red cells, giant platelets, and metamyelocytes on the smear) that reflects the disruption of marrow stromal architecture. The presence of pancytopenia and the absence of iron deficient erythropoiesis are indications for bone marrow aspiration and biopsy.

Anemias caused by ineffective erythropoiesis

The most common and important anemias caused by ineffective erythropoiesis are the macrocytic anemias. Macrocytic (megaloblastic) anemias in older adults are caused by vitamin B_{12} and folate deficiencies. The box below lists the common causes of anemias resulting from ineffective erythropoiesis.

Vitamin B_{12} deficiency (pernicious anemia). Pernicious anemia (PA) occurs most frequently among persons who are over the age of 60 years old and is more common among women. Antibodies against gastric parietal cells and intrinsic factor result in atrophic gastritis and decreased secretion of extrinsic factor, which cause a failure of vitamin B_{12} absorption. PA may be very severe, with its presenting symptoms including weakness and a lemon-yellow discoloration of the skin. Neurological abnormalities, including peripheral neuropathy, ataxia, loss of the sense of position and loss of the upper motor neuron signs, are frequent. Behavioral abnormalities and dementia are well described for patients who have PA. Occasionally there is evidence of a more generalized immunological disorder, manifesting with myxedema, hypoadrenalism, and vitiligo. The diagnosis of PA (or folate deficiency) is suggested by

---

ANEMIAS CAUSED BY INEFFECTIVE ERYTHROPOIESIS

Macrocytic (megaloblastic)
Vitamin B_{12} deficiency
Folate deficiency
Refractory

Microcytic
Sideroblastic
Thalassemia

Normocytic
Stromal
Dimorphic

pancytopenia, macrocytosis, hypersegmented polymorphonuclear leukocytes in the peripheral smear, decreased reticulocyte index, and increased LDH (lactic dehydrogenase) and indirect hyperbilirubinemia. The bone marrow classically shows giant metamyelocytes, hypersegmented polymorphonuclear leukocytes, and enlarged erythroid precursors with more hemoglobin than would be expected from their immature nuclei (nuclear cytoplasmic dissociation). The diagnosis of PA is confirmed by a serum vitamin B_{12} concentration <100 pg/ml. Vitamin B_{12} deficiency also may be caused by diseases of the ileum. The Schilling test distinguishes a deficiency of intrinsic factor (malabsorption corrected by ingested vitamin B_{12} and intrinsic factor) from an abnormality in the ability of the ileum to absorb the vitamin B_{12} intrinsic factor complex (absorption still impaired with intrinsic factor plus vitamin B_{12}). Treatment for PA consists of weekly or biweekly injections of 100 mg of vitamin B_{12} until stores are replenished. A maintenance dose at monthly intervals is then adequate.

Folate deficiency. Epidemiological studies generally have shown an adequate folate nutriture in healthy older persons. Folate deficiency, of sufficient severity to cause anemia in elderly persons, is most frequently found in association with protein energy malnutrition and excessive alcohol consumption. Alcohol and other drugs also are known to interfere with folate absorption and internal metabolism. Vulnerability to deficiency is significantly greater when folate requirements increase as a result of inflammation, neoplastic disease, or hemolytic anemia. The hematological profile is identical to that described for vitamin B_{12} deficiency. The diagnosis is made by the demonstration of significant reductions in the serum (<2 ng/ml) or red cell (<100 ng/ml) folate concentration. Prior to therapy with folate, it is important to exclude vitamin B_{12} deficiency from the diagnosis because treatment with folate can aggravate the neurological abnormalities resulting from reduced vitamin B_{12} concentration.

Other causes. The major causes of ineffective erythropoiesis and microcytosis are thalassemia and sideroblastic anemia. Acquired sideroblastic anemia is primarily a disease of elderly persons. It is a heterogenous disorder characterized by the presence of iron deposits in the mitochondria of normoblasts. The disorder is a consequence of impaired heme synthesis. It usually reflects an intrinsic marrow lesion (idiopathic) but may be secondary to inflammation, neoplastic disease, or drug ingestion. The common finding is the presence of dimorphic red cell populations, one of which is markedly hypochromic while the other is well-filled with hemoglobin. The diagnosis is made by the demonstration of ringed sideroblasts in the bone marrow, as well as the presence of maturation abnormalities of myeloid and erythroid precursors. A fraction of elderly patients with sideroblastic anemia show some response to pharmacological doses of pyridoxine (200 mg 3 times daily). This dose should be given to all patients until it becomes apparent that a rise in hemoglobin concentration will not occur. For those patients who are unresponsive to pyridoxine, the anemia must be treated symptomatically.

Di Guglielmo's syndrome is more common with advancing age, and the presenting symptom is a megaloblastic erythroid precursor. Frequently abnormal sideroblasts also are seen. The peripheral smear usually demonstrates pancytopenia with occasional nucleated red cells or immature myeloid and megakaryocytic precursors. The bone marrow is markedly hyperplastic. It is essential to exclude vitamin B_{12} and folate deficiencies from the diagnosis, and a trial of pyridoxine may be indicated. Treatment is usually supportive. There is some evidence that these disorders are premalignant, evolving rarely into a subacute or acute myelogenous leukemia.

Hemolytic anemias

The causes of hemolytic anemia that have been found for older patients are somewhat different than the causes that have been found for younger patients. Rather than a congenital disorder, autoimmune hemolytic anemia is the most common cause that has been found for elderly persons. The diagnosis is made by a positive Coombs' test. For younger patients, autoimmune hemolysis only rarely is identified. In contrast, for elderly patients the anemia is likely to be associated with lymphoproliferative disorder (non-Hodgkin's lymphoma or chronic lymphocytic leukemia), collagen vascular disease, or drug ingestion. Treatment with corticosteroids and splenectomies are usually effective for patients with red cell antibodies of the IgG type. Patients with red cell antibodies of the IgM type are more likely to be refractory to such treatment.

Microangiopathic hemolytic anemia is a disorder of elderly persons that is of some importance. This disorder usually is associated with severe infection or disseminated neoplasm and manifests not only hemolytic anemia but also disseminated intravascular coagulation. Thrombocytopenia and hemosiderinuria, as well as red cell fragmentation and prolonged partial thromboplastin time, should be suggestive of microangiopathic hemolytic anemia.

REFERENCES

1. Boggs DR, Patrene KD: Hematopoiesis and aging. III Anemia and a blunted erythropoietic response to hemorrhage in aged mice, *Am J Hematol* 19:327, 1985.
2. Garry PJ, Goodwin JS, Hunt WC: A longitudinal study of anemia in the elderly. In Chandra RD, ed: *Nutrition, immunity and illness in the elderly*, New York, 1985, Pergamon.
3. Hill RD: The prevalence of anemia in the over-65s in a rural practice, *Practitioner* 217:963, 1967.
4. Hillman RS, Finch CA: *Red cell manual*, ed 5, Philadelphia, 1985, FA Davis.
5. Lipschitz DA, Mitchell CO, Thompson C: The anemia of senescence, *Am J Hematol* 11:47, 1981.
6. Lipschitz DA et al: Effect of age on hematopoiesis in man, *Blood* 63:502, 1984.
7. Williams LH, Udupa KB, Lipschitz DA: An evaluation of the effect of age on hematopoiesis in the mouse, *Exp Hematol* 14:827, 1986.
8. Yip R, Johnson C, Dallman PR: Age-related changes in laboratory values used in the diagnosis of anemia and iron deficiency, *Am J Clin Nutr* 39:427, 1984.

SUGGESTED READINGS

Hill RD: The prevalence of anemia in the over-65s in a rural practice, *Practitioner* 217:963, 1967.
Lipschitz DA, Mitchell CO, Thompson C: The anemia of senescence, *Am J Hematol* 11:47, 1981.
Yip R, Johnson C, Dallman PR: Age-related changes in laboratory values used in the diagnosis of anemia and iron deficiency, *Am J Clin Nutr* 39:427, 1984.

CHAPTER 47

Oral and dental problems

PATRICK M. LLOYD

KEY POINTS

- A dry mouth is not a normal age-related change.
- Medications used to manage urinary incontinence, depression, hypertension, and other common health problems of older patients increase the prevalence of oral disease and dysfunction.
- Dental caries is the major cause of tooth loss after the age of 70.
- Oral disease in elderly persons is chronic, generally asymptomatic, even in advanced stages, and atypical in presentation.
- Tobacco, alcohol, and age are the three most significant risk factors for oral cancer.
- Preventive measures are the most cost-effective means of controlling dental and oral diseases for geriatric patients.
- Stroke patients who have chewing difficulties, swallowing disorders, or facial paralyses should be evaluated by a prosthodontist.
- Caregivers of cognitively or physically impaired patients need counsel and instruction to safely provide daily oral hygiene care.

CLINICAL RELEVANCE

For the older patient, dentistry's first priority is the alleviation of pain and suffering attributable to oral disease or dysfunction. Providing patients with safe, comfortable, and effective mechanisms for eating, while simultaneously giving them access to a wide variety of foods, promotes patients' well-being and hastens convalescence after surgery, chemotherapy, or other major medical treatment. Interpersonal skills, highly dependent on physical appearance and effective communication, can be enhanced by improving the shape, texture, and color of anterior teeth, by replacing visibly missing teeth, or by providing underlying support to external tissues of the lower third of the face. Clarity of speech can be sharpened by proper positioning of the teeth in relationship to the lips and tongue. The goals of these services are consistent with those of all disciplines involved in geriatrics—maximizing functional performance, fostering independence, and maintaining a high quality of life.

As the ages of patients reach into the eighth, ninth, and tenth decades, the conventional styles of practicing dentistry and the priorities of service undergo complete transformation. General health status, medication profile, functional performance, and cognitive ability enter into the process of treatment planning, delivering care, and maintenance programing. Regular contact by the dentist with the primary care physician is standard to ensure an uneventful and expeditious course of treatment.

CLINICAL MANIFESTATIONS

Tooth loss

Advances in the detection, treatment, and prevention of dental disease have led to unprecedented rates of tooth retention in elderly persons. The percentage of the group aged 65 years and older with all or some of their natural teeth has risen from 40% in 1957 to 60% in 1986, with even higher percentages in the cohort aged 65 to 75 years old.[7]

During the first three decades of life, the primary cause of tooth loss is dental caries. From one's middle 30s to late 50s, periodontal disease is the main reason teeth are removed. After one reaches 60 years of age, tooth decay is again the major cause of tooth loss. But the type and extent of dental decay experienced by older patients are fundamentally different from the type and extent that affect other segments of the population. For the most part, elderly patients experience decay along the edges of restorations and crowns or on the root surfaces of teeth that have become exposed because of gingival recession. Interproximal surfaces are also prone to decay, especially in those instances where the recession has left openings for debris to collect between the teeth. There are four major risk factors that predispose older persons to high rates of dental caries and tooth loss: (1) diminished sensation, (2) gingival recession, (3) oral hygiene, and (4) xerostomia.

Diminished sensation. There is a predictable diminution of innervating tissues within the pulp of the dentition as patients age. A constant deposition of a calcified matrix along the outermost region of the dental pulp throughout the life of teeth reduces the total pulp volume and therefore the number of nerve fibers within the pulp (Figure 47-1).[5] This change substantially reduces an older patient's ability to perceive incipient or even moderate degrees of tooth decay. There is generally no pain or discomfort until considerable damage has occurred.[5] The presenting complaints of older patients differ dramatically from those of younger patients who report

PULPAL CONFIGURATION

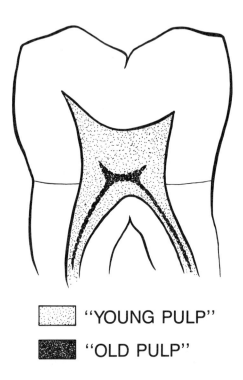

☐ "YOUNG PULP"

■ "OLD PULP"

Figure 47-1 Comparison of total pulp volume in young versus old tooth. The progressive stenosis of pulpal space diminishes nocioceptive information to elderly persons, thereby predisposing the older dentition to extensive caries in the absence of symptoms.

acute, throbbing, and radiating pain. Often, older patients seek treatment because food impacts in carious sites or a fractured tooth is unsightly or lacerates the tongue and buccal or other mucosal surfaces. If the caries has involved the pulp of the tooth, there may be apical abscess formation with resultant drainage or localized swelling. Patients with advanced stages of caries may be febrile and may have asymmetrical facial contours, as well as swallowing discomfort. Should the offending tooth be attached to a bridge or removable partial, it is likely to involve the entire unit. This situation prohibits the patient's use of the prosthesis and further compromises the patient's chewing ability.

   Gingival recession. Gingival recession also contributes to an increased rate of dental caries as a cause of tooth loss in late life. The apical migration of tissues increases the total surface areas of the teeth, which patients have to maintain (Figure 47-2). The roots of the teeth are without enamel covers, making them more susceptible to decay than the other parts of teeth. The surfaces also are irregular—there are grooves

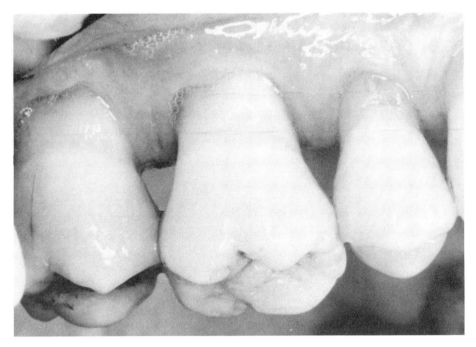

Figure 47-2 Gingival recession, which has resulted in wide open spaces between the posterior teeth, is illustrated in this 72-year-old person.

and concavities where roots join one another. These areas are difficult if not impossible to maintain their being free of food or debris.

Oral hygiene. Another risk for tooth loss is physical or cognitive impairment that interferes with the mechanics of oral hygiene care or the ability to continue a routine practice. Severely physically disabled and cognitively impaired patients depend on well-informed, properly trained, and sympathetic caregivers for daily oral hygiene. Without such special attention, these patients predictably experience dental problems—grossly carious teeth, abscesses, fractures, and gingival tissues become extremely sensitive and bleed profusely on contact.

Xerostomia. A dry mouth had long been considered an expected inconvenience and disability of late life. Salivary glands, like other organ systems, were thought to decline in function as patients age. However, there have been independent cross-sectional and longitudinal studies that report no alteration in the output of these exocrine glands in healthy nonmedicated men and women of any age.[2,8] For both the resting and stimulated states, there was no appreciable change in flow rate or composition.

What then is responsible for this seemingly universal problem in older patients? According to Mandel,[6] the causative factors for disrupting the normal production and

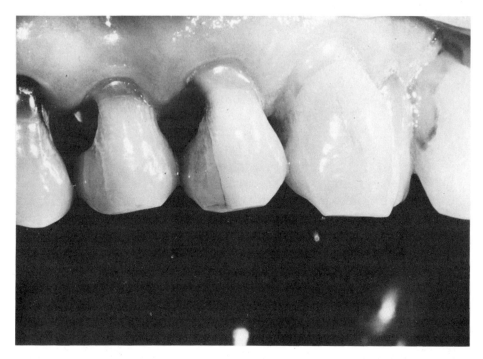

Figure 47-3 The consequences of drug-induced xerostomia in a 79-year-old patient who was free of caries 2 years earlier, before methantheline was prescribed to control urinary incontinence.

flow of saliva are local disease or infection of the gland, systemic illness, direct irradiation, and certain classes of medications. By far the most common cause of dry mouth, particularly in older patients, is medication. Agents used to manage urinary incontinence, hypertension, depression, and other major medical problems that are prevalent among elderly persons modify how salivary glands perform (Figure 47-3). The anticholinergic group is the most frequently reported class of medication that is known to cause dry mouth. (See the box on p. 461.)

The problem of a dry mouth in elderly persons disrupts the normal processes of mastication, deglutition, speech, and oral health. Without an adequate volume of saliva or an appropriate composition of substances within the saliva, patients become less effective and agile in their chewing, swallowing becomes more cumbersome and uncoordinated, and speaking becomes more labored and indistinct. Furthermore, patients have increased rates of tooth decay, gingivitis, mucositis, aphthous ulcer, and soft tissue irritation under removable dental prostheses. Taste acuity may become blunted, which further deprives older persons of the full enjoyment of eating.

CLASSES OF DRUGS CAUSING XEROSTOMIA

Appetite suppressants	Antihypertensives
Anticholinergics	Diuretics
Antiparkinsonians	Narcotics
Anticonvulsants	Hypnotics
Antihistamines	Muscle relaxants
Antidepressants	Tranquilizers
Antispasmodics	Sympathomimetics

Oral cancer

Although accounting for a relatively small percentage of newly diagnosed or fatal cancers, 4% and 2.2% respectively, oral cancer remains one of the most disabling, physically disfiguring, and quality-of-life-compromising forms of cancer to affect patients. The main risk factors for oral cancer are smoking, tobacco, and age, with age increasing the high-risk factor.[9] About 85% of all oral cancers occur in patients who are more than 50 years of age, and the average age of patients at the time of diagnosis is 60 years.

Early carcinomas of the oral cavity are usually painless. Pain is a symptom only after the mucosa becomes ulcerated, the lesion penetrates a neurovascular bundle, or something physically irritates the surface of the lesion (e.g., denture, toothbrush, food). The most common first complaint, the one likely to cause a patient to seek professional care, is that a lump has been discovered. An altered or restricted ability to perform chewing, swallowing, speaking, or breathing may be experienced. Problems positioning dentures or partials also are reported. It may be painful to insert a prosthesis or the occlusion between opposing teeth may be imbalanced because the tumor prevents complete seating of the prosthesis.

The sites where oral cancer is initially identified are generally more posterior in the oral cavity, adding to the delay in patients' seeking treatment. By far the most

Table 47-1 Common sites for oral cancer

Cancer site	Percent of lesions
Tongue	34
Floor of mouth	23
Oropharynx	20
Gingiva	10
Buccal mucosa	6
Palate	3
Lip	4

From Gorsky M, Silverman S: Denture wearing and oral cancer. *J Prosthet Dent* 52:164, 1984.

common site for oral cancer for both men and women is the tongue.[4] (See Table 47-1.) These lesions are located laterally, ventrally, or basally on the tongue, and they often go undetected unless a thorough and detailed oral examination is performed. Self-examination for oral cancer is difficult in the more posterior or recessed areas of the mouth because of the need to simultaneously retract obscuring tissues, accurately direct a focused light source, and get in position for optimal viewing. As a consequence, diagnoses of lesions in the areas amenable to treatment are made during oral cancer screenings, routine dental checkups, or physical examinations. (See Figure 47-4.)

What has perplexed clinicians and often delayed this degree of scrutiny is the similarity between a benign nonthreatening lesion and one that is malignant. Thus, definitive diagnosis of a lesion as an oral cancer is ultimately reached by a biopsy and histological examination. A detailed record of the lesion is invaluable for diagnosis, continued observation, and subsequent referral. A description of the anatomical location and a drawing that maps the patterns and dimensions are essential, as are the distribution of color, presence or absence of hemorrhage, and surface topography. A determination should be made about the duration and sensitivity of the lesion and any associated functional disturbances. Important risk factors (i.e., age, smoking

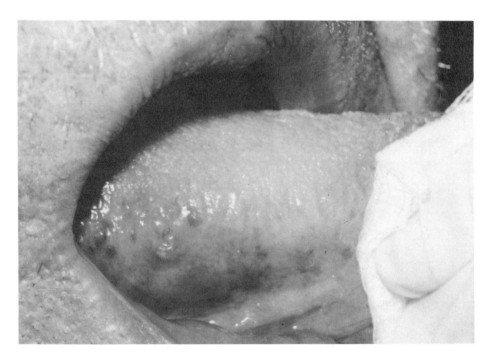

Figure 47-4 Asymptomatic squamous cell carcinoma on the right lateral surface of the tongue of a 69-year-old man who has a 60-pack-per-year history of smoking.

history, alcohol intake, nutritional status, and previous oral or other cancers) should be identified.

DIAGNOSTIC APPROACH

Elderly patients as a group visit their dentists less frequently than do other segments of the population. Less than one third of elderly patients have annual visits and almost one half have not seen their dentists in 5 years. Because of this infrequent contact and because older patients are at the highest risk for many of the most terminal forms of oral diseases, it is critical that non-dental health professionals are competent in providing oral screening assessments. A systematic approach to reviewing the oral statuses of older patients can be readily incorporated, without inconvenience to the practitioner, as part of a routine history and physical examination. This systematic approach is the initial and most important step in the diagnosis of oral and dental diseases.

A health questionnaire that is completed by the patient gives the practitioner historical and contemporary information about virtually every aspect of the patient's lifestyle. Included within the traditional list of illnesses and disorders that cover major body functions should be unique questions that address oral and dental problems. The box below provides an example of the dental and oral health questionnaire. The responses to these questions should be considered within the context of the entire health questionnaire. Oral problems that are identified by the patient through the questionnaire should be considered when the practitioner examines the patient's

---

DENTAL AND ORAL HEALTH QUESTIONNAIRE

1. What is your dentist's name? _____
2. When was your last dental checkup? _____
3. How often do you visit your dentist? _____
4. Do you have partials or dentures? _____
5. Do your partials or dentures function satisfactorily? _____
6. Are your teeth loose? _____
7. Do your gums bleed? _____
8. Is your mouth dry? _____
9. How often do you brush your teeth? _____
10. Can you chew your food well? _____
11. Do you have problems swallowing your food? _____
12. Do you smoke or chew tobacco? _____
13. How much alcohol do you drink? _____
14. Do you get sores or ulcers in your mouth that do not heal? _____
15. Do you get infections in your mouth or on your lips? _____
16. Do you have numb areas in your mouth or on your face? _____

mouth. Correlating a symptom with a clinical finding enhances the diagnostic process.

With gloved hands, a mouth mirror, a point light source, and a gauze pad, the practitioner can conduct a thorough oral examination. To ensure completeness, a consistent sequence should be used when the practitioner examines the patient's mouth. The practitioner should begin the examination with the outermost structures and advance inwardly. Throughout the course of the examination, the practitioner should note surface irregularities, bleeding and painful sites. Anatomical and functional observations should be compared for symmetry. Few significant oral problems are present symmetrically.

Maximal opening of the mouth should be checked by instructing the patient to open the mouth as wide as possible. From the incisal edges of the anterior teeth, the normal maximal opening is approximately 30 to 35 mm or the width of three fingers. Coordinated, bilateral tongue function can be assessed by having the patient protrude the tongue as far forward as possible. Deviation should be checked; the midline should be coincident with that of the overall face. Tongue lateralization skills can be examined by instructing the patient to move the tongue from right to left. If the patient is unable to understand the command, the patient's face should be touched on the side toward which the movement should be directed and the command should be repeated. The patient should be asked to place the tip of the tongue into the buccal vestibules, right and then left. This is a critical movement for food manipulation and bolus construction.

Have the patient remove any dentures or partials and observe the manner in which this is done. Removal should be without pain and difficulty. Fractures, missing teeth, sharp edges, and cleanliness should be noted. The hands-on portion of the examination is begun by inspecting the lips. Bidigitally the substance of the lips is palpated, the buccal tissue is compressed between the thumb and index finger, and the parotid gland is milked. Droplets of saliva should be seen exiting the duct in the middle posterior third of the buccal mucosa.

A thorough inspection of the tongue has long been regarded as an essential component of the physical examination.[1] With the aid of a 2- by 2-inch gauze pad, the practitioner can lightly yet firmly grasp the tip of the patient's tongue, without undue discomfort for the patient (Figure 47-5). Pulling the tongue forward and then rolling it side to side offers a complete and direct view of all sides, especially those areas at high risk—lateral border, ventral surface, and base. The entire tongue can be palpated and checked for consistency and tone.

Although somewhat awkward, visual examination of all intraoral tissue surfaces is essential. Palatal elevation is noted; it should be symmetrical and should elevate sufficiently to seal off the nasopharynx. The tonsillar area also can be inspected during this maneuver. The floor of the mouth is examined by bimanual palpation. One index finger moves throughout the region and intraorally compresses against the other index finger, which is under the base of the mandible. Salivary glands in the floor of the

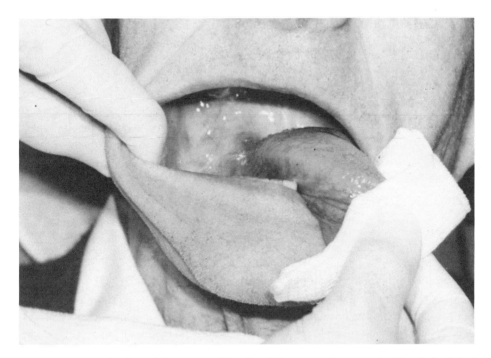

Figure 47-5 Examination of the tongue. The tip of the tongue is grasped with a 2- by 2-inch gauze and is extended to examine the lateral borders fully.

mouth (sublingual and submaxillary) can be milked and checked for patency of the ducts.

The hard palate and the alveolar bone supporting the teeth should be palpated for overt osseous concavities, draining abscess formations, surface nodules, or exposed bones. The practitioner should use the thumb and index finger to grasp the teeth and check them for mobility. Movement along the horizontal plane is generally indicative of periodontal disease with moderate to severe loss of the bones supporting the teeth. However, if the teeth can be compressed into their sockets, this is a much graver situation that necessitates immediate referral to a periodontist. In this case the disease process has extended beyond the area of the periodontium and into the underlying structures. Finally, oral hygiene should be assessed. Teeth should be relatively free of debris. Halitosis, if present, often can be the result of inadequate oral hygiene and frank gingival-periodontal disease. Fractured or severely decayed teeth should be noted. The clinician should inquire as to whether the patient has any pain or discomfort from the affected teeth.

Biopsies of persistent oral lesions should be obtained, depending on the clinical appearances and presenting symptoms of the lesions. An appointment should be arranged with an otolaryngologist or an oromaxillofacial surgeon while the patient is still in the office so that a follow-up visit can be scheduled to discuss the result of the biopsy and necessary treatment. The otolaryngologist or oromaxillofacial surgeon should be given all information that was gathered from the patient's history and physical examination. A complete copy of the pathology report should be requested. The otolaryngologist or surgeon should be consulted after the diagnosis is made to prepare the clinician for the patient's return visit. If the lesion is cancerous, therapies, including surgery, radiation, or chemotherapy, should be considered. The clinician should be prepared to discuss the procedures with the patient.

INTERVENTION

Simple and common oral and dental problems often can be managed by the primary care physician. The box below lists some of these common problems and prescriptions for their therapies.[3]

Education of patients is the most important aspect of managing the problem of a dry mouth. Information about the deleterious effects of xerostomia should come from both the dentist and the physician who has prescribed the medication or medications. A comprehensive oral health care program should be established immediately. This

---

PRESCRIPTION ORDERS FOR COMMON ORAL PROBLEMS IN THE GERIATRIC PATIENT

Oral candidiasis

Nystatin (Mycostatin) oral suspension
100,000 U/ml
Disp: 60 ml
Sig: 5 ml qid; rinse for 2 min and swallow; 1 ml nystatin oral suspension added to water used for soaking acrylic prostheses

Angular cheilitis and cheilosis

Nystatin ointment
Disp: 15 g tube
Sig: to dry affected area, apply ointment after each meal and at bedtime

Gingivitis and stomatitis

Chlorhexidine gluconate (Peridex) 0.12%
Disp: 16 oz
Sig: rinse with 0.5 oz for 30 sec bid and spit out

Localized and generalized mouth pain

Dyclonine HCl (Dyclone) 0.5% 1 oz and diphenhydramine HCl ([Benadryl] over the counter) elixir 12.5/5 ml mixed with Kaopectate (over the counter) 50% mixture by volume
Disp: 8 oz
Sig: rinse with 1 tsp q2h and spit out

Recurrent herpes simplex (orofacial)

Acyclovir (Zovirax) topical ointment 5%
Dips: 15 g tube
Sig: apply to area q2h during waking hours, beginning when symptoms first occur

_____ **SCOPE OF PRACTICE OF DENTAL SPECIALISTS** _____

Endodontist

Evaluation of periapical pain and edema

Diagnosis of atypical or referred dental pain

Treatment of pulpal disease in sclerotic teeth

Surgery of the root end

Oromaxillofacial surgeon

Extraction of teeth in medically compromised or cognitively impaired patients

Revision of bone and soft tissue to improve use of dentures

Biopsies

Placement of dental implants

Assessment and exploration of salivary glands

Treatment of disorders in the temporomandibular joint

Periodontist

Diagnosis of gingival and periodontal diseases

Treatment of medication-induced gingival hyperplasia

Administration of antimicrobial mouth rinses

Surgical repair of gingival and periodontal defects

Placement of dental implants

Prosthodontist

Evaluation of chewing and swallowing disorders

Assessment and construction of complete or partial dentures

Prosthodontics for osteoporotic patients

Restoration of extensively carious or heavily filled teeth

Palliation and prosthetic rehabilitation for oral cancer patients

Restoration of dental implants and prostheses

---

program includes quarterly or more frequent dental examinations, concentrated fluoride solutions (home use of sodium fluoride 1.1% or stannous fluoride 0.4%), saliva substitutes, dietary counseling, noncariogenic lozenges or gums, and vigorous brushing and flossing routines. The goals of the program are to relieve the discomfort of oral tissues, prevent oral infection, and control damage to teeth.

Complex diagnostic and therapeutic dental problems of elderly patients are best addressed by the clinical dental specialties of oromaxillofacial surgery, endodontics, periodontics, and prosthodontics. Consultation with a dental specialist may be obtained by the patient through an outpatient visit to a private office or hospital, depending on the nature of the problem and medical status of the patient. The box above outlines the general scope of practice of dental specialists.

REFERENCES

1. Beaven DW, Brooks SE: *The tongue in clinical diagnosis*, Ipswich, UK, 1988, Wolfe.
2. Chauncy HH et al: Parotid fluid composition in healthy aging males, *Adv Physiol Sci* 28:323, 1981.
3. *Clinician's Guide to Treatment of Common Oral Conditions*, ed 2, The American Academy of Oral Medicine, Fall 1990.

4. Gorsky M, Silverman S: Denture wearing and oral cancer, *J Prosthet Dent* 52:164, 1984.
5. Lloyd PM: Dental pain in the elderly, *Age* 10:70, 1987.
6. Mandel ID: Sialochemistry in diseases and clinical situations affecting salivary glands, *CRC Crit Rev Clin Lab Sci* 12:321, 1980.
7. Meskin L, Brown J: Prevalence and patterns of tooth loss in U.S. adult and senior populations, *Int J Oral Implantol* 5:59, 1988.
8. Ship J, Baum B: Is reduced salivary flow normal in old people? *Lancet* 336:1507, 1990.
9. Silverman S, ed: *Oral cancer*, ed 2, New York, 1985, The American Cancer Society.

SUGGESTED READINGS

Jones J, Mason D, eds: *Oral manifestations of systemic diseases*, ed 2, Philadelphia, 1990, WB Saunders.
Mandel ID: The role of saliva in maintaining oral homeostasis, *J Am Dent Assoc* 119:298, 1989.
Wright JM: Oral manifestations of drug reactions, *Dent Clin North Am* 28:529, 1984.

CHAPTER 48

Peptic ulcer

DAVID LAW

KEY POINTS

- The prevalence, morbidity, and mortality of peptic ulcer disease may be increasing among the elderly population.
- The classic symptoms of peptic ulcer disease may be muted or absent for older adults.
- Nonsteroidal antiinflammatory drugs and cigarettes are important elements in the pathogenesis and management of peptic ulcer disease for elderly patients.

CLINICAL RELEVANCE

Epidemiology

Peptic duodenal ulcer is clearly a disease of the twentieth century, with only rare reports of its occurrence before 1900. The disorder peaked between the 1940s and 1950s, but more recently the total number of reported cases of duodenal ulcers apparently decreased, as well as the total number of complications that require surgery. However, the morbidity and mortality from duodenal ulcer are essentially confined to older patients for whom the disease remains a significant cause of hospitalization, surgery, and death. For elderly persons, there is evidence that the frequency of duodenal ulcer is not decreasing. The lifetime prevalence of duodenal ulcer approximates 10% for men and less than one half of that number for women; however, the hospitalization rates for this disorder show that a greater percentage of women have been affected in recent years.

Peptic gastric ulcer, as opposed to duodenal ulcer, has been a disease of older patients and particularly a disease of older women. Gastric ulcers should be differentiated from pyloric channel ulcers and peptic ulcers of the very distal antrum. These latter two groups behave more like duodenal ulcers than like ulcers of the remainder of the stomach.

For both duodenal and gastric ulcers, the prevalence and severity of complications, including bleeding, perforation, and mortality, are concentrated among the elderly population.

Pathophysiology

For all peptic ulcers, the pathophysiology involves an imbalance between mucosal defense mechanisms and aggressive factors such as acid and pepsin, which endanger the integrity of the gastroduodenal mucosa. Characteristically, patients with peptic duodenal ulcers have higher gastric acid and pepsin secretory rates, which are greater than those found in patients with gastric ulcers, but there are wide variations in both groups.

Extensive investigational evidence exists to implicate a large number of factors, genetic and environmental, in the pathogenesis of peptic ulcer disease. Probably none are as clinically important as three recently emphasized risk factors that impact mucosal defense mechanisms in both duodenal and gastric ulcers: (1) smoking, (2) nonsteroidal antiinflammatory drugs (NSAIDs), and (3) infections with the organism *Helicobacter pylori*.

Smoking. Over the past 15 years there has been increasing evidence that smoking is associated with an increased prevalence of peptic ulcers, that the magnitude of the increase is directly related to the amount of cigarette use, and that both healing and mortality are worse for smokers.[1] These findings are not partial to aged patients but, since many elderly persons continue to smoke, the findings are important components of the occurrence, morbidity, and mortality of ulcer disease for this age group.

Nonsteroidal antiinflammatory drugs. There is now clear evidence that NSAIDs are risk factors for the *most critical complications* from both gastric and duodenal ulcers — bleeding and perforation.[3] NSAIDs inhibit prostaglandin synthesis, and in doing so the drugs may alter the user's mucosal defenses. While the prevalence of these complications in the overall population of users of NSAIDs is small, clinicians, when treating elderly patients who are taking NSAIDs, constantly must be aware of the possible complications. These risks appear to be dose related, worse with increasing age, and more prominent in women.

Helicobacter pylori. This spiral-shaped, gram-negative, ammonia-producing bacterium has been studied extensively over the past 10 years because of its remarkable association with antral gastritis and duodenal ulcer. It is found beneath the mucous layer attached to mucus-producing gastric cells and the tight junctions between them. More than 90% of patients with duodenal ulcer harbor this organism. Koch's postulates have been fulfilled for the etiological role that this organism has in acute antral gastritis, but the processes by which the organism alters mucosal resistance are not yet known. The prevalence of *H. pylori* also increases with age, and it is found among three fourths of healthy Americans by the time they are 75 years old. The exact role that *H. pylori* has in duodenal ulcer is unknown, but eradication of the organism by antibiotics provides a healing rate that is comparable to all traditional ulcer therapies.[2] When compared with traditional therapy, eradication of the organism by antibiotics also markedly decreases the rate of recurrence. Its possible role in gastric ulcer is less clear. The frequency of association of *H. pylori* with elderly patients who have gastric ulcers is about the same for elderly patients who do not have ulcers.

CLINICAL MANIFESTATIONS

The cardinal symptom of peptic duodenal ulcer is a well-localized epigastric or right upper quadrant *pain*, which has a characteristic pattern of chronicity, periodicity, and rhythmicity. Peptic duodenal ulcer disease is a chronic illness, frequently of many years' duration. The disease manifests repeated episodes of distress, lasting weeks or months. These episodes frequently occur at the same time of year for a given patient, and they are characterized by the following pattern during the course of a day: pain, food ingestion, relief, and then pain again a few hours later.

Gastric ulcer characteristically manifests a much less predictable pain pattern— it may have a diffuse location, it may be aggravated by food, and it may be associated with anorexia and weight loss.

Elderly patients, however, frequently do not demonstrate typical symptoms for either type of peptic ulcer disease. Pain may be blunted or totally absent and complications from the disease may be the first manifestations (i.e., bleeding, perforation, or obstruction) in up to 50% of elderly patients who have complications. Pain may be further modified by the use of NSAIDs. For these reasons the practitioner always must be alert to the possibility of an active ulcer in any elderly patient who has a previous history of peptic ulcer disease.

The second most common manifestation of peptic ulcer disease is *bleeding*, which occurs at some time in at least 20% of patients with duodenal ulcers. In elderly patients, bleeding appears to be more frequent and more severe than in younger patients and indeed may be the most common presentation of duodenal ulcer in patients who are more than 50 years old. However, bleeding, like pain, may be less apparent as a symptom and may present instead in the form of resultant anemia and its complications. Thus, when elderly patients demonstrate evidence of decreased cerebral blood flow (e.g., confusion, diminution of cognitive function, or stroke), postural hypotension, or cardiac symptoms such as congestive heart failure or increased angina pectoris, blood loss must be evaluated. If gastrointestinal blood loss is found, peptic ulcer disease must be considered most strongly, even if a patient has no history of pain.

The other acute complication of peptic ulcer disease is *perforation*, and symptoms frequently are modified or even absent for elderly patients. This is especially true for patients who take NSAIDs or corticosteroids. An upright x-ray examination of the abdomen should be obtained for such elderly patients who have blood in the stools and any form of clinical deterioration.

Finally, *gastric outlet obstruction* may manifest with less obvious symptoms in elderly patients. Patients with gradual gastric dilatation may be free of pain, and the condition may manifest itself with only the patients' intermittent vomiting of large volumes of retained foods and fluids, every few days to even as long as a week, and with the patients' being able to eat in between the vomiting episodes. Weight loss usually can be documented.

Functional assessment may show changes in the organ systems that initially are not suggestive of gastrointestinal disease (e.g., cerebral, cardiac, or renal dysfunction). Nutritional impairment, weight loss, vomiting, and functional limitation produced by abdominal pain are associated more obviously with peptic disease and its complications.

DIAGNOSTIC APPROACH

While the physical examination usually is not helpful in the diagnosis of peptic ulcer disease, a history of typical symptoms, as outlined previously, may be very suggestive. Ultimately the diagnosis is made by air-barium contrast x-ray studies or upper gastrointestinal endoscopy. Endoscopy is the most sensitive diagnostic procedure. Either of these procedures necessitates the primary care physician's obtaining consultative assistance from the radiologist or endoscopist.

When the physician documents duodenal ulcer, additional investigation is unnecessary and treatment begins. However, when gastric ulcer is documented, a further definition of the nature of the lesion is necessary. Biopsies and cytology specimens from endoscopy are required to exclude from the diagnosis the presence of gastric cancer, which can mimic benign gastric ulcer. Both diseases may respond initially to treatment by diminution of the ulcer and control of the symptoms, including pain. The opportunity for cure, which is present in some early gastric cancers, may be lost if accurate diagnosis is not pursued rapidly. There are numerous criteria (e.g., age of the patient, environmental factors, size of the ulcer, and location of the ulcer) that alter the likelihood of malignancy in gastric ulcers. However, for the primary care physician who discovers this lesion in an ambulatory patient, the wisest choices are to recognize that 2% to 6% of such lesions are malignant and to opt for consultation with an experienced gastroenterologist for consideration of endoscopy and biopsy.

INTERVENTION

Treatment of active peptic ulcer

Ambulatory treatment is widely accepted for peptic duodenal ulcer and peptic gastric ulcer, provided there is no evidence of malignancy, an adequate support system exists at home, and compliance with treatment is expected.

Over the past 15 years, the role of diet has been greatly downgraded, while the importance of cessation of smoking has been increasingly acknowledged. However, the most profound changes have been in the evolution of drug therapy, from the frequent use of oral acid-neutralizing agents (antacids) in the past to the development of potent acid-secretory inhibitors and medications that promote mucosal defenses against acid peptic disruptions.

Histamine H_2 receptor antagonists. The histamine H_2 receptor antagonists (H_2 antagonists) now constitute the first-line treatment for peptic ulcers. Peptic ulcers in

Table 48-1   Recommended doses of histamine H_2 receptor antagonist drugs

H_2 antagonist	Daily bedtime dose★
Cimetidine (Tagamet)	800 mg
Ranitidine (Zantac)	300 mg
Famotidine (Pepcid)	40 mg
Nizatidine (Axid)	300 mg

★Patients with gastric ulcers should receive full dose daily for 12 wk; patients with duodenal ulcers should receive full dose daily for 8 wk; patients with renal impairments should receive reduced dose.

elderly patients, as well as in the younger patients, should be treated with a full dose of an oral H_2 antagonist given once daily at bedtime. The four most widely used drugs (i.e., cimetidine, ranitidine, famotidine and nizatidine) all have well-established efficacies. There has been extensive clinical experience with cimetidine and ranitidine for elderly patients. While there are some differences in metabolism among these four drugs, they all should be given in reduced doses for patients with renal impairments (e.g., approximately 50% of full dose for those patients with 50% reductions in creatinine clearance [See Table 48-1 for doses of drugs.]).

The drugs are extremely well tolerated, with patients having few side effects. Mental confusion may occur in elderly patients treated with H_2 antagonists, and confusion most notably occurs when these drugs are administered parenterally. It appears to be dose related and reversible. Cimetidine has been reported in this context more frequently than other similar drugs; however, large follow-up studies have not substantiated any greater prevalence of mental confusion associated with the use of cimetidine rather than the use of other drugs. Indeed the safety of these drugs is remarkable, with side effects occurring in less than 3% of patients. Gynecomastia and headache also have been reported. Inhibition of cytochrome P-450-mediated drug metabolism has been documented for cimetidine and to a lesser extent has been documented for ranitidine. Using standard oral doses of H_2 antagonists for outpatients has not caused difficulties in a significant number of patients. However, monitoring blood levels of drugs such as warfarin, phenytoin, or theophylline should be performed for elderly patients who also take H_2 antagonists.

Antacids.   Until the introduction of H_2 antagonists, antacids had been the mainstay of peptic ulcer treatment. Antacids still are prescribed by many physicians and are used as over-the-counter medications by many patients. Within the last decade it has been determined that lower doses of antacids (120 to 180 mEq/day) are just as effective as the standard high-dose regimens. Lower doses decrease the patients' complications from these agents, including diarrhea related to magnesium content and constipation related to aluminum content, as well as phosphate and calcium imbalances. Antacids necessitate at least one dose four times a day, and this dosage is difficult for many elderly patients. This regimen also does not address completely the very important component of nocturnal acid secretion. Antacids are no longer first-line drugs for ulcer therapy, especially for older patients.

Sucralfate. Sucralfate is the basic aluminum salt of a polysulfated disaccharide. It is effective for the treatment of duodenal ulcer. The mechanism of action of sucralfate is neither acid neutralization nor inhibition of acid secretion but enhancement of mucosal defense mechanisms against acid peptic erosion, at least in part, through endogenous prostaglandin effects. Sucralfate may heal ulcers that are not responsive to H_2 antagonists, but it should not be used in conjunction with H_2 antagonists or with antacids because the resulting elevated pH of gastric juice (i.e., reduced acidity) prevents the biological activity of sucralfate. In its full dose (1 g qid 30 to 60 minutes before meals and at bedtime for 8 to 12 weeks) sucralfate may cause two problems for elderly patients. Compliance may be difficult because of the four-times-a-day dosage, but 2 g bid before breakfast and at bedtime appears to be equally effective. Constipation, which occurs in 2% to 3% of patients who take full doses, may become very severe in some elderly patients. Nevertheless, in instances where H_2 antagonists are not tolerated or are ineffective, sucralfate can induce the healing of duodenal ulcer.

Other drugs. Other drugs that are effective for the treatment of peptic ulcer disease include misoprostol (a prostaglandin E_1 analog), omeprazole (a proton pump inhibitor), and certain bismuth compounds such as bismuth subsalicylate or colloidal bismuth subcitrate (mechanisms unclear). At this time these drugs probably should not be initiated by the primary care physician as primary treatment for peptic disease without evaluation of the patient by a consultant.

Treatment and prevention of recurrent ulcer

Because of the increased morbidity and mortality of peptic ulcers in elderly patients, recurrent ulcers demand even more careful evaluation by the primary care physician. Determination of the patients' compliance with instructions and the roles of environmental factors such as the use of cigarettes and NSAIDs, which might be controlled, is essential.

Every effort should be made to have the patients cease smoking. If possible, discontinuing or at least decreasing NSAIDs is preferable; however, many elderly patients literally are dependent on these drugs for an acceptable quality of life. Fortunately, NSAID-associated peptic ulcers, both gastric and duodenal, generally heal when patients take full doses of antacids or H_2 antagonists, even while they continue to take NSAIDs.[2]

For the elderly patient, long-term preventive treatment is preferable when ulcers recur, especially because of the increased prevalence of serious complications, the altered symptoms associated with both the ulcer and its complications, and the combination of comorbidities and diminished physiological reserves that are frequently found in major organ systems. A full course of treatment should be continued until the recurrent ulcer is healed, and then chronic maintenance therapy should be initiated with one half of the full treatment dose.

Because of the possible role of *H. pylori* in chronic peptic ulcer disease, trials are under way to evaluate the effectiveness and feasibility of aggressive multidrug treatment (antibiotics and bismuth compounds) to eradicate *H. pylori* in patients with recurrent duodenal ulcer disease. Preliminary evidence suggests significant reduction in the recurrence rate with continuation of the ulcer-free state while the patient remains free of *H. pylori*.[4] This has the potential to effect major changes in the approaches to the management of recurrent duodenal ulcer and possibly gastric ulcer over the next few years. At this time such treatment is neither approved nor recommended for use by the primary care physician.[5]

REFERENCES

1. Harrison AR, Elashoff JD, Grossman MI: Cigarette smoking and ulcer disease. In *Smoking and health: a report of the surgeon general*, DHEW Pub No PHS 79-50066, Washington, DC, 1979, US Government Printing Office.
2. Marshall BJ et al: Prospective double blind trial of duodenal ulcer relapse after eradication of campylobacter pylori, *Lancet* 2:1437, 1988.
3. McCarthy DM: Acid peptic disease in the elderly, *Clin Geriatr Med* 7(2):231, 1991.
4. Rabeneck L, Ransohoff DF: Is helicobacter pylori a cause of duodenal ulcer?: a methodologic critique of current evidence, *Am J Med* 91:566, 1991.
5. Rauws EAJ, Tytgat GNH: Cure of duodenal ulcer associated with eradication of helicobacter pylori, *Lancet* 335:1233, 1990.

SUGGESTED READINGS

Freston MS, Freston JW: Peptic ulcers in the elderly: unique features and management, *Geriatrics* 45:39, 1990.
McCarthy DM: Acid peptic disease in the elderly, *Clin Geriatr Med* 7(2):231, 1991.
Zakim D, Dannenberg AJ, eds: *Peptic ulcer disease and other acid-related disorders*, Armonk, New York, 1991, Academic Research Associates.

CHAPTER 49

Constipation, diarrhea and fecal impaction

MARY KANE GOLDSTEIN
JOSEPH OLIVEIRA

KEY POINTS

- Constipation and diarrhea are common in elderly persons and require evaluation before treatment.
- Many medications, including laxatives, that are commonly used by geriatric patients cause constipation.
- Fecal impaction may be soft or hard and may be high in the colon or in the rectal vault.
- Fecal impaction may present as acute confusion, urinary retention, or liquid incontinent stool.
- Most constipated patients benefit from more fiber in their diets, but patients with intestinal pseudoobstruction (as occurs in Parkinson's disease and other neurological diseases) are at risk for volvulus and should not be placed on high-fiber diets.
- Diarrhea in patients who receive enteral feeding is not always due to the osmotic load—infectious causes must be considered.

CLINICAL RELEVANCE

Constipation

Precise data on the prevalence of chronic constipation are difficult to obtain because of the great variation in the definition for constipation. Attempts have been made to define constipation in terms of stool frequency, stool size and weight, stool water content, and gut transit time. Normal stool frequency in Western countries is at least three per week for those on low-residue diets and five per week for those on high-residue diets; however, in many parts of the world three per day is more common, so there is clearly a great variation in normal.

Based on self-report, constipation is the most common chronic digestive condition among all age groups in the United States.[6] The prevalence of constipation increases with age throughout adulthood. The prevalence rapidly increases among those who are more than 64 years old, and the prevalence is 4% for those aged 65 to 74 years old and 10.2% for those aged 75 years and older. For the older age groups, constipation is twice as common in women as it is in men and approximately 1.3 times more common among nonwhites than whites. Fecal impaction is particularly common in frail elderly persons, and it is detected in 42% of patients who are admitted to a geriatric ward.[7]

It is clinically important to identify and treat constipation. Urinary tract infections and uninhibited bladder contractions have been attributed to constipation. Fecal incontinence is clearly associated with fecal stasis. Fecal impaction can cause colonic ulceration, autonomic dysreflexia (in spinal cord-injured patients), rectal prolapse, volvulus, and shock from massive fluid loss. The chronic lower abdominal pain of constipation has led to excess surgeries, including unnecessary hysterectomies and appendectomies. Having only three stools per week for a long time is a risk factor for colon cancer. A potentially disastrous complication is stercoraceous perforation of the colon by hard feces.

Constipation often is said to be the cause of hemorrhoids, but this is not supported by epidemiological data. The prevalence of hemorrhoids peaks for those who are between the ages of 45 and 65 years old and decreases thereafter, a contrast to the rapid increase in the prevalence of constipation among those who are more than 65 years old.[1]

A list of the causes of constipation, including medicines, is shown in the box on p. 478. Many of these medications commonly are used for the treatment of older persons. Diuretics deplete fluids and may cause hypokalemia. Adrenergic blockers and calcium channel blockers directly may inhibit colonic motility. Bulk agents with insufficient liquid cause hard stools that are difficult to pass. Chronic use of laxatives that damage the myenteric plexus can lead to *cathartic syndrome*.

Diarrhea

While diarrheal illness is recognized as a serious problem for young children, the majority of diarrheal deaths actually occur among those who are more than 74 years old. Data based on death certificates indicate that 86% of these deaths result from diarrhea that is presumed to be noninfectious. This presumption may be made because of a failure to search for infectious causes, particularly rotavirus.[2] Older persons are at greater risk than are younger persons for serious morbidity from the fluid losses of diarrhea. Maximum concentration ability by the kidney is often impaired, and impaired thirst mechanisms may not lead to the sufficient intake of fluids. Outbreaks of infectious diarrhea are major causes of morbidity and mortality in nursing homes, but in office practices the cases of infectious diarrhea are seen more sporadically.

Diarrhea is the passage of increased stool volume and bulk, usually with a watery component and an increase in frequency. It may be caused by increased secretion of

CAUSES OF CONSTIPATION

Laxative abuse	Colonic and anorectal disorders
Medication	Anal fissure, fistula, or stricture
Aluminum-containing antacids	Appendicitis
Anticholinergics	Colon polyp or stricture
Antidepressants	Colorectal cancer
Antihistamines	Diverticular disease
Antiparkinsonians	Hemorrhoid
Antipsychotics	Hirschsprung's disease
Barium sulfate	Irritable bowel disease
Beta blockers	Megacolon
Bismuth	Volvulus
Calcium channel blockers	Other associated illnesses
Diuretics	Lesion to central nervous system
Metals	Parkinson's disease
• Arsenic	Stroke
• Iron	Diabetes mellitus
• Lead	Hyperparathyroidism
• Other	Hypoparathyroidism
Narcotics	Hypothyroidism
Neurological drugs	Factors associated with aging
Opiates	Inactivity
Diet	Decreased water intake
Lack of fiber, fruits, vegetables, fluids	Psychological factors and illnesses
Foods: high fat content, refined	Anxiety and distress
breads, tea (excess)	Depression
	Psychosis (schizophrenia)

fluid in the intestine, by decreased fluid absorption, or by an intestinal motor disturbance. Medications that can cause diarrhea include laxatives, magnesium-containing antacids, quinidine, propranolol, and digitalis. Artificial sweeteners that are not absorbed (e.g., sorbitol and mannitol) can cause osmotic diarrhea. Some patients seen in ambulatory geriatric care require feeding supplements. Diarrhea occurs in up to 25% of patients receiving enteral nutrition.[5] Some of this diarrhea is due to lactose intolerance, some to high osmotic load, and some to infection. Diarrhea results from bolus feeding of lactose-containing food to lactose-intolerant persons, but the slow rate of presentation of lactose to the intestine with 24-hour continuous feeding does not usually cause a problem.

Inflammatory bowel disease, most prevalent among young adults, also first may present after adults are 50 years of age. For this age group, the presenting symptoms of Crohn's disease most commonly are abdominal pain and diarrhea. Inflammatory bowel disease may be misdiagnosed as carcinoma, diverticulitis, or ischemic colitis. The disease should be considered in the differential diagnosis of older persons with abdominal pain, diarrhea, and weight loss.[4]

CLINICAL MANIFESTATIONS

Constipation

A patient's complaint may consist of change in stool frequency, difficulty in defecation, or sensation of incomplete evacuation. It is important for the clinician to respect the patient's concerns, even when the bowel frequency meets the criterion of more than three per week. When the history is not clear, the patient or caregiver should be asked to keep a record. This is particularly important when the patient is demented.

Fecal impaction may have a subtle presentation. It should be considered when there is deterioration of any patient who is at risk for fecal impaction. The typical symptoms include anorexia, nausea, vomiting, and abdominal pain. Acute confusion and fecal incontinence may be the prominent symptoms. Urinary retention and incontinence may occur from the pressure of the fecal mass. Fever, dysrhythmia, and tachypnea have been reported.

Diverticulitis often occurs with chronic constipation and may be dismissed as discomfort resulting from constipation. The patient typically has left lower quadrant pain and tenderness, a slightly elevated temperature, and an elevated white blood cell count. Life-threatening complications may occur, particularly for the very frail, including perforation of diverticular abscess and obstruction of the colon.

Volvulus is often superimposed against a background of chronic constipation. Patients with histories of physical inactivity, excessive use of laxatives, and use of antiparkinsonian drugs are at risk for colonic volvulus. The patients develop sudden abdominal pain and vomiting. The patients who have volvulus are acutely ill and should be managed in the hospital.

Diarrhea

Diarrhea may be the first symptom of serious underlying illness. Passage of maroon-colored stool signals an ischemic bowel or intestinal bleeding and should be managed in the hospital rather than in the office. A diarrhea of acute infectious origin is easily recognized in most cases by the rapid onset and the associated symptoms of malaise, anorexia, and/or fever. The history may include recent contact with others who have a similar illness, recent ingestion of suspect food, or recent travel. Vomiting suggests food poisoning (staphylococcal toxin), and bloody diarrhea suggests mucosal invasion by pathogens such as *Shigella flexneri*, enteropathogenic *Escherichia coli*, *Campylobacter jejuni*, *Salmonella* sp., or *Entamoeba histolytica*.

Diabetic patients are susceptible to both diarrhea and constipation, which may alternate within the same patient. The incidence of chronic diabetic diarrhea is 10% to 22%.[3] The condition is more common in men than in women. Steatorrhea is common. Most patients have peripheral neuropathies and many have autonomic neuropathies that are demonstrable from the patients' physical examinations. The etiology of diabetic diarrhea is unknown and may vary from one case to another. Some patients have a bacterial overgrowth syndrome.

CLINICAL EVALUATION OF CONSTIPATION AND DIARRHEA

History

Characteristics of the bowel complaint
- Onset: time and circumstance
- Timing of normal versus abnormal stools
- Duration
- Frequency
- Volume of stool
- Consistency of stool
- Relation to food ingestion
- Premorbid bowel pattern
- Associated symptoms: urgency, deferral time (time to access toilet), pain, bleeding, abdominal cramps, rectal sensation of fullness, sensation of passing stool or gas

Other medical history
- Gastrointestinal
- Obstetrical
- Trauma
- Neurological
- Medical conditions causing neuropathy or muscle weakness
- Medications (prescription and over-the-counter)
- Diet: fiber, fruits, vegetables, fluids

Environmental factors

Access
- Restraints or bedrails that inhibit mobility
- Location of bathroom or commode not remembered by patient

Clothing (patient unable to unfasten clothing adequately)
Functional impact
Caregiver history
- Caregiver burden
- Caregiver record

Physical examination

General phsyical examination, including assessment of hydration status
Mental status examination
Abdominal examination
Neurological examination
- Mobility and motor strength
- Signs of autonomic neuropathy
- Sacral reflexes (anal wink and bulbo-cavernosus)
Digital rectal examination
- Inspection for mucosal prolapse or procidentia and signs of inflammatory bowel disease
- Sphincter tone
- Exclude mass and soft or hard impaction
- Occult blood
- Voluntary external sphincter contraction

Adapted from Goldstein MK et al: Fecal incontinence in an elderly man, *J Am Geriatr Soc* 37(10):991, 1989.

DIAGNOSTIC APPROACH

Constipation and diarrhea each may be clinical manifestations in a large number of serious illnesses. For example, an acute intestinal obstruction may be accompanied by constipation or diarrhea. A discussion of all problems that manifest these symptoms of constipation or diarrhea as part of the clinical picture is beyond the scope of this chapter. This chapter focuses only on clinical conditions for which constipation or diarrhea is the major complaint. The general approach to the clinical evaluation of constipation and diarrhea is shown in the box on p. 480. It is particularly important to obtain information from the patient's history and physical examination about concurrent neurological or hormonal symptoms, as well as medications. The rectal examination is an essential part of the evaluation. A complete blood count, electrolyte panel, blood urea nitrogen, serum calcium, thyroid function test, and stool Hemoccult should be performed. A leukocytosis may be seen in fecal impactions. The history and physical examination, together with laboratory studies, usually yield the diagnosis.

Constipation

If constipation is of less than 2 years' duration or if the patient's symptoms have changed during that time, then evaluation for cancer of the colon is mandatory. This evaluation includes either sigmoidoscopy and barium enema or colonoscopy. Patients with leakage of liquid stool or patients who have other symptoms of impaction but with an empty rectal vault should be suspected of having a high impaction. These patients should have abdominal x-rays to locate masses of stool or signs of obstruction. Fecal incontinence with continuous passage of small amounts of stool presents as fecal smearing of the patient's undergarments. The patient may have a daily bowel movement but, because of incomplete emptying, the bowel has a *soft impaction*, which is a large volume of soft fecal material retained in the rectal vault. Thus, the finding of soft stool in the rectum should not be considered to represent *no impaction*. Patients with fecal smearing usually have *fecal stasis*, a large amount of stool in the descending colon, which is seen on the patients' x-rays. In contrast, patients with the less common disorder, irritable colon, have intermittent passage of a stool bolus of normal size.

Diarrhea

Most cases of diarrhea are self-limiting, but some cases are life threatening. Clinical judgment must be used to determine how clear a reasonable diagnosis is from the patient's history (e.g., one day of diarrhea following initiation of lactose-containing formula in bolus feeds for a patient with lactose intolerance) and how aggressive the evaluation of the patient should be. All patients should have a history and physical examination, including a rectal examination. The patient's level of hydration should be established. If the patient is dehydrated, more aggressive management will be necessary. For patients who have diarrhea for more than 1 or 2 days, bloody stool, or fever, stool examination for blood and leukocytes should be performed immediately and stool specimens should be submitted for culture. For patients with significant diarrhea or patients with bloody diarrhea, a sigmoidoscopy should be performed.

If a patient has a chronic diarrhea (more than two weeks' duration), the history should be carefully reviewed for the patient's use of laxative or nonabsorbable osmotic agents, heavy alcohol consumption, and symptoms of hyperthyroidism or Addison's disease (hypoadrenalism). A stool specimen should be examined for ova and parasites. For patients with diabetic diarrhea, islet cell tumor should be considered.

INTERVENTION

Constipation

The patient's history and physical examination may indicate the cause of constipation and thus intervention is relatively clear (e.g., thyroid disease, parathyroid disease, depression, or colon cancer). If possible, adjustments should be made to medications. Those medications with anticholinergic effects should be avoided by the patient, or the dosages of such medications should be reduced by the physician.

When constipation is due to chronic laxative abuse, irreversible neurological damage, or poor colonic motility, a lifelong bowel program must be adopted. For a bowel program to take effect, the rectum and sigmoid colon must be sufficiently cleaned of fecal matter. In some cases this can be accomplished by changes in the diet such as additional liquids and fiber. For patients who do not respond to a change in diet, a hyperosmotic agent such as lactulose or an irritant laxative such as bisacodyl may be used for this initial cleaning of the rectum. For severe cases of fecal stasis, enemas and/or manual disimpaction are necessary. Enemas should be of tap water or standard sodium phosphate, in small volume. Disimpaction usually can be accomplished without anesthesia, but occasionally a pudendal block or general anesthesia is required. With an enema, the material low in the sigmoid is removed but over the course of the next day, fecal material from higher up in the descending colon moves down. It may be necessary to give an enema once a day for up to a week to clear the stasis. During this time, the patient may have frequent leakage of semiliquid stool and may develop worse fecal incontinence. The patient and the caregiver should be warned about these effects in advance and should be reassured that the changes are temporary while the stasis is being cleared. It is usually possible to manage this procedure and its effects at home, perhaps with assistance from a visiting nurse, but occasionally a patient will require admission to a geriatric unit or to a skilled nursing facility for the clearing out phase of treatment. High impactions may require lavage under sigmoidoscopical visualization.

Once patients are ready to start the long-term bowel program, they should be given the instructions that are listed in the box on p. 483. The clinician should go over each step with the patients and their families, explaining the instructions and allowing the patient an opportunity to solve problems at each step and to find socially and culturally appropriate ways to achieve compliance. If the clinician has many patients from a particular ethnic group, then it is efficient to obtain consultation with a nutritionist and other health workers who are familiar with the customs of that group.

One important exception to the recommendation of increased bulk in the diet is the patient who has autonomic neuropathy or intestinal pseudoobstruction. Such a patient is at increased risk for volvulus and must be managed with a combination of suppositories and enemas, as well as avoidance of anticholinergic medications. The clinician should have some understanding of the use of fiber in the diet. There are

**INSTRUCTIONS FOR LONG-TERM
BOWEL PROGRAMS FOR PATIENTS**

Stop use of laxatives except as part of this plan.

Review nonprescription and prescription medications to minimize constipation-causing agents.

Drink warm liquid with breakfast. Take advantage of gastrocolic reflex to defecate after breakfast. Allow adequate time for this.

Never ignore the urge to defecate. If you feel the urge, stop what you are doing and find a toilet. Do not suppress the urge. Be certain that there is quick access to a toilet. Be certain that caregivers understand the importance of a quick response to a request for toileting help.

Walk or perform other exercises for at least 30 minutes each day.

Add several different forms of fiber and roughage to diet, including bran or bulk fiber, fruit fiber such as fresh fruits or dried fruits, and vegetable fiber.

Take adequate liquids. Remember that the level of your thirst may not indicate sufficient liquid intake. You may need to drink water, even when you are not thirsty.

If further stimulation is needed for defecation, use digital stimulation of rectum or glycerine suppository. Time this procedure to take advantage of the gastrocolic reflex (e.g., after breakfast).

Use laxatives only if they are necessary. For very hard stool, use a lubricant (e.g., mineral oil) or stool softener intermittently. Do not use mineral oil if there is a swallowing problem and do not use it continuously. On occasions when the risk of impaction appears high, use an irritant laxative such as bisacodyl or an osmotic agent such as lactulose.

Adapted from Goldstein MK et al: Fecal incontinence in an elderly man, *J Am Geriatr Soc* 37(10):996, 1989.

many different forms of food fiber. One classification calls the major fraction of fiber *non-starch polysaccharide*, which is then subdivided into *cellulose* and *non-cellulose*, the latter including pectin, inulin, guar, and plant gums. Fiber is not completely indigestible, but the amount of digestion varies greatly with the type of fiber. The colon is the major site of degradation of fiber by intestinal microflora. The increased bacterial mass is one of the mechanisms by which fiber increases stool output. Methane and other gases are produced during degradation. These gasses are either passed as flatus or absorbed and breathed out. Bran fiber is not degraded significantly but exerts its effect by holding water and increasing stool bulk. Patients must be instructed to consume sufficient liquid when they use a bran or psyllium supplement. Excessive amounts of fiber in the diet interfere with absorption of minerals and may cause discomfort and bloating.

The squatting position aids defecation. If patients require a toilet with an elevated seat for ease of getting on and off, then a footstool may be used to elevate their feet.

Patients with Parkinson's disease and other neurologic diseases who develop the syndrome of sudden abdominal distention and fecal incontinence require special treatment. They may have a megacolon which is at risk of perforation. They should be managed by someone experienced with the condition. Treatment often includes sigmoidoscopic decompression. Severe, recurrent, fecal impaction or episodes of obstruction may require surgery. The complication rates of such surgery are high.

Diarrhea

Treatment of diarrhea depends on the cause identified in the evaluation. For acutely ill patients, hospitalization is required for hydration and specific therapy.

If diarrhea occurs within 2 days of initiation of enteral feeding, the clinician should dilute the formula, check for the patient's history of lactose intolerance, and switch to continuous rather than bolus feeding. If the diarrhea persists or if diarrhea occurs in a patient who had previously tolerated the feeding, then an evaluation for an infectious cause of the diarrhea should be undertaken.

For patients who have diabetic diarrhea and have no other specific cause for their diarrhea, no treatment emerges as clearly the best. Some patients, presumably those with bacterial overgrowth, show improvement after a 2-week course of broad-spectrum antibiotics. Other patients respond to diphenoxylate hydrochloride with atropine sulfate (Lomotil) and kaolin-pectin (Kaopectate). Clonidine 1 mg/day decreases the frequency of the diarrhea for some patients. Transcutaneous administration of clonidine may prevent hypotensive side effects.

REFERENCES

1. Johanson JF, Sonnenberg A, Koch TR: Clinical epidemiology of chronic constipation, *J Clin Gastroenterol* 11:525, 1989.
2. Lew JF et al: Diarrheal deaths in the United States 1979 through 1987: a special problem for the elderly, *JAMA* 265:3280, 1991.
3. Ogbonnaya KI, Arem R: Diabetic diarrhea: pathophysiology, diagnosis, and management, *Arch Intern Med* 150:262, 1990.
4. Roberts PL et al: Clinical course of Crohn's disease in older patients, *Dis Colon Rectum* 33(6):458, 1990.
5. Silk DBA: Fiber and enteral nutrition, *Gut* 30:246, 1989.
6. Sonnenberg A, Koch TR: Epidemiology of constipation in the United States, *Dis Colon Rectum* 32:1, 1989.
7. Wrenn K: Fecal impaction, *N Engl J Med* 321:658, September, 1989.

SUGGESTED READINGS

Castle SC: Constipation: Endemic in the elderly?, *Med Clin North Am* 73:1497, 1989.
Goldstein MK et al: Fecal Incontinence in an elderly man, *J Am Geriatr Soc* 37(10):991, 1989.
Lew JF et al: Diarrheal deaths in the United States 1979 through 1987: a special problem for the elderly, *JAMA* 265:3280, 1991.

CHAPTER 50

Chronic obstructive lung disease

ADRIAN J. WILLIAMS

KEY POINTS

- Chronic airflow obstruction is a leading cause of death and disability among elderly persons and is both underrecognized and undertreated.
- Cigarette smoking remains the prominent cause of chronic obstructive lung disease, but unrecognized or undertreated asthma is an important subgroup.
- Cough in a nonsmoker is asthma until proved otherwise.
- Spirometry or peak flow measurements are essential in the diagnosis, assessment, and management of chronic obstructive lung disease.
- Pharmacotherapy, including corticosteroids, should be delivered by the inhaled route whenever possible.
- Disturbance of sleep is frequent and control of nocturnal symptoms should be sought.

CLINICAL RELEVANCE

Chronic obstructive lung disease (COLD), also called chronic obstructive pulmonary disease (COPD) or chronic airflow obstruction (CAO), is one of the more common problems of old age. The prevalence of CAO in elderly persons has been increasing since 1971, and in 1981 the disorder was present in as many as 17 million Americans. The incidence of all major forms of CAO is 130/1000 for those who are more than 60 years old, and CAO is listed as the fifth leading cause of death next to infections. The mortality rate stands at 200/100,000 for those aged 65 to 70 years old and 450/100,000 for those aged 75 years and older. The condition may be underdiagnosed for older patients, in part because of the higher prevalence of other diseases such as heart failure but also because of the underutilization of pulmonary function tests as was shown in a recent survey of 199 elderly patients who received day hospital and domiciliary care.[2] One hundred and twenty-one patients had reduced peak flows (70% less than predicted). Eighty-two patients (or nearly 70%) had significant improvements (greater than 15%) after treatment with bronchodilators, but only 6% of these 82 received treatment. Pulmonary function tests must be used to help address this problem.

Definitions and pathogenesis

CAO is not one disease but a group of diseases (therefore a syndrome) that are considered together because they are characterized by decreased expiratory flow in the airways. They produce similar abnormalities of pulmonary function and they are often difficult to distinguish as separate entities either clinically or pathologically. However, there are important implications for management and therefore an effort should be made to distinquish each form of CAO. *CAO* (COPD, COLD) is the term generally used to refer to chronic bronchitis and emphysema, conditions that are characterized by persistent airflow limitation.

Chronic bronchitis. Chronic bronchitis is a daily productive cough that results from hypersecretion of mucus. This cough is invariably due to cigarette smoking (or severe environmental pollution) and is a symptom that can be elicited from cigarette smokers. It is the clinical consequence of an increase in the activity of the protective mucus-secreting apparatus (i.e., mucous glands and goblet cells). Chronic bronchitis is a clinical diagnosis. It may be but is not necessarily associated with airflow obstruction as determined by spirometry. Only 15% to 20% of smokers develop CAO (chronic obstructive bronchitis), while all smokers develop chronic bronchitis.[5]

Emphysema. This form of CAO is due to an increase in the size of the respiratory units or acini and the destruction of alveolar walls. In the most common form of emphysema the destruction centers on the respiratory bronchioles and is therefore *centriacinar*. The severe generalized form of *panacinar* emphysema is an extension of this process into the whole of the acinus. The pathogenesis of this process is thought to be an imbalance between the proteases released in the acinus from leukocytes and macrophages and the protective antiproteases of the body (or antitrypsin), which may be genetically induced or inactivated by release of oxidants from phagocytes or by direct chemical oxidation from cigarette smoke.

Asthma. The clinical definition of *asthma* as reversible airway obstruction is a useful one that helps identify patients at risk, but it is insufficient as the sole framework on which to base treatment. Physiologically, asthma is a problem of bronchial hyperreactivity to a variety of stimuli. Evidence shows that the degree of hyperreactivity correlates somewhat with the severity of disease and that hyperreactivity is favorably influenced by reduced exposure to stimuli and by regular effective treatment. The pathological definition of asthma as chronic eosinophilic bronchitis summarizes this new understanding of asthma as a disease of inflammation and results in important implications for treatment.[4]

The aging lung

Because the lungs are exposed by more than 50,000 breaths/day to a potentially noxious environment, it is perhaps not surprising that aging is associated with substantial changes in the lungs and in lung functions. An understanding of these changes is necessary to understand the impact of CAO.[7]

Mechanical alterations in the lung give rise to characteristic physiological changes. There is a loss of elasticity of the lung partly because of changes in the collagen matrix (an increase in type I collagen and a reduction in type III) and because of reduced alveolar surface area (4%/yr after age 30) and increased size of alveolar ducts and bronchioles. This has been called *senile emphysema* and is most prominent in the apical portions of the lung where gravitational stretching forces are most evident. There are also changes in the chest wall; it becomes stiffer and the respiratory muscles become weaker and less capable of metabolic activity. The consequence of these changes is an increase in resting lung volumes (i.e., functional residual capacity and residual volume because of the closure of "floppy" airways and air trapping) without an increase in total lung capacity. The vital capacity and expiratory flow rate consequently are reduced with aging. The diffusing capacity for carbon monoxide (DLCO) is reduced due to the reduced acinar volume and worsened ventilation-perfusion matching. These changes also produce a fall in alveolar oxygen tension (PaO_2) with age (the predicted normal PaO_2 in torr or mm Hg can be estimated by the formula $100 - [\frac{1}{3} \times age (yr)]$. The control of breathing also is altered, with as much as a 50% reduction in the sensitivity of the respiratory center to hypoxemia, as well as an increase in sleep apneas.

Aging is itself a risk factor for the development of CAO. However, because of the large reserve of lung function, other insults must occur for a clinical effect to be seen. Breathlessness is not experienced until the forced expiratory volume in the first second (FEV_1) is reduced to approximately 1.5 L, a point that is reached, for example, from an FEV_1 of 4 L at age 20 years only after 80 years (at a rate of decline of 30 ml/yr). However, with additional pathology (smoking and asthma are the most important, along with other environmental, genetic, or anatomical abnormalities) this rate of loss of lung function triples and symptoms may develop after only 25 to 30 years and hence are present in the geriatric patient.

CLINICAL MANIFESTATIONS
Diurnal symptoms

The principle symptoms of patients with CAO are cough, sputum production, breathlessness, and wheezing. Chest pain is unusual and hemoptysis, although it is most commonly described as resulting from chronic bronchitis, is uncommon and should be suggestive of another cause. Cough is generally productive and exacerbated by infection or irritants. The cough may be prominent at night and lead to disturbed sleep, and it may be most "productive" when the patient awakens in the morning. Sputum is white (or mucoid) unless it is infected. One important caveat to remember is that cough in a nonsmoker means asthma until proved otherwise. Breathlessness is by far the most important reason for a medical consultation with patients who have CAO. Usually CAO is first noticed by patients when they exert themselves, often when they climb hills or stairs. Progression to disabling shortness of breath is not unusual. The onset of breathlessness signals a major loss of lung function, with the FEV_1 being 1 to 1.5 L. A broad correlation exists between the severity of breathlessness and the FEV_1 but the range may be wide. Wheezing, though not always present, should alert the clinician of the possibility of asthma; however, not all wheezing is asthma. Again, this wheezing may appear or become worse at night because of the normal decline in airway diameter that occurs during the night. Wheezing is more prominent in asthma but it still is a feature of chronic obstructive bronchitis and emphysema.

Nocturnal symptoms

Evidence exists that nocturnal worsening of CAO is serious and is a common occurrence, with as many as 40% of CAO patients awakening every night. The reason for such nocturnal worsening is unclear. The consequences of nocturnal bronchoconstriction include disturbed sleep, hypoxemia, and probable death. There is sleep disruption, which may impair the patient's daytime performance, and sleep deprivation is known to reduce ventilatory drive. The hypoxemia is rarely severe, with saturations ranging from 85% to 95% in stable CAO.

Physical examination

The outward appearances of the chests of patients with CAO may be normal or barrel shaped. Chest expansion is ultimately poor and is associated with subcostal recession in those patients who have significant hyperinflation. There may be a palpable (and visible) tracheal tug in the suprasternal notch. Pursed-lip breathing may be used by severely affected patients as a means to delay the closure of "floppy" airways. Breath sounds are diminished. Inspiratory and expiratory wheezes may be heard, especially from patients who have asthma. However, this wheezing does not grade the severity of the airway obstruction. Clubbing is not a feature of CAO. If it is found, consideration must be given to other conditions that have been associated with clubbing.

Simple clinical features may help the physician to characterize the severity of the older patient's CAO at the time of the office visit. With the patient's increased respiratory distress, breath sounds variably may increase or decrease but tachypnea and tachycardia are inevitable, along with the patient's increased use of accessory muscles, as well as subcostal recession and sleep disturbance.

DIAGNOSTIC APPROACH

History and examination

Patients with CAO usually smoke cigarettes (including elderly patients), but if they have no history of smoking the diagnosis of chronic obstructive bronchitis or emphysema is much less likely (except for those with antiprotease deficiency) than is the diagnosis of asthma. Gradual onset and steady progression of CAO is strong evidence of chronic obstructive bronchitis or emphysema. In contrast, episodical wheezing with some resolution is suggestive of asthma. Childhood respiratory problems are common among patients who have asthma, chronic obstructive bronchitis, or emphysema.

Examination may be helpful in first establishing the diagnosis (e.g., the barrel-shaped chest is pathognomonic of CAO) and in further differentiating the diagnosis if prominent wheezing is heard. Signs useful in predicting the need for hospitalization of the patient are a pulse >120/min, respiration >30/min, and pulsus paradoxus >15 mm Hg.

Laboratory studies

Laboratory tests are essential both to establish the diagnosis and to provide an assessment of the patient's progress. In the office setting these tests can be limited simply to pulmonary function, chest radiograph, and, at specific times, arterial blood gas.

Pulmonary function tests. The diagnosis of chronic airflow obstruction is confirmed by the finding of chronic airflow obstruction. This finding may be achieved by the use of spirometry or peak flow. The simple timed spirogram is suitable for diagnosis and management of patients. Measurements commonly obtained from this plot of volume against time include forced vital capacity (FVC) in liters, forced expired volume in the first second (FEV_1) FEV_1/FVC ratio, and maximum midexpiratory flow rate.

The definitions of normal pulmonary functions for the geriatric population are not without difficulties. The prediction of normal pulmonary functions depends in part on the patient's height, which declines with age, and aging, which mimics the disease under question. It may be that flow rates decline first during middle age because of reduced muscle power and reduced lung elasticity, and then flow rates decline further during old age because of loss of height. Nevertheless, it is usual to accept 80% of the predicted normal measurement as the lower limit of normal for FVC and FEV_1. If the ratio of FEV_1/FVC is less than 0.7, then airway obstruction is confirmed. Severity is defined arbitrarily by the reduction in the FEV_1 (experience of the physician provides the most information). There is a strong predictive value of baseline FEV_1 that can be used to estimate mortality from CAO. The lower the FEV_1 from the mean value of an age-corrected population FEV_1, the higher the death rate from CAO.

Response to bronchodilators. Chronic obstructive bronchitis and emphysema have traditionally been associated with fixed airway obstruction, but absolute irreversibility rarely occurs and, although only small improvements may occur following one's use of a bronchodilator, it may be associated clinically with useful improvements. However, it is mandatory to identify older patients who have significant changes after they use inhaled bronchodilators (i.e., asthma, a potentially treatable disease). Guidelines for what constitutes a clinically significant change have been formulated based on the variability of the test in any one individual. The FEV_1 or FVC may normally change by a maximum of 9.5% between tests so that a change of 10% or greater in either test is statistically significant. However, a change of 15% or greater is more clinically significant and more suggestive of asthma (provided the change is at least 200 ml).

The peak flow meter probably provides an acceptable alternative to the spirogram. This inexpensive and robust device assesses airflow during peak expirations (peak expired flow rate [PEFR]) and is grossly correlated with the FEV_1 (PEFR liter/minute = FEV_1 liter $\times$ 100). The peak flow meter is especially useful for assessing the patients' responses to bronchodilators and for following the patients. Ideally, patients should have their own devices and should record their peak flow rates on a regular basis several times a day (a circadian variability of 20% or greater is consistent with asthma).

Chest radiographs. The chest radiograph is a useful (though not essential) test that provides some evidence for CAO and excludes other problems from the patient's diagnosis (e.g., occupational lung disease, old tuberculosis, or even lung cancer). The radiographic signs for CAO lack sensitivity but are specific. Air trapping leads to a low flat diaphragm, sometimes with a narrow cardiac silhouette. Severe emphysema may be evidenced in one or more lung quadrants by a reduced vascular pattern.

Arterial blood gases. Arterial blood gases are mandatory in the initial assessment of all cyanotic patients and should be obtained for those patients who have substantial symptoms of breathlessness. The value of the study in both instances is to establish the severity of hypoxemia and hypercarbia and to assess the possible intervention with oxygen therapy.

Ear and pulse oximetry measure oxygen saturation and are useful for the broad categorization of patients (e.g., definitely abnormal, 85% or less saturated; probably normal, 94% or more saturated). Oximetry may allow a more complete office assessment and may satisfy the requirements for reimbursement for home oxygen therapy.

Other tests. An electrocardiogram provides additional information about the right side of the heart, but the test is an adjunct to the other studies and is not essential to the evaluation of CAO unless there is a history of cardiovascular disease. Conventional exercise testing is neither easily applied, nor should it be applied, but a functional assessment can be achieved by the 12-minute or 6-minute walk test. This is simply performed by having the patient walk back and forth in the office or a nearby corridor. A clinical assessment of breathlessness before and after the test should be performed.

INTERVENTION

Prevention

Occupational exposures are assumed not to be an issue for elderly patients, but cigarette smoking is of fundamental importance. Although in the early phases of disease the cessation of tobacco smoking is associated with a potential for nearly normal subsequent lung function, by the time the patient's accelerated decline of lung function is reached, recovery is not expected. Cessation of smoking still is valuable because a reduced rate of further decline is likely. Approximately one third of patients are able to cease smoking when breathlessness develops. For other patients, the best supportive therapy during cessation is probably the transcutaneous nicotine patch.

Antibiotics

Occasional winter infections in which sputum becomes purulent are best treated as they occur with courses of antibiotics such as amoxicillin or trimethoprim-sulfamethoxazole. For rapidly recurring infections, monthly cycles of such antibiotics can be used. Otherwise, there is no advantage to prophylactic or aerosolized antibiotic therapy.

Bronchodilator therapy

Bronchodilator therapy for older patients should be primarily through inhalation methods. Under these routes of administration, drug selection and dosage do not differ for older patients. The aim of bronchodilator therapy is to relax smooth muscles in the walls of the airways, reduce gas trapping, and decongest the mucosa. Because the inhalation route of administration is preferable for all bronchodilators, including corticosteroids, attention to details about the use of metered dose inhalers (MDIs) is important. Facileness with MDIs has diminished with the advent of "spacers," which now are recommended. (See Figure 50-1). Allen and Prior[1] studied 30 elderly patients who used MDIs; 60% used the MDI satisfactorily. Several studies have shown the unequivocal benefit of spacers such as the InspirEase or AeroChamber. The exciting development of the breath-activated MDI is likely to help further.

Beta$_2$-Adrenergic agents. The selective beta$_2$ receptor agonist most used is albuterol, which is taken as two puffs two, three, or four times a day or as is necessary to improve breathlessness arising spontaneously after exercise or during infections. Higher doses of inhaled medications can be used for an acute exacerbation of symptoms and can be delivered by a nebulizer. But in the ambulatory setting, care is required to ensure genuine benefit of high doses of medication. This can be achieved by having the patient perform the 6-minute walking test and measuring respirations, pulse and PEFR before and after the test. Side effects of tremors and tachycardia may occur.

Anticholinergic agents. A poorly absorbed derivative of atropine (ipratroprium [Atrovent], 36 to 72 mg qid (18 mg/puff), is useful. Maximum response is seen after

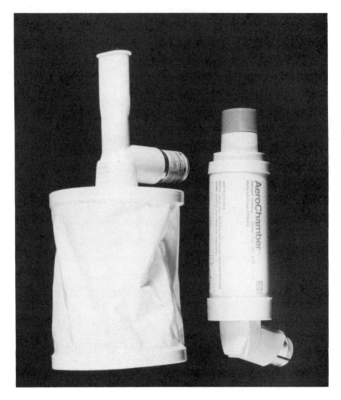

Figure 50-1 Photograph of a metered dose inhaler (MDI) with a spacer. Spacers are tubes inserted between the mouthpiece and MDI to allow large droplets of the medication to be removed. Large droplets result in the inhalation of larger doses of medication but do not necessarily improve therapeutic results.

60 to 90 minutes, with a duration of action of up to 6 hours. Higher doses can be given by nebulizer and are sometimes useful. Additive effects are seen with beta$_2$ agonists (and theophylline). Side effects occur and are especially important among elderly patients. Absorption has been reported to cause urinary retention, and accidental spraying in the eye can precipitate glaucoma. In addition, paradoxical bronchoconstriction has occurred due to muscarinic antagonism of the bronchodilator effect.

Corticosteroids. In cases of bronchial asthma, corticosteroids are critical. For other CAO disorders, the role of corticosteroids is far less clear. In cases of asthma, the antiinflammatory effects of corticosteroids are the crux of modern management. If asthma is confirmed, as outlined previously, the mildest case may be controlled satisfactorily by intermittent inhalations of a beta$_2$ agonists. However, if these drugs are needed regularly *or* if nocturnal wheeze continues to disturb the patient's sleep, then inhaled corticosteroids should be used in sufficient amounts to make the need for albuterol infrequent. The dosage of inhaled corticosteroid should be increased to eight puffs four times a day (with a spacer to minimize oropharyngeal deposition of the drug). Oral corticosteroids are not contraindicated and indeed would be used if control of the asthma is difficult. However, the frequency of serious side effects such as cataract and osteoporosis (10% of asthmatics who take oral corticosteroids experience these adverse effects) is related to the total cumulative dose of corticosteroid.

For chronic obstructive bronchitis and emphysema, there is less uniform response to corticosteroids. Indeed it is likely that only a subset of 25% to 33% of patients with undiagnosed asthma (asthmatic bronchitis) will respond. To detect these patients, it is appropriate to prescribe a trial of corticosteroids. *For stable patients,* 30 or 40 mg of prednisone given daily for 2 weeks, with spirometry before and after, will identify a subset who will then benefit from inhaled corticosteroids (a response of 20% or greater by spirometry is the preferred criterion for success).

Oral agents

Oral therapy with beta₂ agonists and with theophylline is available and may be useful for some older patients, including those who have poor inhaler or spacer techniques or physical disabilities. The sustained-release forms of albuterol (4 mg) and theophylline (200 mg) are preferred. The albuterol can be given at bedtime as sole therapy for mild nocturnal symptoms, as can be the 24-hour preparation of theophylline, which also can provide some benefit during the day. Side effects are more common with such systemic medicines. For theophylline, these side effects include anorexia, nausea, and more serious problems such as dysrhythmias (including multifocal atrial tachycardia for which it may be the main cause).

Treatment of breathlessness

Some patients are anxious about their dyspnea and this exacerbates the sensation of breathlessness. For patients who have dyspnea, tranquilizers, sedatives, and antidepressants have been prescribed, as well as dihydrocodeine and local anesthetics. In general the therapeutic benefit of these agents is marginal and the side effects are considerable.

Oxygen, however, has a well-defined role. It is used as intermittent short-burst therapy and portable oxygen for symptomatic relief of dyspnea and as long-term domiciliary oxygen for chronic respiratory failure.

If oxygen desaturation is linked to exercise and effort dyspnea and *both* are diminished by oxygen, then oxygen may be used intermittently and it usually is prescribed as portable liquid oxygen. Up to 25% improvement in walking distance and relief of dyspnea have been shown.

Nocturnal oxygen also may be indicated for those older patients with demonstrable complications from hypoxemia (polycythemia, cor pulmonale) and without significant diurnal hypoxia (arterial oxygen tension [PO_2] >60 mm Hg), provided sleep apnea has been excluded from the diagnosis. (See Chapter 56.)

Long-term oxygen is appropriate for those patients who have persistent significant hypoxemia (PO_2 <55 mm Hg measured while clinically stable on two occasions separated by 2 to 3 weeks). Such treatment has been shown to increase longevity but perhaps should not be recommended for those who continue to smoke or for those who have another life-limiting condition such as cancer.[8]

Caution must be exercised when oxygen therapy is given to patients with severe chronic hypercarbia (PCO_2 >45 mm Hg). Excessive oxygen therapy may reduce respiratory drive.

Pulmonary rehabilitation

Pulmonary rehabilitation is a multidisciplinary program of physiotherapy, muscle training, and psychotherapy to help a patient return to the highest possible functional capacity.[6] Despite many years of such programs it still is not clear how to use them. Exercise programs and directed breathing techniques may reduce the patient's sensation of dyspnea. Inspiratory muscle training devices are not clearly effective.

Assessment of nutrition and support of the undernourished patient is obviously desirable.[3] Methods to identify those patients who might benefit from nutritional support include measurements of body weight, skinfold thickness, and muscle mass.

REFERENCES

1. Allen SC, Prior A: What determines whether an elderly patient can use a metered dose inhaler correctly, *Br J Dis Chest* 80:45, 1986.
2. Banerjee KD et al: Underdiagnosis of asthma in the elderly, *Br J Dis Chest* 81:23, 1987.
3. Donahoe M, Rogers RM: Nutritional assessment in chronic obstructive pulmonary disease, *Clin Chest Med* 11:487, 1990.
4. Dow L, Holgate ST: Assessment and treatment of obstructive airways disease in the elderly, *Br Med Bull* 40:230, 1990.
5. Fletcher C et al: *The history of chronic bronchitis and emphysema*, New York, 1976, Oxford University Press.
6. Hodgkin JE: Pulmonary rehabilitation, *Clin Chest Med* 11:447, 1990.
7. Knudson R: Physiology of the aging lung. In Crystal RG, West JG, eds: *The lung: scientific foundations*, New York, 1990, Raven Press.
8. Nocturnal Oxygen Therapy Trial Group: Continuous or nocturnal oxygen therapy in hypoxemic chronic obstructive lung disease: a clinical trial, *Ann Intern Med* 93:391, 1980.

SUGGESTED READINGS

Allen SC, Prior A: What determines whether an elderly patient can use a metered dose inhaler correctly, *Br J Dis Chest* 80:45, 1986.
Dow L, Holgate ST: Assessment and treatment of obstructive airways disease in the elderly, *Br Med Bull* 40:230, 1990.
Hodgkin JE: Pulmonary rehabilitation, *Clin Chest Med* 11:447, 1990.

CHAPTER 51

Respiratory infections

PAMELA H. NAGAMI

KEY POINTS

- Pneumonia and influenza together are the fourth most common cause of death for patients aged 65 years old and older.
- The most important factors that predispose elderly patients to acute bronchitis are cigarette smoking and influenza.
- Acute bacterial sinusitis requires early treatment with at least 10 days of appropriate antibiotic therapy and careful radiological follow-up for patients who have air-fluid levels.
- Pneumonia in elderly patients may be atypical, with presenting symptoms that include only tachypnea, low-grade fever, and decreased functional status.
- The decision to treat elderly persons with pneumonia as outpatients must be made only after careful assessment is made of the type of pneumonia, the severity of clinical illness, and the functional statuses and social resources of the patient.

Of all the infections prompting outpatient visits, respiratory infections are the most common. Respiratory syndromes that are well tolerated by younger patients may be life threatening to elderly patients. Pneumonia and influenza together are the fourth most common cause of death for patients aged 65 years and older.[5] In addition, the fiscal impact of respiratory infections is enormous. The direct costs of influenza alone exceed $1 billion per year and may reach $3 to $5 billion per year during epidemic years. These considerations make respiratory infections a special problem for the ambulatory elderly patient, a problem that requires careful individual assessment of each case.

INFLUENZA

Clinical relevance

Influenza is an acute febrile illness caused by infection with a ribonucleic acid (RNA) viruses belonging to one of three genera: influenza A, B, or C. Influenza B and C usually cause mild disease and result in immunity to reinfection. Influenza A produces more severe disease and the virus evades the immune system by changing the proteins of its outer membrane, resulting in recurrent attacks. Between 1975 and 1984, an estimated 10,000 excess deaths were ascribed to influenza and its complications. More than 85% of these excess deaths occurred in patients aged 65 years or older.

Influenza is associated with high mortality in elderly persons because of both its direct and indirect effects. Influenza can cause primary viral pneumonia and, by impairing the function of the cilia lining the bronchopulmonary tree, it may predispose the patient to bacterial pneumonia. In addition, influenza frequently causes death by weakening the patient's general condition. For example, the patient's cardiac and pulmonary conditions may worsen, functional status may diminish, and death may follow weeks to months later.

Clinical manifestations

After an incubation period of 1 to 2 days, influenza begins often abruptly with fever, headache, malaise, and anorexia, followed 1 to 2 days later by rhinorrhea and dry cough (rhinotracheitis). The nasal discharge is usually clear and without the severe obstruction to breathing that is associated with the typical head cold from other viruses. Temperatures of 39° C are not unusual in cases of influenza, and fevers may last for up to 3 days, even in uncomplicated cases. For elderly patients with influenza, fevers usually are present, but temperatures of elderly patients may be lower than those of the younger patients.[3] Otherwise, clinical presentation of influenza for older adults is similar to that for younger adults. However, influenza may be a debilitating disease for elderly patients, even in uncomplicated cases, with full recovery requiring 2 or more weeks. For elderly patients with intercurrent illnesses, debilities following influenza may persist for months.

Pulmonary complications from influenza are common and range from the exacerbation of chronic obstructive pulmonary disease to fulminant bilateral influenzal or bacterial pneumonia. The most common complication affecting elderly patients is acute bronchitis.

Diagnostic approach

Geriatric patients who have mild influenza and have been vaccinated require no specific diagnostic tests. When patients with febrile rhinotracheitis also have pleuritic chest pains, coughs productive of purulent sputum, or signs of consolidation on the examinations of the lungs, chest radiographs and in most cases complete blood counts should be obtained to exclude a complicating pneumonia from the diagnosis. These diagnostic tests also are indicated for elderly patients with severe or prolonged influenza, even if low-grade fever persists.

Intervention

The cornerstone of influenza control for elderly persons is the influenza vaccine. Vaccine-induced immunity only lasts about 6 months, so the vaccine must be administered yearly, preferably in the fall (October and November). The current influenza vaccines effectively prevent severe illness resulting from influenza, even for debilitated elderly patients.[1] In many cases, infection with the virus is prevented altogether or when the virus does occur, it leads only to mild upper respiratory illness.

During community outbreaks of influenza A, severely affected elderly patients may be candidates for therapy with the antiviral compound amantadine. To be effective, the drug must be started within 48 hours of the onset of symptoms. The dose for patients aged 65 years and older is 100 mg by mouth daily for 5 to 7 days. Amantadine is relatively contraindicated for patients with histories of seizure disorders, and the dose must be adjusted according to the package instructions for patients with significant renal impairments. The same dose of amantadine may be administered as prophylaxis against influenza A (not influenza B or C) to unvaccinated elderly persons during an outbreak or to those who are unable to receive influenza vaccines because of allergies. Amantadine may cause agitation and insomnia in elderly patients and should not be viewed as a routine alternative to the much safer influenza vaccine.

Supportive treatment of influenza includes adequate hydration, antipyretics for high fever, and judicious use of antitussives. Antihistamines (because of anticholinergic effects) and decongestants (because of cardiovascular effects) should be avoided or cautiously prescribed for elderly patients. If bacterial bronchitis supervenes, the patient should be treated with a course of antibiotics by mouth as is described in the following discussion.

ACUTE BRONCHITIS

Clinical relevance

Acute bronchitis is an inflammatory condition of the trachea and bronchi and is initiated most often by viral infection (e.g., influenza, rhinovirus). Acute bronchitis is most common among smokers. Attack rates peak in the winter months. Persons at the extremes of life (less than 5 years of age or 65 years of age and older) are most severely affected by acute bronchitis as are patients with underlying chronic bronchitis. Secondary bacterial infections by *Hemophilus influenzae, Moraxella (Branhamella) catarrhalis,* and perhaps *Streptococcus pneumoniae,* commonly occur in elderly persons, particularly among patients with chronic obstructive pulmonary disease.

Clinical manifestations

Acute bronchitis usually begins with prodromal symptoms and signs of a viral upper respiratory infection including coryza, sore throat, and dry cough. The nasal and pharyngeal symptoms subside as the cough becomes the preponderant symptom. Sputum is produced and is initially mucoid, but then it becomes more purulent if bacterial superinfection occurs. There may be low-grade fever, but high-grade fever, rigor, prostration, or pleuritic chest pain are suggestive of pneumonia. Examination of the chest may reveal wheezing and scattered rhonchi without signs of consolidation.

Diagnostic approach

The diagnosis of acute bronchitis is made once the clinical findings have excluded other respiratory infections from the patient's diagnosis. No specific diagnostic tests are indicated for mildly ill geriatric patients with compatible symptoms and signs for acute bronchitis. However, because the clinical presentation of pneumonia may be so indolent in older adults, a chest radiograph always must be obtained to exclude pneumonia from the diagnosis if systemic symptoms (e.g., anorexia, weakness) are present or if there is more than low-grade (over 38.3° C) fever.

Intervention

Prevention of acute bronchitis is best accomplished by yearly influenza vaccination. For patients who develop acute bronchitis, it is important to maintain hydration to prevent dryness and inspissation of bronchial secretions. Cough is the most troublesome symptom and it may be treated with cough suppressants such as dextromethorphan (15 mg q6h). Occasionally, if very severe cough adversely affects the patient (e.g., precipitates angina pectoris), treatment with codeine-containing cough suppressants is necessary. For purulent bronchitis in the absence of pneumonia, a course of oral antibiotics is appropriate. Therapy should be aimed at *H. influenzae* and *M. catarrhalis*. Amoxicillin, 250 to 500 mg by mouth 3 times daily, although a mainstay of therapy, is not active against beta-lactamase-producing strains of these organisms and should be reserved for mildly ill patients. Trimethoprim (160 mg) and sulfamethoxazole (800 mg) by mouth twice a day is safe and inexpensive therapy for patients who can maintain a good fluid intake. A more costly but very effective alternative is amoxicillin-clavulanic acid, 250 to 500 mg by mouth 3 times a day. These latter agents are effective against beta-lactamase-producing strains of bacteria. Erythromycins and tetracyclines, while not reliably active against all the putative agents of acute bacterial bronchitis, are often effective therapies for mildly ill patients.

SINUSITIS

Clinical relevance

Paranasal sinusitis is a common complication of viral upper respiratory tract infections in elderly patients, although in many patients the infection may be unrecognized and self-limiting.[4] Paranasal sinusitis is more common among patients with underlying allergic rhinitis, particularly when there are nasal polyps. Sinusitis can occur when there are maxillary dental infections, nasal foreign bodies and tumors, and nasal fractures. Perhaps the most important predisposing factor is a prior bout of sinusitis, which damages the mucoperiosteal membranes and leads to colonization of the normal sterile sinuses with pathogenic bacteria.

Acute paranasal sinusitis usually occurs during the late stages of a common cold or influenza. The mucosal lining of the sinus becomes inflamed and swollen, and an exudate containing polymorphonuclear leukocytes and bacteria in high titer develops in the sinus cavity. *S. pneumoniae* and nonencapsulated strains of *H. influenzae* account for at least one half of the cases in which diagnosis has been made by percutaneous aspiration of the sinuses. Anaerobic bacteria may be present, particularly in chronic cases of sinusitis and in cases of sinusitis following dental disease. *Staphylococcus aureus*, *M. catarrhalis*, and other gram-negative bacilli are seen in some cases of sinusitis.

Clinical manifestations

In acute paranasal sinusitis the nasal drainage from one naris or both nares changes from clear to purulent brick-colored, and the drainage is sometimes foul smelling or foul tasting. There may be pain in the face, in the maxillary teeth, or in the eye, depending upon which sinus is involved. A deep boring headache is typical of sphenoid sinusitis. These symptoms are accompanied by some fever, anorexia, and malaise. The patient frequently has a nasal and resonant voice, which is recognizable to the experienced practitioner. Suppurative complications of acute sinusitis include orbital cellulitis, frontal bone osteomyelitis, and meningitis.

Diagnostic approach

Based on clinical findings alone, the diagnosis of acute sinusitis cannot be made with precision, therefore, radiographic examination is also necessary. Radiological opacity or an air-fluid level establishes the diagnosis, while mucoperiosteal thickening is suggestive of sinusitis but also is representative of residual damage from past episodes of sinusitis. When ethmoid or sphenoid sinusitis is suspected, a computed tomographic scan of these sinuses is necessary because plain films usually are unrevealing.

The bacterial cause of sinusitis cannot be determined by cultures of nasal pus or exudates that are present at the sinus ostia because of contamination of the specimens by resident floras in the nasal passages. In uncomplicated cases percutaneous puncture of the sinuses is not necessary because patients may be treated with empirical regimens aimed at the usual pathogens.

Intervention

As with acute bronchitis, the most effective preventive measure for acute sinusitis is the yearly administration of influenza vaccine. Avoiding aspirin and nonsteroidal antiinflammatory agents decreases the formation of obstructive nasal polyps in sensitive patients. Prompt attention to dental infections prevents extension to the sinuses.

Antibiotic therapy for acute sinusitis should be directed toward *S. pneumoniae* and *H. influenzae*. In areas of the country where beta-lactamase-producing strains of *Hemophilus* are uncommon, amoxicillin, 250 to 500 mg by mouth 3 times daily, is a good choice. Trimethoprim (160 mg) and sulfamethoxazole (800 mg) by mouth 2 times daily is an acceptable alternative for patients who are able to maintain a good fluid intake. This latter regimen is active against beta-lactamase-producing *H. influenzae* and *M. catarrhalis*. Amoxicillin-clavulanic acid, 250 to 500 mg by mouth 3 times daily, shares the spectrum of trimethoprim and sulfamethoxazole and has good activity against anaerobes that may be present in chronic and recurrent cases of sinusitis; however, amoxicillin-clavulanic acid is a much more expensive antibiotic. Clindamycin, erythromycin, and oral cephalosporins are sometimes used with success in the treatment of acute sinusitis, but these antibiotics are less active against some of the previously mentioned pathogens. Antibiotic therapy should be continued for at least 10 days.

Whenever an air-fluid level persists on the patient's radiographs, despite an adequate course of antibiotics, referral to an otolaryngologist is indicated. Orbital extension, intracranial complications, and sphenoid sinusitis mandate urgent referral to the otolaryngologist or neurosurgeon.

BACTERIAL PNEUMONIA

Clinical relevance

Pneumonia is the fourth most common diagnosis for patients who are admitted to medical wards in the United States. Up to 60% of cases of pneumonia occur in patients 65 years of age or older, and in this age group pneumonia is the leading cause of death due to infection. Mortality is higher for elderly patients than it is for younger patients who are hospitalized for pneumonia (12.8 versus 1.5/100 cases), and mortality is especially high for those with bacteremic pneumococcal pneumonia (57%).

Elderly patients are predisposed to pneumonia for a variety of reasons.[5] Nocturnal aspiration of oropharyngeal contents is common among elderly persons, as well as patients with gastroesophageal reflux, and it increases in the presence of neurological conditions (e.g., dementia, Parkinson's disease), hypnotic drugs, and alcohol. Once aspiration has occurred, the cleansing function of coughing may be less effective for elderly patients because of their blunted cough reflexes and decreased force of coughs. Chronic bronchitis, which is common in elderly persons, predisposes elderly patients to colonization of pathogenic bacteria in the normally sterile airways. Finally, an extremely important predisposing factor for elderly patients who develop pneumonia is influenza.

Clinical manifestations

Pneumonia commonly follows a viral upper respiratory tract infection and is heralded by fever with or without rigors, pleuritic pain in the involved hemithorax, cough, and prostration. For elderly patients the presenting symptoms are often atypical and subacute, especially in patients with cognitive impairments.[2] The fever response may be blunted, pleurisy may be absent, and cough may be absent or weak. In elderly patients with underlying congestive heart failure or emphysema, the auscultatory signs of pneumonia may be absent or masked. However, patients should be observed carefully for tachypnea, a consistent sign of pneumonia among elderly patients. There often is a decline in the patient's functional status, in addition to decompensated cardiac or pulmonary disease, confusion, and falls. Dehydration may be severe by the time the patient seeks medical attention. Even in the absence of specific symptoms and signs, a temperature of 38.3° C or greater in an elderly patient who is seen in the emergency department is highly predictive of a serious bacterial infection such as pneumonia and should prompt a thorough diagnostic workup.

Diagnostic approach

If the clinical findings suggest a possibility of pneumonia, a chest radiograph should be obtained. If pneumonia is confirmed, most elderly patients require hospitalization. (See the box below.) In select circumstances in which the older patient is highly independent and appears relatively well, has a small single-lobe pneumonia, is not hypoxic, has no serious underlying diseases, has adequate support at home, and is able to return for follow-up, the pneumonia may be treated on an outpatient basis.

The most likely causes of community-acquired pneumonia for elderly persons are

---

INDICATIONS FOR ADMITTING ELDERLY PATIENTS WITH PNEUMONIA TO THE HOSPITAL

Immunocompromised, debilitated, or alcoholic
Multilobar involvement
Temperature >38.3° C
Room air Po_2 <70 torr (mm Hg)
Suspected gram-negative enteric, *S. aureus*, or *Legionella* sp. pneumonia
Normal or low white blood cell count with shift to immature forms
Inadequate response to oral antibiotics
Baseline deficits in activities of daily living
Social supports not adequate for treatment at home
Hemodynamic and/or pulmonary instability
Presence of toxicity or sepsis
Inability to drink adequate fluids

S. pneumoniae, 50%; *H. influenzae,* 5% to 15%; *S. aureus,* 5% to 15%; and gram-negative bacilli, 5% to 15%.[5] In patients with chronic obstructive lung disease, *S. pneumoniae, H. influenzae, M. catarrhalis,* and *Legionella* sp. are common pathogens. If aspiration is suspected as a precipitating event, anaerobic bacteria along with *S. pneumoniae* are causative organisms for pneumonia.

Intervention

For outpatient management of pneumonia, baseline complete blood counts, renal function tests, and serum electrolytes should be obtained. Expectorated sputa should be obtained for Gram's stain and culture; however, because of oropharyngeal contamination, such sputa are only reliable in 50% of the cases.

Antibiotic therapy for pneumonia should be guided by the Gram stain and history. If empirical treatment is necessary, antibiotics should be directed against *S. pneumoniae, H. influenzae,* and *S. aureus* unless the history indicates underlying disorders (e.g., chronic lung disease). For patients who are not allergic to penicillin, amoxicillin-clavulanic acid, 500 mg 3 times daily, is a good choice. For those patients who cannot tolerate penicillin but can take cephalosporin, an oral second-generation cephalosporin such as cefuroxime axetil, 500 mg 2 times daily is effective. Trimethoprim (160 mg) and sulfamethoxazole (800 mg) twice daily is a good and inexpensive alternative for patients who are allergic to penicillin, although pneumococcal isolates occasionally resist this agent. Also, clindamycin, 450 mg 3 times daily, or erythromycin, 500 mg (enteric coated) 3 to 4 times daily may be used.

An intramuscular antibiotic may be used as sole therapy or to supplement oral therapy for those patients who receive outpatient treatment of pneumonia. The most cost-effective choice is probably the second-generation cephalosporin cefonicid, given as 1 g (diluted in 2.5 ml of lidocaine, 1% without epinephrine) q24h. Ceftriaxone has a somewhat longer half-life but this advantage is offset by its higher cost. The administration of intramuscular antibiotics allows the patients to be monitored daily, either during visits to the physician's office or during daily visits by a home health nurse who administers the drugs.

The use of intravenous antibiotics as primary outpatient therapy for pneumonia in elderly patients may be feasible under certain circumstances. Cefuroxime, 750 mg to 1.5 g q8h by gravity drip or automated ambulatory infusion pump, is a good choice for empirical therapy. However, elderly patients with pneumonia who are ill enough to require intravenous antibiotic therapy usually should begin therapy in the hospital. Parenteral or oral therapy then can be completed at home.

The duration of antibiotic therapy for elderly patients with pneumonia ranges from 14 to 21 days, depending on severity of illness and presence of underlying chronic diseases. The patients should be reexamined in 2 to 4 days and chest radiographs should be repeated if clinically indicated (fever, pleurisy). After patients complete their antibiotics, final chest radiographs should be obtained at 6 weeks to document resolution of infiltrates.

The convalescence of elderly patients with pneumonia is typically prolonged, and a certain percentage of elderly patients never return to baseline functional status or they die because of underlying diseases that have entered a decompensated phase as a consequence of the pneumonia. Special attention must be directed toward the intake of normal nutrition by the patients and toward the resumption of ambulation. Home visits by physical therapists may be invaluable for assessing the patients' abilities to resume activities of daily living at home and for assisting patients with their rehabilitation.

REFERENCES

1. Barker WH, Mullooly JP: Influenza vaccination of elderly persons: reduction in pneumonia and influenza hospitalizations and death, *JAMA* 244:2547, 1980.
2. Cunha BA, Gingrich D, Rosenbaum GS: Pneumonia syndromes: a clinical approach to the elderly, *Geriatrics* 45:49, 1990.
3. Keating HJ III et al: Effect of aging on the clinical significance of fever in ambulatory adult patients, *J Am Geriatr Soc* 32:282, 1984.
4. McMahan JT: Paranasal sinusitis: geriatric considerations, *Otolaryngol Clin North Am* 23:1169, 1990.
5. Verghese A, Berk SL: Bacterial pneumonia in the elderly, *Medicine* 62:271, 1983.
6. Ziment I: Management of respiratory problems in the aged, *J Am Geriatr Soc* 30 (suppl 11): S36, 1982.

SUGGESTED READINGS

Yoshikawa TT: Approach to the diagnosis and treatment of the infected older adult. In Hazzard WR et al, eds: *Principles of geriatric medicine and gerontology*, ed 2, New York, 1990, McGraw-Hill.
Slavin RG: Management of sinusitis, *J Am Geriatr Soc* 39:212, 1991.
Siegel D: Management of community-acquired penumonia in outpatients, *West J Med* 142:45, 1985.

CHAPTER 52

Cardiac Problems

GEORGE E. TOFFET
ROBERT J. LUCHI

KEY POINTS

- Goals of rate control for older patients with atrial fibrillation are resting ventricular responses of 60 to 90 beats/min that increase with modest exertion (walking 100 feet) to less than 100 beats/min.
- Appropriate pacemaker insertion increases survival and improves quality of life for elderly patients with sick sinus syndrome.
- For older patients with arteriosclerotic heart disease or cardiomyopathy, ventricular ectopy is associated with increased mortality; for those without heart disease, this arrhythmia is thought to be innocuous.
- The diagnosis of diastolic dysfunction or combined systolic and diastolic dysfunction is crucial to the management of congestive heart failure for elderly patients.
- Atypical presentation of myocardial ischemic pain is common among elderly persons. If patients have episodical difficulties of any kind, consideration should be given to myocardial ischemia as its cause.

DYSRHYTHMIAS

Atrial fibrillation

Clinical relevance. The incidence of atrial fibrillation (AF) in community-dwelling persons 75 years of age or older is approximately 11%. The prevalence of AF increases with age.[7] AF is an important precipitating cause of congestive heart failure (CHF) and increases the risk of stroke fivefold in the absence of rheumatic heart disease (RHD) and twentyfold in the presence of RHD. Furthermore, the impact of AF on the risk of stroke increases as one ages.

Clinical manifestations. Although AF can be asymptomatic for most patients, AF produces a variety of symptoms, including palpitations, weakness, dizziness or syncope, and dyspnea, and can precipitate heart failure or myocardial ischemia. Falls and confusion may be manifestations of low cardiac reserve and cerebral hypoperfusion. The patient's physical examination is characterized by an irregularly irregular heartbeat with varying intensity of S_1 (first heart sound) and pulse volume. In cases of AF, ventricular filling is not uniform; some ventricular systoles are not appreciated as a peripheral pulse because of the low volume of blood that is ejected. Because of this *pulse deficit* (i.e., the difference in heart rate that is determined by auscultation and palpation of a peripheral pulse), measurement of heart rate for a person with AF should be determined only by auscultation of the heart.

Diagnostic approach. Clinical suspicion of AF is confirmed by electrocardiography (ECG). AF is characterized by the replacement of P waves with fibrillatory waves, irregular in amplitude and rate, that usually exceed 400/min. The ventricular response is completely irregular. Common causes of AF are some drugs and alcohol. Almost any acute illness may produce AF, especially acute infection, pulmonary embolus, and myocardial ischemia. Thyroid function tests are obtained routinely since hyperthyroidism may produce AF without any other manifestations of thyroid hyperfunction.

Echocardiography provides significant information relevant to the cause and helps to direct therapy. The degree of left atrial enlargement is inversely proportional to successful return to sinus rhythm. Atrial or ventricular thrombi can be visualized by echocardiography. If thrombi are seen, they can add to the urgency of anticoagulation. Holter monitoring may be necessary to document whether AF is persistent or paroxysmal and to determine if potentially proarrhythmic drugs (digoxin, class I antiarrhythmics) used to treat AF are causing significant ventricular dysrhythmias or atrioventricular (AV) conduction disorders.

Intervention. Patients who have AF and rapid ventricular rates and who cannot be controlled with the drugs that are mentioned on the following pages, those who have significant underlying heart disease (especially valvular heart disease) or the Wolff-Parkinson-White (WPW) syndrome, and those for whom electrical cardioversion is indicated are usually referred to cardiologists. Patients with paroxysmal AF followed by symptomatic bradycardia or long pauses and those with persistent AF and very slow ventricular responses (in the absence of drugs affecting the conduction system) are candidates for pacemaker placement.

Cardioversion (i.e., reversion to sinus rhythm) can be accomplished by chemical or electrical cardioversion. If the onset of AF has precipitated angina pectoris, CHF, or hypotension, urgent *electrical cardioversion* should be considered. Elective cardioversion should be considered for those patients with a reasonable chance of return to sinus rhythm. Successful conversion to sinus rhythm is most likely when AF is less than 6 months in duration and left atrial size is normal or only modestly increased. Cardioversion is almost never successful when AF has persisted for years and when left atrial size is markedly increased. Relative contraindications to cardioversion are digoxin toxicity, sick sinus syndrome (SSS), and recurrent AF after prior cardioversion. Anticoagulation is necessary when AF has been present for more than 5 days and maintained for 3 weeks before cardioversion and for a longer interval (4 to 6 weeks) thereafter. The greatest risk of embolic event is during periods of change in rhythm.

Chemical cardioversion is attempted with quinidine, propafenone, or procainamide after adequate control of the ventricular rate with digoxin or verapamil.[1] Attempting chemical cardioversion before adequate control of the ventricular rate may precipiate rapid supraventricular tachycardia. Simultaneous administration of verapamil and quinidine has been reported to produce hypotension, so this useful combination necessitates staggered oral doses. Quinidine increases serum digoxin concentration; therefore, the digoxin dose should be reduced prior to quinidine administration and should be adjusted subsequently, according to serum digoxin concentrations. Propafenone has beta-blocking activity that slows AV conduction. These agents may have to be continued indefinitely to maintain sinus rhythm.

The goals of *controlling ventricular response* are resting ventricular responses of 60 to 90 beats/min that increase with modest exertion (walking 100 feet) to less than 100 beats/min. If an asymptomatic older patient has AF and a controlled ventricular rate without medications, drug therapy may not be needed; however, some clinicians administer digoxin to prevent the patient from developing a rapid ventricular response, which may occur under stress. Rate control is most often attained with digoxin alone; if it is not controlled, verapamil or beta blockers may be added. A change in the patient's rhythm during the course of digitalization should be investigated by ECG and consideration should be given to digoxin toxicity. For those patients who have paroxysmal AF with rapid ventricular rates, digoxin may be given to control ventricular rates. Occasionally, digoxin may prevent the recurrence of paroxysmal AF. Table 52-1 summarizes the drugs that are used for the treatment of AF.

Prevention of systemic embolization by *anticoagulation* is indicated for those patients whose AF cannot be converted to sinus rhythm. Warfarin (Coumadin) is the drug of choice. Significant decrease in the risk of stroke can be accomplished by increasing prothrombin time merely 1.2 to 1.5 times the control value. However, the risk of full anticoagulation for elderly patients is not trivial and further data are needed on the efficacy and benefit of anticoagulation. The efficacy of aspirin has not been clearly documented for elderly persons with AF, but aspirin may be more appropriate for persons who should not or refuse to take warfarin.

Once ventricular rate is well controlled, the patient or caregiver can monitor weekly apical heart rates when the patient is at rest and after exertion. Persons who take warfarin for anticoagulation therapy require diligent monitoring of prothrombin time. More than 50% of those patients who have successful cardioversions return to AF within 1 year, despite therapy to maintain sinus rhythm. Increased age is associated with reversion to AF.

Table 52-1   Drugs for treatment of atrial fibrillation

Drugs	Pharmacological changes with age/adverse effects	Precautions and recommendations
Maintaining sinus rhythm		
Quinidine	Clearance may be delayed	Monitor serum levels (1.5-3 μg/ml); drug increases digoxin level
Propafenone	Beta-blocking effect; decreased renal excretion	Avoid for patients with COPD; drug is proarrhythmic; drug increases digoxin and metoprolol levels
Procainamide	Decreased renal excretion; increased levels of nitrogen-acetyl procainamide (NAPA); 90% develop (+) antinuclear antibody; few develop lupuslike syndrome	Monitor levels of drug and active metabolite NAPA (procainamide 4-8 μg/ml; NAPA <8 μg/ml)
Controlling ventricular response		
Digoxin	Decreased volume of distribution; decreased renal excretion; levels increased by quinidine, verapamil and propafenone	Toxicity and low serum levels may occur; anorexia and confusion common with age; avoid for patients with hypertrophic cardiomyopathy and WPW syndrome
Verapamil	Liver metabolism of drug unchanged with age; may increase digoxin level	May decrease inotropic effects; use with caution for patients with low output CHF; may cause constipation; use for patients with hypertension or hypertrophic cardiomyopathy; combine with digoxin for patients with difficult rate control
Atenolol, Metoprolol	CNS side effects (depression, visual hallucinations, nightmares); symptomatic bradycardia; poor tolerance	$Beta_1$ selectivity not absolute; use with caution for patients with pulmonary disease or PVD; combine with digoxin for patients with difficult rate control

Sick sinus syndrome

SSS encompasses persistent sinus bradycardia, apparent sinus arrest or exit block, combined sinoatrial (SA) and AV conduction disturbances, and altered paroxysmal atrial tachycardia with slow atrial or ventricular rhythm (tachycardia-bradycardia syndrome).

Clinical relevance. The incidence of SSS is 2% in persons with known or suspected heart disease. Fifty percent of pacemakers implanted in persons aged 65 years and older are for symptomatic bradyarrhythmias associated with SSS.

SSS encompasses a heterogenous group of bradyarrhythmias involving defects in impulse generation by the SA node, conduction through the atria, and conduction through the AV node. Progressive fibrosis accompanied by ischemia or infiltrative processes such as cardiac amyloid causes destruction of the cardiac conduction system. As a part of "normal" aging, up to 90% of the SA nodal cells that are present when one is 20 years of age are dead when one is 75 years of age.[4] Those cells that are present are often isolated and their intrinsic function may not be normal.

Clinical manifestations. Symptoms of SSS are most often those of transient decreased perfusion (i.e., dizziness, light-headedness, or syncope). Angina pectoris or dyspnea from CHF may be present in persons with coronary insufficiency or impaired ventricular function. Some patients only report palpitations or are asymptomatic despite severe conduction pathway disease. Patients with underlying conduction disease may have their symptoms exaggerated by beta receptor blocking drugs, calcium channel blocking drugs, digoxin, or other drugs acting on the cardiovascular conduction or autonomic nervous system.

Diagnostic approach. Findings from the ECG may be normal or reveal sinus bradycardia. Less frequently, supraventricular tachycardia alternating with bradycardia, pause resulting from SA arrest, or SA exit block are seen. The ECG often shows other signs of conduction pathway disease. Fifty percent of patients with SSS also have first- or second-degree AV heart block. Many have coexistent bundle branch blocks.

Diagnosis is made by continuous ambulatory ECGs (Holter monitors) and observations of the arrhythmias of SSS. Correlation of symptoms with findings is critical for confirmation of diagnosis and for selecting proper treatment. SSS should be differentiated from carotid sinus hypersensitivity.

Intervention. Because definitive therapy often requires pacemaker placement, cardiology consultation should be obtained after Holter monitoring documents a dysrhythmia that is associated with symptoms. If symptoms do not occur during ambulatory ECG monitoring, then cardiac electrophysiological testing may be indicated. The role of drugs that are used to treat patients with the bradycardia of SSS is limited. Hydralazine or nifedipine may induce a reflex tachycardia that temporarily improves symptoms, but these agents cannot be recommended for definitive treatment.

The role of the primary care physician is to make a systematic examination for drugs that can decrease sinus node function (i.e., selected eye drops, sympatholytic agents, vagotonic agents, clonidine, and lithium, in addition to cardiac medications). The response of symptoms to the withdrawal of these agents should be assessed.

If tachycardia persists after pacemaker placement, calcium channel blockers, beta blockers, digoxin, or other agents for rate control may be required. The diseased conduction pathway may be exquisitely sensitive to the suppressive effects of drugs, so doses should be prescribed cautiously.

Even for those persons aged 80 years or older, the survival rate after appropriate pacemaker placement for symptomatic SSS is good. Though there is a modest increase in mortality in the first year after placement, subsequently the survival of patients is not different from age-matched controls. The survival is primarily determined by atherosclerotic (arteriosclerotic) heart disease (ASHD), which frequently accompanies SSS.

Ventricular premature beats

Clinical relevance. For persons aged 80 years or older who have no evidence of heart disease, 96% have ventricular premature beats (VPBs) that are found after 24-hour continuous monitoring.[2] However, multifocal VPBs are seen only in 18%, couplets in 8%, and ventricular tachycardia in 2%. In the Baltimore Longitudinal Study, 80% of patients aged 60 to 85 years old who had been vigorously screened to exclude coronary disease from their diagnoses showed VPBs after they were monitored. Of those patients, 35% had multifocal VPBs, 11% had couplets, and 4% had ventricular tachyardia (VT). There are further increases in the prevalence of ectopy when elderly persons exercise. Thus, ventricular ectopy may be a "normal" finding among elderly persons. However, for an unscreened population in which the prevalance of arteriosclerotic heart disease (ASHD) is high, the presence of VPBs is associated with poorer survival and may be a marker for coronary artery disease. In the absence of ASHD, there is no real morbidity or excess mortality associated with VPBs. Even complex ventricular ectopy in asymptomatic patients without clinical heart disease has no effect on their survival. In contrast, when patients are known to have ASHD or dilated cardiomyopathy, VPBs are an independent risk factor for death.

Clinical manifestations. Depending on the number, duration, and frequency of VPBs, as well as the presence of coronary heart disease, CHF, or cerebrovascular disease, patients may be asymptomatic or may experience dizziness, syncope, stroke, chest pain, dyspnea, palpitation, or CHF.

Diagnostic approach. Ventricular ectopy, which is characterized by premature cardiac sounds that often are followed by a compensatory pause, may be found upon cardiac auscultation. An ECG easily confirms the diagnosis of the arrhythmia if it is present at the time of the test. Otherwise, diagnosis necessitates continuous Holter monitoring.

Intervention. Management and further evaluation of the patient with *multiple complex* VPBs along with organic heart disease requires the consultation of a cardiologist. Patients with syncope or falls from VPBs, as well as runs of VT, also may benefit from the cardiologist's expertise. The decision to perform invasive electrophysiological studies usually is made after one or more trials of antiarrhythmic agents. Table 52-2 summarizes treatment recommendations for VPBs.

Nevertheless, the primary care physician contributes significantly to the initial management of older patients who have VPBs. Many medications can increase the frequency of ventricular ectopy, including digoxin, theophylline, tricyclic antidepressants, and classic antiarrhythmic drugs. The clinician should consider the need for these drugs. Other factors that should be addressed by the primary physician are stress, caffeine intake, cigarette abuse, and sedentary lifestyle. Optimizing pulmonary function for patients with chronic lung disease and optimizing cardiac function for patients with CHF also decreases ectopy. Hypokalemia and hypomagnesemia should be considered as potential causes of VPBs, especially for those patients who take digoxin.

Table 52-2   Treatment of ventricular ectopy

Patient status	Treatment
Asymptomatic with no heart disease	Treatment not indicated
Asymptomatic with heart disease	Treat if VPBs >120/hr, couplets or runs of VT; use quinidine or procainamide; follow drug levels and do Holter monitoring
Symptomatic with no heart disease	Treatment not indicated if only occasional palpitations or light-headedness; treatment may be required for symptom control if complaints are frequent or serious (e.g., syncope)
Symptomatic with heart disease	Treat in consultation with cardiologist especially if VPBs are complex

Frequent follow-up is necessary during changes in a patient's therapy. This follow-up includes ambulatory ECG monitoring to assess the efficacy of treatment in suppressing ectopy.

Prognosis depends on the status of the underlying heart. If the patient has low ejection fraction or coronary disease, VPBs bring increased probability of death. Treatment of the VPBs may not alter that probability. For the disease-free older person, ventricular ectopy, even when complex, is thought to be innocuous.

CONGESTIVE HEART FAILURE
Clinical relevance

The incidence of CHF (new cases/1000 community-dwelling individuals) increases exponentially from 1 to 1.8/1000 for those aged 45 to 54 years old to 50/1000 for those aged 85 years and older. The incidence of CHF among community-dwelling elderly persons is 7% to 8% for those aged 75 and older.[5] The prevalence of CHF also increases dramatically with age. Because persons with CHF may have very poor exercise tolerance, there can be a profound effect on quality of life. Older persons with CHF have a poor prognosis; 30% have a first-year mortality and 50% have a third-year mortality. CHF is the most frequently recorded discharge diagnosis for Medicare patients. The health care costs related to CHF exceeded $1 billion in 1981.

Age-related changes in the cardiovascular system result in compromised physiological reserves. Significant decreases in adrenergic responsiveness, calcium homeostasis, and diastolic function, as well as increases in left ventricular (LV) wall thickness, occur. Forty percent of men 75 years of age and older have CHF with normal left ventricular ejection fractions (LVEF), which suggests that their CHF is due to diastolic dysfunction. The remainder have decreased LVEF and their CHF is probably the result of combined LV systolic and diastolic dysfunction. The distinction between

CHF secondary to diastolic dysfunction as opposed to systolic and diastolic dysfunctions is important when physicians choose therapy for CHF.

Clinical manifestations

The typical clinical features of CHF (exertional and rest dyspnea, paroxysmal nocturnal dyspnea [PND], peripheral edema, fatigue) are often absent in elderly patients. Instead, poor systemic perfusion may result in confusional states, ischemia of the extremities, lethargy, or uremia. Restlessness may predominate instead of dyspnea or PND. Physical examination may reveal rales or pedal edema but these are not specific for CHF. However, a jugular venous distention, hepatojugular reflux, and third heart sound (S_3) remain important confirmational signs of CHF. The chest x-ray is valuable when findings are positive; however, x-rays may be difficult to obtain for frail older persons, or once x-rays are obtained, they may be difficult to interpret for various anatomical and practical reasons.

Diagnostic approach

Two-dimensional echocardiography with Doppler is an essential part of the initial investigation to evaluate the left ventricular systolic and diastolic functions and valvular function. This is the best noninvasive way to determine whether or not systolic dysfunction is present. A major goal for the physician is to identify and correct the precipitating factors by completing a history and physical examination and by obtaining laboratory tests, including complete blood count, chemistry panel (e.g., SMA-20), thyroid function, ECG, and ambulatory ECG. The clinician also must evaluate the patient's compliance with medication and diet regimens. There should be a systematic review of all cardiodepressant, proarrythmic, or sodium-retaining medications.

Intervention

Dietary sodium restriction is a vital part of the therapeutic regimen. Restriction of sodium chloride (NaCl) in the range of 4 g/day is tolerated by most patients. If this degree of salt restriction is not tolerated, NaCl is restricted to the extent possible. Care must be taken to prevent undernutrition. (See Chapter 45.)

Diuretics are essential for decreasing congestion in both normal and low LVEF patients. Diuretics should be used judiciously and with an awareness to the functional urinary incontinence they may produce. The angiotensin-converting enzyme (ACE) inhibitors improve quality of life and extend life expectancy in those patients with CHF and low LVEF. Except for the first dose, which may cause hypotension (hypotension may be prevented by decreasing the doses of diuretics and other drugs that can produce this condition), ACE inhibitors are fairly well tolerated by older patients. Digoxin is a useful drug, within narrow limits. For patients with sinus rhythm and preserved LVEF, digoxin is *not* indicated. For those patients who have a sinus rhythm

Table 52-3 Drugs for treating congestive heart failure

Drugs	Pharmacological changes with age/ adverse effects	Precautions and recommendations
Furosemide	Duration of action is longer; lower peak serum level	Reduced serum and total body potassium; dehydration; urinary incontinence
Enalapril, Lisinopril, Captopril	Decreased renal excretion; longer duration of action	Hypotension (especially if patient is hypovolemic); renal insufficiency; hyperkalemia
Digoxin*	Requires lower dose; decreased renal excretion; decreased volume of distribution	Digoxin toxicity common; digoxin antibodies for life-threatening toxicities

*See Table 52-1.

and low LVEF, an S_3, and a dilated ventricle, digoxin may improve CHF symptoms. Maximum increase in LVEF in elderly patients is achieved at an average serum concentration of 0.8 ng/ml. Digoxin also is indicated if atrial fibrillation is present as described above. Patients with CHF and normal LVEF may benefit from diuretics and sodium restriction; it is not clear if these patients benefit from vasodilators. If echocardiography demonstrates hypertrophic cardiomyopathy, beta receptor blocking drugs or verapamil may be useful. (See Table 52-3 for drug information and precautions.)

Rehabilitation. A short period of bed rest is indicated during the outpatient treatment of those who have CHF and rest dyspnea. Thereafter, bed rest is not helpful because it increases debility, venous thrombi, and pulmonary emboli. Modest exercise, usually walking, decreases the patient's chances of thrombi and emboli and may promote a sense of well-being. Exertion should be stopped when dyspnea develops or when the heart rate exceeds an individually determined heart rate.

Preventive measures. Prevention of exacerbations of CHF requires vigilance by the patient (or caregiver) and the physician. The precipitating factors of CHF must be anticipated and treated promptly. Compliance with diet and drug regimens must be maintained. Education of the patient and family about possible consequences of nonprescription drugs such as nonsteroidal antiinflammatory drugs, which may lead to fluid retention, is important.

The prevention of CHF per se requires the identification of risk factors such as ventricular hypertrophy, diabetes mellitus, hypertension, cigarette abuse, hypercholesterolemia, and obesity. Though aggressive treatment of these presumed risk factors seems to be indicated, there is as yet no specific evidence that their treatment will decrease the incidence of CHF among elderly persons.

Follow-up. Frequency of follow-up varies from weekly to monthly visits, depending on the severity of the CHF and presence of other complicating problems (e.g. renal insufficiency). Weights can be monitored daily at home by most patients. Care givers can be taught to recognize early signs and symptoms of CHF, as well as supervise compliance with diet and medication. Monitoring of serum electrolytes and magnesium, serum digoxin level, and renal function are performed as needed and are especially important when alterations in the medical regimen are made.

ATHEROSCLEROTIC HEART DISEASE

Clinical relevance

Atherosclerotic or arteriosclerotic heart disease (ASHD) is the most common category of heart disease afflicting elderly persons and, for this age group, is the leading cause of death for all U.S. ethnic groups.[6] The incidence of ASHD increases with age in both sexes until age 75. After age 75 the incidence of ASHD decreases somewhat for men but continues to increase for women.

Myocardial ischemia results when myocardial demand outstrips the delivery capacity of diseased coronary arteries because of atheromatous plaques and/or thrombi. Ischemia impairs myocardial systolic and diastolic function and is a common cause of cardiac dysrhythmias. Myocardial ischemia may not produce symptoms (silent ischemia) or it may cause chest pain (anginal syndromes) or symptoms other than chest pain (i.e., dyspnea [anginal equivalents]).

Clinical manifestations

The two clinical syndromes of importance in the outpatient care of elderly patients are *stable* and *unstable angina pectoris*. Classic *stable angina pectoris* presents as retrosternal discomfort, which is brought on by exertion and relieved by rest, with radiation to the left shoulder, arm, and jaw, or to the upper abdomen. The discomfort is commonly described as pressure, squeezing, or tightness, usually lasting 5 to 10 minutes. Relief by sublingual nitroglycerin or its equivalent occurs in 1 to 2 minutes. *Unstable angina pectoris* is defined as any one of the following:

1. New onset angina at rest or brought on by minimal exertion
2. Significant change (usually doubling) in frequency or intensity of previously stable angina
3. Severe prolonged (more than 20 minutes) chest pain, incompletely relieved by nitroglycerin, accompanied by reversible ECG signs of myocardial ischemia and normal levels of serum cardiac enzymes (MB creatine kinase [MB-CK])

Atypical myocardial ischemic pain is common among elderly patients. Chest discomfort may be replaced by dyspnea, faintness, weakness, confusion, palpitation, nausea, vomiting, episodic sweating, increased agitation, or increased salivation. Demented patients may not be able to recall their symptoms but caregivers' observations may alert the physician that something is amiss. *If a patient is having episodic difficulty of any kind, give consideration to myocardial ischemia as its cause.*

Diagnostic approach

Classical stable angina pectoris. Physical examination that is done during the course of acute myocardial ischemia may reveal tachycardia, increased blood pressure, accentuated fourth heart sound (S_4) gallop, or new systolic murmur. ECG during ischemia shows a new ST segment depression (or occasionally elevation) or a new dysrhythmia or conduction abnormality. An ECG performed in the interval between anginal episodes often is unchanged. If the patient is ambulatory, walking the patient at a comfortable pace may bring out an anginal attack at which time the diagnosis is strengthened by rapid relief of the patient's symptoms through sublingual administration of nitroglycerin. In more difficult cases, stress testing is essential. The stress may be induced by exercise; however, if musculoskeletal impairment or poor conditioning limits the patient's ability to exercise, stress may be induced by drugs (e.g., adenosine or dobutamine reactive hyperemia test). It is recommended that the patient be monitored both by ECG and radionuclide scintigraphy during stress testing.

Unstable angina pectoris. Diagnosis of unstable angina pectoris mandates urgent admission of the patient to a monitored bed to exclude myocardial infarction from the patient's diagnosis or to confirm myocardial ischemia as the origin of the patient's symptoms and treatment. If the patient refuses hospitalization, treatment should be applied as energetically as practical in an outpatient, home, or nursing home setting.

Intervention

Nonpharmacological treatment includes control of risk factors (i.e., hypertension, hypercholesterolemia, hypertriglyceridemia, diabetes mellitus, smoking, stress, and lack of exercise). Factors that may precipitate myocardial ischemia (e.g., anemia, hyperthyroidism) should be diligently sought and appropriately treated. Aspirin in a dose of 325 mg/day is given to those patients who have no contraindications. More recent evidence suggests that low doses of aspirin, 160 mg/day, may be equally effective.

Nitrates. Nitrates are the mainstay of treatment.[9] The mechanism of their action in anginal syndromes is complex. Multiple preparations are now available, from the traditional rapidly acting sublingual tablet to slow release (24-hour) transdermal patches. For older patients, taking sublingual tablets seems to be as easy as using nitroglycerin spray to control acute attacks and to prevent occasional attacks precipitated by predictable exertion. For more sustained prophylaxis, the transdermal disk preparations are generally preferred to nitroglycerin ointments and to isosorbide dinitrate. Symptomatic orthostatic hypotension is an especially common side effect for elderly patients because of their poor compensation for orthostatic stress. Drugs with hypotensive potential should be stopped or the dosage should be reduced if possible. The first few doses of nitrates, regardless of preparation, must be taken while the patient is seated or recumbent to prevent orthostatic dizziness or syncope. The patient's tolerance to the antianginal effects of continuously acting transdermal preparations can be prevented by removing the transdermal patch for 4 hours out of each 24-hour period. Abrupt withdrawal of nitrate therapy may result in coronary artery spasm and rebound angina. Since nitroglycerin tablets lose potency over time, they routinely should be replaced every 3 months.

Calcium channel blockers. Calcium channel blocking drugs differ significantly in their side effects and in the way they reduce myocardial ischemia. Verapamil has the greatest effect on the sinus node and conduction system and therefore is particularly useful for treating a patient who has angina pectoris and a supraventricular dysrhythmia when the latter is not sufficiently well controlled by digoxin. (See Table 52-1.) Verapamil decreases myocardial contractility and therefore should be used cautiously for the patient who has reduced LVEF. Nifedipine does not have an action on the cardiac conduction system; it is a powerful systemic arterial vasodilator. Because nifedipine does not depress sinus node or conduction tissue activity, it is better tolerated than verapamil by patients with bradyarrhythmias. Nicardipine has less peripheral but greater coronary artery vasodilation. Diltiazem's effect on cardiac conduction, myocardial contractility, and peripheral artery vasodilation are intermediate between verapamil and nifedipine.

Beta receptor blocking drugs. Beta receptor blocking drugs reduce myocardial oxygen consumption by decreasing heart rate and myocardial contractility. These effects are especially beneficial in cases of exercise and stress-associated anginal syndromes because blood pressure decreases during exercise, which further decreases the afterload. Side effects include bradycardia, fatigue, poor exercise tolerance, blunted response to hypoglycemia, bronchoconstriction, depression, visual hallucinations, nightmares, and precipitation or worsening of CHF. (See Table 52-1.) Beta receptor blocking drugs should be used with caution for patients who have impaired myocardial contractility, AV conduction disturbance, significant bradyarrhythmia, or chronic obstructive lung disease.

Revascularization. To improve quality of life or to reduce the likelihood of premature death, revascularization is indicated for those patients willing to accept its risks. Angioplasty is relatively well tolerated by appropriately selected elderly patients and if successful, angioplasty abolishes or greatly reduces the frequency of anginal attacks.[3] Coronary artery bypass grafting prolongs the lives of patients who have triple vessel disease and those who have multiple vessel disease and impaired left ventricular systolic function. Operative mortality increases progressively with age, degree of left ventricular functional impairment, and number of associated medical conditions. Although operative mortality in carefully selected septuagenarians and octogenarians reportedly ranges from 8% to 10%, coronary artery bypass grafting should be used judiciously for the treatment of frail elderly patients.[8]

Rehabilitation. Patients must be encouraged to return fully to their previous levels of activity. Aerobic exercise (30 minutes' duration with 5 minutes of warm-up and cool-down) at least 3 times/wk to a heart rate determined by exercise stress testing is important. For many patients, walking is preferred to jogging. Water aerobics are prescribed for those patients with arthritis of the lower extremities. For patients with considerable debility, range of motion and muscle strengthening exercises and gait retraining must be undertaken before aerobic exercise can begin. Resumption of sexual intercourse should be encouraged as myocardial ischemic pain is brought under control. Nitroglycerin, 0.4 mg sublingually, taken prophylactically before sexual intercourse may be useful. Advance directives should be discussed with the patient, family, or surrogate decision maker.

REFERENCES

1. Bolognesi R: The pharmacologic treatment for atrial fibrillation, *Cardiovasc Drugs Ther* 5:617, 1991.
2. Fleg JL: Ventricular arrhythmias in the elderly: prevalence, mechanisms, and therapeutic implications, *Geriatrics* 43(12):23, 1988.
3. Jeroudi MH et al: Percutaneous transluminal coronary angioplasty in octogenarians, *Ann Intern Med* 113:423, 1990.
4. Lev M: Aging changes in the human sinoatrial node, *J Gerontol* 9:1, 1954.
5. Luchi RJ, Taffet GE, Teasdale TA: Congestive heart failure in the elderly, *J Am Geriatr Soc* 39:810, 1991.
6. Luchi RJ, Woolbert SC, McIntosh HD: Atherosclerotic heart disease. In Luchi RJ, ed: *Clinical geriatric cardiology*, Edinburgh, 1989, Churchill Livingstone.
7. Martin A, Camm AJ: Cardiac dysrhythmias. In Luchi RJ, ed: *Clinical geriatric cardiology*, Edinburgh, 1989, Churchill Livingstone.
8. Merrill WH et al: Cardiac surgery in patients age 80 years or older, *Ann Surg* 211(6):772, 1990.
9. Shub C: Stable angina pectoris. III. Medical treatment, *Mayo Clin Proc* 65(2)256, 1990.

SUGGESTED READINGS

Luchi RJ, Taffet GE, Teasdale TA: Congestive heart failure in the elderly, *J Am Geriatr Soc* 39:810, 1991.
Martin A, Camm AJ: Cardiac dysrhythmias. In Luchi RJ, ed: *Clinical geriatric cardiology*, Edinburgh, 1989, Churchill Livingstone.
Merrill WH et al: Cardiac surgery in patients age 80 years or older, *Ann Surg* 211(6):772, 1990.

CHAPTER 53

Hypertension

ROBERT M. PALMER

<table>
<tr>
<td>KEY POINTS</td>
<td>
<ul>
<li>Hypertension is the most important treatable cause of heart failure and stroke.</li>
<li>Clinical trials have demonstrated the effectiveness of antihypertensive therapy for both diastolic and systolic hypertension.</li>
<li>Multiple blood pressure measurements should be obtained before drug therapy begins.</li>
<li>Drug therapy is initiated with low doses of thiazide diuretics, beta blockers, angiotension-converting enzyme inhibitors, or calcium channel blockers.</li>
<li>Medication compliance is enhanced by once-daily doses, written instructions, and family involvement.</li>
<li>The goals of therapy are a diastolic pressure of 80 to 85 mm Hg, a systolic pressure of 140 to 160 mm Hg, and the prevention of adverse drug effects.</li>
</ul>
</td>
</tr>
</table>

CLINICAL RELEVANCE

Epidemiology

The influence of age on blood pressure is demonstrated in population prevalence studies. Systolic blood pressure increases linearly with aging, up to 75 years; the rate of increase is steeper for women than men. In contrast, diastolic blood pressure increases slightly until age is 55 to 60 years and it plateaus or decreases slightly thereafter. After 75 years of age, the relationship between blood pressure and age is less certain and is confounded by selective mortality, comorbidity, and treatment of hypertension and other cardiovascular disorders.

The Joint National Committee on Detection, Evaluation, and Treatment of High Blood Pressure defines *hypertension* as a systolic blood pressure ≥160 mm Hg and/ or a diastolic blood pressure ≥90 mm Hg, based on the average of two or more readings on two or more occasions. *Borderline systolic hypertension* is a systolic blood pressure ≥140 mm Hg, but <160 mm Hg. *Isolated systolic hypertension* (ISH) is a systolic pressure ≥160 mm Hg with a diastolic blood pressure <90 mm Hg. *Diastolic hypertension* is further divided into mild (90 to 104 mm Hg), moderate (105 to 114 mm Hg), and severe (≥115 mm Hg) categories. Although office readings obtained with blood pressure cuffs are recommended for blood pressure screening, home and ambulatory readings are sometimes useful.

In community surveys, more than half of Americans aged 65 years and older have borderline or elevated systolic and/or diastolic blood pressures. However, when measurements of blood pressure are repeated on different days, only about 10% to 15% of elderly patients have diastolic hypertension and 10% to 15% have ISH. The prevalence of ISH increases with advanced age, and ISH occurs in 15% to 20% of Americans aged 80 years and older.

Numerous cross-sectional and longitudinal studies demonstrate the role of hypertension as an independent predictor of cardiovascular and cerebrovascular complications in middle-aged and older persons. In particular, elevated blood pressure increases the risks of myocardial infarction, congestive heart failure (CHF), angina pectoris, stroke, and transient ischemic attack. Hypertension is also a risk factor for occlusive peripheral vascular disease, atrial fibrillation, and vascular dementia.

Despite the traditional emphasis on diastolic blood pressure, prospective studies reveal systolic hypertension as a stronger independent predictor of cardiovascular morbidity and mortality. The risks of hypertension are increased when left ventricular hypertrophy is diagnosed by an electrocardiogram or echocardiogram. These epidemiological findings underscore the significance of hypertension in old age and antiquate the notion that higher systolic blood pressure is a normal consequence of aging.

Surprisingly, the relationship between blood pressure and the risk of cardiovascular disease and mortality is not well established in studies of people aged 75 years and older. Indeed, elevated blood pressure in the very old may serve as a marker of relatively good health, as is suggested by data from community populations that show a paradoxical (inverse) relationship between blood pressure and mortality.[4] However, the relationship between age and mortality is confounded by the high prevalence of comorbid conditions, particularly dementia, malnutrition, and occult malignancies, all of which reduce life expectancy.

Pathophysiology

Essential hypertension. The pathophysiology of essential hypertension differs between young and old patients. While salt sensitivity, obesity, and insulin resistance play important roles in the pathophysiology of essential hypertension, changes in vascular structure and function assume heightened importance as one ages. Hypertension causes changes in the arterial tree that parallel changes seen in the usual aging process. Loss of elasticity in arterial connective tissue results in increased peripheral vascular resistance, decreased aortic compliance, and increased resistance to systolic ejection, as well as compensatory responses, including left ventricular hypertrophy. The increase in peripheral vascular resistance also may result from hypertension or changes in sympathetic nervous function. Beta receptor sensitivity and vasodilation decrease as one ages, while alpha-adrenergic vasoconstriction is unaffected. Few studies compared young and elderly hypertensive patients with respect to hemodynamic differences. One study showed age-related differences in patients with established essential hypertension who had been matched for several important variables. Cardiac output, heart rate, stroke volume, and intravascular volume were significantly lower in the elderly group (> 65 years of age versus < 42 years of age); whereas total peripheral resistance and left ventricular mass were higher.[5]

Isolated systolic hypertension. ISH is usually caused by progressive arterial stiffness that is associated with aging and accelerated by environmental (life-style) influences. For some patients, ISH represents "burned out" essential hypertension (i.e., the stiffened left ventricle cannot maintain high diastolic blood pressure). Elevated systolic pressure further damages the arterial vessels and ultimately leads to the complications of stroke, heart failure, peripheral vascular disease, and nephrosclerosis.

Clinical trials

Despite the epidemiological evidence of the cardiovascular risks associated with hypertension, the effectiveness of antihypertensive treatments in reducing the inci-

---

RESULTS OF EUROPEAN WORKING PARTY
ON HIGH BLOOD PRESSURE IN THE ELDERLY

Double-blind, randomized, placebo-controlled trial
Patients more than 60 years of age; mean age, 72 years old
Mean blood pressure 183/101 mm Hg
Active treatment: hydrochlorothiazide 25 mg plus triamterene 50 mg daily
Mortality reduction by active treatment
• Total mortality: not significant
• Cardiovascular: 27%
• Cerebrovascular: 32%
Primary benefits
• Reduction in fatal myocardial infarction
• Incidence of severe congestive heart failure reduced
• Incidence of nonfatal strokes reduced
No benefits to subjects (mostly women) aged 80 years or older at time of entry to study

---

Modified from Amery A et al: Mortality and morbidity results from the European working party on high blood pressure in the elderly trial, *Lancet* 2:1349, 1985; Amery A et al: Efficacy of antihypertensive drug treatment according to age, sex, blood pressure, and previous cardiovascular disease in patients over the age of 60, *Lancet* 1:589, 1986.

RESULTS OF SYSTOLIC
HYPERTENSION IN THE ELDERLY PROGRAM

Multicentered, double-blind, randomized, placebo-controlled trial
Community-dwelling well elderly subjects aged 60 years and older; mean age, 72 years
  old
Mean blood pressure 170/77 mm Hg
Active treatment: Chlorthalidone 12.5 to 25 mg/day; step-two drug, atenolol 25 to 50
  mg/day or reserpine 0.05 to 0.1 mg/day
Results of active treatment
• Stroke decreased by 36% over 5 years
• Reduction in cardiovascular events, especially left ventricular failure
• No difference in overall deaths from all causes
Serious side effects uncommon

Modified from SHEP Cooperative Research Group: Prevention of stroke by antihypertensive drug treatment in older persons with isolated systolic hypertension, *JAMA* 265:3255, 1991.

dence of morbid complications for patients aged 65 years and older only recently has been demonstrated in major intervention trials. The European Working Party on High Blood Pressure in the Elderly (EWPHE) and the Systolic Hypertension in the Elderly Program (SHEP) have been the most influential of these trials.[1,2,8]

The results of these studies are shown in the boxes on pp. 519–520. The SHEP study showed the benefits of drug therapy for the "well elderly." However, the results are difficult to generalize to the treatment of the very old, frail, or chronically ill elderly patients. Neither the SHEP nor the EWPHE study was designed to define the optimum drug therapy for hypertension. The effectiveness of drug therapy of diastolic hypertension was confirmed in a randomized clinical trial in Sweden, where overall mortality was reduced by active treatment.[3]

CLINICAL MANIFESTATIONS

Patients with essential hypertension remain asymptomatic until complications supervene. Nonspecific symptoms (e.g., headache, dizziness, and epistaxis) often are attributed incorrectly to hypertension. Indeed the development of symptoms indicates the presence of a target organ complication, a severe degree of hypertension, or a secondary cause of hypertension. Virtually every organ system can be affected by hypertension. Clinically, symptoms related to cardiovascular, neurological, and renal complications are most common.

An inventory of all hypertension-related symptoms is beyond the scope of this chapter. However, a few clinical features should be mentioned. Hypertensive hypertrophic cardiomyopathy should be considered for elderly patients who have hypertension with dyspnea and chest pain.[9] Therapy differs for these patients. Presenting as vascular dementia, cognitive impairment may be the first manifestation of hypertension in older adults. (See Chapter 35.) Renal effects of hypertension, especially renal impairments, must be closely monitored because of the preexisting effects of aging on renal function.

In accelerated hypertension (diastolic blood pressure ≥120 mm Hg), patients may have acute confusion (hypertensive encephalopathy), acute renal failure, and congestive heart failure. Although essential hypertension appears to be the most common cause of accelerated hypertension, secondary causes, particularly renovascular and renal parenchymal diseases, must be considered.

DIAGNOSTIC APPROACH

Blood pressure measurement

The diagnostic approach to the elderly patient with elevated blood pressure includes a careful evaluation of cardiovascular risk factors, a targeted physical examination, and a cost-effective laboratory evaluation to assess comorbid conditions and secondary causes of hypertension. The standard guidelines for the accurate measurement of blood pressure apply to the elderly patient. Appropriate techniques are important to minimize measurement error and to improve diagnostic precision. Because of the high prevalence of postural hypotension in elderly patients, blood pressures should be measured while the patients are in a sitting position and 1 minute after assuming a standing position.

Variations in blood pressure are common and related to circadian rhythm (lower in early morning), timing of the last meal (wait at least 30 minutes after previous meal), drug-blood pressure interactions (including over-the-counter medicines), and altered blood pressure homeostasis.

Some patients have pseudohypertension (due to thickened or hardened brachial or radial arteries) in which the intraarterial pressure is lower than the cuff-measured pressure. Pseudohypertension should be suspected when patients have persistently elevated blood pressures in the absence of complications from hypertensive target organs, when patients fail to respond to antihypertensive medications, and/or when pulseless brachial or radial arteries are palpable (Osler's maneuver).[6] Despite its appeal, however, the Osler's maneuver is highly subject to observer error and bias and is not reproducible with accuracy.

Finally, the diagnosis and monitoring of hypertension can be aided by ambulatory blood pressure measurements. Ambulatory measurements are most helpful when physicians evaluate asymptomatic patients who have variable office blood pressure readings and when either the diagnosis of hypertension or the response to treatment is uncertain.

Evaluation

The basic evaluation of hypertension differs little between young and old patients. The diagnosis of hypertension is made only after multiple blood pressures have been obtained on several visits (at least three to six determinations for asymptomatic or mildly hypertensive and/or previously normotensive patients). The medical history should include information about prior hypertension; cardiovascular, cerebrovascular, or renal diseases; cardiovascular risk factors, including hyperlipidemia, cigarette smoking, and diabetes mellitus; and nutritional problems such as obesity and salt and alcohol ingestion. The history also should include a review of activities of daily living, cognitive function, depression, and sexual dysfunction—factors that may influence the choice of therapy. The psychosocial histories of older patients are particularly important. For example, patients who are dependent in activities of daily living or are cognitively impaired may be unable to adhere to drug therapy. Therefore, reliable family support is necessary to ensure that patients comply with medications and to monitor drug therapy.

The only significant causes of secondary hypertension in the elderly patient are either renal parenchymal or renovascular diseases in the presence of an abdominal aortic bruit. Endocrinological causes such as Cushing's disease and pheochromocytoma appear to be exceedingly rare. The evaluation of these diseases during routine screening is unwarranted.

The physical examination should focus on the presence of hypertensive complications and should uncover comorbid conditions that influence the selection of antihypertensive treatments. The cardiovascular and eye (funduscopic) examinations are particularly important.

Laboratory studies

The basic laboratory evaluation for elderly hypertensive patients differs little from that which is done for younger hypertensive patients. The basic studies include complete blood count, urinalysis, and serum levels of electrolytes, glucose, creatinine, uric acid, calcium, and albumin as well as blood urea nitrogen. An electrocardiogram and, for most patients, a chest x-ray are useful baseline studies. Additional laboratory studies are guided by the likelihood of secondary causes of hypertension.

INTERVENTION

Therapy for either diastolic or isolated systolic hypertension should be initiated only after the patient is evaluated carefully, with particular emphasis on target organs and the hypertensive complications of stroke, heart failure, renal insufficiency, and peripheral vascular disease. The impact of therapy on the patient's quality of life should be considered with regard to activities of daily living, sexual function, exercise tolerance, mood and cognition, and general well-being. When prescribing medications, physicians should consider adverse effects that occur frequently among older patients (e.g., sedation, postural hypotension, dry mouth, constipation, electrolyte disturbance, and glucose intolerance).

Both drug and non-drug therapies are helpful. Initial management of asymptomatic or mildly hypertensive patients (diastolic blood pressure 90 to 100 mm Hg; systolic blood pressure 160 to 170 mm Hg) includes weight loss for obese patients, reduced consumption of alcohol (e.g., one or two drinks per day), aerobic exercise (e.g., walking, biking), and low-salt diet. Although recent studies have shown beneficial effects of salt restriction and aerobic exercise for elderly hypertensive patients, few clinical studies have examined the long-term safety and effectiveness of non-drug therapies. Nevertheless, a trial of non-drug therapy is a reasonable alternative or adjunct to drug therapy for many asymptomatic and borderline hypertensive patients.

Drug therapy for hypertension is indicated for most elderly patients whose diastolic blood pressures remain ≥90 to 95 mm Hg after multiple readings, especially when there are multiple cardiovascular risk factors or hypertensive complications. The appropriate prescribing of medications requires an understanding of the age-related

Table 53-1 Precautions and recommendations for prescribing drugs for ambulatory elderly patients

Drugs	Pharmacological changes with age/adverse effects	Precautions and recommendations
Thiazide diuretics (hydrochlorothiazide)	Dose-response curve flat at doses >25 mg daily; adverse metabolic effects (hypokalemia, hyperglycemia) increase	Use low doses (≤25 mg daily); monitor electrolytes and serum glucose; add potassium (K+) chloride if K+ <3.5 mEq/L
Beta blockers	Reduced renal clearance of atenolol and nadolol; reduced hepatic clearance of propranolol and metoprolol; bronchospasm; heart failure; aggravation of peripheral vascular disease	Reduce dose for impaired renal function; monitor for bradycardia and adverse drug interactions; side effects may be less common with cardioselective agents (e.g., atenolol) in low doses
ACE inhibitors	Reduced renal clearance; risk of functional renal failure; skin rash; cough; angioedema; drug interactions (loop diuretics and NSAIDs)	Use lower doses for elderly patients; avoid excessive diuresis and concomitant use of NSAIDs
Calcium antagonists	Decreased elimination of diltiazem and verapamil; decreased atrioventricular conduction (less in elderly patients); constipation (verapamil); decreased heart rate (verapamil, diltiazem); ankle edema (especially nifedipine)	Use low doses; check electrocardiogram for heart block; high-fiber diet with verapamil; support hose for edema

alterations in disposition of antihypertensive drugs (Table 53-1), the risks of specific adverse drug effects and drug interactions, and the costs of drug therapies. There are no clinically important differences in the blood pressure response to thiazide diuretics, beta-blockers, angiotensin converting enzyme inhibitors (ACE) and calcium channel blockers.

First-step therapies (monotherapies) for hypertension

Thiazide and related diuretics. Traditionally the thiazide diuretics (Tables 53-1 and 53-2) have been regarded as the first-step treatment for hypertension. At equivalent doses, the thiazide and related diuretics (e.g., chlorthalidone) are equally effective in the treatment of elderly hypertensive patients. Adverse metabolic effects are uncommon with low doses.

Beta blockers. Despite the proven effectiveness of beta blockers, they are not generally recommended as first-step treatment for older patients because of the risks of serious adverse effects, especially age-related changes in cardiac contractility and heart rate that cause bradycardia, fatigue, and left ventricular systolic dysfunction.

ACE inhibitors. The ACE inhibitors are generally well tolerated by elderly patients. The antihypertensive efficacy of ACE inhibitors is greatly enhanced by the addition of a diuretic. Some of the currently available ACE inhibitors are prodrugs (e.g., enalapril), which must be converted to active metabolites. Duration of action also differs among these drugs (e.g., captopril has a short half-life; lisinopril has a long half-life). Adverse renal effects may occur in some elderly patients. The most annoying side effect of ACE inhibitors is a chronic nonproductive cough. The more serious side effects of angioedema and neutropenia are uncommon. Drug interactions can be problematic. (See Table 53-1.) Despite these caveats, the ACE inhibitors are probably the preferred first-step therapy for the treatment of hypertensive patients who have diabetes mellitus or heart failure resulting from systolic dysfunction.

Calcium channel blockers. Three groups of calcium channel blockers (Tables 53-1 and 53-2) are commonly used to treat hypertension and are equally efficacious. The prototype drugs are verapamil, diltiazem, and nifedipine. Calcium channel blockers are effective in treating unstable angina, reversing left ventricular hypertrophy, and improving renal hemodynamics in diabetic nephropathy.[7] The calcium channel blockers are generally well tolerated by elderly patients. Compared to the short-acting preparations, the newer long-lasting (sustained release [SR]) forms improve patients' compliance with medications and decrease the incidence of side effects. The nifedipine tablet has smoother and better pharmacokinetic properties than the nifedipine capsule, thus permitting a single daily dose and smoother blood pressure response.

Specific recommendations (Table 53-2). Despite the proliferation of new antihypertensive drugs, the office management of hypertension can be successfully achieved with a few specific agents. For example, most mildly hypertensive patients can be managed with either a diuretic (hydrochlorothiazide), a beta blocker (atenolol), an

Table 53-2   First-step therapy (monotherapy) for hypertension in elderly patients

Drug	Initial dose	Usual maximum dose
Diuretics		
Hydrochlorothiazide	12.5 mg qd	25 mg qd
Indapamide	1.25 mg qd	2.5 mg qd
Furosemide	20 mg bid	40 mg bid
Beta blockers		
Atenolol	25 mg qd	50 mg qd
Nadolol	20 mg qd	40 mg qd
Metoprolol	50 mg qd	200 mg qd
ACE inhibitors		
Captopril	12.5 mg bid	50 mg tid
Enalapril	2.5-5 mg qd	20 mg qd
Lisinopril	2.5-5 mg qd	20 mg qd
Calcium channel blockers		
Verapamil (sustained release)	180 mg qd	360 mg qd
Diltiazem (sustained release)	180 mg qd	360 mg qd
Nifedipine XL (gastrointestinal therapeutic system)	30 mg qd	60 mg qd

ACE inhibitor (lisinopril), or a calcium channel blocker (nifedipine XL). The first-step therapies, with the possible exception of the calcium channel blockers plus thiazide diuretics, have an additive effect when they are combined. Blood pressure is controlled adequately with a single agent in about half of the mildly hypertensive patients and in about 80% of the patients treated with two drugs (e.g., thiazide plus ACE inhibitor; calcium blocker plus beta blocker). Low doses of drugs used in combinations are likely to cause fewer side effects than large doses of single agents.

Other medications. The alpha-adrenergic receptor blockers (e.g., prazosin), centrally acting alpha agonists (e.g., clonidine), and nonspecific vasodilators (e.g., hydralazine) have been shown to reduce blood pressure in elderly hypertensive patients. However, the peripheral alpha receptor blockers increase the risks of postural hypotension, syncope, and presyncope, which severely limit the utility of these drugs for the treatment of elderly patients. These side effects also can be seen with the alpha-beta blocker labetalol. The centrally acting alpha agonists often cause symptoms of sedation and dry mouth, which may prove intolerable to very old patients. Symptomatic hypotension and rebound hypertension following abrupt cessation of therapy are also common. The transdermal therapeutic systems may be better tolerated, but side effects are still problematic. The vasodilator hydralazine is a time-honored second- or third-step drug. However, when compared with calcium channel blockers and ACE inhibitors that act as specific vasodilators, hydralazine potentially has more side effects, including symptomatic hypotension, fluid retention, and provocation of angina pectoris. Reserpine is an inexpensive and time-honored agent, but it may induce or exacerbate depression and psychomotor slowing in frail patients. Although reserpine in low doses has been used safely in both the Veterans Administration cooperative studies and the SHEP study, the high risk/benefit ratio in most old patients probably precludes its widespread use.

Office monitoring

Patients with hypertension should be monitored at periodic intervals. Patients are usually seen every 2 to 4 weeks until their blood pressures are adequately controlled. Thereafter, visits every 3 to 4 months are sufficient. Laboratory chemistries should be obtained at least every 3 to 6 months, when patients take ACE inhibitors or thiazide diuretics. Laboratory studies are required less often for patients taking calcium channel blockers because these agents have no adverse metabolic effects. Beta blockers and diuretics alter serum lipids and justify an annual reevaluation of serum cholesterol and triglycerides.

The goal of blood pressure treatment is to reduce the risks associated with hypertension. For diastolic hypertension, the optimal diastolic blood pressure is probably 80 to 85 mm Hg; for ISH, a blood pressure of 140 to 160 mm Hg is desirable. A safe slow reduction in blood pressure helps the physician to prevent side effects and to maintain a good quality of life for the older patient. Treatment is most likely to be effective when a therapeutic relationship is established with the primary physician and when the patient and family are actively involved in the treatment plan.

REFERENCES

1. Amery A et al: Mortality and morbidity results from the European working party on high blood pressure in the elderly trial, *Lancet* 2:1349, 1985.
2. Amery A et al: Efficacy of antihypertensive drug treatment according to age, sex, blood pressure, and previous cardiovascular disease in patients over the age of 60, *Lancet* 1:589, 1986.
3. Dahlot B et al. Morbidity and mortality in the Swedish Trial in Old Patients with Hypertension (STOP-Hypertension). Lancet 338:1281, 1991.
4. Mattila K et al: Blood pressure and five year survival in the very old, *Br Med J* 296:887, 1988.
5. Messerli FH et al: Essential hypertension in the elderly: haemodynamics, intravascular volume, plasma renin activity, and circulating catecholamine levels, *Lancet* 2:983, 1983.
6. Messerli FH, Ventura HO, Amodeo C: Osler's maneuver and pseudohypertension, *N Engl J Med* 312:1548, 1985.
7. Schulman SP et al: The effects of antihypertensive therapy on left ventricular mass in elderly patients, *N Engl J Med* 322:1350, 1990.
8. SHEP Cooperative Research Group: Prevention of stroke by antihypertensive drug treatment in older persons with isolated systolic hypertension, *JAMA* 265:3255, 1991.
9. Topol EJ, Traill TA, Fortuin NJ: Hypertensive hypertrophic cardiomyopathy of the elderly, *N Engl J Med* 312:277, 1985.
10. Wikstrand J et al: Antihypertensive treatment with metoprolol or hydrochlorothiazide in patients aged 60 to 75 years, *JAMA* 255:1304, 1986.

SUGGESTED READINGS

Applegate WB: Hypertension in elderly patients, *Ann Intern Med* 110:901, 1989.

Applegate WB, ed. Hypertension, *Clin Geriatr Med* 5(4):639, 1989.

The 1988 Report of the Joint National Committee on Detection, Evaluation, and Treatment of High Blood Pressure, *Arch Intern Med* 148:1023, 1988.

Working Group on Hypertension in the Elderly: Statement on hypertension in the elderly, *JAMA* 256:70, 1986.

CHAPTER 54

Peripheral vascular diseases

HIEP PHAM
BRUCE E. ROBINSON

KEY POINTS

- The classical signs of acute arterial occlusion are the five p's (pain, pallor, paresthesia, pulselessness, and paralysis).
- Medical management of intermittent claudication consists of risk factor manipulations, tobacco elimination, regular walking, and pentoxifylline.
- Screening for abdominal aortic aneurysm should be considered for those patients with risk factors (included male sex, age 50 years or more, hypertension, and family histories of aneurysm) and evidence of atherosclerotic complications elsewhere.
- The complications of chronic venous insufficiency include acute deep venous thrombosis, varicose veins, superficial thrombophlebitis, stasis dermatitis, edema, and ulcers.

ACUTE ISCHEMIA

Clinical relevance

Sudden interruption of the blood flow to the extremities can be caused by embolism, thrombosis, trauma, vasospasm, or iatrogenic factors. The major cause of acute arterial occlusion is arterial embolism. The majority of emboli (up to 80%) originate from the heart, with the remainder deriving from large proximal arteries. Atherosclerotic complications (e.g., cardiomyopathy with atrial fibrillation) now are fourfold more common than rheumatic valvular disease as sources of embolism. Silent myocardial infarction has been reported to be the source of emboli in 11% of older patients.

Clinical manifestations and diagnostic approach

Acute arterial vascular occlusion is signaled by the acute onset of severe pain in 60% of patients, acute numbness and coldness in 20% of patients, and subacute or silent presentations in the remaining 20% of cases. The extent of ischemia depends on the site of occlusion and the presence of collateral circulation. After approximately 8 hours of ischemia, muscles and nervous tissues suffer permanent damage, whereas it may require several more hours before the skin may show signs of damage or demarcation. The first sign of severe tissue ischemia is the loss of fine touch and proprioception. With the loss of motor function and presence of anesthesia, ischemia is considered irreversible and amputation is necessary.

The differential diagnosis of an acutely painful and discolored leg should include arterial thrombosis, arterial embolism, arterial spasm, deep venous thrombosis, trauma, vasculitides, and iatrogenic causes such as postcatheterization obstruction and dissecting aneurysm. A careful history and physical examination usually leave one cause as the dominant possibility, with noninvasive testing (described later in this chapter) available for confirmation.

The physical signs of acute arterial occlusion which are present depending on the severity and stage of the occlusion. Initially, part of the affected limb appears pale or slightly cyanotic and is cool to the touch. When the classical signs of the five *p*'s (pain, pallor, paresthesia, pulselessness, and paralysis) of acute arterial occlusion are present, the disease is at the advanced stage. Doughy firmness of the muscle indicates the presence of more severe ischemic changes, and nonblanching cyanosis of the skin may signal permanent damage to the skin. Cardiovascular examination may reveal the cause and the source of the arterial occlusion. Doppler arterial studies are necessary in localizing the site of the obstruction and the degree of arterial obstruction.

Intervention

The initial treatment of acute arterial occlusion is anticoagulation, regardless of the choice of surgical procedure (i.e., thrombectomy or embolectomy). The treatment or correction of the underlying cause of the acute arterial occlusion is essential to prevent recurrences.

CHRONIC OCCLUSIVE DISEASE

Clinical relevance

The older patient who has limited tolerance for activities because of pain in the lower extremities is often seen in geriatric outpatient settings. Because peripheral arterial occlusive disease without symptoms is common among older persons, other conditions capable of producing the clinical symptoms should be considered and the natural history of the disease explained to the patient prior to surgical referral.

Clinical manifestations

The characteristic clinical presentation of intermittent claudication is pain, cramp, or fatigue in the muscles of the lower extremity. Each symptom is related to sustained exercise and can be relieved by a brief period of rest. The location of the pain suggests the site of the lesion; for example, calf pain suggests superficial femoral artery occlusion; thigh and calf pain suggests iliofemoral occlusion; and hip and buttock pain suggests aortoiliac occlusion. The physical examination of the patient with symptoms of claudication systematically should evaluate the pulses of both the upper and lower extremities and the neck, as well as the aortic pulsation of the abdomen. The absence of the dorsalis pedis pulse may be a developmental variant in some individuals. The popliteal pulse is difficult to palpate in some obese persons. Chronic ischemia characteristically produces reduced muscle mass, loss of soft tissue resulting in prominent bony protrusions, thin skin, absence of hair, and thickened, dystrophic toenails. Unfortunately, these signs are common among older patients without arterial disease. More helpful are the changes in color and temperature; for example, the color of the feet is often pale or mottled and the toes may be cool. Capillary refilling and venous filling will be retarded when there is significant ischemia and both should be compared between the extremities. The foot that is affected by chronic ischemia exhibits pallor when it is elevated 30 degrees above the horizontal, and there is marked rubor with dependency. Cracks in the plantar skin, indolent superficial ulcerations, and delayed healing in response to minor trauma are additional findings that correlate with impaired circulation.

Diagnostic approach

When the cause of symptoms is in doubt, treadmill exercise testing reproduces the symptoms and better defines the clinical manifestations.

The ankle/brachial index is the simplest and most useful noninvasive measure of the integrity of arterial circulation of the lower extremities. Significant arterial occlusive disease is reflected by an ankle/brachial index lower than 1.0; claudication can be expected in the range of 0.5 to 0.9, and rest pain can be expected below 0.4. Elderly patients with severe arterial calcification have unreliable ankle/brachial index readings, and more sophisticated noninvasive approaches are necessary. The combination of segmental arterial pressure, wave form recording, and arterial plethysmography is considered reliable as an indicator of the location and severity of disease. Lumbar spinal stenosis is particularly common in older persons and produces exertional pains, cramps, or fatigue in the legs. The discomfort of spinal stenosis also is relieved by rest. Electrography and nerve conduction study following exercise are sensitive to symptomatic spinal stenosis.

> ──────── **ADVICE FOR PATIENTS WITH ARTERIAL INSUFFICIENCY** ────────
>
> Stop tobacco use in any form
> Walk to tolerance: 30 minutes 3 to 7 times per week
> Choose well-fitted, comfortable, protective footwear
> Inspect your feet nightly for blisters, corns, calluses
> Seek immediate podiatric attention for lesions of feet
> Avoid going out in extreme cold
> Check temperature of bathwater with hands
> Institute weight reduction if obese
> See your doctor immediately for numbness, prolonged pain, ulceration, or discoloration
>   of your feet

Intervention

Treatment of intermittent claudication begins with control or modification of the risk factors associated with occlusive disease. (See the box above.) Cessation of tobacco use in any form decreases the acceleration of atherosclerotic disease and may result in improvement for some patients. For those older patients with abnormal lipid profiles, diet modification and drug therapy also should be considered. Long-term control of hypertension and diabetes mellitus also is important in the medical management of peripheral vascular disease.

A systematic program for walking or other exercise may significantly improve the symptoms of intermittent claudication. Exercise theoretically enhances collateral circulation and thus improves circulation to the affected muscle groups.

Pentoxifylline improves filterability and viscosity of the blood by increasing red blood cell deformity and decreasing plasma fibrinogen and platelet aggregation. Several double-blind controlled trials of pentoxifylline consistently have shown that this drug is significantly more effective than placebo in increasing walking distance and decreasing the time from onset of pain. The side effects of pentoxifylline include gastrointestinal symptoms (nausea, vomiting, and bloating) and dizziness and necessitate the discontinuation of the drug in about 3% of the patients. The recommended dosage of pentoxifylline is 400 mg 3 times a day. The benefit of the drug may not be noticeable until after 4 to 8 weeks of medical therapy.

ABDOMINAL AORTIC ANEURYSM

Clinical relevance

A true abdominal aortic aneurysm (AAA) is a localized dilatation of the abdominal aortic wall by more than 3 cm. All three layers of the vessel (intima, media, and adventitia) are involved. A false aneurysm is essentially a perforation of the aorta with subsequent hematoma formation limited by adventitia or surrounding vascular tissues. Most AAAs are a complication of atherosclerosis. Other less frequent causes include trauma, infection, syphilis, cystic medial necrosis, inflammation, and Marfan's syndrome.

The incidence of AAA has been estimated at 10 to 20/1000 population. In patients with known peripheral vascular disease, the prevalence of AAA has been reported to be nearly 10%. Factors associated with increased risk of aneurysm include age more 50 years, male gender, history of hypertension, family history of aneurysm, and clinical evidence of atherosclerotic complications elsewhere.

Clinical manifestations

Most patients with AAAs are asymptomatic unless there is bleeding, dissection, rupture, or impending rupture. Symptoms may include mild to severe abdominal and/or low back pain. Through routine physical examinations, many AAAs are detected as pulsating abdominal masses. Ectatic abdominal aortas without aneurysm also may be palpable and may be confused with AAAs.

Diagnostic approach

Lederle, Walker, and Reinke[2] argue for AAA screenings every 2 to 3 years for all persons more than 50 years of age because the prevalence of AAA in persons of this age group is 3%, and surgery is effective in reducing AAA mortality. Physical examination is sufficient for screening older persons with abdominal girths of less than 100 cm (40 inches). However, in those with larger girths, screening by abdominal ultrasound is recommended. Ultrasonography is inexpensive and highly reliable in terms of sensitivity and specificity. Efforts at aneurysm detection should be recommended even more strongly to those elderly persons with risk factors for aneurysm.

Intervention

For persons in whom an aneurysm is identified, careful counseling is necessary to determine who should be referred for vascular surgical evaluation because there are some differences of opinion on candidates for surgical management. The natural history of the asymptomatic aneurysm between 3.5 and 6.0 cm is a critical factor in the decision for surgery. Nevitt, Ballard, and Hallett[3] found that the diameter of aneurysms increased by a median of 0.21 cm/yr, and only 24% of aneurysms had an expansion rate of 0.4 cm or more/yr.

The risk of rupture relates primarily to the size of the aneurysm, with a clear increase in risk for sizes larger than 5 cm. It is reported that there is a rupture risk of approximately 5% for AAAs smaller than 5 cm in diameter, 16% for those 5 to 6 cm, and 76% for those larger than 7 cm. However, in some autopsy series, nearly 30% of rupture deaths were caused by aneurysms smaller than 5 cm. Nevertheless, the same population-based study by Nevitt, Ballard, and Hallett[3] found cumulative incidence of rupture was 6% after 5 years and 8% after 10 years; there were no ruptures in 5 years for patients with aneurysms less than 5 cm in diameter, and ruptures were found in 25% of those with aneurysms of 5 cm or more. Symptoms such as hypogastric or low back pain, if due to aneurysm, suggest that rupture has occurred or is imminent. One third of those patients with unoperated symptomatic aneurysms die within 1 month and 80% die within 1 year.

The overall risk of death from aneurysm resection is estimated at 2% to 7%. The risk of aneurysm resection in the individual is determined by comorbid conditions and not by age. Reported series of resections, including resections for patients more than 80 years of age, have found little difference in mortality because of age. Therefore, in patients with *asymptomatic* AAA, it would seem reasonable to observe aneurysms smaller than 4 cm with periodic ultrasonograms at 3-month intervals for the first year and every 6 to 12 months after the expansion rate is estimated. Aneurysms between 4 and 5 cm are somewhat controversial, with continued medical surveillance suggested by some and resection suggested by others. In patients with acceptable surgical risk, resection of AAAs larger than 5 cm would be recommended. However, even in this group, the natural history of these lesions would permit long-term survival for most of those patients affected by AAA.

CHRONIC VENOUS INSUFFICIENCY

Clinical relevance

Chronic venous insufficiency occurs as a consequence of venous flow disturbances, which are most often caused by venous valvular defects and occasionally by venous obstruction. The most common complaints of patients with chronic venous insufficiency are the unsightly engorgement of the lower extremity veins, swelling that progresses with dependency and is relieved with lower limb elevation, and heaviness and aching of the legs that is relieved with elevation or walking. The clinical diagnosis of venous hypertension is based on the presence of venous varicosities and characteristic skin changes in the lower legs and feet such as brawny edema, brownish pigmentation, subcutaneous fibrosis, and atrophy. The classic ulcer of chronic venous hypertension most commonly occurs on the medial and occasionally on the lateral side of the leg and rarely is circumferential.

Clinical manifestations, diagnostic approach, and intervention of complications

Acute deep venous thrombosis. When the onset of leg swelling is unilateral or relatively acute, the diagnosis of acute deep venous thrombosis must be considered. However, leg edema in many older persons is asymmetrical and factors other than venous thrombosis can cause a sudden change in the extent of edema. Historical associations should be sought for the swelling and the clinical factors that predispose the patient to deep venous thrombosis (i.e., recent immobility, cancer, infection, and congestive heart failure are associated with venous thrombosis). An evaluation should be made for other symptoms and signs of acute deep venous thrombosis of the leg, including fever, pain, tenderness, palpable cords, pain with dorsiflexion at the ankle (Homans' sign), and changes in color or temperature. However, such changes are not found in all patients with deep venous thrombosis and in many the swollen limb is the only clue.

Diagnosing or excluding deep venous thrombosis has been made safer and easier by the availability of duplex Doppler ultrasonography and venous impedance plethysmography. Both techniques demonstrate excellent (greater than 90%) sensitivity and specificity for significant deep venous thrombosis but are insensitive to small clots in the calf veins; however, the clinical significance of such clots is in doubt. If calf vein clots are suspected, a noninvasive study should be repeated in 4 to 7 days to exclude from the diagnosis involvement of the deep venous system.[1] When the diagnosis of deep venous thrombosis is made, hospitalization for anticoagulation is indicated.

Varicose veins and superficial thrombophlebitis. The most common sequela of uncontrolled chronic venous insufficiency is that of varicose veins. Varicose veins are visibly dilated superficial veins that may be produced either by valvular incompetence of the superficial veins themselves or by high transmitted pressure through perforator veins from the deep venous system. About 60% to 75% of patients with varicosities report that family members have the same affliction.

One of the most common complications of varicose veins is superficial thrombophlebitis. While this condition is associated with connective tissue diseases and advanced stages of malignancies, it is most often present with no underlying illness other than chronic venous insufficiency. The involved vein is hard, cordlike, and tender to the touch. Edema is usually not present, and erythema is minimal unless it is due to associated cellulitis. Most commonly, superficial thrombophlebitis is a local event only; however, it is occasionally associated with low-grade fever. The treatment of localized superficial thrombophlebitis should include elastic compression stockings and nonsteroidal antiinflammatory medications. If the thrombophlebitis is extensive and expands, bed rest, limb elevation, and warm compresses, as well as daily reevaluation, are recommended. When superficial thrombophlebitis is extensive or extends above the lower thigh, pulsed Doppler ultrasound of the extremities should be performed to exclude from the diagnosis extension of the process into the deep venous system. Significant fever may indicate bacterial endovascular infection, requiring hospitalization.

Stasis dermatitis, edema, and venous ulcers. Stasis changes in the skin of the lower legs are the next most common manifestations of chronic venous insufficiency. The changes of chronic venous hypertension range from edema to thick hard subcutaneous tissue and skin that has brownish pigmentation and/or is dry, hairless, atrophic, eczematous, and ulcerated. The clinical appearance of stasis dermatitis is similar to that of contact dermatitis, superficial fungal dermatitis, peripheral arterial disease, and bacterial cellulitis. These conditions also can occur concurrently and should be considered when the patient initially comes to the physician's office because of these symptoms or when the condition fails to respond to therapy for stasis.

The essential part of either surgical or medical management of the complications of chronic venous hypertension is the control of edema. Patients with edema should interrupt prolonged periods of limb dependency with periods of gravity drainage. This ideally can be done with 10 minutes of limb elevation for every 2 hours of limb dependency. To be effective, the legs must be raised above the level of the heart and not simply propped on a stool. To accomplish nocturnal gravity drainage, the foot of the bed can be elevated 6 inches. A graded elastic stocking with a minimum pressure of 40 mm Hg at the ankle should be worn at all times when the patient is upright. Stockings should be replaced every 3 or 4 months because of the loss of a tight fit. In general, if the stockings are comfortable, they are probably too large and need to be replaced.

For acute exacerbations of stasis dermatitis with weeping inflamed skin, the previously described pressure-relieving measures can be combined with moist compresses of mild astringents such as Burow's solution. When the weeping has resolved, low-potency corticosteroid creams (such as hydrocortisone 1% or triamcinolone .025%) can be used alone or mixed with zinc oxide paste. Warm compresses increase itching, and topical antibiotics may be allergenic and therefore are not recommended.

Venous ulcers are common complications of stasis dermatitis. All venous ulcers heal if the superficial venous pressure can be satisfactorily controlled either by limb elevation or adequate compressive devices. Recently developed ulcers with slough can be treated with moist saline gauze and compressive elastic bandages that are changed three or four times a day. The frequent changing of the dressing provides debridement of the wounds. For epithelizing chronic venous ulcers, the Unna boot provides continuous compression, protection, and topical treatment of the wound. The Unna boot is a gauge dressing impregnated with gelatin, zinc oxide, and Caladryl that is applied from the toes to the knee after the ulcer initially has been cleansed; the boot is then overwrapped with an Ace bandage. It should be changed every few days initially weekly when the course of the lesion is determined. Unna boots are not recommended for patients who have ulcers with signs of infection or peripheral arterial disease.

Occlusive dressings also have been shown to accelerate healing of chronic venous ulcers. They are produced in different forms and textures such as foams (Synthaderm), films (Opsite), hydrocolloids (Duoderm), and hydrogels (Vigilon). The most important point is not to prematurely remove the dressing since this can remove the newly formed epithelial surface of the wound. The occlusive dressings should be left on until fluid starts to leak from the sides of the dressing. This may occur from hours to days after application. For patients who have ulcers with signs of severe dermatitis

ADVICE FOR PATIENTS WITH
CHRONIC VENOUS INSUFFICIENCY

Elastic support is needed for a lifetime

Elevate legs 30 minutes 3 times a day or 10 minutes every 2 hours

Avoid prolonged standing or sitting; walk around at least every 15 minutes

When legs swell or skin gets red and scaly, increase the elastic support and elevation

Exercise regularly; walk, swim, jog, or cycle

Seek physician's advice for increased redness, pain, swelling, warmth, or ulceration

Small cuts or scrapes can lead to serious ulcers—be careful

Control of edema through compression or elevation is an essential part of either surgical
or medical management of complications from chronic venous hypertension

and patients who are likely to remove the dressings, adherent occlusive dressings such as Duoderm or Opsite should be avoided, but the nonadherent dressings such as Vigilon or Synthaderm are recommended. Topical kesanterin, topical zinc oxide, and oral zinc sulfate (220 mg 3 times/day) also have been shown to accelerate the ulcer healing process.

The box above summarizes general recommendations for patients with chronic venous insufficiency.

REFERENCES

1. Huisman MV et al: Management of clinically suspected acute venous thrombosis in outpatients with serial impedance plethysmography in a community hospital setting, *Arch Intern Med* 149:511, 1989.
2. Lederle FA, Walker JM, Reinke DB: Selective screening for abdominal aortic aneurysms with physical examination and ultrasound, *Arch Intern Med* 148:1753, 1988.
3. Nevitt MP, Ballard DJ, Hallett JW: Prognosis of abdominal aortic aneurysms: a population-based study, *N Engl J Med* 321:1009, 1989.

SUGGESTED READINGS

Nevitt MP, Ballard DJ, Hallett JW: Prognosis of abdominal aortic aneurysms: a population-based study, *N Engl J Med* 321:1009, 1989.

Walsh DB et al: Peripheral vascular disease in the geriatric patient. In Reichel W, ed: *Clinical aspects of aging*, ed 3, Baltimore, 1989, Williams & Wilkins.

CHAPTER 55

Eye disorders

MARY ELINA FERRIS

KEY POINTS

- Increased age is accompanied by decreased visual acuity, increased rates of blindness, and other eye disorders.
- Keratitis or "dry eye" is the most prevalent ocular disorder in elderly persons; medications are a frequent cause.
- In the United States, macular degeneration is the leading cause of irreversible visual loss, followed by glaucoma.
- Glaucoma screening for elderly patients is controversial but still recommended by ophthalmologists.
- Age-related changes in the lens of the eye result in greater need for artificial illumination and less ability to visually adapt to darkness.

Many age-related changes in the eye and surrounding tissues combine with disease to result in visual impairment. *Impairment* generally implies blindness in one or both eyes or trouble seeing even with glasses, which occurs in one out of every seven persons aged 75 years and older. These complaints increase with age as shown in Figure 55-1. More than 50% of legally blind persons in the United States are elderly persons, and more than one half of all new cases of blindness each year involve persons aged 65 years or older.[6] Functional abilities and quality of life are extremely dependent on preservation of vision in elderly persons who also may suffer losses in the other senses.

Many of these eye disorders may first be detected in the primary care office, and early intervention or referral may result in significant preservation of sight and quality of life. Several of the disorders, particularly in the external eye, may be treated completely in the primary care office.[4] Even for those problems referred to the ophthalmologist, ocular medications and systemic illnesses may influence other aspects of the elderly person's care, necessitating knowledge of these eye disorders by the primary

537

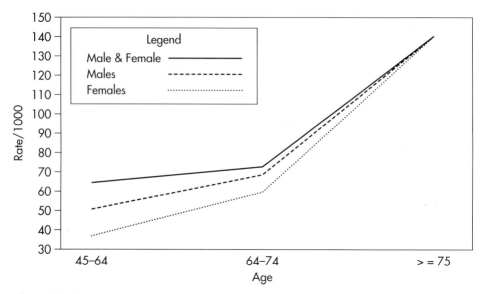

Figure 55-1 Rate of visual impairment by age and sex. (*Modified from data from US Department of Health and Human Services: Current estimates from the national health interview survey: United States 1983, US Public Health Service Pub No 86-1582, series 10, No 154, Hyattsville, Md, 1986*)

care provider. The following sections describe age-related external eye disorders and visual disorders. Visual manifestations of systemic diseases also can be significant in elderly persons and are described within these sections.

AGE-RELATED EXTERNAL EYE DISORDERS

Senile ptosis, entropion, ectropion, pterygium, pinguecula, and keratoconjunctivitis sicca

Clinical relevance. With aging, a variety of changes occurs in the eyelid, conjunctiva, and cornea that can affect function and quality of life for elderly persons. Starting from the outer structures, a *ptosis* (drooping of the eyelid) may interfere with vision. This condition may be acquired with aging, accompanied by a loss of tone in the levator muscle and thinning of the lids, or it may result from diseases such as third cranial nerve palsy, Horner's syndrome, myasthenia gravis, or trauma.

With age, the eyelids may develop *entropion* (border turned inward) and *ectropion* (border turned outward) from spasticity of the eyelid retractor muscles, which exposes the conjunctiva or physically irritates the conjunctiva and cornea. The position of the tear punctum may become altered and interfere with tear drainage, causing tears to spill onto the cheeks (epiphora).

The conjunctiva changes with age, causing *pinguecula* (hypertrophic degenerated connective tissue that is yellow or elevated) on either side of the cornea. Pinguecula can be irritated by outdoor exposure. *Pterygia* are growths of pinguecula that can encroach on the cornea from either side and even interfere with vision. They are thought to be associated with cumulative exposure to ultraviolet light.

The *dry eye* (keratoconjunctivitis sicca syndrome) is the most common eye complaint among elderly persons, causing a mild chronic irritation or an incapacitating burning sensation. There is a natural decrease in basal tear secretion with age, but reduced tear production can be affected by other drugs or systemic diseases as shown in the box below. A study of 103 female elderly residents in a retirement home revealed 26% had dry eye complaints; 50% of those who had dry eye complaints were taking medications that reduced tear production.[5] Although collagen vascular diseases such as Sjögren's syndrome have been associated with dry eyes, they are much less common than age-related changes (e.g., only 2% of the patients in the above study satisfied criteria for Sjögren's).

Eye blinking, which is vital for distribution and pumping of tear drainage, may be reduced in Parkinson's disease and may further aggravate dry eye symptoms. Herpes zoster (shingles) also may cause a keratitis of acute onset and requires ophthalmological evaluation.

Clinical manifestations. Typically the patient experiences a feeling of dryness, a gritty irritation, and a sensation of a foreign body or even severe pain in the eye as a result of the above conditions and disorders. Constant irritation may lead to recurrent infections, with conjunctival reddening and discharge. Chronic tear leakage can cause crusting and may macerate surrounding skin. Embarrassment and outdoor irritation may cause the elderly person to withdraw and avoid social contact.

Arcus senilis may be noted in elderly patients as a ringlike opacity around the periphery of the cornea caused by deposition of phospholipids. It can be associated

---

CONDITIONS AFFECTING TEAR PRODUCTION

Drugs

Antihistamines
Anticholinergics
Antihypertensives
Phenothiazines

Systemic diseases

Lupus erythematosus
Sjögren's syndrome
Polyarteritis nodosa
Sarcoidosis

Table 55-1   Artificial tears

Types of ocular lubricants	Examples
Short-acting artificial tears	Hydroxypropyl methylcellulose (Isopto Tears)
Long-acting ointments	White petrolatum and mineral oil (Lacri-Lube)
Sustained-release tear insert	Lacrisert

with familial hypercholesterolemia but also can be seen with normal aging. If asymmetrical, it could be the result of severe unilateral carotid disease.

Diagnostic approach. A thorough clinical evaluation of the eye and surrounding tissues guides the physician to the correct diagnosis.[3] The eyelids also should be inspected for infections and dermatological malignancies, the latter occurring most frequently near the lower lid and inner canthus. Crusting on the lids and lashes is usually a sign of bacterial infection, which can be chronic if caused by underlying staphylococcal or seborrheic blepharitis.

Pupillary size and reaction should be checked with a penlight, including the clarity of the corneal reflex. A hazy reflection indicates a more serious condition that necessitates referral. Small pupils with red eyes suggest iritis, and midsize pupil dilation with pain is highly suggestive of acute closed-angle glaucoma.

Fluorescein staining of the conjunctiva viewed with blue or ultraviolet light (Wood's lamp) may detect corneal abrasions, a particular risk in exposed or dry eyes. A slit lamp evaluation also may be useful to evaluate the cornea and conjunctiva, especially for foreign bodies. The slit lamp may reveal the absence of a tear meniscus on the lower lid margin consistent with the dry eye syndrome.

Tear evaluation can be done with Schirmer's test, which uses a special strip of filter paper placed in the lower conjunctival cul-de-sac for 5 minutes after a drop of local ophthalmological anesthetic (e.g., tetracaine or proparacaine HCl) is administered. If the moistened exposed portion of the paper is less than 10 mm, the result of the test is considered abnormal.

Intervention. Eye lubricants are the mainstay of treatment for many external eye disorders of elderly patients. Saline drops provide temporary relief but are very short acting; as a result, preparations have been developed to add large molecular weight polymers that increase viscosity and duration. Many lubricants are sold over the counter as "artificial tears," which may be selected and combined based on their duration of action in the eye as shown in Table 55-1. Patients should be cautioned that sensitivity to preservatives in artificial tears such as thimerosal and benzalkonium have been reported. Some products are available without such additives (Murocel and Muro Tears).

Prior to the patient's beginning a regimen of lubricants for disorders such as entropion, ectropion, or keratitis, bacterial infection may necessitate treatment with topical antibiotics such as sodium sulfacetamide. Education of patients must be done to encourage their compliance and coping with these chronic conditions and to encourage the patients be alert to changes in their chronic dry eye symptoms that could indicate a developing infection. If patients frequently need to wipe tears away, the clinician should encourage "blotting" to prevent further stretching of the lax eyelid and worsening of the problem.

Other treatments include therapeutic soft contact lenses for ptosis and for keratitis to hold the tear film against the cornea. However, contact lenses also may cause abrasions in dry eyes and should be used with care. Environmental changes to increase humidity or even occlusive ocular patching may improve symptoms. Punctal occlusion by the ophthalmologist may enhance moisture retention by preventing tear drainage in dry eyes.

Removal of irritating eyelashes and eyelid reparative surgery may help symptoms associated with ectropion and entropion. Soft conforming contact lenses also have been used to protect the eyes from lashes turned inward.

Surgical treatment for pterygia is often followed by recurrence and can result in scarring, which limits ocular mobility. Local vasoconstrictor drops (0.12% phenylephrine) three times a day often shrink the tissue and reduce irritating symptoms.

Chronic eye irritation that does not respond to the usual conservative measures outlined above should be referred to the ophthalmologist to consider other rare causes such as Fuchs' epithelial-endothelial dystrophy, which is seen in older females as progressive corneal edema.

AGE-RELATED VISUAL DISORDERS

Cataracts, macular degeneration, glaucoma, and diabetic retinopathy

Clinical relevance. Many elderly persons have a variety of age-related visual deficits. Near vision deteriorates in almost all elderly persons as a result of structural changes in the lens and surrounding tissue, leading to the loss of accommodation (presbyopia) and the need for reading glasses. The lens becomes more yellow, allows less light transmission, and filters out bluer colors. Lens changes also may cause stray light to scatter and decrease resistance to glare, which can be a hazard to night driving. Peripheral field defects may be present in up to 13% of persons aged 65 years and older, many of whom are unaware of these problems.

The risk of being "blind" (corrected vision to 20/200 or field defect of 20% or greater) is nearly 10 times greater for those aged 65 years and older, who account for 50% of all legally blind Americans. It is no wonder that many elderly persons fear visual loss in their later years, and many even underreport visual symptoms as a result. Disease can further worsen visual changes, with cataracts and macular degeneration increasing with one's advancing age. The risk for cataracts increases with age-related changes in the lens, diabetes mellitus, environmental exposure (ultraviolet rays, microwaves, infrared waves), and medications, especially corticosteroids. While cataracts are the most prevalent cause of blindness worldwide, macular degeneration is the leading cause of irreversible visual loss in the United States.

The macula is the part of the retina most vulnerable to degenerative disorders. It is responsible for fine details and color vision. Thirty percent of adults aged 65 years and older have some loss of macular function, and macular degeneration (visual loss of at least 20/40) is present in 8% to 11% of persons aged 65 to 74 years old and 20% of those aged 75 years and older. The degree of retinal involvement does not necessarily correlate with impairment of visual acuity.

Glaucoma is the second leading cause of new blindness in the United States, and it affects 2% of the population more than 40 years of age. The most common type is open-angle (90% of cases), which progresses without symptoms until irreversible visual field losses occur. Closed-angle glaucoma has a peak incidence among persons 70 years of age. Certain groups (i.e., elderly persons, African-Americans, diabetics, persons with myopia, and those with family histories of glaucoma) are more at risk for glaucoma.

Diabetes mellitus is responsible for 10% of cases of blindness in persons aged 65 years and older. Some studies have suggested age-related increases in the retinopathy rate of older diabetics, particularly in association with long duration of the disease. Diabetes also increases the risk for cataracts, glaucoma, and retinal detachments.

Medications and nutrition also may affect vision in elderly persons (Table 55-2). It is prudent to inventory all prescription and nonprescription drugs when acute visual changes in this group are considered.

Clinical manifestations. Patients with cataracts generally complain of painless progressive loss of vision that may affect one or both eyes. Initially the cataract may be *immature*, with clear lens cortex remaining, but when the entire lens becomes opacified

Table 55-2 Medications and vitamins affecting vision

Agent	Effect
Drugs	
Acetazolamide	Transient myopia
Chloroquine	Blurred vision; pigmentary degeneration of macula
Corticosteroid	Cataracts and glaucoma (usually if taken more than 2 years)
Digitalis	Blurred or strange colors (reversible with smaller dose)
Ethambutol	Diminished vision and color discrimination; inflammation of optic nerve
Phenothiazine	Pigmentary retinopathy
Sulfonamide	Transient myopia
Thiazide	Transient myopia
Vitamin deficiencies	
A	Night blindness
B (thiamin, niacin)	Loss of central vision

Table 55-3   Clinical manifestations of cataracts

Location or stage of cataract	Symptoms
Posterior subcapsular	Near vision acuity reduced
Nuclear	Distance vision acuity reduced; worsened by night and bright daylight
Advanced	Total visual impairment

it is termed *mature* (or *hypermature* if lens protein leaks through the posterior capsule and causes an inflammatory reaction). Symptoms may differ depending on the location of the cataract (Table 55-3).

Macular degeneration causes a slow central vision loss that can be painless over many months or years. Patients may note loss of fine discrimination when they read; for example, while peripheral vision remains intact. If patients note a persistent glare after they have gazed at a bright object or that straight lines appear wavy, the examiner should be alert to the possibility of this disease. Patients with macular degeneration are often given Amsler grids to check their vision daily and report new vision changes (Figure 55-2).

Severe eye pain, redness, blurred vision, headache, nausea, and vomiting in an elderly patient is suggestive of acute closed-angle glaucoma. In early cases of glaucoma the patients' symptoms may be most noticeable in a darkened room when their eyes are stressed to accommodate to the darkness. Other causes of eye pain to be considered for elderly persons include conjunctivitis, corneal abrasions, iritis, sinusitis, and disorders of the optic nerve.

Sudden visual losses present an emergency situation that may be due to eye disorders or systemic diseases. Retinal detachments, which are more common among elderly persons because of changes in the vitreous humor of the eye or after cataract surgery, include a variety of often transient presenting symptoms (i.e., lightning flashes and/or a "curtain" drawn over the eye with or without floaters in the eye). Spontaneous loss of vision in one or both eyes may be due to transient ischemic attacks or temporal arteritis. If the deficit persists, there may be hemorrhage or central retinal artery occlusion. Visual loss that is centrally located may indicate macular or optic nerve disease. In any case urgent ophthalmological evaluation is indicated.

Diagnostic approach. Examination of the eyes should be a routine part of geriatric care, not only to detect changes in vision and new disease, but also to reassure elderly patients who are generally very fearful of blindness. Although there has not been rigorous proof of the benefits of detecting early visual impairment, there is a common belief among many clinicians that correction of deficits prevents injury and promotes independent living. Standard vision tests with the Snellen eye charts should be done separately for each eye while the patients wear their current glasses. Reading ability (near vision) can be evaluated with a Jaeger near reading chart. Adequate lighting must be provided for both of these vision tests to ensure accurate results.

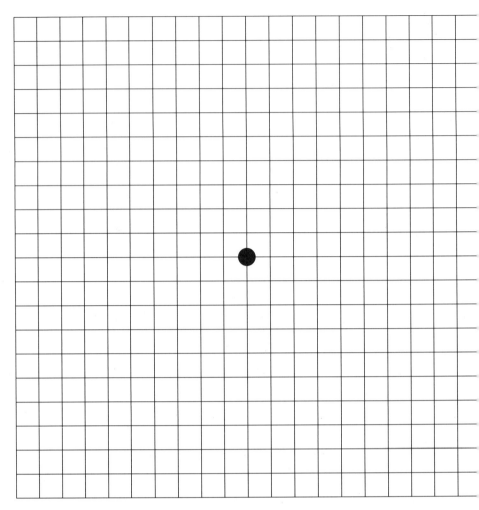

Figure 55-2 Amsler grid. While wearing glasses, if these are worn, patient examines the Amsle grid with each eye. Grid is placed on wall or desk at comfortable distance normally used fo reading.

The pinhole test may be a useful screening maneuver to distinguish changes i vision resulting from refractive error versus more serious disease. If Snellen testin; reveals diminished vision (when patients wear their glasses, if that applies), ask th patients to repeat the test as they look through a pinhole opening in a piece o cardboard. If vision improves significantly with the pinhole, the problem is mos likely refractive and does not originate from the lens, retina, or optic nerve. This i because the pinhole constricts incoming light to a narrow bundle and prevents th blurring caused by nearsightedness or farsightedness. This technique can identif

Table 55-4 Techniques for glaucoma detection

Technique	Findings in glaucoma
Intraocular pressure testing	Ocular hypertension if >21 mm Hg; glaucoma often at 35 mm Hg
Funduscopic examination	Optic nerve abnormalities: cupping, pallor, hemorrhage
Peripheral field testing	Visual field defects

accommodative errors such as myopia or presbyopia that respond to a prescription for new glasses.

Visual inspection may reveal lens abnormalities such as cataracts. Generally an opacity in the lens will be seen, which in advanced stages prevents the examiner from visualizing the retina altogether. Early stages of cataracts can be seen from a distance with the ophthalmoscope focused on the lens or even grossly can be seen by altered light reflection.

Glaucoma may be detected with three techniques as described in Table 55-4. Intraocular pressure can be evaluated with tonometry, either the handheld Schiötz or the more sophisticated applanation technique through a slit lamp. When using the Schiötz device, the examiner first places a drop of local ophthalmological anesthetic (e.g., tetracaine or proparacaine HCl) in each eye and instructs the supine patient to stare straight ahead at the ceiling. The device is gently applied to the cornea and a reading is made from the dial. Unfortunately, many false negatives and positives occur when tonometry is used for glaucoma screening. Contraindications to using the Schiötz include any disruption in the cornea such as active infection, injury, or past disease that would distort the result. Even without these instruments it is possible to make an assessment of intraocular pressure by manually pressing or ballotting the eyeballs to compare rigidity between them. Acute closed-angle glaucoma is accompanied by very high intraocular readings (normal is 10 to 21 mm Hg).

Funduscopic examination with the ophthalmoscope is useful to detect not only glaucomatous changes, but also retinal changes of macular degeneration, diabetes mellitus, and arteriosclerotic disease. Cataracts may interfere with this examination, but if the examiner can visualize the retina by using the ophthalmoscope, it is unlikely that the cataract is causing a severe obstruction to visual acuity. Pupil dilation significantly aids the examiner, but it should be used with great caution if the patient has to drive afterward or has an intraocular lens that may dislocate. It is also prudent to avoid dilation if there is a personal or family history of glaucoma, since dilation may precipitate an acute angle-closure glaucoma in up to 50% of patients with this disease.

Funduscopic findings in macular degeneration include drusen and abnormalities in the macular area, possibly with hemorrhaging or scarring. Diabetic retinopathy may be seen as hemorrhage, neovascularization, and other vascular abnormalities. Ophthalmologists further elucidate these disorders by using fluorescein angiography.

Peripheral fields can be assessed by the confrontation test in which the patient looks straight ahead while the examiner's fingers move at the periphery. More accurate testing is available with automated devices that randomize light sources and record responses mechanically, but these are rarely available in the primary office. While peripheral vision testing is useful to explain falling problems or visual disabilities that do not improve with glasses, it is not very useful to detect glaucoma since visual field losses usually develop late in the course of the disease.

In fact, the report from the U.S. Preventive Services Task Force[7] in 1989 does not recommend any routine tonometry for open-angle glaucoma screening because of inaccuracies in the above screening tests and unproven benefits of early detection of glaucoma. Nonetheless, the belief that early treatment of glaucoma may preserve sight underlies the continued recommendation of the American Academy of Ophthalmology and the American Optometric Association that elderly persons should have annual tonometry.

Intervention. Although many definitive treatments of eye disorders in elderly patients necessitate ophthalmological referrals, the primary care clinician nonetheless can provide a crucial link for the patient between different therapies and services, particularly those that support the patient and help the patient to cope with the loss of visual acuity.

Surgical removal of cataracts is the definitive treatment for this problem. More than one million cataract operations are performed in United States annually. While in the past surgery was postponed until the cataract was mature or significantly interfered with life, techniques have improved in safety now (local anesthesia, outpatient surgery) such that earlier removal is recommended.

Cataract surgery is indicated when the visual impairment compromises the patient's ability to function, and outcomes of at least 88% improvement to an acuity of 20/40 can be promised. Preoperative office evaluation of the patient for eye surgery should include attention to stabilization of underlying medical problems such as angina, diabetes mellitus, and pulmonary disease.[1] Particular risks for ocular surgery and preventive measures are shown in Table 55-5.

After cataract surgery, patients need compensation for their missing lens either

Table 55-5   Risks and preventive measures for successful eye surgery

Risk	Prevention
Coughing	Narcotic cough suppressants; consider general anesthesia
Bleeding	Evaluate aspirin usage; stop anticoagulants prior to surgery
Hypertension (mm Hg diastolic >110)	Control blood pressure; clonidine seems particularly useful

Table 55-6 Precautions and recommendations for prescribing drugs for ambulatory elderly patients

Drugs	Pharmacological changes with age/adverse effects	Precautions and recommendations
Fluorescein sodium	Hypersensitivity: (mainly with IV dose) hives, bronchospasm hypotension, shock	Use with caution when there is history of asthma; local tissue damage; if extravasated, urine fluorescence in 24-36 hr
Ocular lubricants (over the counter)	Transient blurred vision; mild discomfort; eyelash stickiness; photophobia; hypersensitivity; eyelid edema	Use with caution when patients drive: blurred vision; avoid corneal abrasions when inserting medications; frequent instillations may necessitate enthusiastic compliance; NOTE: the preservative benzalkonium chloride should not be used with soft contact lenses
Phenylephrine 0.12% (over the counter)	Hypersensitivity; rebound congestion	Contraindicated in narrow-angle glaucoma; use with caution in other chronic diseases; NOTE: the preservative benzalkonium chloride should not be used with soft contact lenses
Pilocarpine HCl	Accommodative spasm; allergic conjunctivitis; headache; nausea; vomiting; ocular pain; tachycardia	Decreased visual acuity with cataract; risk of retinal detachment; may precipitate asthma; use with caution in cardiac disease
Sodium sulfacetamide	Hypersensitivity; Stevens-Johnson syndrome; headache; blurred vision	Microorganism resistance possible; purulent discharge blocks activity
Topical anesthetics		
Tetracaine or proparacaine HCl	Transient stinging, burning; conjunctival redness; keratitis and scarring; rare systemic toxicity	Avoid prolonged use; no eye rubbing while in effect; use with caution in cardiac disease; use with caution in hyperthyroidism
Pupil dilating		
Tropicamide 0.5%	Blurred vision; fast acting	Dislocates intraocular lenses; can precipitate glaucoma
Phenylephrine 10%	Easily reversed	

with new implanted intraocular lenses, glasses, or contact lenses. Sun protection also is recommended, particularly to screen ultraviolet rays. Postoperatively, it is important to note that patients may have opacification in their posterior lens capsules after cataract removal. This opacification may be treated, with good results, by the ophthalmologist using laser therapy.

Emergency treatment for closed-angle glaucoma can be instituted even before the patient is seen by the ophthalmologist, particularly if the clinician detects elevated pressure accompanied by a red eye. Pilocarpine 2% drops should be placed in the affected eye every 15 to 30 minutes for several doses. Ongoing treatment for open- and closed-angle glaucoma may involve many medications, including diuretics, beta blockers, and anticholinergics, that cause systemic side effects. Even medications exclusively prescribed for the eye lead to systemic absorption and side effects.

Therapy for macular degeneration includes magnification and improvement of other obstacles to vision such as cataracts. For later stages of macular degeneration, treatment is similar to that for diabetic retinopathy, with laser photocoagulation often being very important. Early referral to an ophthalmologist is important so that timely and maximal treatment can begin.

Emotional and practical support are clearly important for patients with eye disorders. While 12% of blind persons (visual acuity <20/200) see nothing, 75% of the persons in this category can recognize people and objects. *Low vision aids*, which include a variety of magnifying devices on stands and special lighting and magnified televisions, are becoming more widespread and frequently available.[2] Rehabilitative services such as mobility training, vocational rehabilitation, and social service assistance should be recommended. Agencies such as the American Foundation for the Blind can provide counseling and valuable resources such as books recorded on cassette tape. Seeing Eye dogs are difficult to train for elderly persons and in many cases are not necessary.

Finally, certain precautions should be practiced when ocular agents are prescribed for older patients. These are summarized in Table 55-6.[8]

REFERENCES

1. Adler AG, Kountz DS: Eye surgery in the elderly, *Clin Geriatr Med*, 6(3):659, 1990.
2. Bailey OD: Low vision and the elderly patients, *J Am Optom Assoc* 59(4):307, 1988.
3. Ehrlich DR, Keates RH: What to do when the elderly patient complains of external eye problems, *Geriatrics*, 33(7):34, 1978.
4. Miller D: *Ophthalmology: the essentials*, Boston, 1979, Houghton Mifflin.
5. Strickland RW et al: The frequency of sicca syndrome in an elderly female population, *J Rheumatol* 14:766, 1987.
6. U.S. Department of Health and Human Services: Current estimates from the national health interview survey: United States 1983, US Public Health Service Pub No 86–1582, Series 10, No 154, Hyattsville, MD, 1986.
7. U.S. Preventive Services Task Force: Guide to clinical preventive services: an assessment of the effectiveness of 169 interventions, Baltimore, 1989, Williams & Wilkins.
8. Woodard DR, Woodard RB: *Handbook of drugs in primary eyecare*, Norwalk, Conn, 1991, Appleton & Lange.

SUGGESTED READING

Adler AG, Kountz DS: Eye surgery in the elderly, *Clin Geriatr Med* 6(3):659, 1990.

CHAPTER 56

Sleep disorders

HELENE EMSELLEM

KEY POINTS

- "Normal" sleep changes with aging and age-related changes may contribute to undesirable sleep patterns.
- The prevalence of sleep disorders increases with advanced age.
- Sleep disorders in elderly persons are treatable.
- The diagnosis of sleep disorders in elderly persons may be complicated by the presence of concurrent diseases; nevertheless, the sleep complaint should be addressed.
- Thorough evaluation to ensure proper diagnosis of the sleep disorder is critical to prevent initiation of inappropriate and potentially harmful therapy.
- Overnight polysomnography to monitor sleep and a daytime multiple sleep latency test to evaluate wakefulness are helpful adjuncts to the diagnosis of sleep disorders.
- Prior to prescribing a sedating medication, reconsider the possibility of obstructive sleep apnea.

CLINICAL RELEVANCE

The quantity and quality of nighttime sleep are key determinants of the quality of one's daytime functioning. Although sleep complaints are pervasive in the general population, the prevalence and intensity of sleep disturbance increase with advanced age.[2] One half of Americans aged 65 years and older experience sleep disruption, and an even greater percentage of institutionalized elderly persons have sleep complaints.

Several factors are responsible for this dramatic increase in sleep-wake complaints as people age. First, there are "normal" physiological changes in sleep that occur with aging and impact negatively on sleep. The most striking change is the *increase in spontaneous arousals* that disrupt sleep continuity. To awaken in the morning and feel well rested, a person must cycle through the five stages of sleep in an orderly sequence, with minimal arousals, and spend a certain percentage of total sleep time in each of the sleep stages. Repeated awakenings disrupt this internal "architecture" of sleep, causing unrestorative sleep and daytime complaints. Another age-associated change in sleep is a dramatic *decrease in slow wave sleep.* Although a universal phenomenon, its normality is questionable in view of the large number of complaints of unrestful nighttime sleep in the geriatric population. Slow wave sleep is thought to play a significant role in the physically rejuvenating aspects of sleep. Furthermore, sleep is *more fragmented* for elderly persons who tend to sleep for shorter periods, napping during the daytime rather than consolidating sleep into one nocturnal period. Thus normal physiological changes in sleep may prevent restful nighttime sleep and contribute to sleep-wake complaints in elderly persons. In addition, medical complaints (e.g., pain, nausea) and side effects from drugs disrupt normal sleep patterns in older adults. Furthermore, primary sleep disorders (e.g., obstructive sleep apnea, periodic leg movements) frequently increase among the geriatric population.

DIAGNOSTIC APPROACH

The evaluation of a sleep-wake complaint requires a complete history and physical examination. The patients' sleep-wake schedules, including arousal, daytime functioning, falling asleep, and sleeping itself, are reviewed. If the sleep patterns and problems are not clearly defined at this point, the physician may request the patients to keep sleep logs recording the time when they go to bed, time when they fall asleep, time, duration, and reason for arousals, and time when they wake up in the morning. If the patient is sleepy during the day, a record of daytime naps is also helpful. Routine laboratory investigation should include complete blood count, serum electrolytes, blood glucose, erythrocyte sedimentation rate, and thyroid function studies. In endemic areas, serological studies for Lyme disease may be appropriate. Brain imaging studies and electroencephalograms (EEGs) are not routine parts of the evaluation. If the cause of the sleep disorder is not apparent after the initial thorough evaluation, referral to a sleep laboratory or to a clinician who specializes in sleep problems may be warranted. The following information is a description of some of the more specialized studies performed in sleep laboratories.

Polysomnography is the overnight recording of EEG, eye movement, limb movement, muscle tone, electrocardiogram, and respiratory parameters (nasal and oral airflow, chest and abdominal movements, and oxygen saturation). A standard polysomnogram provides information about the sleep architecture, including the time that it takes to fall asleep (sleep latency), total sleep time, and sleep stages. The number, type, and duration of disordered breathing events are recorded and a respiratory disturbance index (apnea + hypopnea index) is calculated to reflect the number of disordered breathing events occurring per hour. A respiratory disturbance index of below 5 is normal. An index of 5 to 15 is abnormal, although the clinical significance of this range is not clear regarding benefits from treatment. These patients should be carefully observed over time. An index above 15 is abnormal and is an indication for treatment.

The presence and degree of daytime sleepiness may be assessed with a multiple sleep latency test (MSLT). Every 2 hours beginning at 9 AM the patient is given a 20-minute opportunity to sleep. The average latency to sleep onset for the 5 naps is calculated and the number of naps with rapid eye movement (REM) sleep is noted. Normal values for the MSLT have been determined; an average sleep latency of 10 minutes or more with REM sleep on no more than 1 nap is considered to be normal. An average sleep latency less than 5 minutes with REM sleep recorded on 2 or more naps is consistent with a diagnosis of narcolepsy. Patients with sleep latencies between 5 and 10 minutes meet criteria for a diagnosis of excessive daytime sleepiness and an underlying cause should be sought.

CLINICAL MANIFESTATIONS AND DIAGNOSTIC APPROACH FOR SPECIFIC CAUSES OF INSOMNIA

A complaint about sleepiness or wakefulness is best evaluated clinically in reference to the sleep-wake schedule. The symptom *insomnia*, inability to sleep, may be manifested (1) at sleep onset, (2) during the night with multiple nighttime arousals disturbing sleep continuity, or (3) in the early morning with an early morning awakening.

Sleep onset insomnia

To fall asleep at a predetermined time each evening, the brain stem mechanisms that initiate sleep must be triggered by body temperature and internal hormonal rhythms. These internal rhythms are entrained to the external day-night cycle. The entire system is subject to permeation by behavioral reinforcement.

Psychophysiological insomnia. Psychiatric disorders such as agitated depression, psychosis, and anxiety disorder may be associated with difficulty initiating sleep. In normal patients psychophysiological insomnia may develop as a manifestation of negative conditioning to the bedtime environment. Patients invariably report improved sleep in unfamiliar settings such as hotel rooms. A total preoccupation with falling asleep develops and the cycle may be difficult to break without the initiation of behavior modification techniques. Individuals prone to somatization of tension are thought to be more susceptible to developing this disorder.

Restless leg syndrome. Restless leg syndrome increases with one's advanced age and should be considered for the elderly individual who has sleep onset insomnia. It is a poorly understood sensorimotor disturbance of the limbs, characterized by the onset of an uncomfortable sensation in the lower legs and culminating in the irresistible urge to move the legs while the individual is at rest. The sensation is described as a building tension, creepy-crawly feeling, or tingling. Leg movement relieves the sensation only to have it recur. The symptom may be present during the day when the individual sits quietly, but it is most evident at bedtime when the individual attempts to relax and go to sleep. History is often adequate to confirm the diagnosis. There is a continuum between the restless leg syndrome and the nocturnal disorder periodic leg movements of sleep.

Inadequate sleep hygiene. Poor or inadequate sleep hygiene may contribute to difficulty falling asleep and may be a factor in sleep onset insomnia for elderly persons. This is most frequently caused by haphazard and irregular nappings. An essential element of good sleep hygiene is a regular sleep-wake schedule. Regularity reinforces the internal body temperature rhythms and sleep onset mechanisms. Napping, although necessary for some individuals, must conform to a schedule and must be minimized to preserve the integrity of nighttime sleep. Also, the time one spends in bed waiting to fall asleep should be minimized to prevent a secondary psychophysiological insomnia. Careful history may reveal other factors contributing to sleep onset problems such as a poor eating schedule and environmental issues.

Hypnotic-dependent sleep disorder. The use of hypnotic agents for sleep onset insomnia for more than 3 weeks invariably induces tolerance. Increasing the dose improves the situation only transiently, and tolerance and sleep onset difficulties recur. Although sleep onset is initially hastened by these agents, disruption of sleep architecture occurs with reduced slow wave and REM sleep time. As the dose increases, daytime symptoms develop, including sleepiness, cognitive impairment, visual-motor problems, nervousness, and irritability, related to the cumulative deleterious effects of the sedative hypnotic agent. Unguided attempts by the patient to stop the medication exacerbate the symptoms because withdrawal takes place and reinforces the psychological dependency.

Nighttime awakenings

Arousals after the initiation of sleep may be attributed to environmental factors such as a loud noise, major psychiatric disease, medical illness such as paroxysmal nocturnal dyspnea, or an intrinsic sleep disorder. Benign prostatic hypertrophy precipitating arousals to void, antiasthmatics containing the stimulant theophylline, and diuretics controlling congestive heart failure are just a few examples. Whatever the underlying cause, repeated arousals disrupt the continuity of sleep and decrease the total sleep time. The resultant chronic sleep deprivation leads to irritability, inattention, prolonged motor reaction time, memory difficulty, and excessive daytime sleepiness or fatigue.[7] These symptoms may be misinterpreted as depression or dementia. This diagnostic pitfall may be particularly troublesome because many antidepressants exacerbate other sleep disorders. The box on p. 553 summarizes suggestions for good sleep hygiene.

Periodic leg (limb) movements of sleep. Periodic leg movements of sleep (PLMS) is a pathological disorder that frequently increases as people age, and it is characterized

_____ **SLEEP HYGIENE SUGGESTIONS FOR ELDERLY PERSONS** _____

Establish a regular bedtime and wake-up time.

Set aside time in the evening for relaxation and thinking. Consider keeping a "worry" diary of problems, plans, and solutions.

Avoid alcohol, caffeine, and nicotine—they all disrupt sleep.

Minimize awake time in bed—reserve the bed for sleep and sexual activity.

Create an optimal sleep environment, with special attention to noise, temperature, and light.

Hunger disturbs sleep; maintain a regular eating schedule and include a light evening snack, if necessary.

Avoid napping; if napping is necessary, restrict naps to a fixed time and duration.

Exercise daily to the extent possible; avoid exercise just prior to bedtime.

Review sleep-wake side effects of medications with the prescribing physician.

Maximize daytime exposure to bright light.

by repetitive stereotyped movements in the limbs during sleep.[1] Normally there is inhibition of motor activity during sleep and therefore very little movement. In PLMS, motor signals "escape" from the brain stem and activate the muscles of the legs, causing stereotyped stretchinglike movements of the feet and toes that may be barely detectable. There may be an associated brisk myoclonic jerk of the leg; thus, the original term for this disorder is *nocturnal myoclonus*. Each leg movement may cause an arousal or several arousals and thus disrupt sleep. A patient with PLMS may have unexplained nighttime awakenings, daytime sleepiness, or both. PLMS is *not* an epileptiform disorder, and there appears to be a continuum between the restless leg syndrome during wakefulness and PLMS. Nearly all patients with restless legs have PLMS as well. There is also an association between PLMS and metabolic disorder, obstructive sleep apnea, and REM behavioral disorder, described in the following sections.

The diagnosis of PLMS may be suggested by the patient's history, but overnight monitoring of sleep by polysomnography is necessary to confirm and quantitate the magnitude of the problem. It is essential to exclude from the diagnosis concurrent sleep apnea because agents used to treat PLMS (e.g., clonazepam) may exacerbate underlying apnea. The underlying pathophysiological mechanism has yet to be elucidated.

Obstructive sleep apnea. Obstructive sleep apnea (OSA) affects approximately 6% of the population, with an average age of onset occurring during the fifth decade and a dramatic increase in prevalence occurring with aging. The impact of OSA on the already fragile sleep of elderly persons is significant. Epidemiological studies are necessary to assess the extent of OSA in older adults and to define limits of normal for this age group.

OSA is characterized by repeated episodes of upper airway closure during sleep. With the onset of sleep, there is muscle relaxation throughout the body.[3] The majority of the airway is protected from collapse; the palate is bony and the trachea has cartilaginous rings. The pharynx is entirely muscular and relies on muscle contraction to maintain patency. Muscle relaxation at sleep onset may result in partial closure of the airway at the level of the pharynx, causing turbulence of airflow and snoring. A continuum has been postulated to exist between benign snoring secondary to partial airway collapse and varying degrees of OSA.

The clinical hallmarks of OSA are loud snoring coupled with excessive daytime sleepiness. Repeated arousals disrupt the normal cycling between the five stages of sleep, and in severe cases there may be a total absence of slow wave and REM sleep. The patient may be consciously aware of awakenings or simply may wake up in the morning exhausted. Repeated oxygen desaturation secondary to apnea may predispose the patient to nocturnal cardiac arrhythmia. Hypertension is a common complication.

Central sleep apnea. Central sleep apnea is characterized by repeated episodes of cessation of respiratory effort during the night. The airway does not obstruct; rather, the brain fails to stimulate the respiratory musculature. Central apnea is a rare disorder among the young and middle-aged, but it frequently increases with aging and associated cardiovascular and cerebrovascular disease. In contrast to patients with OSA, patients with central apnea rarely snore but may arouse themselves when airflow resumes. Nighttime awakenings and/or daytime sleepiness are the cardinal symptoms. The diagnosis requires an overnight polysomnogram and treatment modalities are limited.

Sleep bruxism. Grinding of the teeth at night is a movement disorder that may contribute to nighttime sleep disruption. Clinical criteria for the diagnosis have not been firmly established, but evidence of significant tooth wear coupled with overnight polysomnography documenting bruxism and arousal is necessary.

REM Behavioral Disorder. REM sleep is a remarkable stage characterized by the presence of awake-frequency brain rhythms, total body paralysis, and intermittent bursts of conjugate eye movements associated with dreaming. The cortex is active during REM sleep but no memories are formed. The purpose of REM sleep and dreaming is unknown; nevertheless, it is clearly necessary because REM sleep deprivation leads to sleepiness, irritability, poor attention, and impaired performance.

The REM behavioral disorder (RBD) is a disorder of elderly persons (average age of onset occurs during fifth to sixth decade). It is an unusual syndrome characterized by the lack of muscle atonia (paralysis) during REM sleep.[6] In RBD, movement is possible during REM sleep and patients may literally act out their dreams. This can be dangerous to the patients and to bed partners. Unless injury occurs, arousals during the active REM sleep of RBD are infrequent and daytime function is not impaired. The limited epidemiological data that exist suggests that 50% of patients with RBD have an underlying degenerative neurological disorder such as Parkinson's disease, Alzheimer's disease, or progressive supranuclear palsy. Evaluation should include a complete neurological examination, magnetic resonance imaging (MRI) scan of the head, and in some cases lumbar puncture. Diagnosis of RBD requires an overnight sleep study.

Other causes. Nighttime awakening in older adults can be precipitated by a variety of underlying medical conditions (e.g., gastroesophageal reflux, dementia, Parkinson's disease, and various pain syndromes, including fibromyalgia).[5] Diagnostic approaches should be appropriate to the suspected underlying disease.

Early morning awakening

Advanced sleep phase syndrome. Beyond the age of 65, there is a tendency to fall asleep earlier and wake up earlier in the morning (i.e., an advanced sleep phase syndrome). This "natural" phenomenon may create the impression of an early morning awakening and be misinterpreted as depression. Wakefulness in the early morning hours is less socially acceptable than staying up late at night. The sleep phase may be adjusted by therapy with bright lights, but data are lacking regarding the efficacy of this therapy modality for elderly persons.

Depression. A cardinal symptom of depression in all age groups is the inability to perpetuate sleep in the early morning hours. The early morning awakening associated with depression must be differentiated from the advanced sleep phase syndrome, intrinsic sleep disorders such as OSA or PLMS that cause arousals in the early morning hours, and side effects from medication or other diseases.

Excessive daytime sleepiness

Excess daytime sleepiness may be a result of sleep disruption from any of the previously mentioned disorders of nighttime sleep or may be a symptom of a primary disorder of wakefulness. An individual with OSA or PLMS may be unaware of the partial arousals caused by the disorder and may awaken feeling tired and unrested. A similar fatigue or sleepiness is seen in individuals with respiratory disease and nocturnal oxygen desaturation. Patients may not be able to distinguish between sleepiness and fatigue. The distinction between these disorders and depression may be particularly difficult. An overnight polysomnogram to document nighttime sleep, followed by a daytime MSLT to quantitate the degree of daytime sleepiness, is essential.

Narcolepsy. Narcolepsy is a disorder characterized by the tetrad of daytime sleepiness, cataplexy, sleep paralysis, and hypnagogic hallucinations. Patients experience repeated daytime episodes of sleepiness often associated with REM sleep. Following a nap, the patient is refreshed, only to become overwhelmingly sleepy again 2 to 3 hours later. There is a strong genetic factor and nearly 100% of patients have the HLA-DR2 or HLA-DQw1 phenotype. The onset is usually in adolescence and symptoms may persist lifelong, although diagnosis may be delayed.[4] The onset of symptoms

Table 56-1 Causes of insomnia in elderly persons

	Insomnia			Excessive daytime sleepiness
Cause	Sleep onset problems	Nighttime awakenings	Early awakenings	
Advanced sleep phase syndrome			+ + + +*	
Central sleep apnea		+ +		+ +
Dementia	+ +	+ + + +	+	+ + +
Depression	+ +	+	+ + + +	+
Fibromyalgia		+ +		+ + +
Hypnotic-dependent sleep disorder	+ + + +	+ +		+ +
Inadequate sleep hygiene	+ + +			+
Narcolepsy		+		+ + + +
Obstructive sleep apnea		+ +		+ + + +
Pain	+ +	+ + +	+	+
Parkinsonism and movement disorders	+ +	+ +		
Periodic leg movements of sleep		+ + +		+ + +
Psychophysiological insomnia	+ + + +			+
REM behavioral disorder		±		
Restless leg syndrome	+ + + +			+
Sleep bruxism		+ +		+
Sleep-related asthma		+ +		
Sleep-related gastroesophageal reflux		+ +		+

*Range of involvement; +, minimal involvement; + + + +, major involvement.

in elderly persons is suggestive of "symptomatic" narcolepsy, and neurological evaluation to exclude from the diagnosis the presence of a degenerative disease or structural lesion is necessary.

Table 56-1 summarizes the major sleep disorders and causes of sleep disruptions in elderly persons.

INTERVENTIONS

Table 56-2 summarizes interventions for causes of insomnia.

Table 56-2 Treatment approaches for insomnia

Sleep disorder	Treatment
Psychophysiological insomnia	Develop sleep log; sleep behavior modification; environmental changes; occasional short-acting hypnotics
Restless leg syndrome	Same as periodic leg movements of sleep
Inadequate sleep hygiene	Avoid or minimize naps or schedule naps; change environmental factors
Hypnotic-dependent disorder	Substitute long-acting sleep benzodiazepine such as clonazepam and gradually withdraw medication; sleep behavior modification
Periodic leg movements of sleep	Clonazepam 0.25 mg at bedtime; may need dose increase every 2 weeks (0.25 mg to maximum of 2 mg); controlled use of codeine and propoxyphene (addictive potential)
Obstructive sleep apnea	Continuous positive nasal airway pressure (CPAP); dental devices to reposition tongue and jaw
Sleep bruxism	No good data for elderly patients; possible bite plates and clonazepam
REM behavioral disorder	Clonazepam; start at 0.25 mg/day
Gastroesophageal reflux	Treat reflux

REFERENCES

1. Ancoli-Israel S et al: Sleep apnea and periodic movements in sleep in an aging population, *J Gerontol* 40:419, 1985.
2. Dement WC, Miles LE, Carskadon MA: White paper on sleep and aging, *J Am Geriatr Soc* 30:25, 1982.
3. Kaplan J, Staats BA: Obstructive sleep apnea syndrome, *Mayo Clin Proc* 65:1087, 1990.
4. Kelly JF, Lowe DC, Taggart HM: Narcolepsy in the elderly: a forgotten diagnosis, *Age Ageing* 16:405, 1987.
5. McCain GA, Scudds RA: The concept of primary fibromyalgia (fibrositis): clinical value, relation and significance to other chronic musculoskeletal pain syndromes, *Pain* 33:273, 1988.
6. Schenck CH et al: Rapid eye movement sleep behavior disorder: a treatable parasomnia affecting older males, *JAMA* 257:1786, 1987.
7. *The International Classification of Sleep Disorders, Diagnostic and Coding Manual*, Rochester, Minn, 1990, American Sleep Disorders Association.

SUGGESTED READINGS

Prinz PN et al: Geriatrics: sleep disorders and aging, *N Engl J Med* 323(8):520, 1990.
McGinty D: Sleep disorders in the elderly: rationale for clinical awareness, *Geriatrics* 42(12):61, 1987.

Index